THE

HOMŒOPATHIC

MATERIA MEDICA,

Arranged Systematically and Practically

BY

A. TESTE,

Graduate of the University of Paris, and Member of the *Société Gallicane* of Homœopathic Medicine, etc.

TRANSLATED FROM THE FRENCH, AND EDITED

BY

CHAS. J. HEMPEL, M. D.

Fellow and Corresponding Member of the Pennsylvania Homœopathic College; Honorary Member of the Hahnemann Society of London, &c.

PHILADELPHIA:
PUBLISHED BY RADEMACHER & SHEEK, 239 ARCH STREET.
NEW YORK:—WILLIAM RADDE, 322 BROADWAY.
ST. LOUIS: J. G. WESSELHŒFT, 79 MARKET STREET.
1854.

KING & BAIRD, PRINTERS, No. 9 SANSOM STREET.

EDITOR'S PREFACE.

The work which is here offered to the public, is not the production of a trifling mind, but of a man who made it his business to reflect deeply on the present character of the Homœopathic Materia Medica. He felt, with a host of other intelligent practitioners, that the present arrangement of our drug-symptoms, which constitute our guides in the use of drugs as remedial agents, is exceedingly arbitrary and complicated, and that it is therefore eminently desirable to simplify the Materia Medica, by expunging all such symptoms, or even drugs, as have proved useless in practice, or by substituting for the present incoherent arrangement of our materials, a system of symptomatic relations based upon subjective analogies. Pursuing this mode of investigation, Teste was gradually led to arrange the principal remedies of our Materia Medica into twenty classes, which he terms groups. Each group is headed by a leading remedy or type, to which the other members of the group are related, not only by a similarity of symptoms, but likewise, by the internal affinities of the drug-diseases which these remedies are respectively capable of exciting in the healthy organism.

The plan of presenting our drugs as a coherent series of groups, is somewhat novel, but neither fanciful nor repulsive to the reason. On the contrary, it is fair to inquire: If all the creations of nature constitute orders of varieties, why should medicinal substances form an exception to this general law? And if it should be true that drugs and their effects upon the healthy body, likewise constitute a generalization of natural phenomena, would not this simplify their study and their application to the treatment of disease? The first question, then, would be, to investigate the law under which drugs and their dynamic properties are combined into a series; a knowledge of this law would imply, or lead to, a knowledge of their orderly application in the treatment of disease, and would put a stop to the unjustifiable abuse which many homœopathic practitioners are guilty of, in prescribing a number of remedies not only successively, but simultaneously, in a case where one or two only, would prove amply sufficient in the hands of a scientific physician. Teste is one of the few inquirers in our School, who consider it their duty to simplify the Materia Medica by expunging all that seems unworthy of confidence, and classifying all our reliable drugs and symptoms in accordance with the unmistakeable analogies which the proving of these drugs upon the healthy, has revealed to us. The present work gives us the results of our author's investigations and discoveries in this direction. Whether he has discovered the whole truth, or only a part thereof, experience will decide. This much is certain: that his work is a treasure of interesting facts, observations and reasonings, and that every physician will find it to his interest and to the eminent advantage of his patients, to study the present work with care and attention.

A most interesting portion of the work are the contributions from Old-school literature. A history of the empirical use of the drug is given in every case, and it will be uniformly found, that, wherever a drug had the reputation of being a specific in a certain disease, and really did effect, striking, rapid and permanent cures, such a result was invariably attributable to the homœopathicity of the drug-action with the nature of the malady.

Speaking of the homœopathicity of a drug to a disease, the reader will not fail to observe that, according to our author's mode of viewing it, a drug is only homœopathic to a disease when the drug-disease is analogous to the natural malady. Both the primary and the secondary action of the drug must correspond to the primary and the secondary action of the natural malady. An inflammatory fever, for instance, first commences with a chill; this is its primary symptom. The bounding pulse, the hot and dry skin, constitute symptoms of vital reaction, and the drug which is to be truly homœopathic to this disease, must not only have the chill, but likewise, corresponding symptoms of reaction, or commonly termed, secondary symptoms. It is well known that Aconite has both the chill and the heat and dryness of the skin, together with the bounding pulse, and that it is, therefore, equally homœopathic to the primary as well as to the secondary symptoms of fever. In the books, Aconite is generally recommended for the secondary symptoms only, namely, for the bounding pulse, heat and dryness of the skin, thirst, etc. It might therefore seem, if we were called to a patient who was still under the influence of the primary chill, as though Aconite could only be administered upon the principle of *contraria contrariis*; but this would simply be a seeming antagonism; for Aconite would not only hasten the vital reaction, but might have to be continued after this reaction had fully set in, until the primary as well as the secondary phenomena of the natural malady should have been subdued. A similar rule applies to the use of every other drug in our Materia Medica, and can, of course, only be properly applied where both the primary and the secondary action of the drug is positively known. It is our author's aim to furnish many useful hints, instructive suggestions, and positive indications concerning this important point in the pharmaco-dynamics of our school.

One word as regards the translation. I have

endeavored as much as possible, to preserve the expression of the original, except where a strictly literal rendering of the text was incompatible with English grammar and a correct and fluent style. In all such cases, I have deemed it my privilege so to modify the original text, as would leave the author's meaning unimpaired, and, at the same time, be considered an acceptable phraseology in our own language.

It may be proper to state in this place, that the business of translating is not as easy of accomplishment as some may be disposed to imagine. The several extracts which Teste was obliged to make in the course of his work from other authors, and more particularly from Jourdan's translations of Hahnemann's Organon, and his Materia Medica, contain a number of important errors. In his preface to Aconite, for instance, Hahnemann mentions as one of the most characteristic indications for the use of Aconite, "*ein agonizirendes Umherwerfen.*" The meaning of this is, "a tossing about as if the patient were in great agony:" but in Jourdan's translation, as well as in various English publications, it is rendered, "a tossing about such as characterizes Aconite." The translators were evidently misled into this absurd mistake by the apparent similarity of the spelling of "*agonizirendes*" and "Aconite;" not to mention a variety of equally interesting misapprehensions of Hahnemann's text. Being perfectly acquainted with

Hahnemann's original expressions, I have, of course, avoided a repetition of all such errors. In connection with this subject, I must be permitted to state that several reviews of Teste's work have been recently laid before me, which are filled, from beginning to end, with the most absurd misconceptions of the author's meaning, and evince a shocking ignorance of his language. *Ne sutor ultra crepidam!*

With these brief remarks, I recommend this work to the careful study of the profession, and sincerely trust, that it may stimulate others to similar efforts in the noble task of imparting to our art a universally acknowledged scientific basis.

CHARLES J. HEMPEL.

NEW YORK,
January, 1854.

To Doctor Petroz,

I HUMBLY DEDICATE THIS BOOK TO YOU, MY TEACHER AND FRIEND;

TO YOU WHO HAVE DONE SO MUCH
FOR THE PROPAGATION OF A DOCTRINE
THE TRUTH OF WHICH HAS BEEN SO
OFTEN AND SO LOUDLY PROCLAIMED

BY YOUR SUCCESS IN THE TREATMENT OF DISEASE;

TO YOU WHOM I DO NOT HESITATE TO REGARD AS THE MOST
EXPERIENCED OF ALL HOMŒOPATHIC PRACTITIONERS,

AS A MOST SKILLFUL DIAGNOSTICIAN,

AND, IN ONE WORD,

AS ONE OF THE GREATEST PHYSICIANS OF OUR TIME.

ALPHONSE TESTE.

INTRODUCTION.

THE Homœopathic Materia Medica differs from the Materia Medica of the Old School, particularly in this, that it is susceptible of being constituted as a science, which is, in some respects, independent of the other branches of the healing art; by which is to be understood, that the Homœopathic Materia Medica contains, within itself, its primary facts or fundamental principles, its laws of development and practical application, in one word, the reason of its own existence.

But, inasmuch as every science necessarily implies the idea of multiple and correlative definitions, or propositions which are methodically developed out of, and therefore depending upon, each other, it is impossible that a science should exist without a system.[1]

Hence, the Homœopathic Materia Medica cannot become a science, in the true acceptation of this term, except by first being systematised; otherwise, it would

[1] I have defined the term "*system*" as follows: "A complete series of beings or facts compared amongst each other by their common properties, and disposed, either agreeably to the unchangeable order of nature, or in such a manner as to form the terms of a progression, which can be continued, by the reason, beyond the limits of positive observation.—(Encyclopedia of the XIX. century, article SYSTEM.)

simply be an assemblage of incoherent facts which would exclusively appeal to the memory, and being increased in number from day to day, would necessarily be forgotten after a while, at least in a great measure, and would thus remain a dead letter in the archives of our science.

Indeed, at all times physicians have felt the necessity of systematically arranging the elementary facts of therapeutics, and hence it is, that the systematic arrangement of the Materia Medica has always been an object of the efforts of the most eminent practitioners.

They, as well as we, understood by systemisation, or systematical arrangement of the Materia Medica, the logical classification of drugs. But previous to the reform, which was introduced by Hahnemann, every classification of this kind was radically impracticable. The principal obstacles to the practical application of these classifications were the following:

1. A vague and even erroneous notion of the drug in general.

2. Ignorance of the law governing the true relation between the drug and the disease; and, for the same reason,

3. Ignorance of the law which governs the relations of drugs to each other; and lastly,

4. Blind, absolute and final submission of therapeutics to the abstract speculations of general pathology.

This last point alone would have been sufficient to ruin at once, and from its very foundation, every attempt to achieve a systematic arrangement of the Materia Medica. Indeed, how was it possible to conceive a permanent order in the science of therapeutics, when every hypothesis which gave rise to a new system, became for the pathologist a new source of indication?

The complete absence of a fixed point of comparison, which might have served as a basis for a somewhat satisfactory classification of drugs, is clearly manifest in all the works on Materia Medica, which have been published from the time of Dioscorides until now. In one treatise, the various drugs are arranged with reference to their physical properties; in another, with reference to their physiological properties, although almost entirely unknown; or even, to their therapeutic properties, concerning which, erroneous notions only, generally prevailed. At last, as if in despair, their classification as drugs, is entirely discarded, and their medicinal history is given empirically, without any other order being assigned to them, than the kingdom, class, family, species, or, in one word, the category to which they belong in natural history.

Let us observe, however, that, howsoever negative, in a therapeutic point of view, at least, this last mode of classification may have been, it was nevertheless, for the very reason that it was such a perfectly negative system, the least deficient that had been followed so far. For the very reason, however, that it was a tacit protestation against the various pathological systems, no school could adopt it without forswearing its principles. This is the reason why, since Murray's[1] *Apparatus medicaminum*, which all modern innovators reject as a shapeless

[1] Murray et Gmelin, *apparatus medicaminum tam simplicium, quam præparatorum et compositorum*, Gœttinguæ, 1796, 8 vol. in 8.

compendium of empirical prescriptions, the spirit of classification has again prevailed in the Materia Medica. Indeed, it was impossible that Rasori and Broussais, those modern hippocratists, (although Broussais, especially, by referring every species of disease to one and the same circumstance, an irritation, rejected both pathology and therapeutics,) should not have had their respective systems of Materia Medica, as the Galenists, Paracelsus, Stahl, Brown, etc., had had theirs in regular succession.

God be praised! we have every reason to believe that the Materia Medica has been forever freed from these dangerous wanderings in the regions of speculation.

A precise and lucid perception of the character of a drug, obtained by observations on the healthy organism, and serving as a guide in the appreciation and observation of the phenomena of disease.

Evident and incontestable proofs of the curative virtues of the drug in a given case of disease.

Hence the determination of a fixed, unchangeable relation between the phenomena of the disease and the action of the drug.

This it is that we owe to the immortal founder of homœopathy; these are the great truths which a change of systems will never overthrow, and which will prove permanent acquisitions to the healing art.

And yet, in spite of these lucid, positive and eminently suggestive facts, there still exist homœopathic physicians, who regard the systemization of our Materia Medica as something impossible. I go farther; I believe that Hahnemann himself would have rejected all ideas of a systematic arrangement of our Materia Medica, as something conflicting with the fundamental axioms of homœopathy. But such a rejection would simply have been the extreme consequence of his own absolute principles, with which it must be confessed, he finds himself, every now and then, in direct antagonism. Let me endeavour to explain this. Hahnemann's doctrine, rests almost entirely upon the following four propositions:—

Diseases are dynamic alterations of the healthy life-principle.

Drugs are likewise dynamic modifiers of the healthy life-principle, and, by reason of the principle subsequently expressed, dynamic modifiers of disease.

Likes cure likes, or *similia similibus curantur.*

Every disease is necessarily and rigorously individual.

Let us examine these four propositions as briefly as possible.

A. Hahnemann, who was a declared spiritualist in philosophy, was a vitalist in physiology, and hence in medicine. That is to say, instead of holding with Descartes and Stahl, to the doctrine of a human dualism, he distinguishes in man, three substantial principles, namely: matter, the soul proper, and another substance, immaterial like the soul, a sort of intermediate principle between the soul and body, to which he refers all diseases, and all our vital functions.

The general idea of this hypothetical force, is, however, not any newer in medicine than it is in philosophy. Hippocrates, and all the vitalists, except Stahl, and his exclusive followers, admit something similar in their doctrines. "In health," says Hahnemann, "the vital force which dynamically animates the material body, exercises an unlimited power. It preserves every part of the organism in an admirable vital harmony, as regards sensation and action, so that the spirit which resides in us, and which is endowed with reason, is able to freely employ these living and healthy instruments, for the purpose of accomplishing the high end of our existence."[1]

The vital force, therefore, whose physiological mission is as lucidly as possible expressed in this paragraph, represents very nearly the sentient soul of Buffon and of the *spiritualistic* opponents of Descartes.[2]

[1] *Exposition of the homœopathic doctrine*, or *Organon of the healing art*, Paris Edition, 1845, p. 108.

[2] Hahnemann's vitalism differs from that of Hippocrates, and more particularly from that of Stahl, who regarded the soul as the only vital principle in man, in this, that his vital force, so far from being an intelligent substance, and capable, if left to itself, of bringing about salutary crises in diseases and curing them, is, on the contrary, "this gross nature which cannot, like an intelligent surgeon, bring together the gaping lips of a wound and unite them by the first intention; which, in a case of fracture, no matter what quantity of osseous matter this force may cause to shoot out, is nevertheless unable to set and adjust the two ends of the bone; which, not knowing how to tie a wounded artery, allows a man full of life and strength, to succumb to the loss of his blood; which is ignorant of the art of replacing in its normal situation the head of a bone that had been displaced by a luxation, and which, in a very little while, renders the reduction even impossible in consequence of the swelling which it causes all around; which, in order to get rid of a foreign body that had been forcibly introduced into the

"In disease," adds Hahnemann, "this spiritual force, which is active in itself, and universally present in the body, is the only one which, at first, perceives the dynamic influence of the agent hostile to life. Having been disturbed by this perception, this force becomes capable of communicating to the organism the disagreeable sensations which it experiences, and of driving it to those unusual actions which we call diseases, etc."[1] And further on. "It is only the disturbed vital force that produces diseases, etc. etc." . . . .

. Whence it follows that every disease which is inaccessible to the mechanical processes of surgery is not, as the allopathists define it, something distinct from the living organism, etc.[2]

Is this theory correct, or is it a specious sophism? God alone knows. To me it seems, at least, certain, that there exists no doctrine which is as plausible, and which can be as satisfactorily brought to bear upon an explanation of the pathological facts as well as of the most abstract combinations of medical philosophy. Hahnemann, who starts from this irrefutable principle, to which we shall have occasion to

cornea, destroys the whole eye by suppuration; which, in strangulated hernia, has no other means of removing the obstacle than gangrene and death; which, in dynamic diseases, frequently causes such changes of form as render the situation of the patient much more unpleasant than before, etc." (Organon, p. 31.) This shows that, so far from reducing the physician to the role of a mere-expectant observer, as was the case with the system of the *naturalists*, who, at most, had no other object in view, in the treatment of disease, than *to aid nature*, Hahnemann's vitalism imperiously requires an active system of therapeutics.

[1] *Organon, loc. cit.*

[2] *Id. p.* 109.

revert more than once, that a dynamic force can only be modified by another dynamic force, and vice versa, quotes for the corroboration of his theory, and as a proof of the dynamic character of our diseases; those which are so often seen resulting from purely moral emotions, a great joy, a chagrin, a fear, etc., all of which are evidently immaterial causes of disease. But in order to show in the most conclusive manner, if not the initial, at least the indispensable part which the vital force acts in all our diseases, is it not sufficient to allude to the complete inertia of all morbid agents in their action upon the dead body, that is to say, upon the body after the vital principle has left it?

It should be mentioned that Hahnemann does not define disease as some independently existing being or state; and in this he is right, for an absolute definition of disease could only be a sophism or an error.

Hahnemann's doctrine is, indeed, a condemnation of all such definitions proposed either before or after him by the system-makers. These theorists deduce their general idea of disease almost invariably from some contingent truth which is falsely taken for the absolute truth. To consider *spasm* or *atony*, an *excessive* or *deficient excitability*, *hyposthenia* or *hypersthenia*, the *irritability* or the *contractility of the muscular fibre* as so many absolute principles of disease, is, in my opinion, as far from the truth, as to define color in this abstract manner: color is the red; color is the blue; color is the yellow; color is the violet, etc. Homœopathic physicians certainly accept spasm, atony, the various degrees of excitability, hyposthenia or hypersthenia, the irritability and contractility of the muscular fibre, as physiological and pathological facts, but they believe that Hoffmann, Brown, Rasori and Broussais, have each taken some particular and purely contingent manifestation of the vital force for a fundamental principle and the elementary basis of their respective systems. And, in this respect, they maintain, and justly too, that all those systems, which seem more or less specious, if judged with reference to each other and the consistent facts upon which they are primarily based, are nevertheless false in their totality, absurd before the tribunal of the searching reason, and disastrous in the treatment of disease.

But, if Hahnemann, in order to avoid an useless bandying of theories, does not stop at defining the nature of disease, he gives us of diseases the correct and happy definition which we have cited as one of the corner-stones of his doctrine. Yes, this simple formula: diseases are dynamic and virtual alterations of health, contained within itself the programme of an immense revolution in the domain of medical philosophy.

We have seen what Hahnemann understands by the dynamism of disease; we have now to agree about an understanding of the term "virtuality" or inherent force.

By the virtuality of disease we have evidently to understand the special and totally distinct character of the disturbance which constitutes the malady.

Since we have to admit that the symptoms, which are the only perceptible manifestations of diseases, are necessarily subordinate to their inmost nature, that is to say, their virtuality, it follows from this, that every disease necessarily manifests itself to the observer as a particular assemblage of symptoms. But is it not exceedingly probable that every disease, by reason of its inherent force or virtuality, must, in its manifestations or materializations, if we may so express ourselves, affect certain organs or systems in preference to others? At any rate, it cannot be denied that the observation of pathological facts, and more particularly of epidemic diseases, seems every day to confirm this hypothesis. Albeit a disease no matter howsoever local it may appear, confessedly affects the whole organism, because the vital principle is an indivisible whole, yet I cannot help thinking that a disease, without losing any thing of its dynamic nature, or of its universal presence in the organism, manifests a more or less marked tendency super-induced by its inherent force, to assume a distinct form in one part of the animal economy rather than in another.

I trust that no one will do me the injustice to confound this theory with that of the organists; for the dynamic nature of diseases is certainly not impaired in the least, by attributing to them an *elective sphere*, not of activity, but of manifestation. We shall soon discover that the same theory is applicable to the effects of drugs, or to what we shall hereafter designate as *drug diseases*. Unless we accept the doctrine of a distributing force, which is inherent in the diseases, as well as the drugs, I confess that the former would seem to me nothing but impalpable myths, and the doctrine of drugs a pure chimera.

Most, or, at least, a great many of the substances which we regard as drugs, are susceptible of affecting the animal economy in three different ways, namely :—

1. Mechanically.
2. Chemically.
3. Dynamically.

The *mechanical action* of a drug, whether applied to the surface of the body, or introduced into the intestinal canal, or any other natural passage, is determined by the same conditions that govern the action of any other inert substance placed in a similar situation, namely: volume, density, weight, shape, or in one word, its physical properties. Drugs can only exercise a mechanical action, when employed in massive doses; this is so evident, that it seems useless to dwell at length upon this point.

The *chemical action* of drugs consists in the chemical reaction, which they exercise on the material elements of the organism, with which they are brought in contact. Does it not follow from this definition, that the chemical action of drugs is no less than their mechanical action, subordinate to their ponderable quantity? Wherein, indeed, consists the chemical action of a drug, if not in the atomic displacements and transformations, in other words, in the combinations which take place between the molecules of the material drug, and those of the living tissues, or of those tissues which the chemical agent had succeeded, by its presence, in depriving of their vitality, and decomposing them? This shows that the molecular affinity operates in this case without the aid of the vital force, or, rather, against it. But who is not acquainted with the existence of the well-established law, that every chemical combination between the atoms of bodies, rests upon definite and invariable numerical relations, so that each quantity of a given re-agent, as regards volume and weight, can only saturate a determinate quantity of the substance with which it is capable of forming a new compound? Hence it follows, that, in order to effect perceptible chemical modifications in the organism, a drug has to be employed in a corresponding quantity.

Nevertheless, it is not always easy to distinguish the chemical action of drugs from their dynamic action, of which we shall speak presently, inasmuch as the massive doses which are indispensable to the production of chemical results, are not always an obstacle to the manifestation of dynamic effects.[1]

It is in the *dynamic action* of drugs that their inherent force exclusively consists. This action bears only upon the vital force, and manifests itself exclusively in the living organism.

The important and fundamental distinction of the action of drugs on the organism, into mechanical, chemical, and dynamic, is not new in medicine. Strange, it is precisely the materialists, (Rasori, for instance,) who have endeavored to establish it.

[1] This result takes place in the cauterizations effected by means of the corrosive sublimate, the arsenic-ointment, &c. The chemical wound sometimes shows itself complicated by frightful symptoms induced by the inherent dynamic force of these agents. The redness, the vesicles, &c., which, according to my own experience, are caused by the application to the skin of the twelfth attenuation of Rhus toxicodendron, cannot, certainly, be regarded as chemical effects.

Admitting, however, this distinction, these philosophers have, on the one hand, failed in profiting by it, owing to their inability, from ignorance, to separate the dynamic properties of drugs from their chemical and physical effects; and, on the other hand, what ideas they had of the dynamic action of drugs, were limited, false and confused. The followers of Rasori, for instance, who affect to prescribe only dynamic remedies, employ, nevertheless, mercury, acids, stibium, etc., in enormous doses, and more than sufficient to give rise, in the organism, to chemical reactions, and even to purely mechanical disorders, the simultaneous effects of which, disturb, alter, and disguise, most frequently, the dynamic phenomena. It is, moreover, known how the inherent medicinal action of drugs is understood by the School of Rasori. It is denied, or nearly so; that is to say, although allowing to the modifying agents, which it calls dynamic, a special action on such and such tissues or systems, it limits this action to two opposite directions, and classes all drugs under two general heads, as *hyposthenisants* or *hypersthenisants*. The fundamental conception of Rasori, would be incompatible with any other mode of viewing the action of drugs.

It is then exclusively to the founder of homœopathy, that belongs the honor, if not of having discovered the dynamic drugs, but, at least, of having taught us the means of distinguishing their morbific force from their mechanical and dynamic properties.

B. Hahnemann saw from the first, that there was but one way of attaining this end, the extreme reduction of the doses. He instituted experiments in conformity with this idea, and it may be said, that his success went far beyond his hopes. It is more than probable, indeed, that he was only gradually led to the employment of infinitesimal doses, and that he had not even suspected at first, that the millionth, trillionth, or even decillionth portion of a grain of some substance which was often found to be inert in massive doses, became endowed, when thus reduced quantitatively, with the extraordinary power of which he then found it possessed. Carried away by this discovery, which was the most astonishing he had yet made, he was led to think that the inherent power or principle of the drug might perhaps be separated from the material envelope; a hypothesis which, in his judgment, changed all remedial agents to purely dynamic forces.

This hypothesis agreed perfectly with his opinions concerning the nature of diseases, and the known causes of several of them. "The causes of disease cannot possibly be material, since the least foreign substance introduced into the bloodvessels, however mild it may appear to us, is suddenly repulsed by the vital power, as a poison; or, where this does not take place, death itself ensues. Even when the smallest foreign particle chances to insinuate itself into any of the sensitive parts, the principle of life, which is spread throughout our interior, does not rest until it has procured the expulsion of this body, by pain, fever, suppuration, or gangrene."[1] This is, indeed, in the doctrine of Hippocrates, the general theory of disease, which, according to this great observer, is nothing else than a reaction of the

[1] Organon, p. 34, American Edition.

organism against a material foreign principle. Hahnemann says, moreover, "What nosologist has ever seen one of those morbid principles, of which he speaks with so much confidence, and upon which he presumes to found a plan of medical treatment? Who has ever been able to exhibit to the view, the principle of gout, or the virus of scrofula?" And further on, "Even when a material substance applied to the skin, or introduced into a wound, has propagated disease by infection, who can prove (what has so often been affirmed in our works on pathogeny,) that the slightest particle of this material substance penetrates into our fluids or becomes absorbed?" . . . . . . "How much of this material principle — what quantity in weight, would be requisite, for the fluids to imbibe, in order to produce, in the first instance, syphilis, which will continue during the whole term of life, etc.?" Final conclusion of Hahnemann: virus, miasms, in one word, most of the causes of our diseases, are immaterial, that is to say, purely dynamic agents, like the diseases themselves, and therefore, capable of being perfectly assimilated to the moral causes whence the diseases so frequently result.[1] Evidently, Hahnemann here goes too far.

Now can we admit, with him, that a foreign substance, even the mildest, cannot penetrate into the

[1] Hahnemann goes so far in his views concerning assimilation that, in his memoir on the effects of coffee, in the organon of the healing art, he speaks of coffee, mercury and *chagrin* as things belonging to the same category. "Coffee," says he, "is the substance which, next to mercury and chagrin, contributes most towards spoiling the teeth."

blood-vessels, without being immediately expelled by suppuration or gangrene at the risk of life, when we see madder (which is a foreign principle, not very hurtful, it is true, still not assimilable,) penetrate so far into the tissues of animals which had been fed on this root, that its presence can even be discovered in the bones to which it imparts a red color? But this is trifling. Who does not know that, in many cases of poisoning with arsenic, the poison has been discovered by Marsh's test, not only in the intestinal canal, the liver, spleen, bladder, &c., but also in the blood, the muscular tissue? In all such cases, the poison had passed through all the ramifications of the vascular apparatus without occasioning either suppuration or gangrene, or even immediate death. I have seen a gilder who had left his shop for upwards of six months, and who had, of course, ceased to be exposed to the vapors of mercury, but whose body was still impregnated with this poison to such an extent that every time he took a hot vapor bath, the mercurial emanations which this bath occasioned, literally whitened a gold ring which this patient carried on his finger. A perceptible quantity of mercury must, therefore, have been absorbed, and must have remained, for six months, at least, in the body of this unfortunate workman, without occasioning either gangrene, suppuration, or any other febrile phenomenon; for the symptoms of my patient presented the following group: nocturnal bone-pains, alternate anorexia and canine hunger; irregular periodical paroxysms of neuralgia in the left half of the cranium and face; trembling of the limbs; slight swelling at the left elbow; general emaciation, (not very considerable) and lastly, every now and then, involuntary jactitation of the lower limbs, in different directions, and of a more or less peculiar and odd character. We are compelled to admit that, if this observation does not altogether invalidate the doctrine of a complete disengaging of the inherent toxical forces from their material agents, it shows, at least, beyond a doubt, that these latter are absorbed. Facts similar to those which we have quoted, abound in the annals of medicine, as is well known.

Upon what grounds, in fact, is the immateriality of viruses, miasms, and of the causes of diseases in general, based? Upon facts which are more than doubtful, and which, so far from proving the conclusions which are drawn from them, simply exhibit the imperfection of our senses, and of our artificial means of investigation. Who has seen, exclaims Hahnemann, who has touched, weighed, the syphilitic virus, the marsh miasm, etc.? Nobody, assuredly. But who sees, by a bright sky, the watery vapor, of which the atmosphere consists in a great measure? Who suspected, before Lavoisier, that the air had weight? Who suspected, previous to the decisive experiments of modern chemists, that particles of copper, iron, sulphur, phosphorus, etc., etc., although invisible, impalpable, imponderable, are constantly floating in the air we breathe? In support of Hahnemann's dynamism, which is a sort of universal pneumatism, existing independently of the material element, the fact is often cited that a grain of musk may for ten years, without losing an atom of its weight, give out its penetrating and distressing emanations, causing dizziness, sick headaches, spasms and other unpleasant accidents in thousands of individuals; whence the conclusion is derived that the odor of musk is a purely dynamic substance. Such a proof, however, to men who, like us, are used to prescribe day after day, as efficacious agents, the millionth, trillionth, decillionth, portion of a grain, seems really puerile. Admitting that a grain of musk loses every day a decillionth, or, if you please, a thousand decillionth portion of its weight, that is to say, a thousand medium homœopathic doses, must it not be evident to every one who has some idea of numbers, that the total loss which this grain of musk would undergo in the course of a thousand years, would still remain inappreciable by the most delicate of our instruments of weight?

As regards homœopathic attenuations, which, for want of a better term, we have agreed to call dynamisations, no matter to what an extent they may be continued, even the highest must still contain some material portion of the original drug, unless we assume that matter ceases to be divisible beyond a certain point. I assert even that there exists an undeniable relation between the dynamic activity of a drug and its material quantity. If this were not so, we should have to admit, which we happily need not, that a poison which, like arsenious acid, for instance, is capable of causing death *dynamically*,[1]

[1] I say dynamically, for the symptoms which are produced by certain poisons when given in massive doses, are evidently of the same nature as those which are produced by their dilutions, and differ from the latter only by their greater intensity. This is so true that even the traces of the chemical action of arsenic are often inappreciable in the organs of individuals which had been poisoned by this metal.

when given *in small quantities* of the crude substance, would be just as deleterious in the thousandth attenuation as it was before undergoing the process of dynamisation.[1]

But if the dynamic activity of a drug depends, in a measure, upon the number of its material atoms,

[1] The absorption of the material drug, does, in reality, not invalidate the dynamic power inherent in the material constituents, and by which the drug acts upon the vital force. In analyzing chemically the different parts of the human body, various and irregularly distributed quantities, according to the nature of the analyzed tissues, of a large number of the material agents which we employ as dynamic remedies, have been discovered in them, a curious fact which may one day shed light on the practice of homœopaths. We read in J. Müeller :—"The elements of the human body and of the superior animals are oxygen, hydrogen, carbon, nitrogen, sulphur, (especially in the hair, albumen and cerebral substance,) phosphorus, (principally in the bones, teeth, cerebrum,) chlore, fluor, (especially in the bones and teeth,) manganese and silicium, (in the hair,) iron, (principally in the blood,) the black pigment and the crystalline body. (*Manual of Physiology*, vol. I., p. 2.) Finally, according to the same author in the *Comptes rendus de l'Académie des Sciences*, Vol. XII., p. 1076, and foll., it is maintained that the human body, in its normal state, contains arsenic and even some other metals. I am persuaded that, with more perfect means of analysis, we should find not only the simple bodies mentioned by Müeller, but also a large number of other substances, and more particularly of such as constitute, if not our drugs, but their active elements. Is it not worthy of remark, on the one hand, that, in the normal development of the individual, certain principles should be directed towards certain regions or organs in preference to others, and, on the other hand, that clinical experience should show, that a given drug is especially efficacious in those cases where the disease manifests itself more especially in the regions and organs where this agent naturally exists in the healthy organism? The principal therapeutic properties of sulphur, manganese, silicia, phosphorus, lime, &c., seem to tend to confirm this proposition.

it depends still much more upon the degree of attenuation to which the atoms have been reduced. We do not yet know, and we may probably never know, the relation which exists between the progressive diminution of the dynamic power of a drug consequent upon the quantitative reduction of its volume, and the equally progressive augmentation of the same power occasioned by the atomic attenuation of the drug from dilution to dilution. What is certain is, that, if the effects of these two opposite causes do not reciprocally counter-balance each other, (if they did, a poison, as we said before, would be just as dangerous in dilution as in the mother-tincture, or in massive doses of the crude substance) the diminution of the drug action by quantitative reduction, becomes the less perceptible, the more the mechanical operations by which the diminution is effected, are multiplied. There are even physicians, and I am one of them, who pretend to have observed, in *certain* patients and *certain* maladies, that the dynamic power of the highest attenuations manifests itself more promptly, and, therefore, more efficaciously, than that of the lower.

Be this as it may, I am fully convinced that the dynamic power of drugs (which I desire to be distinguished from the morbific force inherent in each drug respectively) is strictly subordinate to the spontaneously or artificially developed attenuation of their molecules. This is the reason why all naturally inert substances, or substances of a doubtful activity, such as marble, charcoal, lycopodium, etc., are fixed, insoluble, tasteless and inodorous, whereas substances that are naturally medicinal, such as arsenic, phosphorus, ambra, moschus, most of the acids and poisonous plants, have, generally speaking, a taste and odor, and are more or less volatile.[1] Whence I do not hesitate to infer, that it is simply by breaking the cohesion of inert substances, and by attenuating more and more their atoms, that the Hahnemannean dynamisation transforms these substances into therapeutic agents.

Miasms, those subtle emanations, which Hahnemann represents as purely dynamic forces, are, probably, nothing else than the material effluvia of

[1] It is worthy of remark that several substances which, in their natural state, are inert and inodorous, become odoriferous after acquiring medicinal properties by the artificial division of their molecules. "Horn, ivory, bones, the lime-earth impregnated with petroleum," says Hahnemann, (Materia Medica Pur., vol. I., p. 79,) "are inodorous in themselves, but, as soon as they are filed or rubbed, they spread an odor, which, finally, becomes even intolerable." "It is true," says Hahnemann in another place, "that a substance which is naturally poisonous, may not have any smell," and, in support of this assertion, he quotes the fox-glove and the anemone of the meadows, which are well known as deleterious plants, but, at the same time, have no odor. But because a substance is not odoriferous, does it, therefore, follow, that it is not volatile, or not even diffusible upon being introduced into the animal economy? What is an odor, if not a perception caused by the special action, upon the olfactory nerve, of the substance which produces it? In experimenting with a drug it is quite possible that the most powerful agents may be incapable of producing among their symptoms a peculiar smell. Mercury, for instance, is inodorous. But this does not hinder its volatility, which is so great that it can be distilled at a moderately elevated temperature. We know from the accidents which are occasioned every day among the workmen who, by their business, are exposed to mercurial emanations, that, although almost without any smell, mercury is nevertheless one of the most frightful poisons with which we are acquainted.

organic substances in a state of decay, dynamized by nature, and floating through the atmosphere which becomes their vehicle, together with the gases produced by the putrid fermentation that gives rise to the effluvia.

In my opinion, therefore, there is no radical difference between miasms and drugs. Both are *germs*, or, in order to avoid a dubious metaphor which might be taken literally, causes of diseases, the legitimate effects of which can be compared amongst each other. In one word, I regard a dynamic drug, as a *fixed miasm*, or, if you choose, a *virus*, which a physician makes use of in case of need, in order to produce a malady which shall be capable of neutralizing another one, precisely as he would use for a similar end, the typhus, small-pox, cholera-miasm, if he could seize and handle it according to his own pleasure.

Nevertheless, Hahnemann protests against this assimilation of drug diseases to miasmatic diseases. But the difference which he establishes between these two classes, seems to me without any real foundation.

"The physical and moral powers, which are called morbific agents, do not possess the faculty of changing the state of health unconditionally; we do not fall sick beneath their influence, before the economy is sufficiently disposed and laid open to the attack of morbific causes, and will allow itself to be placed by them in a state where the sensations which they undergo, and the actions which they perform, are different from those which belong to it in the normal state. These powers, therefore, do not excite disease in all men, nor are they at all times the cause of it in the same individual.

"But it is quite otherwise with the artificial morbific powers which we call medicines. Every *real* medicine will at all times, and under *every* circumstance, work upon every living individual, and excite in him the symptoms that are peculiar to it, (so as to be clearly manifest to the senses, when the dose is powerful enough,) to such a degree, that the whole of the system is always (*unconditionally*,) attacked, and, in a manner, infected by the medicinal disease, which, as I have before said, is not at all the case in natural diseases.

"It is, therefore, fully proved by every experiment, and observation, that the state of health is far more susceptible of derangement from the effects of medicinal powers, than from the influence of morbific principles and contagious miasms; or, what is the same thing, the ordinary morbific principles have only a conditional, and often very subordinate influence, while the medicinal powers exercise one that is absolute, direct, and greatly superior to that of the former."[1]

These remarks, as is easily seen, proceed rather from a preconceived idea, than from actual observation. Hahnemann, supposing that drugs effected their cures, by substituting for the natural maladies, artificial diseases, which were at the same time more intense and less permanent than the former, found himself obliged to admit, in order to justify his theory, that the medicinal forces possessed an activity far superior to that of the natural morbific

[1] *Organon*, p. 108, American edition.

agents. But, on the one hand, this pretended substitution of a drug disease for a natural malady, does not bear a moment's examination, as everybody knows now-a-days, except the Allopaths, who, by a strange singularity of reasoning, have appropriated to themselves the only error which Hahnemann has probably committed.[1] And, on the other hand, experience has, long since, refuted the facts upon which the three paragraphs of the Organon which I have quoted, are based.

1. If it be true, according to Hahnemann, that the morbific agents do not possess an absolute power of altering the healthy functions, and that they make us sick, only in so far as the organism is predisposed for the reception of their disturbing influence; it is likewise true, according to all careful observers, that, when some violent epidemic, like the cholera, for instance, manifests itself, all those who, by reason of some pre-existing, generally chronic, affection, or in consequence of extraordinary physiological or hy-

[1] This theory of substitution necessarily implies the doctrine of *medicinal aggravations*. For, how could a disease be more powerful than the one which it replaces, without, at least, a momentary aggravation of its symptoms? Now let me ask, what practitioner has not frequently seen the most painful maladies, neuralgias, for instance, disappear almost *instantaneously* without the slightest appearance of an aggravation of the pains, under the influence of a well-selected remedy? I go farther, I am persuaded that the medicinal aggravation only takes place in cases where the prescribed remedy is only *imperfectly* homœopathic. But it is useless to combat a theory which Hahnemann himself abandoned when he had become enlightened by experience. The method of substitution now-a-days has remained the exclusive property of Messrs. Trousseau and Pidoux, to whom, I doubt not, a *medicinal aggravation* is never wanting.

gienic measures, do not possess a sort of immunity against the prevailing disease, are, more or less, at extremely various degrees, it is true, affected by the epidemic.

2. It is likewise an established fact, at least, for every physician who has devoted himself with more or less systematic perseverance to the proving of drugs with infinitesimal doses, that these drugs do not affect all provers, either in the same manner, or with the same degree of intensity; and that it frequently happens that persons are completely insensible to the action of the drug, apparently, at least.[1] Hence, we are obliged to conclude, that the influence of drugs, as well as that of any other morbific cause, is only perceived on condition that a sort of peculiar receptivity should pre-exist, or, in other words, that the organism should be endowed with a certain aptitude, to be impressed by the action of the drug.

It may, therefore, be doubted whether the human organism is, as Hahnemann believes, possessed of a greater degree of willingness to be disturbed by medicinal, than by natural morbific agents, such as contagious miasms.

Lastly, as regards the preponderance which Hahnemann attributes to the action of the drugs over that of the natural morbific causes, this portion of his doctrine of substitutions, is undoubtedly, that which bears less than any other, the double criticisms of reason and experience. What! because belladonna prevents scarlatina, shall we therefore infer that this

[1] Nevertheless, when these persons are sick, they become sensible to such small doses of the drug, as would not have produced any *perceptible* effect upon them during health.

drug acts with more certainty or energy, than the scarlatina virus? "In order that drugs should be able to preserve the organism from an epidemic malady, their power to modify the vital force must be superior to that of the epidemic."[1] Not in the least. The drug and the contagious miasm are two principles which neutralize *each other;* for, if belladonna prevents the *effects* of the scarlatina-virus, the virus, in its turn, opposes the development of the symptoms inherent in the belladonna,[2] which would only manifest themselves in case the virus should not yet have been absorbed. Does the vaccine, which is a preventive against small-pox, possess in a higher degree than the disease, the power of modifying the vital force? Nobody believes this. A single objection is sufficient to reject this erroneous hypothesis; if the vaccine prevents the development of small-pox, does not, on the other hand, the small-pox miasm prevent the development of the vaccine virus? It is not then from the relative superiority of their dynamic power, that the natural or artificial morbific agents derive their efficacity against diseases similar to those which they themselves would produce, if allowed to act alone, without being irresisti-

[1] Organon, p. 120, note.

[2] Is it not moreover evident that an individual who takes a drug, or is inoculated with a virus, vaccine for instance, voluntarily favors the absorption of the modifying agent, whereas he generally uses every effort in order to withdraw himself from the influence of the epidemic miasm? At a time when the inoculation of the small pox virus was still the fashion, it frequently happened, especially in the country, that children were sent in the very midst of the epidemic, where they became infected with the virus without it having been necessary to inoculate it.

bly opposed in the development of their natural effects, by the presence of these very maladies.

We consider it, therefore, an established fact, *that there is no essential difference between the dynamic drug and the contagious miasm, no essential difference between the drug disease and the natural malady.* Accordingly, nature itself sometimes employs one disease in order to blot out a pre-existing analogous malady; so that the former becomes, with reference to the latter, a real drug disease, in other words, one of those salutary infections, of which our drugs constitute the *viruses.* Hereafter, I shall have occasion, more than once, to return to this doctrine concerning the assimilation of drug diseases with natural maladies; for this is one of the fundamental facts upon which my systematic arrangement is founded.

C. *Similia similibus curantur.*—"There have been physicians from time to time," says Hahnemann, in his Organon, p. 100, who have suspected that drugs cured diseases by virtue of the power with which they were endowed of producing analogous morbid symptoms. "The term *suspected* does not express the exact truth. The law of similia has been clearly expressed: first, by Hippocrates, or, if you choose, by one of the authors of the Hippocratic collection; secondly, by Paracelsus; thirdly, by Stahl.[1] But,

[1] Hippocrates, after having explained the rules of healing *by contraries,* says: "Another proceeding: the disease is produced by similars, and by similars which the patient is made to take, he is restored from disease to health. Thus, that which causes strangury where there is not any, removes strangury where it exists; a cough, as well as a strangury, is caused and removed by the same substances." (Works of Hippocrates, translated by Littre, Vol. VI.,

although the application of this law, which is the most general and the best proven in medicine, has been, on several occasions, crowned with success in the hands of Old School practitioners, the law had, nevertheless, a very limited bearing, owing to the paucity of their observations concerning the physiological properties of drugs, on which account the law became fruitless in the immense majority of

p. 335.) Stahl is still more explicit: "The rule which is admitted in medicine, of treating diseases by contraries or by remedies which are opposed to the effects of these maladies, is completely false and absurd. I am persuaded, on the contrary, that diseases yield to agents which determine a similar affection, (*similia similibus*,) burns by the heat of a stove near to which the parts are held; congelations by the application of snow and cold water; inflammations and contusions by the application of spirits. I have removed a disposition to acidity by small doses of sulphuric acid, in cases where a quantity of absorbing powders had been employed without any benefit." (J. Hummel, *Comment de arthrit. tam tartarea quam scorbutica*, etc. Buding, 1738, in 8vo., p. 40–42.) Hahnemann, who relates this passage, and who, after having mentioned Hippocrates, quotes, as having made more or less similar assertions, Boulduc, Detharding, Bertholon, Thoury, Stœrck, says nothing of Paracelsus. And yet, of all his scientific predecessors, Paracelsus, is the one whose ideas Hahnemann has most faithfully adhered to. His hypothesis of a double immaterial principle in man; the cure of diseases by substances which are capable of causing similar diseases in the healthy organism; the material reduction of these substances to the highest possible degree, (*quintessences*); all this may be found in the book of Paracelsus, which is entitled *Archidoe.* What then was wanting in order that this extraordinary man should have founded the doctrine which emanated from Hahnemann? Only one thing, but an immense and fundamental thing, a thing which all his successors, from Van Helmont to Tommasini, have failed to perceive, and which will forever constitute the great glory of Hahnemann: the physiological proving of drugs with infinitesimal doses.

cases. Indeed, with the exception of certain specific virtues which were attributed rightly or wrongly to a small number of therapeutic substances, whose mode of action on the animal economy was totally unknown, all that was known of the properties of drugs was, that some caused vomiting, others a diarrhœa, some acted on the urine, others caused sweat, etc. It was, moreover, known, it is true, that vomiting had been seen arrested by emetics, a diarrhœa by purgatives, an excessive secretion of urine or sweat by diuretics or diaphoretics. But, after all, vomiting, diarrhœa, diuresis, or sweating, are symptoms which are common to a great many diseases, and could only, in very few cases, be looked upon *as idiopathic maladies.* The manufacturers of systems even, who, in their theories, endeavored to refer the numberless diseases to which man is subject, to one or two fundamental elements, were obliged to admit that these diseases, in spite of the pretended sameness of their natures, nevertheless, manifested themselves in forms that were as numerous as diversified, and whose *similars* were as unknown in therapeutics, as their *contraries* were unknown in pathology. The *similia similibus,* as well as the *contraria contrariis,* was frequently without any meaning to a practitioner who had occasion to apply it. It is by pursuing a steady course of experimentations for thirty years, that Hahnemann succeeded in organizing a complete Materia Medica, and fecondating a law, which others, as he himself admits, had undoubtedly divined before him, but which had remained until then, an empty and unmeaning formula.

To discover in the physiological and dynamic

effects of drugs, representations of the diseases, or, in other words, series of symptoms which corresponded to the perceptible manifestations of the natural diseases, this was the thought which guided Hahnemann in his work. The conviction which had induced him to impose upon himself this immense task, reposed upon innumerable facts which, although due to chance, were not the less conclusive for all that. Unfortunately, the method which he pursued, in collecting and arranging the results of his provings, was, in my opinion, essentially defective. This method evidently emanated from the paradoxical distinction, which, as I have shown above, he supposed existed between the drugs and the miasms, or the natural morbific agents. Hence it followed, that Hahnemann, unwilling to recognise every drug as the principle of some essential affection, in the same sense as the miasms of variola, whooping-cough, marsh fevers, etc., constituted each the principle of some other essential affection, did not care, as he certainly should have, to give us a picture of his drug diseases in their unitary completeness. His provings are nothing more than mere *lists of symptoms.* But a mere list of symptoms, were it ever so complete or numerous, is not the image of a disease. We shall return to this important subject bye and bye.

Be this, however, as it may, it having been shown by Hahnemann, that the law of similitude was the basis of the *specific action* of drugs, which had remained unexplained until then, it necessarily happened that a portion of his disciples forsook the principle of an absolute individualization of diseases, which will be examined hereafter, and looked upon the proving of drugs simply as a means of realizing the old utopia of Sauvages, and of the nosologists of his School, namely, to place after the name of every malady, the name of its *specific remedy.*[1]

In conformity with this notion, the followers of the Homœopathic specific system, not perceiving that all attempts at founding therapeutics upon the constantly varying data of pathology, led them back into the erroneous fancies of the past, and resulted in building upon sand, conceived the project of doing, by means of the physiological proving of drugs, for each malady, considered as a concrete and definite being, what, three centuries ago, chance, in their opinion, had done for syphilis, and what, since then, the same chance (in spite of many contradictory facts,) had done for chlorosis and the marsh fevers. "Let *stomatitis, gastritis, enteritis, ascites, coryza, pulmonary catarrh, pneumonia, pleuritis, articular rheumatism, sciatica,* etc., have each their specific remedy, as syphilis has its, and medicine will, hereafter, be the most positive of all sciences." We may as well admit that there is perhaps, not one among us, who, when first commencing to practise homœopathy, did not, for some weeks at least, hug this chimera, natural fruit of the prejudices which had been inculcated by our former teachers. Unhappily, when, at a later period, enlightened by meditation and a more thorough study of things, we again examined with a calm judgment, this doctrine which had seemed to us so simple, so correct and comprehensive, we soon

[1] Paracelsus and many others, had entertained the same idea, which was superseded by the *methodical nosology.*

discovered, that insurmountable obstacles opposed its realization.

When I mention the terms *gastritis, enteritis, bronchitis, ascites, catarrh, rheumatism*, etc., I feel very well that I use a deficient language, which is constantly rendered unintelligible by the almost unlimited multiplicity of acceptations belonging to each of these technicalities. It is useless to state in proof of the constant identity of this or that disease, to which I give the name which the school has sanctioned, that the pathologists of every age and period have given of every malady a similar description, it does not require a long experience to perceive that all pathologists may have been misled by the same illusion. At least, I have become satisfied by positive proofs, that a morbid condition, which is called alike, requires, in many cases, a different treatment.

And what intelligent homœopath, after having practised his art for two or three years, feels disposed to admit, for example, that there exists a specific remedy for rheumatism, for bronchial catarrh, for diarrhœa? Do we not know from our Materia Medica, that almost all our drugs produce conditions which are so nearly alike, that if our pathologists had to give them a name, the same name would have to be chosen for all of them? And has not every physician on the other hand, had many opportunities of convincing himself at the sick-bed, that each of their drugs cured only, at least, in a prompt and certain manner, a particular shade; a purely individual symptom of these pretended maladies?

All this, however, is only the weak side of the specific doctrine; for it has also a specious truth in its favor; let us examine the doctrine in its favorable aspects, in order to do it full justice.

Although it frequently happens that the mere names of diseases mislead the practitioner much more frequently than they enlighten him, we are, nevertheless, obliged to acknowledge that this is not always so. When I say *croup*, *measles*, *purple-rash*, *scarlatina*, *variola*, *itch*, *typhus*, *yellow-fever*, *plague*, *cholera*, and various other maladies, I am certain that each of these diseases, so far from awakening in the minds of those who hear these names, a vague symptomatic abstraction, as is the case when we say *angina*, *catarrh*, *ascites*, *rheumatism*, etc., presents, on the contrary, the fixed image of a pathological state, which scarcely ever varies in its manifestations, and is, therefore, always, or nearly always, identical. I repeat, *almost always*, not in every case, for after all there does not seem to be anything absolutely true in pathology; an absolute pathological truth seems to be a mere fiction, a sort of ideal, whose realization seems incompatible on the one hand, with the infinite diversities of the human organism, and, on the other hand, with the constant change of conditions in which the morbific cause, be it ever so unchangeable itself, is obliged to act at more or less prolonged intervals. This is the reason why one variola epidemic is not exactly like another, one scarlatina epidemic not exactly like another, etc. Nevertheless, it is incontestably true, that all epidemic diseases, be they observed in any country or at any period, preserve, if not all their symptoms, at least all those which belong to them characteristically. Hence, the same drug, or rather the same series of drugs, have been found applicable to most of the cases of a particular epidemic. Consequently it was in itself a rational proceeding to look for a *specific* remedy or a specific mode of treatment in this or that epidemic. Even Hahnemann had sometimes to resort to such a proceeding.

But if this be the plausible side of the specific doctrine, it is not the less true that in order to have a perfectly legitimate basis of existence, this doctrine should, above all things, have demonstrated the validity of the following two principles:

1st. Essential sameness or symptomatic invariability of all diseases.

2d. Essential sameness of the physiological effects of all drugs.

We shall find out presently, in examining Hahnemann's opinions concerning the individualization of diseases, to what an extent all diseases, whether natural or medicinal, may be considered *essential*.

D. "Every physician," says Hahnemann, "adopting a treatment of such a general character, however unblushingly he may affect to be an homœopathist, is and will always remain, a generalizing allœopathist; *as without the most especial individualization, homœopathy has no meaning*."[1] This maxim rigorously excludes empiricism of whatever name, and upon whatever data it be based, and in this respect, I consider the maxim just, and accept it explicitly. But is it, as has been supposed, the negation of diagnosis or prognosis; in one word, does it imply the complete upsetting of pathology? Such a conclusion seems to me to go beyond Hahnemann's own ideas.

[1] Organon, p. 28, note.

It is true, this great observer lays it down as a principle, (to which he did not always adhere as rigorously as he ought to have done,) that every case of disease has its individual shades, which require a particular treatment; in consequence of which he protests against every treatment which is simply based upon the *general character* of diseases. But does this authorize us to believe that he denied the existence of these general characteristics? On the contrary, the more we study his writings, the more we become convinced that he firmly believed in the existence of types in pathology. And a proof that he believed in them is this, that he takes care to describe them whenever an opportunity offers; the following quotations which have been extracted at random, are more than sufficient to justify this assertion.

"In a sudden affection of the stomach," says, Hahnemann, "with frequent nauseous eructations, as of spoiled food, (sulphuretted hydrogen,) accompanied with depression of mind, cold at the feet, hands, etc., physicians, till the present time, were in the habit of attending only to the degenerated contents of the stomach. A powerful *emetic* must fetch it out entirely," etc. Then follows a judicious criticism of the processes to which allœopathic physicians have recourse under similar circumstances, after which Hahnemann adds: "These gastric affections of dynamic origin are commonly produced by a disturbed state of mind, (grief, fright, anger,) cold, exertion of the mind or body immediately after eating, and sometimes even after a temperate enjoyment of food." What is this gastric affection, the symptoms of which are described by Hahnemann with so much precision, the habitual causes of which he indicates, and to which he seems to think every body is more or less liable? He does not name it, I admit; but what matters it, provided it is true that he regards this affection as a type? Well, this is undeniable; for notwithstanding the absolute principle of individualization which he had laid down a moment ago, he indicates *specifically*, perhaps too much so, the remedy indicated by the general malady which he had just described. "If, instead of those powerful and often injurious evacuating medicines, the patient should only smell once of a globule of sugar the size of a mustard seed, impregnated with the thirtieth dilution of pulsatilla, which infallibly restores the order and harmony of the whole system, and that of the stomach in particular, then he is cured in the space of two hours." Here, then, we have pulsatilla mentioned as the real *specific* of a certain disease of the stomach, to which pathologists might undoubtedly have assigned a general appellation without incurring the censure of Hahnemann.

"It is the custom," says Hahnemann, in another place, "at the present day, when gastric acid becomes superabundant, (which is frequently the case in chronic diseases,) to administer an emetic to relieve the stomach of its presence. But the following morning, or a few days after, the stomach contains just the same quantity, if not more; on the other hand, the pains cease of themselves, when their dynamic cause is attacked by an extremely small dose of dilute sulphuric acid, or with another antipsoric remedy, homœopathic with the various symptoms."[1] In this

[1] Organon, p. 31.

passage Hahnemann is a little less explicit than in the passage previously quoted. Nevertheless, he leaves us to infer, that in certain cases at least, *acidity of the stomach* may constitute a disease for which sulphuric acid is the best remedy. Pathologists might therefore mention acidity of the stomach, as a typical form of disease, without disagreeing with the founder of homœopathy.

But more than all this. Does not Hahnemann mention the *goïtre*, the *spasmodic gastralgia*, the *epidemic whooping-cough*, *croup*, *measles*, *scarlatina*,[1] etc., as typical diseases, which can therefore be defined and described in general terms without reference to any particular case? And lastly, *syphilis*, *sycosis*, and *psora*, these three pillars of the Hahnemannian pathology, are they not alone sufficient to show how little founded is the reproach which has been visited upon our illustrious teacher, that he denies the existence of definite diseases, and thus repudiates the whole past of medical experience?

But if Hahnemann does not reject the essential nature of diseases, or at least of some of them, as a principle, he denies, and justly, the complete identity, in different persons, of such and such a morbid condition, which is generally designated by the same name, whence he concludes, that, at least, in the vast majority of cases, (and I should not hesitate to say in all cases,) every disease, if observed with sufficient attention, constitutes a true individuality, the treatment of which, in order to be strictly homœopathic, requires to be conducted in a special manner.

[1] See his memoir: the belladonna, a preventive against scarlatina.

It does not seem difficult, for that matter, to account for the undeniable tendency which is inherent in some maladies, (epidemics, for instance,) to adopt essential and generic characteristic signs. This tendency arises from the peculiar character of the forces which produce them. This now has to be explained.

Among the causes of disease, some act upon us mechanically and physically; hence, they have no specific character. Such causes are, external injuries, dampness of the atmosphere, changes of temperature, draughts of air, etc.

Other causes act dynamically and specifically, such as viruses and miasms.

Each of the causes belonging to the first class, may, according as the individual is predisposed, give rise to pathological affections which are very different among each other. A draught of air, for instance, may occasion a coryza, a pleurisy, a rheumatism, etc. Is it not evident that, in such a case, the malady, which is subordinate to the age, sex, constitution, temperament, idiosyncrasy of the patient, to his hygienic habits, his degree of vitality, the greater or less degree of congenital or acquired, habitual or momentary irritability, or atony of this or that part of his organism, must necessarily present, in every individual, not only a peculiar degree of intensity, but also a peculiar development and combination of the symptoms? It seems to me, that these facts are confirmed by every day's experience, notwithstanding all that has been said, and can be said, in favor of the essential character of diseases. The plan of classifying diseases, in accordance with the physical causes which produce them, would therefore seem purely chimerical, and, on the other hand, it would seem absurd, to regulate, in accordance with mere names, the treatment required by each malady.[1]

In *miasmatic diseases*, on the contrary, the inherent force of the cause governs the individual physiological conditions among which it acts, so positively, that, whatever these conditions may be, the effects produced, will always consist of certain functional or determinate organic disorders, much more changeable in their degree of intensity than in the mode of their development.

Hence, of all known diseases, the so-called miasmatic or epidemic diseases would undoubtedly be those whose generic character it would be the most easy to establish, and which could be most readily subjected to the exigencies of a methodical classification.

But miasmatic and dynamic diseases being, as was shown above, strictly corresponding[2] to each other,

[1] Evidently the choice of the remedy is subordinate, both to the symptoms of the disease, and *to the pre-existing physiological condition of the patient.* The remedy which would unite the greatest number of chances of success, would be the one which, in a healthy individual, having as nearly as possible the same age, sex, and temperament of the patient, had produced a disease similar to the one with which the sick person is affected.

[2] Monsieur Orfila, in his letter of the fourth of January, 1853, to the president of the Académie de Médecine, in order to announce to this learned body the presents which he offered to it, and the prize which he instituted, goes so far as to propose the following subject, as the subject of a prize-essay: An investigation of the subtle poisons, whose absorption engenders epidemic diseases. "For thirty years," writes Orfila, "I have taught in my lectures, that intermit-

it follows that drug diseases, which are comparable to natural diseases, (for this constitutes the foundation of the Homœopathic doctrine,) are, at least, as much as the latter, comparable to each other, and susceptible, therefore, of being classified with reference to their reciprocal analogies and dissimilarities. The systemization of the Materia Medica is entirely included within this last proposition.

But before exhibiting the grounds upon which we propose to base our realization of this idea, let us resume what has been said so far.

1. All diseases, whether natural or medicinal, are, according to the happy definition of Hahnemann, virtual and dynamic alterations of the health.

2. The effects of drugs are (contrary to Hahnemann's opinion,) neither more nor less absolute, more nor less constant than those of the other (dynamic) causes of the diseases to which man is subject.

3. That the law of similarity, *similia similibus*, which is the reason of the specific action of remedial agents, not to be understood, however, in the sense of some homœopathic physicians, for their specificism is an erroneous deduction, is so much the more productive of happy results the more strictly it is applied to the *totality* of the two diseases which are intended to neutralize each other.

tent fevers, typhus, contagious and eruptive phlegmasias, dysentery, puerperal peritonitis, cholera, diphtheritis, etc., are specific diseases, which are occasioned by a poison that has developed itself in the animal economy, or has been introduced from without, into the respiratory passages, to be finally mixed with the blood," etc., (Bulletin de l'Académie de Médecine, Vol. XVIII., p. 307). I am of Orfila's opinion, but I do not believe that a chemical analysis will ever enlighten us concerning the inmost nature of miasms.

4th, and lastly, that of all diseases those which are least subject to the principle of absolute individualization established by Hahnemann, are epidemic and medicinal diseases, which nevertheless, does not prevent either from presenting marked differences in single individuals; so that the same morbific cause (this point is of great importance for us, as will soon be seen,) even when of a dynamic character, produces by its action, upon different individuals more or less dissimilar effects, whereas, different morbific causes, acting equally in different mediums, seem on the contrary, capable of producing in certain cases, effects that are more or less similar.[1]

Without insisting any further on these propositions, which in a treatise of medical philosophy, would undoubtedly require very long commentaries, let us at once enter upon an examination of the question which constitutes the special object of this work, namely: the classification of drug diseases, or which is the same, of drugs.

And to begin, is it not evident that in order to compare long diseases between themselves and to classify them afterwards, the first requisite is that they should be known? Now, do we know them? or how ought we to proceed to acquire this knowledge in case we should not yet possess it? An imposing question, for it not only implies criticism, but also, as we shall see presently, a thorough remodelling of the

[1] This is precisely the reason why the drug which acts best in epidemics, is but seldom the same for all patients. But there certainly exists a relation between all the drugs which succeed by turns in combatting one and the same essential malady: the formation of my groups rests principally upon this consideration.

immense labors of Hahnemann; for I make bold to affirm that, up to this moment, drug-diseases are, for the most part, only very little known to us.

Hahnemann has collected the pure effects of a hundred drugs, with a perseverance that is above all praise, and often with an acuteness of observation that was peculiar to him. But as I have already stated on a previous page, a series of symptoms juxtaposed at random, that is to say, according to an arbitrary rule, and which, in most instances, inverts the natural order in which the symptoms originally developed themselves, does not by any means, exhibit the image of a disease. This is so true, that if we would isolate the symptoms of a most perfectly defined and characteristic malady, typhus, for instance, as has indeed been done until now with all drug-diseases, we should have great difficulty in recognizing the original malady.

Every disease presents, independently of its mere symptoms, a special mode of development which imparts to it a characteristic distinction from all other diseases, and, in a great measure, gives its symptoms their true meaning. In other words, every disease, whether natural or medicinal, has its own course, its own phases of invasion, growth, condition, decrease and termination, and, in my opinion, it is only by an exact description of these different periods, that it becomes possible to give a true idea of the whole disease. There does not exist anything like it in our systems of pathogenesis,[1] immediate or

[1] Hahnemann, it is true, states *sometimes* in his *Materia Medica Fura,* in how many hours or days such and such a symptom has

consecutive, principal or accessory, constant or exceptional symptoms, all, generally, are classed alike, and occupy the same rank, what was to be done, in order to avoid this unpleasant confusion? Precisely that which I invite my colleagues to do with me.

Let us suppose, that we can count upon the aid of fifteen or twenty provers of both sexes, intelligent and devoted.[1] Each of these provers, trying upon himself, in previously determined conditions, the same drug in the same attenuation,[2] has only to note faithfully, from hour to hour, and from day to day, the symptoms which he perceives in himself, in order to be able, after a certain period, to furnish for the study of others, the complete *history* of the drug disease, at least with reference to his age, sex, tem-

manifested itself. But it is evident that neither he nor his disciples have made it a rule to proceed in this manner, which would, moreover, have been insufficient. The frequently admirable abstracts of morbid conditions which are often quoted in this work, and which Hahnemann places in front of his provings, in his work, entitled, *Doctrine and Homœopathic treatment of chronic diseases,* abound, to be sure, in characteristic traits; but they are not, and could not be, the synthetic images of drug diseases, such as I understand them. As regards the duration of the effects of drugs, which depends upon the vitality of the prover, upon the nature of the drug, and upon its degree of dynamization, it has frequently been fixed very arbitrarily.

[1] It is an organized Homœopathic society that is capable of accomplishing such a work, which, if carefully done, would redound to its glory.

[2] This condition is so much the more important, as the course of drug diseases is, to my certain knowledge, subordinate to it. I have become convinced, for instance, that drug diseases, if produced by the same drug, run their course the more rapidly, the higher are the attenuations which had been used for the proving.

perament, etc., conditions which should be scrupulously mentioned in front of his report.

Let us now suppose, that these fifteen or twenty individual observations, instead of being all mixed up in one incoherent list, according to the common usage, are arranged and combined by an experienced nosographist, a generalizing mind, another Hahnemann, provided nature were a little more prodigal of men of such calibre; is it not true, that, by this means, we shall arrive at the true synthesis of a drug disease, the imaginary type of which will be found sketched in the general synopsis, and will be necessarily elucidated by the fifteen or twenty individual observations that have served to establish it, and to represent all its shades?[1] Let us suppose, moreover, that the same method of investigation is successively applied to all drugs, and the Materia Medica will then become a true nosology, *entirely independent of the old pathology*, and thenceforth susceptible of a systematic arrangement in the closet of the physician.

We readily comprehend the immense advantages which would result to practitioners from such a revision of the Materia Medica. The more immediate of these advantages seem to emanate from the following considerations.

All drugs, whatever may be the special nature of their action, give rise in every part of the organism where this action manifests itself, to two orders of symptoms, which are generally, if not always, opposed to each other. Hahnemann attributed no other

[1] This is precisely the method which all good nosographists of every age have followed.

symptoms to the drugs directly, except those which he had seen develope themselves under their influence, and which he therefore called *primary symptoms*, whereas, he considered as simple reactions of the organism, all those symptoms that succeeded the former, and which he therefore designated as *secondary*. I shall not stop to inquire how far this theory of organic reactions is founded. This is purely speculative, and I attach only a mediocre importance to it. But the fact itself, is undoubtedly, one of the most interesting which the founder of Homœopathy has observed; and the striking contrast which it implies, seems to merit a profound study. It would be curious to know how far the secondary symptom is always the *contrary* of the primary, and how this contrary is understood and realized by nature in certain cases. What we know positively, is, that such a drug which *primarily* causes diarrhœa, is *secondarily* followed by constipation, whereas, such other drug gives rise to phenomena of an inverse order. One drug, *first* occasions a stoppage in the nose, and a dry cough, *afterwards* a fluent coryza and bronchial catarrh, whereas, another drug causes precisely the reverse symptoms. Here is a drug which *first* slackens, *afterwards* accelerates, the circulation, whereas another occasions first an increased speed, and afterwards an increased slowness of the pulse; opium *first* makes one drowsy, *afterwards* wakeful, whereas coffee makes one wakeful *first*, and *afterwards* puts one to sleep, etc. Since I have named two drugs, the alternate effects of which are generally known, at least in their totality, I will avail myself of them in order to show how important it is for us to discover

4

by pure experimentation the opposite effects of all therapeutic agents. This simple proposition which seems to me self-evident, *that natural maladies, as well as drug-diseases, have their primary and their secondary symptoms,* would render all demonstration superfluous, for, if this be true, who does not comprehend that it is not sufficient that a drug, in order to be really homœopathic to a given disease, should be capable of producing symptoms similar to those of the natural malady; but that the alternate effects of the drug and those of the disease must develop themselves in the same order. For instance,

Somebody complains of sleeplessness; he is restless, talkative, the cheeks are flushed, the extremities cold, etc. Is it *coffee* that he should take? Perhaps. . . In questioning him we learn that this state of agitation has *followed* a sort of *coma,* or even somnolence only, which had lasted one or two days, etc. Well, on this simple hint, I affirm that it is not coffee that he must have, *opium* alone will quiet him, and will restore his sleep; I say this from my own experience. Another patient, on the contrary, is sad, depressed in spirits and strength, drowsy; he is moreover costive, chilly, irritable, etc.; but this group of symptoms was ushered in by an excess of foolish mirth. Hence, I conclude that, notwithstanding these present symptoms, it is coffee he must have, and not by any means, opium. I need not say why. These cases evidently imply a general rule, and explain the fact that in a *number of cases* where not coffee or opium, but the foxglove,[1] especially in

[1] I scarcely need remark, that in either of these cases, the remedy should be indicated by more symptoms than I have deemed necessary to mention.

phthisis, or musk, belladonna, henbane, etc., were given, and effected a cure, the *contraria* principle may have *seemed* to succeed, but where in reality the cures were effected in conformity with the law *similia similibus*. This shows how valuable for the homœopathic physicians would become all indications derived from a historical report of drug diseases, with an accurate distinction of the primary and secondary effects of drugs.

Unfortunately the elements of such a scientific organization of our Materia Medica were wanting; for, I regret, the history of drug diseases, as I understand them, is only confessedly and obscurely perceived from the provings in our possession. It seems therefore as though the classification which I offer, were rather premature. However, I may do myself the justice to believe that, in reference to the totality of the effects of each of the drugs of which I have spoken in this work, I possess notions sufficiently correct, not to have committed any considerable errors in the formation of my categories or *groups*, according as either term has been adopted by me. Besides the provings, which I have subjected to a careful study, I have consulted the following sources in the arrangement of my materials: 1st. The natural history of drugs. 2d. Their known effects on animals of different species. 3d. Lastly, and principally, the history of their empirical applications.

1. *Natural History*.—By the natural history of the drugs I do not here mean the designation of the kingdom whence they are drawn, nor of the family, genus, etc., to which they belong in the systems of naturalists. Although I have deemed it necessary to mention

these indications in front of the history of every drug, yet I think that they are only of secondary importance to the physician. What is, in my opinion, of far greater importance to a practitioner is, that he should be acquainted with the regions of the globe whence the drugs are obtained, and with the special nature of the localities which produce them spontaneously. I say *spontaneously*, for every body knows that plants can be, and are transplanted every day, and that those which grow spontaneously in the South, can be made to grow in the North; that plants which naturally prefer a damp and marshy soil, can be made to grow in a dry soil; that those which are met on slopes and mountain-plains, can be made to grow in valleys and low regions, and vice versa. But independently of the well known fact that drugs which have been thus transplanted, lose either totally or partially the medicinal properties of which we know they are possessed, it is really only by studying their geographical and topographical conditions that we can hope, as we shall soon see, to discover certain special peculiarities of their destination. I am unable to say how far the outlines which I am going to offer, are founded and new as scientific facts, but they undoubtedly deserve to be taken into consideration.

The more we investigate the general relations of our reputed drugs with the diseases to which man is subject, the more we are struck by the curious circumstance that it is precisely in the districts where certain pathological affections prevail, we meet, by some admirable arrangement of the Creator, an abundance of the substances which are most capable of curing them. This coincidence may only be the necessary result of climacteric, hygrometric or telluric influences which, acting simultaneously upon the plants, animals and men of one and the same region, create in them certain elements of similitude, of which the *similia similibus* explains to us the consequences in the pathological order. Let this coincidence be accounted for in any manner you please, what seems to me irrefutable is, that it exists. To cite a few examples, the *bitter-sweet,* which is so often successfully given for the effects of a temporary or prolonged stay in a cold and damp atmosphere, prefers damp and cool localities. The *wolf's-bane,* on the contrary, which grows on mountain-tops, corresponds, as is well known, to inflammatory fevers and acute phlegmasias, to which the inhabitants of mountainous regions are particularly exposed in consequence of the habitual vigor of their constitution and their sanguine temperament. Whilst the *nux vomica* which is so often given with success for dysentery and bilious affections, grows in the East-Indies, the classic home of these kinds of affections, we derive from the north-east of Europe where the scrofula is indigenous, the *wild pansy* whose efficacy in this disease has been so often verified. *Copaiva* is perhaps the only remedy with which the plica polonica has ever been cured, and this drug is nowhere more abundant than in Poland. The *cedron,* which is an admirable antidote against the poison of the crotalus and the coral snake, grows almost exclusively in regions inhabited by these dangerous reptiles, etc. But should we conclude from these facts which it would be easy for me to multiply to an infinite extent, that each of our drugs is exclusively adapted to the endemic maladies of the countries whence it is obtained, or at most to individuals whose constitution is identical with that which is generally possessed by the inhabitants of these countries? This question, however strange it may seem at first, is nevertheless of a high interest. Without undertaking to answer it for the present, I propose it as a subject of study for homœopathic physicians, who will undoubtedly agree with me, even without much thought or experience concerning this subject, that the natural history of drugs, if studied from the standing-point which I have selected, will most probably furnish us useful and precious inductions.[1]

2. *Known observations and effects of drugs on animals of different species.*—In relating the observations of toxicologists, or the accidental cases of poisoning, I take care, as is seen, to add the words "*of different species*," for it is upon this distinction that the practical value of this question depends.

It is strange that, in experimenting with poisons on animals, physiologists, albeit they must have observed a difference in the effects of the poisons according as they were administered to cats, sea-hogs, goats, rabbits, birds of prey, fowl, etc., should never have taken the trouble to investigate the causes

[1] Example; *arsenic* and *veratrum* have both frequently cured the cholera, the principal symptoms of which they contain. But what class of patients have been principally cured by veratrum *which comes from the north of Europe and grows on mountain tops?* Patients with a sanguine temperament, quick, lively, and not having been weakened by a long attack, like those who were principally cured by arsenic.

of their difference. To say, in general terms, that animals, to whatever species they may belong, whatever climate they may inhabit, on whatever food they may live, resist the deleterious action of any poison the better the more vigorously they are organized, would be to assert a thing which is contradicted by experience. Indeed, I intend to show hereafter, and more particularly in speaking of pink-root, arsenic, the nux vomica, etc., that certain species of animals resist certain poisons *the less the more vigorous* these animals are. Now, inasmuch as, on the one hand, these poisons constitute those of our drugs which we employ most frequently, and inasmuch as, on the other hand, I am compelled to recognize the existence of evident physiological analogies between the idiosyncratic varieties of the human species and the principal types of the animal series, from the carnivorous inhabitant of the desert to the peaceful ruminator of our stables; it is easily seen how the proving of the same poison on different species of animals may have suggested to me every now and then a variety of useful hints.

3. *Empirical application of drugs.*—In every age physicians have constituted two classes of minds, speculative and practical. The former, who are disposed to indulge in abstract generalizations, have almost always been mediocre practitioners. The latter, on the contrary, who do not attach much importance to systems, and never submit to them blindly, do not recognize any other truths but those of an immediate and evident use, without even always caring to know upon what grounds their usefulness is

founded. All great practitioners have been, and probably always will be more or less *given to empiricism.* Some among them (and I might mention one or two instances) seem to be endowed with a sort of intuition, that is to say with a faculty which is neither the judgment nor the memory, and which suggests to them, in all difficult cases, the best method of treatment without they themselves ever being able to account for the reasons of their proceeding. Be this as it may, all the true observations of the Old School emanate from this latter class.

Among these observations, there are many which it would seem could not have been arrived at, except by pure experimentation, and which, obtained as they were by intuition, or an *a priori* mode of reasoning, must appear strange and even incomprehensible to homœopathic practitioners. We may remark in passing, that allœopathic physicians even are not aware of the mine of this kind of wealth, which is buried in the annals of their own doctrine. They are lost truths to most of them, and this need not astonish us, since these truths are not furnished with a suitable *criterium* in their estimation. But it is easily perceived why such documents should have been invested with the highest interest to me, and why I should, therefore, have considered it my duty to collect as many of them as possible.

In the first place, I was sure that I should find in them a new and striking confirmation of the homœopathic principle; for an appreciative comparison, such as I have instituted at the head of every drug, of the successful cures which have been effected by empiricists and homœopathists in the same cases, shows that they must result from the same law, *the law of similitude.* I may safely defy any serious and sincere physician who has read my book, to doubt the reality and immutability of this law. But independently of this proof which must seem superfluous to any one who has practised homœopathy for some weeks only, the empirical traditions of the old school offered to me inductions of a different kind, and which were more directly connected with the special object of my work. Is it not, indeed, evident, that the cure of certain pathological conditions, or, if you please, of certain symptoms, by means of a given drug, authorized me to attribute to this drug physiological effects, which, if not similar, were at least analogous in such a manner that, if pure experimentation had henceforth become the beacon light of therapeutics, clinical experience might, in its turn, be appealed to, in order to confirm the results obtained by our physiological provings? And besides, in verifying, according to the reports of faithful observers, the authentic cures, by means of a certain number of drugs, of various pathological conditions, but which are sufficiently similar to justify a belief in their identity, how could the idea have escaped me that these drugs are possessed of analogous properties?

In this way I found even in allœopathic traditions, that is to say, in the records of clinical experience, and independently of all pathogenetic investigations, the first data for a logical systemization of our Materia Medica.[1] Why should I hesitate to admit it? The

[1] In proportion as opportunities offer, I shall indicate the sources

work which I here offer to the public, rests in a great measure upon such data carefully weighed, compared with each other, and verified in the crucible of pure experimentation.

Thus, having devoted several years to the task of collecting as complete and accurate facts as possible concerning each of our drugs, I then proceeded to collate, and, finally, to class them.

After this, the determination of a certain number of *types*, around which *analogous* drugs could be grouped, became the object of my endeavors. This method which has been invariably followed by the naturalists ever since its first adoption by Antoine Laurent de Jussieu, was the only one that corresponded to my views.

If various considerations did not impose upon me the necessity of suppressing the purely analytical labors of my work, in order to leave only its conclusions, as it were, it would be seen after how many long and painful gropings, I was finally induced to adopt the following twenty types.[1]

where I have obtained the documents in question. I have rejected as not proving any thing, and as devoid of all true meaning, all clinical records tainted with poly-pharmacy or compound drugging. Unfortunately they constitute the majority. How much is it to be regretted that a number of great practitioners should not have been able to resist the temptation of compounding their drugs! This abuse alone would have sufficed to prevent the old school therapeutics from ever becoming a science.

[1] It is not by any means by design that I have adopted this number. After many modifications, by addition and substraction, this number was found to be the number of drugs to which I had given a preference without counting them.

1. Arnica montana,	11. Chelidonium majus,
2. Mercurius solubilis,	12. Acidum muriaticum,
3. Sulphur,	13. Lycopodium clavatum,
4. Arsenicum album,	14. Zincum,
5. Pulsatilla,	15. Aconitum napellus,
6. Sepia,	16. Conium maculatum,
7. Causticum,	17. Thuya occidentalis,
8. Ipecacuanha,	18. Chamomilla vulgaris,
9. Bryonia alba,	19. Atropa Belladonna,
10. Dulcamara,	20. Ferrum metallicum.

These twenty drugs are so arranged, agreeably to the order indicated by the general relations which the various groups that are governed by these remedies, respectively occupy towards each other.

These groups are as follows :—

GROUP I.	*Type.*	Arnica montana.	
	Analogies.	Ledum palustre.	Rhus toxicodendron.
		Croton tiglium.	Spigelia anthelmia.
		Ferrum magneticum.	
GROUP II.	*Type.*	Mercurius solubilis.	
	Analogies.	Argentum foliatum.	Creosota.
		Arsenicum album.	Plumbum.
		Sulphuris acidum.	Stannum.
		Mercurius corrosivus.	Nitri acidum.
		Crocus sativus.	
GROUP III.	*Type.*	Sulphur.	
	Analogies.	Croton tiglium.	Lobelia inflata.
		Mercurius corrosivus.	Mercurius solubilis.
		Bovista.	Asterias.
		Æthusa.	Cicuta virosa.
		Creasota.	Ratanhia.
GROUP IV.	*Type.*	Arsenicum album.	
	Analogies.	1st series (1).	Veratrum album.
		Argentum.	Zincum.
		Mercurius.	Lycopodium.
		Nux vomica.	Colocynthis.
		Sepia.	Copaivæ balsamum.
		Alumina.	Plumbum.
		Indigo.	Bryonia alba.
		Sulphur.	Cina.

		Lachesis.	Carbo vegetabilis.
		Ferrum metallicum.	Bismuthum.
		Petroleum.	Nux moschata.
		2d SERIES. Belladonna.	Bryonia.
		Carbo vegetabilis.	Opium.
		Capsicum.	Aconitum.
		Cedron.	Thuya.
		3d SERIES. Argentum.	Ferrum metallicum.
		Zincum.	Opium.
		Plumbum.	Arnica.
		Capsicum.	
		4th SERIES. Lobelia.	Sepia.
		Alumina.	Ferrum.
		Sulphur.	Argentum.
		Mercurius solubilis.	Merc. corrosivus.
GROUP V.	*Type.*	Pulsatilla.	
	Analogies.	Silicea.	Graphites.
		Calcarea carbonica.	Phosphorus.
		Hepar sulphuris.	
GROUP VI.	*Type.*	Sepia.	
	Analogies.	Copaivæ balsamum.	Alumina.
GROUP VII.	*Type.*	Causticum.	
	Analogies.	Cocculus.	Nux vomica.
		Coffea cruda.	Staphisagria.
		Corallia rubra.	Arsenicum.
GROUP VIII.	*Type.*	Ipecacuanha.	
	Analogies.	Pulsatilla.	Silicea.
		Nux vomica.	Dulcamara.
		Arsenicum.	Bryonia.
		Chelidonium majus.	Spongia tosta.
		Iodium.	Zincum.
		Chamomilla.	Ignatia.
		Phosphorus.	Belladona.
		Felix mas.	Antimonium
		Tartarus emeticus.	[crudum.
GROUP IX.	*Type.*	Bryonia alba.	
	Analogies.	Allium sativum.	Lycopodium.
		Colocynthis.	Nux vomica.
		Digitalis.	Ignatia.
GROUP X.	*Type.*	Dulcamara.	
	Analogies.	Sulphur.	Chelidonium.
		Corallia.	Pulsatilla.
		Bryonia.	Calcarea carbonica

GROUP XI.	*Type.*	Chelidonium majus.	
	Analogies.	Capsicum.	Viola odorata.
		Hepar sulphuris.	Corallia rubra.
		Allium sativum.	Cannabis indica.
		Dulcamara.	Cina.
		Digitalis.	Bryonia alba.
		Pulsatilla.	Silicea.
GROUP XII.	*Type.*	Acidum muriaticum.	
	Analogies.	Agnus castus.	Hyoscyamus niger.
GROUP XIII.	*Type.*	Lycopodium clavatum.	
	Analogies.	Natrum muriaticum.	Antimonium
		Viola tricolor.	[crudum.
GROUP XIV.	*Type.*	Zincum.	
	Analogies.	Plumbum.	Colchicum.
		Sambucus.	Arsenicum.
		Argentum.	Drosera.
		Nitri acidum.	Ferrum metallicum.
		Mercurius corrosivus.	Platina.
GROUP XV.	*Type.*	Aconitum Napellus.	
	Analogies.	Cocculus.	Cannabis.
		Chamomilla.	Conium.
		Dulcamara.	
GROUP XVI.	*Type.*	Conium maculatum.	
	Analogies.	Jatropha curcas.	Chamomilla.
		Phosphoris acidum.	Senega.
		Solanum nigrum.	Cantharis.
GROUP XVII.	*Type.*	Thuya occidentalis.	
	Analogies.	Platina.	Bismuthum.
		Castoreum.	
GROUP XVIII.	*Type.*	Chamomilla vulgaris.	
	Analogies.	Gratiola officinalis.	Helleborus nigra.
		Viola tricolor.	
GROUP XIX.	*Type.*	Belladonna.	
	Analogies.	Agaricus.	Lachesis.
		Cedron.	Stramonium.
		Opium.	Opium.
		Arnica.	Clematis erecta.
		Ruta graveolens.	Tabacum.
		Aurum.	Camphora.
		Cannabis.	Hyoscyamus.
		Bryonia alba.	

GROUP XX.	*Type.*	Ferrum metallicum.	
	Analogies.	Plumbum.	Magnesia muriatica
		Phosphorus.	Ratania.
		Carbo animalis.	Bovista.
		Pulsatilla.	China.
		Zincum.	Baryta carbonica.
		Secale cornutum.	Cuprum.

Each of these twenty groups represents a series of drugs, or rather of drug diseases, which resemble each other more or less, by their course and symptoms, if they develope themselves in physiological conditions that are similar; or, which offer, in certain cases, the appearances of an almost complete similarity, if they develope themselves in physiological conditions that are different.[1] Hence, we may infer, that diseases occasioned by the drugs of one and the same group, may, to a certain extent, be abstractly considered as the various shades of one and the same malady, the most acute form of which, (almost in every group,) would be represented by the *type*. I have described at the head of each group, under the title of "*common characteristics*," the principal symptoms, but not the course (this I found impossible,) of this artificial malady which any other member of the group is likewise capable of producing with more or less completeness.

In perusing the preceding list of my groups, the same drug will be found mentioned in several

[1] Ipecac., and tartarus emet., for instance, if proved successively, and at convenient intervals, by the same prover, would probably point in this individual to two distinct maladies, and yet evidently analogous to each other; whereas ipecac., if given to a little child, and tartarus emet., if given to an adult, might produce, in these two individuals, two apparently such similar diseases that a nosographist might not hesitate to give them the same name.

groups. A moment's reflection will suffice to show that this could not be otherwise. Who does not know that every malady, whether medicinal or otherwise, may not, according to the light in which it is viewed, be compared, and, in certain respects, be considered similar to other maladies which are notoriously dissimilar among each other?[1]

The order according to which the drugs in each group are arranged, expresses their degree of affiliation with the typical drug.

With every drug, I have combined its natural and therapeutic history, and its recent applications as derived from the pathogenetic provings. As regards the pathogeneses themselves, I shall only relate my own, or such as exist only in works of small circulation, and shall, for all other provings, refer the reader to the special works, where they may be found, and which works are in the hands of all Homœopathic physicians. I need scarcely observe, that I have not been able to class all the drugs now known; this was impossible, for the simple reason, that I did not possess sufficient data for the accomplishment of such a task. This is the reason why such substances as manganese, mezereum, and several others, have been omitted in my work for the present; they are in pretty general use, it is true, but my information concerning their therapeutic value was not suffi-

[1] *Scarlatina*, for instance, might be at the same time classed among the *anginœ* and the acute *cntaneous diseases*. It is true that, in order to be classed logically, it should be placed in the first rank of dermatoses, and in the last rank of anginæ: considerations of this kind have always guided me in the classification of drug diseases.

ciently positive to permit me to receive such drugs among my categories.

Lastly, among the general observations belonging to each group, I have indicated the *diseases corresponding* to the drugs of which each group is composed. But to be of any real value, this co-relation should be preceded by an almost total revision and remodelling of our pathological sciences; I therefore attach no very great importance to this part of my work for the present.

Nevertheless, the practitioner will often find useful indications in the relations which I have established. This, at least, is my firm belief. All things considered, my work, whatever time and labor I may have bestowed upon it, is only an incomplete sketch of such an one as the vastness of the end which I have proposed to attain, would render necessary. If it should fulfil no other use, may it, at least, have this good, to inspire some day, a man of genius, with the thought of more worthily accomplishing my task!

February, 1853.

THE HOMŒOPATHIC MATERIA MEDICA;

ARRANGED SYSTEMATICALLY AND PRACTICALLY.

GROUP I.

TYPE; ARNICA MONTANA.

ANALOGOUS REMEDIES:

LEDUM PALUSTRE.
CROTON TIGLIUM.
FERRUM MAGNETICUM.
RHUS TOXICODENDRON.
SPIGELIA ANTHELMIA.

COMMON CHARACTERISTICS.

FEELING of weariness and soreness all over, as after great fatigue, or as from some external violence.

Rush of blood to the head, as in apoplexy.

Stupefying headache, with shuddering, sensation of coldness or actual coldness all over, except about the head, face, and sometimes the hands and feet.[1]

Pressive, cutting, burning, or lancing pains in the outer parts of the head, especially at the temples, in the parietal regions, and at the occiput.

Swelling of the bulbs of the eyes, with or without lachrymation.

Red, erysipelatous swelling, or else paleness of the face; obstinate nose-bleeding.

Pressive, contusive, cutting, tearing pains, which are sometimes frightful, especially at the nape of the neck, loins, shoulders, hands, in the fingers, legs, feet, and big toes.

Pain in the joints, as if sprained or dislocated.

Numbness and paralytic weakness of the limbs.

Red swelling of the fingers and hands.

[1] Except, perhaps, in the case of Spigelia.

Red, blueish swelling, or infiltration without swelling, of the big toe, the instep, ankle and leg, up to the knee.

Formications in the skin.

Acute inflammations of the skin, adopting the following forms:—phlegmon, erysipelas, pustules or vesicles, which are filled with a clear liquid, that is either colorless, or else is slightly tinged like amber.

Effusion of blood under the epidermis (ecchymosis), petechiæ.

Red or colorless, but always painful swelling of the subcutaneous glands.[1]

Mouth dry, hot, the tongue being covered with a kind of pellicle, under which a number of small vesicles are seen, similar to those which, at the same time, are noticed on the skin.[2]

Anorexia, thirst, bitter taste of the food, loss of taste, bilious eructations, and vomiting; vomiting of blood.

Tingling, burning, pinching, or cutting pains in the stomach and bowels.

Painful engorgement of the liver and spleen; jaundice, intermittent fever.

Constipation, sometimes with tenesmus, or alternating with diarrhœa; small, slimy, sanguineous stools, or consisting of pure blood, accompanied with a violent cutting colic.

Spasmodic cough, which is sometimes very violent.

Agitation of the blood in the chest; hæmoptysis.

Sensitiveness of the chest to contact; pressure on the chest; dyspnœa; violent shootings in the chest and region of the heart.[3]

Irascible temper; moroseness or imaginary apprehensions; attack of fainting, as after a fall or hæmorrhage.

Drowsiness in the day time, without being able to sleep; sleeplessness in the evening, in bed; dreams about quarrels, murders, fires.

[1] Except, perhaps, in the case of Spigelia.

[2] I have noticed this symptom, which explains a great many others, more particularly in the case of ledum, rhus and croton.

[3] Especially in the case of Spigelia.

Intermittent neuralgic pains, sometimes recurring at long intervals.

Aggravation of the symptoms in the evening, at night, in artificial warmth, *and during motion*, (especially in the case *of arnica*,) sometimes during rest (particularly in the case of *rhus* and *spigelia*.)

CORRESPONDING MALADIES.

Traumatic lesions of every variety, even burns of the different degrees. Active hæmorrhages. Simple and phlegmonous erysipelas: (especially of the face.) Zona. Pemphigus. Eczema. Urticaria. Anthrax. Boils. Acne. Wens. Warts. Parotitis. Articular rheumatism. Gout. Muscular rheumatism. Cerebral congestion and paralysis of the extremities. Traumatic or rheumatic cataract. Neuralgia. Angina. Bronchitis. Pneumonia. Hepatitis. Traumatic affections or affections consequent upon the retrocession of an acute eruption upon the skin, (acne or eczema,) etc., etc.

The six remedies which compose this group, possess such symptomatic affiliations amongst each other, that, in many respects, they seem to represent the shades of one and the same malady. However, they are far from producing, in the same degree, under perfectly identical circumstances, the symptoms which have been classed under the head of *common characteristics;* nor are they in the same degree or indiscriminately, adapted to the diseases which we have just now named as corresponding to them. In giving the history of each drug, the physiological and pathological conditions upon which its use depends will be mentioned. What I may affirm, however, even now, is, that it frequently happens that several among them may, in the same individual and in the same malady, be successively indicated. This remark is, indeed, applicable to almost every one of the twenty groups which I have adopted.

The remedies of the *Arnica* group, which are truly sovereign in a large number of acute affections, occupy, moreover, (and more particularly those last named,) an important rank in the treatment of chronic maladies. I ought to observe, however, first, that with the exception of spigelia and the magnetic iron, which constitute the transition-points between this group and the following, they exercise only a very limited action upon the osseous system; second, that their feeble power to alter the nature of the secretions, renders them almost entirely inefficacious in degenerations of tissues. It is thus that, among cutaneous diseases, they only reach those which manifest themselves in the simple forms of erythema, phlogosis of the dermis or of the subcutaneous cellular tissue, pustules and colorless vesicles; or, lastly, the warts and callosities, which, as is well known, emanate from an excess of local secretion of the epidermis-matter, induced by some mechanical cause.[1]

The remedies of the Arnica group only respond to a small portion of the series of known cutaneous disorders. It is among the symptoms of *Mercurius* and *Sulphur* that we have to look for its completion. Let me state that, among cutaneous diseases, I include all those which, by their nature, are susceptible of invading every part of the organism, but the primary seat of which *seems* to be the skin.

From such considerations, upon which the contiguousness of my first three groups is based, emanates the line of demarcations which I draw between the members of the *Arnica* and those of the *Bryonia* group, whose action seems to me to proceed inversely to that of the former; that is to say, from the centre to the periphery, and not from the periphery to the centre.

Finally, it may be well to allude to a few relations existing between the *Zincum* and *Arnica* group, which, perhaps, may be of use to practitioners.

Arnica Montana, *leopard's-bane.*—A species of the genus *Arnica*, family of the radiata, class syngenesia polygamia superflua.

This aromatic plant was described for the first time with correctness by Tabernæmontanus, naturalist of the sixteenth

[1] Callosities, corns and warts, are concretions of dried serum, but not sensibly altered in its composition.

century. It grows on the high mountains of the south of Europe and in the plains of the north of France, where some varieties of it exist, distinguished by the large size of its leaves, the height of its stems, etc. It has black, thin, fibrous roots, which emanate from a sort of rhizoma; single stems; leaves oval, and marked with lines, entire, opposite on the stem; flowers radiate, large and of a beautiful yellow color; fruit with plumose tufts, enclosed in a common double calice or involucrum.

Notwithstanding the acrid and bitter taste of this plant, it does not, according to Linné, exercise any deleterious action on herbivorous animals: "Oxen and goats," says he, "eat it with pleasure."[1]

The *arnica* of Bohemia was the one which was formerly the most valued.[2] It was prescribed in the shape of infusions, decoctions, and locally. The root, stem, and blossoms were successively given a preference by physicians, who, however, gave up the root for good, for this reason, that it rapidly loses its taste and aroma by drying. It is this root, but fresh, that is used for homœopathic preparations.[3]

Empirical applications.—For a long time already popular empiricism had used the properties of arnica, when a Belgian physician, named Fehrius or Fehr, drew the attention of his colleagues to this plant. The facts which were published by this physician, tended to show that the arnica, whether used externally or internally, was a specific remedy for *sanguineous effusions, sugillations, ecchymoses,* etc.[4] A large number of German, Swedish, and French practitioners, among whom we distinguish Buchner, Schulz, Rosenstein, de la Marche and Collin, confirmed Fehr's observations with great readiness, and the use of arnica soon became very extensive. According to Murray it was successfully used against the following maladies: *external lesions, such as are*

[1] *Flora sulcica*, p. 295.
[2] De la Marche, dissert. de arn. veræ usu, p. 14.
[3] See Hahnemann, Mat. Med. Pur., vol. I.
[4] Murray, *apparat. medicam.*, vol. I., p. 158.

caused by a blow, a fall, a contusion, etc.; a certain form of *fall pleurisy; cachexia; œdema; atrophy; traumatic peri-pneumonia; suppression of the menses, or lochia; uterine hæmorrhage; calculous nephritis; gout; muscular contractions; gangrene; jaundice* caused by contusions; *paraplegia; hemiplegia; paralysis of the bladder; amaurosis*, caused by a cerebral affection.[1]

The pathogenesis of the arnica explains to us the cause of these successful applications, which were purely accidental, and which, being deprived of a fixed principle, must have remained without result to the healing art until homœopathy was discovered.

More fortunate than Borda and the Berlin physicians, who regarded the arnica as a calming agent in inflammations of the lungs,[2] Stoll used it with success in certain forms of dysentery, especially in *epidemic dysentery*,[3] and cured with this drug several cases of *intermitting fever*, a circumstance which induced this celebrated physician to term it the *quinquina of the poor*, a designation, however, which it does not seem to deserve.

Lastly, at a more recent period, *arnica* has been lauded as a remedy for *spasms, convulsions, tetanus*,[4] *convulsive cough, trembling*, and even for the *itch*.[5] It is true, that in the last named disease, care was had to add a good dose of sea-salt to the decoction of the plant, which was prescribed in lotions, so that it would be difficult to say to which of these two agents the removal of the psoric eruption was due, which is of very little consequence so far as we are concerned; for the result of such a system of medication could only be pitiable.

After having passed in review the cases where the arnica

[1] Murray, apparat. medicam,, vol. I., p. 158.

[2] *Flora ticinensis*, vol. II., 1823.

[3] Stoll, Med. Prat., vol. I., p. 129; vol. II., p. 52 and 376. Stoll was right. Without being a specific remedy, the *arnica* as well as *rhus tox.*, its analogous remedy, corresponds to several symptoms of this disease.

[4] *Arnica* may have been successfully employed in tetanus caused by traumatic lesions.

[5] *Revue medicale*, vol. XXII., p. 336.

had effected cures, Murray mentions the accidents which it is capable of producing when administered out of season, or in too large doses. He says that it has occasioned vomiting, anxiety, sweats, an aggravation of pain around injured parts, (*which, however, never lasted long,*) sensitiveness of the abdomen, weakness of the senses and nerves, tingling, lancing and burning pains, or shocks resembling those produced by the electric fluid. Hence Murray concludes, but wrongly, that the presence of fever forbids the use of arnica. Be this as it may, nothing can be more correct than his observations, which, however, have been taken from Plenck, Diltney, Schulz, Collin, and from several other authors.[1]

The arnica is undoubtedly one of those drugs, the therapeutic properties of which have been most justly valued by alloeopathic physicians. This is so true, that a complete collection of all the cases in which it was successfully employed by them, would almost furnish the complete pathogenesis of the drug. Was it mere accident that led empiricism to these successful applications of the arnica? I confess that I feel disposed to view them in the light of the maxim of Jamblicus: "Medicine is the daughter of dreams." But how is it possible that, in spite of such precious traditions, the arnica should have fallen into such a complete disuse that it is not even any longer mentioned in the modern systems of alloeopathic Materia medica?[2] Do systems enjoy the privilege of blotting out facts which they are unable to explain?

Homœopathic applications.—See the pathogenesis of *arnica* in Hahnemann's Materia Medica Pura, Vol. I.[3] It is enough to read this pathogenesis, in order to perceive how far the law of similitude explains and justifies the surname of

[1] Like external lesions of some magnitude, the arnica seems at first to impede or circumscribe the circulation; but this phenomenon, which almost always precedes the traumatic fever, is of short duration.

[2] Especially in that of Messrs. Trousseau and Pidoux.

[3] The pure effects of arnica are so well known by all Homœopathic physicians, that I do not deem it necessary to indicate them, as I shall hereafter do with other remedies.

panacea lapsorum, which was formerly given to the arnica by those who used it empirically.

The sphere of *arnica* comprises, then, all *traumatic lesions*, (*contusions, cut and torn wounds*,) with their immediate consequences, (*internal* or *external hæmorrhages*, *fractures*, *luxations*, *sprains*, *traumatic fever*, *syncope*, *tetanus*, *paralysis*, *pneumonia*, *hepatitis*, etc., etc.,) or their remote consequences, (*partial emaciation*, *neuralgia*, *intermittent fevers*, *encysted tumors*, etc., etc.) But since we now cure these maladies also by *ledum*, *rhus*, and other analogous remedies, it is important to determine the cases where arnica deserves a preference.

The arnica is particularly adapted to sanguine, plethoric persons, with lively complexions, and disposed to cerebral congestions. It acts but feebly on persons that are positively debilitated, with impoverished blood, and soft flesh. This may be the reason why it is eaten with impunity by herbivorous animals, as Linné remarks. It does not do them any harm, and probably, would not do them any good in diseases where it might otherwise seem indicated The case would be different in regard to *spigelia*, whose general action, which tends to depress vascular action, is, so to say, diametrically opposite to that of arnica. The latter would destroy life by exciting the vital force to excess, whereas the former would produce death by depressing the vitality.[1] Hence I conclude, as a general rule, that *arnica* is particularly useful in the inflammatory period of the maladies to whose symptoms it corresponds.

This drug acts principally on the muscles and the cellular tissue. Hence the *boil* is the one of all cutaneous affections which arnica most readily occasions, and, of course, cures. Hence again, it is more particularly adapted to the treatment of *phlegmonous erysipelas* and *deep burns*, than to that of *simple erysipelas* and *superficial burns*, diseases in which *rhus* generally deserves a preference. It is evident that, in such cases, the alternate use of these two drugs must be frequently indicated.

[1] This kind of contrast will be met with in a good many of our groups.

From the fact that *arnica* frequently cures *acne* and *boils*, independently of any traumatic cause, we infer that it likewise cures internal maladies which emanate from the retrocession of these cutaneous efflorescences. I have treated a man of 30 years and a sanguine temperament, in whom the formation of boils constituted a veritable diathesis. For months a large number were seen in the face, on the neck and shoulders. Afterwards they disappeared in order to give place to an intense angina. This process had been going on for several years. I prescribed arnica, which arrested in a few days the throat-disease, and the boils which had disappeared when this disease set in, have not reappeared since. This fact is another proof of the importance which the historic development of the disease possesses for the physician. I doubt not that, by carefully investigating the antecedents of arnica, one would have hit upon some cutaneous affection which arnica cures, and the previous existence of which would have accounted for the efficacity of arnica in the pretended *fall pleurisies*. We may be allowed to ask in this place whether the pleurisies were any thing else than simple pleurodynias, accompanied by pulmonary engorgement.

Every body knows what success has been obtained with the arnica in the homœopathic treatment of *gout*, (especially of the foot;) *idiopathic rheumatism*, that is to say, a rheumatism which is not preceded by the affection of some viscus, and of certain kinds of *neuralgia*, (especially of the head,) characterised by the cutting, tearing, or wrenching pains which the arnica produces.

Arnica may, after *rhus*, prove useful in the painful engorgements of the subcutaneous glands, and even of the vesical glands in persons with a lymphatico-sanguine temperament, but not really scrofulous. It is especially in individuals thus constituted that *arnica* has effected cures of *intermittent fever* combined with hypertrophy of the liver or spleen, which was painful to contact.

In its general action *arnica* exhibits some distant points of similarity to the action of *Belladonna.* It is one of those drugs, small in number, the external use of which is allowed in homœopathic treatment (only in traumatic, or strictly local affections.) But it must not be supposed that, in such cases, it is absolutely necessary to employ the mother-tincture. Experience has demonstrated to me that the sixth, twelfth, and fifteenth alcoholic attenuations of arnica, spigelia, colchicum, were, as a general rule, preferable, both externally and internally, to the mother-tinctures of these drugs.

"Camphor," says Hahnemann, "is the antidote of arnica when administered in large doses and in cases where it was not homœopathic. Wine aggravates its hurtful effects." Positive experience has convinced me that, in many cases at least, cocculus indicus antidotes arnica much better than camphor.

Ledum palustre, *wild rosemary.* Genus *ledum,* family *rhodoracea,* Class decandria monogynia.

This bush, which is also cultivated in gardens, grows in the damp regions of the north of Europe, in the mountains of Vosges, etc. Except by the goat, it is not eaten by animals, on account of the strong and resinous smell of its leaves, which keeps off the lice, prevents floors from getting mouldy, and it is said, imparts to Russian leather the particular odor of which it is known to be possessed.[1]

Empirical applications.—The *medical history* of ledum is very brief. Scarcely any other than the Swedish physicians, have endeavored to employ this drug. A decoction of it was used to free oxen and pigs from their lice; a practice, which

[1] Mèrat and Delens, *Dict. universel de mat. médic. et de thérap. générale.* Paris, 1832, vol. IV., p. 82. Murray disputes this peculiarity; he says of it: "Oleo hujus et cortici betulæ albæ olim creditum corium russicum odorem suum specificum debere, sed testis autopes gravis nuper declaravit ledum omitti." (Pallas, *travels,* vol. I., p. 46, and vol. II., p. 189.) The truth is that Russian leather owes its odor to the birch-bark which is used in tanning it, instead of oak-bark.

has led me to a very curious application of ledum. Linné, to whom we are indebted for a knowledge of this fact, informs us, that the same decoction, if taken internally, has cured *violent headaches*, and a species of *angina*, against which other medicines had been used with much less effect.[1] Westring, likewise, praises ledum highly in a very *fatal epidemic and contagious angina*, characterized by a convulsive cough, rapid and considerable swelling of the cervical glands, which was very painful, and accompanied with a slow fever.[2] Rosenstein, Scopoli, and Jacquin, relate similar facts. Some of the symptoms of ledum account for this success.

"This plant," say Mérat and de Lens, "if applied in the form of a lotion, cures the *itch* and *scald head;* it is supposed to be possessed of narcotic properties, and of the faculty of quieting exanthematic fevers, etc."[3] If these observations were a little more precise, they would be correct. Ledum, indeed, cures neither the itch nor scald head; but it destroys the acarus and lice, and, by this means, may sometimes have facilitated the removal of these eruptions. Without being a *narcotic*, properly speaking, *ledum* has *stupefying* properties, like all its analogues. And like these, it has acute cutaneous symptoms, which, blindly applied, may have given rise to the idea, which was admitted much too generally, however, that ledum possesses *calming* properties in the treatment of exanthematic fevers.

Be this as it may, the Allœopathic traditions concerning ledum, are evidently exceedingly vague and scanty. Indeed, this drug had almost been lost sight of, when Hahnemann published its pathogenesis.[4]

Homœopathic applications.—"Although the action of ledum upon the healthy organism," says Hahnemann, "has not as yet been studied in anything like a complete manner; the symptoms which we know of this drug, are sufficient to show that it is scarcely of any use except in chronic maladies,

[1] Linné, *Flora laponica*, p. 121. [2] Dissert. de led. palustre. [3] Loc. cit.
[4] See Dr. Roth's Mat. med. pura, vol. I., p. 106, and following.

which are principally characterized by cold, and a deficiency of animal heat."[1]

Doctor Roth, who has drawn from various sources a few additions to Hahnemann's pathogenesis, expresses himself as follows, in regard to the action of this drug: "If we would believe what the various authors say of the medicinal virtues of ledum, we might feel tempted to class this drug among those that offer resources against a large number of maladies; but in verifying the sources of these assertions, we will find ourselves disabused."[2]

The former of these two opinions, which was admitted by its author to have been premature, has, to some extent at least, been refuted by experience. As regards the opinion of Doctor Roth, it simply goes to confirm a thing that we had been aware of for a long time past, namely, that the Allœopathic physicians, whose assertions have been collected by our learned colleague, have never had the least suspicion of the true properties of ledum, and have, therefore, been unable, to avail themselves of them in practice.

Ledum, whose sphere of action is contiguous to that of arnica, and is frequently identical with it, seems to me to exercise a special action on the capillary system in parts of the body where the cellular tissue is wanting, and which present in most men a resisting and dry texture, such as the fingers and toes. It is perhaps for this reason, that it acts better on the small than on the large joints. Be this as it may, I have become convinced by numerous facts, that in the treatment of *traumatic whitlow*, in persons of a sanguine temperament, it is incomparably superior to arnica.

A remarkable fact, and which I believe I have been the first to point out, is this, that ledum is to wounds inflicted *with pointed instruments*, what arnica is to contusions.

Guided by a few of its cutaneous symptoms, which seemed to me to agree with the use that was made of this drug in domestic practice at the time of Linné, I commenced with

[1] Mat. med. pura, vol. II. [2] Loc. cit., p. 141.

trying it against mosquito bites, and the result astonished me. A single teaspoonful of a tumblerful of water, in which a few globules of the fifteenth dilution of ledum had been dissolved, quieted completely, in a few minutes, I might even say, in a few seconds, the itching caused by the bite, without any external application being necessary. From mosquito bites, I passed to the stings of bees and wasps, etc., as soon as an opportunity was offered, which, happily, was not very long. Here the result was less prompt, but still very satisfactory. In the space of two years which followed these first trials, I treated with ledum in the most satisfactory manner, 1st, several *whitlows*, which had been caused by pricks with the needle, or by stings of insects; 2d, a violent *bite of a water-rat* at the index-finger of the right hand, in a young man who was catching crabs; 3d, a serious wound in a young lady, who fell with an *embroidering needle in her hand*, which was pierced through and through. No hæmorrhage had resulted from this accident; but I observed in the patient this intense cold which accompanies and characterizes the ledum fever. In from six to seven days the patient was cured.

I have strong reasons to think that ledum is less adapted to the acute arthritis of the large joints, than to the *gout* proper, when it had been seated for a long time in the toe or finger-joints, without causing a swelling of the hand or foot. Ledum is particularly indicated when the violent tensive or tearing pain in one of the small toe or finger-joints, is accompanied with a circumscribed redness and little swelling, general coldness, great depression of spirits, and a sediment of uric acid in the urine.

It is known that ledum produces, and, therefore, cures in some cases an *obstinate swelling* of the feet.

The action which this drug exercises on the skin, differs from that of the arnica in this, that the former causes not so much a boil as a sort of blueish or violet-colored tuberosity, especially on the forehead, and an *eczematous eruption, with a tingling itching*, that spreads over the whole body, penetrates into the mouth, probably also into the air-passages, and occasions a spasmodic cough which is sometimes very violent, and which might be mistaken for *whooping-cough.* The same phenomenon takes place with rhus and croton. In a gouty subject, I have seen cough precede by two days the breaking out of vesicles upon the skin, which could not fail to suggest the use of ledum. These vesicles which had probably existed on the bronchial mucous membrane, before showing themselves in the face, on the shoulders, etc., became quite apparent on the tongue, where they might be traced to the root of this organ.

The ledum eczema, and in this it acts like the rhus and croton eczema, is frequently seen concentrated on one leg, or (which is less frequently the case,) on both legs, at one and the same time. It then shows itself from the instep to the rotula, in the shape of a blueish, hot, rough surface, with or without itching or swelling, but very tenacious. The cure of this unpleasant eruption almost always requires the alternate exhibition of ledum, rhus and croton; we need not recur to it in speaking of these two latter drugs. According to Hahnemann, camphor antidotes, wine heightens the effects of ledum, like those of arnica. *Rhus tox.*[1] is, however, the principal antidote of ledum.

Rhus toxicodendron, *poisonous sumach.*—Genus *rhus,* family terebinthaceæ, class pentandria trygynia.

Rhus toxicodendron which, according to Bosc, is identical with the rhus radicans of Linné, is a bush which grows in North America, on the borders of rivers or in marshy districts, and grows very tall in a soil which suits it. Its lateral branches are numerous and tufty; leaves indented and pubescent, flowers hermaphrodite; fruit, like that of every other species of rhus, small black berries.

[1] I had not yet discovered this peculiarity when I indicated (in my treatise *on children's diseases*) the alternate use of *rhus* and *ledum* against eczema. This treatment has been successful in several cases; but I now believe that the treatment would still be more successful, if the two remedies were given at longer intervals than I have indicated.

The odor which emanates from this bush, is not very strong. The juice of its leaves blackens the hand like caustic; nevertheless, according to the report of Barton and W. Bartram, cows and horses eat them without being in the least incommoded by them.

"In handling this plant, it produces blistering effects upon the skin, which are very remarkable, as has been witnessed by Gouan and Amoreux. Sometimes the head swells to double its size; this happened three times in succession to the celebrated Fontana, while he was experimenting with rhus.[1] Doctors Roth and Doxet have published in the *Homœopathic Gazette, of Paris*, several observations which confirm the facts cited by Alibert. It is known, moreover, that it is not by contact alone that the sumach causes these accidents. To be attacked with them, it is sufficient to inspire the air impregnated with its emanations. The results of the inhalation of the atmosphere of *rhus toxicodendron*, develop themselves in a few hours, and sometimes in a few days; they consist of itching, swelling, redness, pain and pustules, which are more or less vesicular, on the part which had been in contact with the plant, and even on those parts of the body which had not been in contact, like the face, scrotum, eyelids, etc. They are generally accompanied with fever, malaise, oppression lasting for several days, etc. A fatal case is mentioned, where a person touched the several parts after having handled branches of this bush."[2]

In 1825, Lavini, published some remarkable observations concerning the inoculation of the juice of rhus. To the first phalanx of the index-finger, he applied two drops of the juice, and left them for two minutes only in contact with the epidermis. *Twenty-five days* after this, the following symptoms suddenly showed themselves: great heat in the mouth and throat; rapid and considerable swelling of the left cheek, the upper lip and eye lids. In the night following, swelling of

[1] *New elements of Therapeutics*, etc., vol. I., p. 456.

[2] Merat and Delens, *Diction*, *de Mat. Med.*, vol. VI., p. 82.

the forearms to double their natural size; dry, tense, and burning skin, intolerable itching, etc.[1]

Empirical applications.—The old school has endeavored to improve the powerful properties of Rhus, but blindly as usual.

Dufresnoy, army physician and professor of botany in Valenciennes, employed it with success against *tetters* and *paralysis*. Of the twelve observations which he published in 1788, seven refer to cutaneous affections, and the rest to paralysis consequent on convulsions.[2]

Similar results were obtained by several physicians of Brussels, among others by Verdegen, Kok and Van Baerlem.[3] Poutingon, professor at the school of Montpelier, cured with this plant, a paralytic patient in a fortnight, and Gouan cured in a similar manner, and in a few weeks, a young lady afflicted with hemiplegia. Several almost similar facts are contained in the manuscript notes which Dr. Petroz has furnished me. Lastly, ever since the year 1793, Alderson published in England, seventeen observations which went to prove the efficacity of *Rhus* against *paralysis*, and in general against all affections characterized by a sinking of the apparatus of locomotion.[4]

In spite of all these successful trials, the sumach shared, in France at least, the fate of the arnica.[5]

It was lauded to the skies, it was said to have wrought miracles, and after that it was abandoned, more perhaps than arnica, because it was more dangerous. It is well known that one of the problems which the allœopathic healing art has been endeavoring for some time past to solve is, to find remedies which would not hurt, even if given out of season; in other words, remedies that are not remedies.

[1] *Journal de chimie médicale*, June, 1825.

[2] Anc. Journal de Médecine, vol. LXXX., p. 136.

[3] Alibert, *ouvrag. cit.* vol. I., p. 459.

[4] *An essay on rhus tox.* in 8°. Lond. 1793.

[5] *Rhus tox* is frequently used by the German allœopathic physicians; but among the French allœopathic physicians I only know (Dr. Bretonneau of Tours) who has made use of it recently.

Hahnemann, to whom we are indebted for the pathogenesis of rhus,[1] says that the effects of this drug and those of bryonia are analogous. It is, indeed, true, that except the differences which Hahnemann indicates, this analogy exists if we simply compare their symptoms according to the regions, organs and tissues that are respectively affected by these drugs. But, in order to reduce this analogy to its proper value, it suffices to contrast the symptoms of these two drugs with reference to the mode in which they develope themselves. If we succeed in fixing the true starting point and mode of development belonging to the respective series of their symptoms, we cannot fail to recognise that they develope themselves in opposite directions as it were. Let us remark, in passing, that the same observations are applicable to spigelia and digitalis, which, in my first attempts at systemization, I endeavored to unite under the same general view.

Homœopathic applications.—There are few drugs whose effects are better and more characteristically known than those of rhus. Every symptom almost reveals the action of a corrosive caustic, which, on account of its extreme sùbtlety, shows a tendency to invade large surfaces, rather than to penetrate deeply into the tissues. Hence the acute pains and the ataxic effects caused by rhus, and which constitute phenomena that so frequently accompany the affections which resemble those occasioned by the action of rhus, such as burns, erysipelas, erythematous enteritis, etc. Although rhus, like arnica and ledum, acts principally upon the head and the organs of locomotion, yet it differs from arnica in this, that it affects the integuments and membranes, rather than the cellular tissue and the muscles, and from ledum in this, that its effects tend to spread, instead of confining themselves to narrow spaces. The following are the pathological conditions, which, according to the pathogenesis and the

[1] See the pathogenesis of *rhus tox*, in the third volume of his Mat. Med. Pura.

clinical observations of the Homœopaths, this drug has the best chance of curing.

Sense of fulness about the head, worse when stooping, sensation in the brain as if bruised or fluctuating. Stupefying headache, such as exists in acute fevers, or as is caused by intoxication with brandy, with redness or livid paleness of the face, margins around the eyes, pointed nose, comatose drowsiness, occasional reveries, delirium, coldness of the body, numbness of the limbs, general sinking of strength, frequent and depressed pulse. *Acute hydrocephalus; serous and sanguineous apoplexy. Paralysis. Epistaxis.* Tingling in the hairy scalp, at the forehead, nose, and in the whole face. Cracking and ulceration of the vermilion border of the lips. Hot swelling of the upper lip. *Burning pustules around the mouth, followed by crusts which resemble dried honey.* Heat and smarting all over the face. Bloating and deformation of the face. *Parotitis.* Enormous swelling of the whole head. Itching of the skin of the trunk and extremities, especially of the hairy parts; it is at first a tingling, afterwards a burning itching, and is made worse by scratching. *Burns* (see page 74); *chilblains. Consequences of sunstroke,* (even in cases of *meningitis,* as we know from experience). *Erysipelas, pemphigus, zona, eczema.* (see page 78.) Hot and painful engorgements of the subcutaneous glands. Rheumatic pains, which are sometimes very violent, and always spread over a large surface, at the nape of the neck, loins and extremities. *Gout,* (especially when characterized by cutaneous symptoms.) *Hydrarthrosis. Warts* on the hands. Red or colorless infiltration of the extremities with burning pain. *Erythematous gastritis* and *gastro-enteritis,* with hot mouth, as if burnt, keen desire for cold drinks, red and dry tongue, and covered with a sort of false membrane, beneath which vesicles are perceived; tingling in the œsophagus and stomach; sense of burning at the stomach, nausea, vomiting, dull colic, or *pinching* pains, or prickings in the abdomen, which is hot, tense, tympanitic, but only moderately sensible to pressure; constipation followed by, or alternating with, serous diarrhœa; scanty and red urine; frequent and depressed pulse, nosebleed; coma and other ataxic phenomena.

Have we to conclude from this, that rhus tox. is particularly indicated in *typhus?* I think not. Although it is more than probable that rhus develops in the gastro-intestinal mucous membrane, symptoms similar to those which it produces on the skin, that is to say, extensive erythematous inflammations, with raising of the epithelium by means of pustules or serous vesicles, yet pathological anatomy forbids assimilating these phenomena to the organic lesions of typhus. These, like the variola-pustules, to which they have been compared, run a fixed course, and are possessed of essential characteristics, to which rhus corresponds only in rare and exceptional cases, as for example, in the typhus of 1813, against which, Hahnemann states rhus was found efficacious. It is quite natural that this drug should be successfully employed in certain forms of *very acute enteritis*, complicated with ataxic symptoms. But these forms of enteritis, which are falsely termed *typhoid enteritis* by modern Allœopaths, differ essentially from true typhus. In the former, the ataxic symptoms constitute sympathetic effects of the acute inflammation of the skin and mucous membranes, when this inflammation affects a large number of the nervous papillæ, which are spread over these surfaces; whereas, in typhus, adynamia, coma, etc., seem to constitute the fundamental character of the disease. It is, therefore, only now and then, that rhus will be found really indicated in typhus.

What I have said of ledum (see page 78,) concerning its use in acute affections of the air-passages, is likewise applicable to rhus and croton tiglium; cases may occur, however, where these drugs may be specifically indicated in what is vaguely termed *angina*, *bronchitis*, or *pneumonia*.

Rhus is often indicated after *arnica*, as *spigelia*, *zincum*, and *colchicum*, are often indicated after rhus.

The maladies to which it is best adapted, are such as occur most frequently in the spring, rheumatism, gout, erysipelas, eczema, etc. Most of its symptoms, like those of arnica, ledum, etc., are aggravated by artificial heat, sometimes by motion, but more frequently by rest; they are most fully manifested in the evening and at night.

Rhus is antidoted by *Bry.*, *Camph.*, *Coff.*, *Sulph.*, but especially by *Ledum.*

Croton Tiglium.—Genus *Croton*, family euphorbiaceæ, class monœcia monadelphia.

The fruit of this tree, which grows in the East-Indies, consists of small, oblong, blackish and rugose seeds, which are known in commerce under the name of croton tiglium, or pineus nucleus Moluccanus. A yellowish oil is extracted from them, of a nauseous odor, an acrid, burning, horrible taste, and which Allœopathic physicians pretend to use as a drastic and rubefacient.

Empirical applications. — Although mentioned in the Materia Medica of Ferrein, which was published in 1770, yet this oil, which was imported in Europe by a merchant of the East India Company, named Cromwell, was scarcely used in France previous to 1824, if we may credit the report, which, on the 13th of January, 1824, was read by M. Friedlander, before the Royal Academy of Medicine.[1]

Like the juice of rhus, the croton, if applied to the skin, causes a vesicular eruption, and, having been absorbed, a similar eruption on the mucous membranes of the intestines, or at least of the rectum. "It often happens," say Messrs. Trousseau and Pidoux, "that the person who has to make the frictions, is attacked with a vesicular eruption on the face although these parts had not been touched by the oil. Doctor Ernest Boudon, has seen an eruption develope itself on the scrotum, when different parts of the body were rubbed with the oil. It is probable that this eruption arises from the oil having been transferred to these parts."[2] These gentlemen,

[1] Journ. compl. des, sc. méd. vol. XVII. p. 340.

[2] Traité de thérapeutique, vol. I. p. 627.

who cannot deny the facts, do not seem to comprehend that an eruption may be produced without any direct application of the irritating agent to the real part.

The negroes of Bourbon employ the croton against dropsy, a practice which the English and French physicians have hastened to imitate. This drug is used as a drastic for *lead-colic ; tænia*, which it is said to kill, which must sometimes be of dangerous consequences to the patient; and lastly, as a derivative (in the shape of an embrocation,) in acute and chronic *cystitis*, and in *urethritis*. Happily, the blessings which a wise use of the croton is capable of rendering, are proportionate to the dangers which this agent exposes patients to, when treated by the opponents of Homœopathy.

I know of no other pathogenesis of the croton than that published by Jahr, to which the reader is referred.[1]

Homœopathic applications.—But few Homœopaths so far seem to have employed the croton. In Beauvais' Clinique, not a single case treated with croton can be found. I am, perhaps, one of the first, who has employed it in infinitesimal doses.

The croton is a precious drug, whose effects are intermediate between those of rhus and sulphur.[2] I have proved it on myself for a few days only. For want of precise indications, I only use it in very few cases; but since these cases occur most frequently in practice, the consequence is, that, in reality, I employ the croton, perhaps, more frequently than any other remedy.

The itching which is caused by the croton, is, at first, less burning than tingling, (the contrary takes place with rhus ;) there is, to my knowledge, at least, no more intolerable itching than this. It resembles perfectly the itching which is caused by the powder sold by certain jugglers, under the name of *scratching powder*. But this itching

[1] Nouveau manuel de méd. homœop., 5th ed. Paris, 1850, vol. I. p. 275.

[2] There is another drug with which I have made a few experiments, and which probably occupy the same rank as rhus, croton, and perhaps even sulphur: it is the *essential oil of the cashew nut.*

changes to a burning pain, like the itching of Rhus, if the drug is taken in large doses or applied externally. Then the skin becomes inflamed, red, burning-hot, and a yellowish and coagulable serum exudes from it, especially in the palms of the hand, at the genitals, on the abdomen, chest, between the shoulders and behind the ears. Small vesicles, resembling those of urticaria, break out on the inflamed parts, and this eruption may spread rapidly over the whole body.

Guided by a knowledge of the phenomena, which I knew resulted from the alloeopathic use of the croton, I first tried it homœopathically, but without much success, in *erysipelas*, and afterwards with very great success in, 1st, *urticaria*,[1] especially when the skin of the abdomen was the seat of the disease; 2d, against *large copper-colored spots*, likewise on the abdomen, itching, especially all around, and resembling very nearly *hepatic spots*, which the patient, (probably correctly,) took for syphilitic spots, although sepia, mercurius, sulphur, sulphuric and nitric acid had no effect upon them; 3d, against small *red blotches*, not very apparent, on the thighs, abdomen and genitals, *of upwards of fifteen years standing*, and causing an intolerable itching, especially at the vulva, in the case of a young lady who was driven to despair by them; 4th, against recent itch in a great many persons, but conjointly with *lobelia inflata*, and *mercurius corrosivus;* 5th, in the case of a little girl of four years old, of a delicate, cachectic, and essentially psoric constitution. After a vesicular eruption on the chest and neck, and which, I was told, had disappeared of itself in three or four days; the child was attacked with a fetid coryza, or rather, discharge from the nose, which had remained ever since, a period of two years, without interruption. During the winter season, this discharge became less copious and fetid, but as soon as the hot weather set in, it returned with all its unpleasant features. *Sulph.*, *Merc. salub.*, *Calc. carb.*, which I tried first, had no effect whatsoever. The eruption which had

[1] In my treatise on *diseases of children*, I have mentioned *ledum* for urticaria; this is either a misprint or a lapsus pennæ; it should be *croton*.

existed previous to the discharge, led me to try croton, but with very little hope. The result was contrary to my expectations; in less than a fortnight, the symptoms lost three-fourths of their intensity, although we were in mid-summer, at which period the symptoms had always been the most troublesome. It took about six months to complete the cure. *Croton*, *Lob. infl.*, *Kreasot.*, prescribed alternately, and at convenient intervals, were the only remedies employed.

The most decisive result which I have yet seen of the croton, is the following:—

In the month of March, 1850, I was consulted by a merchant of about forty years old, and very fleshy, who, for fifteen years past, had been subject to attacks of the gout, which returned invariably every spring. Only twice, at an interval of four years, the attack had not come on at the usual period; but without being of any use to the patient, who, in the place of the gout, was troubled with a most fatiguing and obstinate exanthem. This exanthem consisted in an intense redness of the whole body, accompanied with a burning itching, especially in the hollow of the hands, at the chest, and behind the ears. These parts were the seat of a yellowish, plastic exudation, emanating from a multitude of small vesicles, in close contact with each other, and which were only distinctly perceived in places where they were less numerous, and where a greater degree of resistance on the part of the epidermis, imparted to them a certain persistence. Each time when this eruption broke out, it remained three months, in spite of purgatives, the baths of Barèges, and a season spent at the baths of Aix, in Savoy. At the period when I saw the patient, he had neither his gout nor his eczema, but a dry, racking, almost convulsive and unceasing cough. The skin was rather hot, he was thirsty, had a little headache, heat in the chest, without dyspnœa; sometimes, especially in the evening, but only for a few days, he showed a tendency to syncope, which was a very remarkable circumstance in a person as robust as he was; there was little or no fever, (the pulse was from 60 to 65 in the minute). I first prescribed *Nux vomica*, then *Bryonia*, *Coral.* and some other drugs, but all in vain, for at the end of three weeks there was no change whatsoever. Weary of waiting any longer, and it must be admitted that the patient had sufficient reasons of growing tired of my treatment, he took it into his head one day to suspend my treatment, and to swallow, of his own accord, three or four tablespoonfuls of the *sirop of white poppy*, before going to bed in the evening. The effect of this preparation was really curious, and was not slow in manifesting itself. The cough ceased entirely for some hours, and then returned with the same intensity. But during this intermission, the malady had come out upon the skin, and, at day-break, the patient found himself covered from head to foot with this horrible eczema which he had been afflicted with before. I must say, that I scarcely recognized him, and that I found him in a state of anxiety and despair, which it is impossible to describe. From experience, he knew that the prospect before him was three or four months of intolerable tortures. In this condition I gave him the croton, and in less than five or six days there remained not a trace, either of the cough or the eruption; the horrible itching disappeared almost on the same day.[1]

What is remarkable in this case is, that the same malady is presented under three different forms: *gout*, *eczema*, *bronchitis*, and that this multiform malady yielded to the same drug. I doubt not, that croton, if given in time, would have prevented the exanthem, and cured the cough from the commencement.

It is to be hoped that a great many facts similar to the preceding one, will soon determine the practical value of the somewhat vague indications which the pathogenesis of croton seems to contain.

[1] This patient having left Paris, I do not know whether his cough, his eczema or his gout have returned. Unfortunately such a thing is not impossible. It is even probable that the principle of his disease still exists; nevertheless, I am persuaded that at the period when I treated him, croton oil would have cured him of his gout as well as of his bronchitis, for a time at least.

According to the statement of a very conscientious and intelligent person, who has had the kindness to prove a great number of drugs for me, dulcamara is the antidote of croton.

Spigelia Anthelmia, pink-root. — Genus Spigelia, family gentianeæ, Class pentandria monogynia.

This small annual plant, which grows in almost all the countries of South America, has black, hairy roots, an almost simple stem, terminating in four lanceolate leaves, out of which starts a thin, elongated spike, loaded with a multitude of greenish blossoms, which furnish a big lobular fruit. When recent, it exhales a poisonous and fetid odor. Its leaves have a nauseous taste, which remains a long time in the mouth.

Spigelia is a violent poison. The cattle that eat of it, perish with horrible pains. It causes vomiting, dizziness, stupor, dilatation of the pupils, subsultus tendinum, pulsations in different parts of the body, and an excessive dyspnœa, which increases until death.[1]

From the period (1739,) when Patricius Brown first promulgated in Europe the properties of this powerful drug, until the period when Hahnemann studied it systematically, physicians contented themselves with slavishly imitating the negroes of Jamaica, and using it solely for worms. In the numerous treatises on Materia Medica, from that of Bergius to that of Trousseau and Pidoux, who, bye the bye, omit this drug altogether, I have not met with any other application of spigelia. It is true, that it possesses vermifuge virtues, which are much more powerful than those that have been attributed to many other plants, for undeniable cures have been made with it. I would even add, that, among its symptoms, there are many that correspond to the sudden changes which the presence of entozoa in the digestive canal frequently determines. But independently of its not always being the most convenient vermifuge, this restricted use of

[1] Coxe, *Americ. dispens.* p. 128.

spigelia would deprive us of a drug whose homœopathicity in many diseases is self-evident, and where no other drug could replace it. "The astonishing and diversified virtues of spigelia, show that it has a far higher destination than to cleanse the bowels of worms."[1]

Homœopathic applications. Spigelia is probably less frequently employed than it should be.[2] There are few diseases, however, which are as common as those of which it presents the symptoms. It would seem as though the pathogenesis of this drug represented in a chronic form, all the pathological affections whose acute form is found among the symptoms of *arnica.* I earnestly call the attention of my colleagues to this comparison, which, so far from being purely speculative, as might be supposed, is simply a rigorous deduction, on my part, from numerous and closely observed clinical facts. *Spigelia* is indicated by the following physiological conditions and symptoms:—

Sense of weariness all over, with a sensation of coldness or real coldness of the body; heat about the head or face only; every motion, such as a step, is painfully felt in every limb. *Headache, which deprives one of sense, with vertigo, as though one would fall,* especially in the morning, after rising, and sometimes periodical; *neuralgia;* with pulling, pressive pains, or shootings in the frontal eminences, penetrating far into the brain; also *at the occiput, in the left parietal region;* pain at the sinciput, in contracting the muscles of the face; excessive *sensitiveness of the hairy scalp,* when touching it, drawing it into wrinkles, or when simply touching the hair; *rheumatic ophthalmia, profuse lachrymation* with or without pain, especially of the left eye; vanishing of sight; blurred vision; *dimness of the crystalline lens, rheumatic cataract* (of the left eye); ulceration of the eye-

[1] See the pathogenesis of *Spigelia* in Hahnemann's *Materia Medica pura,* vol. III.

[2] In Beauvais' Homœopathic Clinique, we find only twenty-two cases treated with *Spigelia,* namely, six cases of *ophthalmia,* three of *toothach,* three of *prosopalgia,* one of *carditis,* one of *syphilis, orchitis, cataract, cephalalgia, paralysis, convulsions, grippe, fever and ague,* and *worm-fever.*

lids, agglutination of the eye-lids by a viscous gum; *prickings in the lids;* paralysis of the upper lid; tingling in the inner ear; *otalgia; passing deafness; facial neuralgia;* exostosis at the forehead and zygomatic bone; *neuralgia at the lower jaw*, radiating to the nape of the neck and temple; digging pain in the carious teeth; pressive *odontalgia* from within outwards, with a sensation of coldness at the teeth; *aggravation by cold water*, and *suspension of the pain during a meal*, coming on especially in the *morning*, afternoon, and at night. Yellow, pale, or earthy color of the skin; such an extreme sensitiveness of the skin, that the slightest blow causes acute pain; *cutaneous neuralgias aggravated by cold water: carbuncle* (after *arnica*). Rheumatism at the nape of the neck, with painful numbness, which the lying on the back renders intolerable. *Violent shootings in the walls of the chest*, especially the left side, under the clavicle, or *on a line with the heart;* painful *contraction of the muscles of the chest;* stitches in the region of the diaphragm. *Rheumatism, with pain as if sprained*, in the shoulders, wrists, in the finger-joints, hip, knee, and in the joint which the big toe forms with the first metatarsal bone; pressive, pulling, or cutting pains in the extremities lengthwise; *trembling of the upper extremities;* contraction of the flexor muscles of the fingers; burning itching in the palms of the hands; *cold, viscous sweat in the hollow of the hands;* sub-cutaneous tubercles in this part; contusive pain at the knee; pulling in the legs from below upwards, with heat in the feet, or from above downwards, with coldness of the feet; *sprain at the foot;*[1] burning pain at the instep (without redness); deep-seated and lancinating pain at the sole of the foot, when resting the body upon it.

Dry, pale, and cracked lips; sensation of dryness and of *prickings as with pins*, in the mouth, although it is filled with a tenacious and nauseous saliva; coated tongue; fetid

[1] In sprains, *Spigelia* is often indicated after *arnica*. In the case of an old maid troubled with bad humors, I have employed it even externally with the most satisfactory results; arnica had remained without effect.

breath; sensation as if a half-fluid body were ascending towards the throat; *anorexia* or *bulimy*, tingling in the œsophagus; nausea in the morning and afternoon; bilious vomiting; neuralgic pains at the stomach; *sensation of a lump in the umbilical region*, as *if rolled upon itself; pinchings* or cutting pains in the abdomen; *swelling of the abdomen;* lancing pains in the abdomen, with falling back of the head, and loss of sense; noisy and sometimes painful borborygmi in the abdomen; emission of flatulence which has the smell of rotten eggs; tension in the groin; *hernia inguinalis*, hard stool, like sheep's dung, and enveloped in a quantity of mucus; mucous diarrhœa, with tenesmus; tingling and prickings in the rectum; *discharge of ascarides;* copious and frequent emissions, especially at night, of a watery or whitish urine.

Tingling in the wind-pipe; chronic hoarseness; catarrh of the air-passages, with fever, heat of the skin, but absence of thirst and sweat; violent cough, with or without expectoration, and sometimes accompanied with a violent dyspnœa, which increases most while the chest is bent forwards; painful angina and bronchitis, *alternating with the rheumatic pains in one shoulder*, and sometimes co-existing with these pains. *Stitches at the heart; palpitations of the heart*, especially in the morning, while sitting quiet; a sort of shuddering at the heart; sensible decrease in the number of the beats of the heart; fever, with predominance of coldness; habitual chilliness; violent gaping; drowsiness in the daytime; sleeplessness in the evening, before midnight; disturbed, unrefreshing sleep, full of disquieting dreams; sour sweat during sleep; quotidian intermittent fever, commencing in the morning with a shuddering, followed by a dry heat, with absence of thirst. Anxious sadness; forebodings of unpleasant occurrences; depression of spirits even to suicide. *Marked predominance of the pains in all the organs of the left side.*

Spigelia, which ought, perhaps, to terminate the series in which I have placed it, presents some of the symptoms which characterize the drugs of the following group, namely:—Foulness of the breath and secretions; *blackish* pustules on the skin; general languor and prostration; depression of the pulse; aggravation of the pains in the cold, and especially in cold water; tendency to softening of the bones; striking action upon the periosteum; aggravation of the symptoms during rest, at night or in the morning, or sometimes about two o'clock in the afternoon; production of entozoa; and lastly, predominance of its action upon the left side of the body. It will be seen afterwards, how much importance I attach to this latter consideration.

All this shows, that as a general rule, spigelia is principally indicated in chronic affections, or in recent affections of debilitated, pale, thin, or bloated persons, complaining of chilliness, and disposed to rheumatic pains, without heat or swelling of the affected parts.

This drug is often indicated after *arnica;* after spigelia we often have to give *Zinc. Arsenic,* and sometimes *Digitalis* in affections of the heart.

Cocculus and *Camphor* antidote spigelia.

Ferrum magneticum;—*sesquioxyde of iron: magnetic iron.*

In the Allœopathic materia medica, there reigns such a confusion concerning the compounds of iron, that it is absolutely impossible to find out what statements refer to one or the other of these compounds. Formerly, the so-termed *eau de boule de Nancy* was used in *muscular pains,* in *paralysis, contusions, sprains,* etc., that is to say, in affections to which the magnetic iron seems especially to correspond. But this preparation, which is an impure tartrate of iron, is only remotely related to our ferrum magneticum. In this instance, therefore, empiricism is dumb, or, at any rate, has to be considered so by us.

Jahr, this clever and indefatigable compiler, who has already rendered great service to the cause of homœopathy, gives us in the last edition of his Manual, the synopsis of a pathogenesis of the magnetic iron, (Gaspari's,) to which I refer the reader. This synopsis, short and incomplete as it doubtless is, deserves nevertheless to be read and studied.

In some of the symptoms which the magnetic iron produces on the head and eyes, this drug seems to be somewhat analogous to pulsatilla, or rather graphites; all its other symptoms justify the place which I have here assigned to it. I am convinced (and my clinical observations confirm me still more in my belief) that the primary action of *Ferrum magnet.* takes place on the organs of locomotion, and gives rise to general and partial effects, which, by a process of reasoning, may be ranked with those of arnica, and still more with those of rhus and spigelia.

Until now I have employed this drug in a very small number of cases only, with the following results :—

1st. In a case of chronic rheumatism of the nape of the neck, in an old man with bad humors and an irritable disposition, (after Spig.) 2d. In a case of *compound capsular cataract*, in a gouty patient; the patient was not cured, but considerably relieved. 3d. In a case of rheumatism of both thighs, and coming on after violent exercise; the patient was a servant, and was obliged to rub every morning the floors of a suite of large rooms. I treated him at two different periods for the same disease. The first time I gave him *Ferrum magneticum* after *arnica*, but the second time, four or five months after, I gave him Ferrum at once, and the effect was speedy and marked. 4th. Lastly, in a case of mercurial neurosis, in an individual who was very sensitive to medicine, and in whom ferrum developed some of its symptoms almost instantaneously with an incredible vehemence. One of the symptoms which had induced me to prescribe it in this case, was a painful contraction of the posterior cervical muscles, and against which none of the remedies which I had tried, had had any effect. *Ferr. magn.* was given in the sixth dilution, four globules in a tumblerful of water, two table-spoonfuls every day. The first table-spoonful, which was taken in the morning, seemed to produce a sensible improvement; but, a quarter of an hour after the second dose, which was taken at four o'clock in the afternoon, the sight became dim; a halo of fire, red and violet, was seen first in front of the right, and afterwards in front of the left eye; soon after, this halo, which formed a circular zigzag-shaped line, became narrower and narrower, and finally produced such a complete blindness, that the patient assured me he was unable to distinguish night from day-light. This condition, which was undoubtedly very alarming, considering that my patient's eyes were very weak, lasted about an hour, and did not pass off entirely until after a meal. This accident was followed by other much more distressing and alarming phenomena. Towards eight o'clock in the evening, the pain in the nape of the neck, which first was seated on the left side, passed to the right side, invading the whole extent of the trapezoid muscle, where it became literally frightful. For two days and nights, this patient who was a brave and strong man, and whom I had seen bear the most painful surgical operations without uttering a sound, suffered to such an extent, that he uttered heart-rending cries. *Camphor*, which was given as an antidote, seemed to aggravate this frightful pain; nor were *Puls.* or *Bry.* any more efficacious; *rhus tox.* effected some relief. This drug, however, did not prevent the recurrence, *for eight days in succession*, of the visual phenomena, although with less intensity than the first time, and at irregular intervals, generally towards six or seven o'clock in the morning, and *sometimes even at night, in perfect darkness.*

A drug which is capable of causing such violent symptoms, must necessarily contain great curative virtues. I therefore recommend to my colleagues the study of magnetic iron, whose pathogenesis requires, above all things, to be completed.

I am not yet acquainted with the true antidote of this drug.

GROUP II.

TYPE: MERCURIUS SOLUBILIS.

ANALOGIES: ARGENTUM FOLIATUM. ARSENICUM ALBUM. SULPHURIS ACIDUM. MERCURIUS CORROSIVUS. CROCUS SATIVUS. KREOSOTA. PLUMBUM. STANNUM. NITRI ACIDUM.

COMMON CHARACTERISTICS.

It is worthy of remark, that several of the substances which compose this group, are, in their natural state, possessed of the power of preserving organic matter from decomposition,[1] and yet exercise an exactly opposite effect

[1] It is known that arsenicum and corrosive sublimate are employed for this purpose by stuffers and naturalists. Kreasot is used for a similar purpose, (in smoking the meat). The soluble salts of silver and lead, especially the nitrate of lead, according to a note which was communicated to the Academy of Sciences by Monsieur Le Maître de Rabodanges, (in the sitting of the 8th of June, 1846,) likewise enjoy the property of preserving animal matter. The *smoking liquor of Libavius* which, when crystallising in damp air, forms the *tin-butter* of the ancient chemists, and which is an escharotic, together with arsenicum, corrosive sublimate, the nitrate of silver, etc., was recommended by Vicq. d'Azyr as an antiseptic in exhumations, etc. And lastly, saffron serves to preserve meat from putrefaction. As regards nitric and sulphuric acid which, on account of their extraordinary affinity for water, carbonise, it is true, organic products, they are both of them possessed of antiseptic properties, and, indeed, justly. This is the reason why, according to Gmelin, (App. Med., vol. II., p. 36,) sulphuric acid was even yet employed at the end of the last century on board ships to keep the water sweet. It ought to be remarked that several substances, as far as their dissolving action on the organic products is concerned, possess properties which are diametrically opposite to those of arsenic, corrosive sublimate, kreasot, etc. I may cite, among others, oxalic acid. "This acid," says Giacomini, "when introduced into a stomach taken from a dead body, dissolves all its coats in a few hours; on the contrary, if injected into a living stomach, it does not extend its action beyond the mucous coat, and the corrosion does not take place until after death." (*Traité philos. et expér. de Mat. Med.* et de Therap., frunst., from the Italian by Mojon, p. 15.)

upon the living tissues, a fact upon which their common pathogenetic phenomena and their common therapeutic action depend. Thus all have the following leading symptoms:

Suppression, or more frequently increase of all the secretions, with putrid alteration of the secreted substances.

Foulness of the mouth and breath: putrid taste, like foul flesh in the throat; intolerable odor of the fæces, and often even of the pus discharged from the ulcers; fetid smell of the sweat and sometimes of the urine.

Bloating and softening of the flesh, with tendency to decomposition; nocturnal bone-pains.

Softening, interstitial distention, friability, dry caries of the bones.

Depression of the vital action; cadaverous coldness, general or partial; apparent or real mortification of the extremities, or stinging heat, followed by profuse sweat.

Predominance of action on the left side of the body, that is to say, on the side which is the weakest side of most persons.

Deep derangements of the nervous action; great disorders of the intellectual and moral sphere; weakness of the senses, as at the approach of death.

Sort of violent oscillations of the vital principle; opposite effects in all the functions; paralytic numbness, or frightful pains, with involuntary motions; ravenous hunger, or else anorexia; unquenchable thirst, or else adipsia; comatose somnolence, or else sur-excitation of the whole organism, which absolutely prevents sleep; exaltation of the sexual desire, or else complete extinction of the sexual powers, etc.

Lastly, production of intestinal worms and other parasites.[1]

[1] This is the reason why all these substances are *anthelmintic*. All their symptoms are, so to say, signs of putrid decomposition.

CORRESPONDING DISEASES.

Syphilis.—Itch.—Variola.—Cutaneous affections, such as erysipelatous, gangrenous, squamous, papulous, etc.—Scurvy.—Scrofula.—Acute and chronic arthritis.—Bone-pains.—Exostosis.—Dry and humid caries.—Production of abnormal tissues.—Inflammations of viscera.—Catarrhal affections.—Passive hæmorrhages.—Ascites.—Albuminuria.—Diabetes.—Weakening and loss of the senses.—Weakening of the intellectual faculties.—Mania.—Dementia.—Idiocy.—Atrophy of one or several limbs.—Neuroses of the most diversified and strange kind.—Frightful neuralgia.—Worm affections, etc.

An absence of the excitement naturally occasioned by light and the business of the day, external cold, (especially when accompanied with dampness,) rest, and finally, lying upon the affected parts, are conditions which favor the essentially dissolvent action of mercury and its analogies.

A characteristic phenomenon of this action, and which the practitioner should well keep in view, is its predominance on the left side, which circumstance seems to me to be founded on a general law.

I here give my observations on this subject without any commentary; I believe they are worthy of notice.

The general idea of Rasori, if not of Brown, was correct; there are drugs which excite, and drugs which depress the vital action, *stimulants* and *counter-stimulants*.[1] In other words, as I remarked in speaking of Spigelia, there are poisons which kill by exalting, and poisons which destroy life by depressing the vital forces. The drugs of which we speak, belong essentially to this latter category, whereas, pulsatilla, bryonia, veratrum, and more particularly nux vomica, might be considered as the types of the opposite category, if we leave their specific properties out of consideration. I ought to remark, that every drug belongs, more or less, to one or the other of these two classes, although I have

[1] Rasori and his disciples, operating upon the sick organism, have not been able to define either class; their observations almost always implied opposite truths.

not always been able to determine the fact with correctness. Hence results the general co-relation existing between such and such a drug, and such and such a temperament.

But what I desire more particularly to prove here, in order not to be obliged to refer to this point again, hereafter, is that certain phenomena are connected with the predominance of the action of the drug on this or that side of the body. Thus, from the fact that a drug acts *primarily* and in a marked manner, on the right side of the body, we have a right to conclude *à priori:* 1st, that the symptoms which it produces, are aggravated by light, heat, the open air, and exercise; 2d, that they will be mitigated, on the contrary, by silence, cool air, darkness and rest; 3d, that in the fevers which it causes, a quick and full pulse will prevail; 4th, that in lying down, the pains will be principally felt in parts which do not serve as points of support; 5th, that from the first, an aversion to food, or, at any rate, a speedy satiety will be noticed, but never, except in a few extraordinary cases, which it would be easy for me to account for, that extreme hunger, which shows a pressing want on the part of the organism to repair its exhausted condition; 6th, that if the drug produces amenorrhœa or dysmenorrhœa, these symptoms will never be accompanied with an impoverished condition of the blood, which, if its course is sluggish and painful, will not be any the less rich in fibrin, and will, on the contrary, pass off in black and resisting coagula, as is the case with pulsatilla; 7th, lastly, that cachexia and adynamia are not the general effects which the drug tends to produce, which might likewise occasion as serious disorders of a reverse character.

The *contrary* of all the accidents which have just been enumerated, takes place but in endless degrees and shades, with every drug which acts primarily upon the left side of the body.

In this respect, every careful observer will find, that there is no difference between natural and drug-diseases. Among the former, so far as their organic manifestations are concerned, several seem positively to develope themselves from left to right, whereas, others proceed in the opposite direction, which simply means that there are diseases, which *essentially exalt*, and diseases which *essentially depress* the vitality; the former was denied by Brown, the latter by Broussais.[1] These considerations are not, by any means, devoid of interest. To prove it, I will content myself with relating the following fact.

In 1848, a patient, whose physician I had not yet become, lost his left eye in consequence of frightful neuralgic paroxysms which were seated in the bottom of the orbit, and it was supposed, proceeded either from an old syphilis, or, which seems to me much more probable, to judge from what I now know of the case, from some allœopathic mercurial treatment, which he had undergone some years before, and which had been carried to the last degree of insane violence; that is to say, the treatment was continued all the time, for no other reason than for the purpose of removing mercurial symptoms which were incessantly reproduced, and which were mistaken for *syphilis* for the whole of *six months*. In 1850, the neuralgia first showed itself at the bottom of the right eye. This was assuredly an exacerbation of the genuine disease. Whether syphilitic or mercurial, the disease had not ceased to exist: it proceeded *normally*, that is to say, from the left to the right, to its work of destruction. The paroxysms lasted three days, almost without an interruption, and were complicated with the most violent ophthalmia.

In a consultation, *Calcarea carb* was proposed. Isolatedly considered, the symptoms pointed to this remedy: I accepted it, less, however, from conviction, than from deference to the eminent colleague who had advised it. The patient took it, and the pains subsided almost instantaneously. It will be seen hereafter, that the action of Calcarea proceeds in an

[1] In support of my theory, the statistics of venereal hospitals may be consulted, and it will be seen how many organs or functional lesions (neuralgia, amaurosis, deafness, etc.,) after a venereal affection, were more frequently observed on the left than on the right side.

opposite direction to that of Mercury; hence, I had to conclude that my theory was wrong. Unhappily for the patient, this was not the case. After forty-eight hours of suspension, or rather repression, the paroxysms returned with greater violence than ever.

Free to do as I pleased, I followed the idea which I have developed in the preceding paragraphs, and selected *arsenic* accordingly. The result was permanent and decided. Not only was the paroxysm arrested, but alarming symptoms of amaurosis which had been setting in for a long time previous, and were similar to those that, in 1848, preceded the loss of the left eye, were gradually dissipated.

I shall not dwell upon this point any longer.

The energetic, deep, and persistent action of Mercury and its analogies, shows satisfactorily that the diseases which they are specifically called to combat, are such as deeply invade the organism, undermine it without mercy, and tend to dissolve it. But independently of these diseases, which, according to an expression of Broussais, are essentially and primarily chronic, there are others of an acute character, but which nevertheless require to be treated with the drugs of which we are speaking. Thus, certain exceedingly acute rheumatic diseases, with redness and swelling of the affected joints, tearing pains, profuse sweat, sour or fetid odor, etc., frequently yield only to *Merc. sol.* or *corr.* The same remark applies to certain kinds of *ophthalmia*, *hepatitis*, etc.; it is not, therefore, indispensably necessary that a disease should present a *specific* character in order to render the employment of the drugs of this group necessary. It is sufficient that the disease should have the prominent symptoms, from whatever cause it may otherwise have emanated, or whatever be its inmost nature.

All the drugs of this group are anti-syphilitic. This proposition alone would suffice to destroy *the specific system* which, owing to the radical impossibility of generalizing its fundamental principles, never has had any serious chance of existence.

It is worthy of remark, however, that Hahnemann, whose genius swept every existing medical doctrine, and overthrew all existing systems, seems to have remained more or less undecided all his life, as regards the specific system. Not only does he seem to accept the exclusive efficacy of mercurius in syphilis, in other words, its *absolutely specific action in the disease*, as an immutable, absolute fact; but he pursues even to the remotest corners of medical ontology, his inquiry into the general relations existing between such and such a disease which he discovers, or fancies he discovers, and such and such a drug that cures it. Is not *thuya* his specific remedy for *sycosis? sulphur* for *psora?* It is true, in the treatment of sycosis, he alternates *thuya* with *nitric acid*,[1] without, however, accounting for the homœopathicity of this proceeding, which snatches from thuya a considerable portion of the prestige of its specificity in this disease. It is likewise true, that, compelled to admit that *sulphur* will not cure all non-syphilitic diseases, he declares that "the cure of an inveterate psoric disease can never be accomplished by *sulphur* alone."[2] But as regards the want of success which is frequently encountered in the mercurial treatment of syphilis, Hahnemann does not seem willing to doubt the specific character of mercury in this disease which, however, is of a very remote origin, except when complicated with psora. "Wherever such a complication does not exist, an infinitesimal dose of the best mercurial preparation is sufficient to cure forever, and thoroughly, the whole syphilitic disease."[3] It is moreover evident, that even at the time when Hahnemann first published his Materia Medica Pura, he looked upon *mercurius* and *thuya* as exclusively endowed with the property of curing syphilis and sycosis,—mercurius the former, and thuya the latter; and this is the reason why these two otherwise long-acting drugs are not classed among his *anti-psorics*. The following passage from the Materia Medica Pura shows that my statement is correct:—"To administer the smallest dose

[1] *Chronic Diseases*, vol. I. [2] Ibid. [3] Ibid.

of pure mercury prepared in the manner which I have just described, Homœopathy must, in the first place, have recognized the indispensable necessity of employing it in a given case of chronic disease, UNLESS *this remedy should be* ABSOLUTELY *indicated by a case of pure syphilis, not complicated with psora, for in such a case a single infinitesimal dose is sufficient* to annihilate the CHRONIC MIASM."[1]

Hahnemann's specificism assuredly differs from that which some German homœopaths are endeavoring to introduce now-a-days, for it leaves a vast majority of all diseases beyond the reach of its influence. But for all that, it is a form of specificism which carries with it several serious defects which I have to point out.

1. It tends to impart false notions to homœopathic physicians, with respect to these two drugs, and, by making them believe that mercury cures exclusively *syphilis*, and thuya, *sycosis*, leads them to the opinion that they exercise only a very equivocal action in other chronic diseases.

2. It seems to place mercury, thuya, and even sulphur, beyond the pale of the law of similitude. At least it seems indisputable, that such is the idea which a great many homœopaths attach to Hahnemann's notion of the specificity of these drugs. How many among them, for instance, when mercury does not help in a case of inveterate syphilis, at once jump at the conclusion that there must be some psoric complication, and, upon the strength of this supposition, prescribe sulphur empirically, without its being at all indicated by the symptoms! And, by a legitimate reciprocity, how many, in a case of refractory psora, jump at the inference that it is a complication of disguised syphilis, and blindly prescribe mercury!

3. Lastly, by attributing the failures of mercury in syphilis to psora, Hahnemann affirms that mercury is not only the *best*, but the *only* remedy for syphilis, which is a very serious error. It is from such an error that the forcible concessions

[1] *Mater. Med. Pura*, vol. III.

which Hahnemann has made to the specific system, emanate; for, if we admit that a disease without regard to its duration, course, symptoms, the idiosyncracy of the patient, etc., can only be combated by a single remedy, it is evident that the name of the disease is sufficient to indicate the treatment, and that a comparison of its symptoms with those of the drug, must be superfluous. All this is different if, instead of one, we admit several anti-syphilitics. The mere name of the disease ceases to indicate the treatment; we have to observe symptoms, and the law of similarity again reigns supreme.

In this sense, therefore, I had a right to say that my general principle "*all the drugs, belonging to the group mercury, are anti-syphilitic*," overthrows the sophisms of the specific system; for, by upsetting the specificity of mercury in syphilis, the whole edifice of the specificists falls to the ground.

Mercurius. *Hydrargyrum, Argentum vivum, Argentum liquidum, Argentum fusum, Argentum mobile, Aqua argentea, Aqua metallorum, Aqua sicca, Proteus, Chamæleon minerale, Servus fugitivus, Illusor chymicorum, Impostor chymicorum, Azoph, Zaibar, Zabach,*[1] *Mercurius solubilis,* black oxide of mercury.

This metallic poison which is ranked by modern allœopathic physicians among their alteratives, a term the real meaning of which I do not believe I have ever properly understood, is so much the more frightful in its operations, that its effects do not always show themselves immediately after its introduction in the organism. It was not used as a drug before the fifteenth century. It is generally attributed to J. Wid-

[1] Gmelin, *apparat. medic. corpora. metallica.*, vol. II., p. 1.: "Mercury is indebted for its many appellations to—1st. The mysterious and cabalistic part which the seekers of the absolute and the philosopher's stone caused it to act for so many centuries; 2d. The fact that physicians had made it a rule to hide from their patients its real name which would have (justly) frightened them, or whose real name they (the physicians) desired, from other motives, to keep secret."

mann, whose treatise on syphilis was published in 1497.[1] Shortly after, mercury became the subject of a multitude of publications which spread its use, until the whole of Europe had become the theatre of its ravages. "If I except blood-letting," says Hahnemann, "the external purgatives, the abuse of opium as an anodyne or as a means to procure artificial sleep, and to arrest diarrhœa and spasms, or the abuse of cinchona in suppressing typical fevers, or strengthening in cases where weakness is solely caused by the continuance of the malady or an exhausting treatment, there is no remedial agent employed by allœopathic physicians, which has more contributed to shorten life, than their much vaunted calomel and corrosive sublimate."[2]

Empirical applications.—Since there is scarcely a single important disease for which mercury has not been used, either on the supposition of some latent syphilis, or because it was simply intended to try it at random, it is easily comprehended what enormous accidents must have resulted from such deplorable abuses. But, on the other hand, such blind trials must have at times led to cures, and, indeed, a knowledge of the pure effects of mercury explains to us, now-a-days, the reasons why it acted successfully in some cases. In analyzing the long chapter which Gmelin devotes to mercury, we find that it was more particularly used in most of the diseases whose symptoms are represented in our provings. These are, among others, *syphilis*, (primary and secondary,) *angina*, *scurvy*,[3] *scrophula*,[4] *catarrhal inflammations of the eyes*, *amaurosis*, *inflammations of the lungs and bowels*,[5] *hepatitis*,[6]

[1] *Tract de pustulis et morbo qui vulgato nomine mal de Frangos appellatur.* Ju. 4, 1497. The Arabs had employed mercury before Widmann, but only externally, in lepra.

[2] Materia Medica Pura, vol. III.

[3] Kramer, dis. epistol. de scorbuto, 1737.

[4] Borden, recueil des pièces qui ont concouru pour le prix de chirurgie, (1759,) vol. III., p. 80.

[5] F. Lind, London Medical Journal, vol. VIII., and Hamilton, Medical Commentaries, collected and published by A. Dunken, vol. XI.

[6] Clarke, Medical and Philosophical Commentaries, by a Society in Edinburgh, London, 1777, vol. V.

dropsy, dysentery, worm affections, variola,[1] *anthrax, carbuncle, plague,*[2] *rheumatism, gout, cutaneous diseases, whether syphilitic or no, elephantiasis,*[3] *plica polonica, spina ventosa,*[4] *rickets and every other disease of the bones, metritis, venereal and non-venereal hydro-sarcocele, hysteria, epilepsy, mania, tetanus,* and lastly *rage.*[5]

Although physicians, when they effected a cure of one of the above-mentioned diseases, rarely failed to attribute it to the removal of a disguised syphilis by means of mercury, it must not be supposed, on that account, that they ever dreamed of investigating the reasons of the anti-syphilitic specificity of this drug. They supposed that mercury cured syphilis, by carrying off the syphilitic virus during the process of salivation. It was quite an event when, in the sixteenth century the discovery was made that mercury will cure syphilis without the patient being salivated. One error, however, being substituted in the place of another, it was supposed that the sweat, the diuresis, or the diarrhœa which followed the exhibition of mercury, replaced the absent salivation; the gross humoralism which prevailed at that period, did not allow of another explanation.

The numberless accidents which were caused by mercury, revealed in the meanwhile its physiological action in almost all its various shades, and with tolerable clearness. An almost complete pathogenesis of this agent, might be obtained by collecting the effects of a certain number of mercurial intoxications which are so frequently observed, and involuntarily produced by physicians. This pathogenesis, like that which has been obtained by the pure provings, would represent the primitive and secondary symptoms of syphilis in their totality, and with tolerable correctness. What is the

[1] Th. Dinsdale, *present method for the inoculating of the small pox*, 1767, in 8vo., p. 17.

[2] Schreiber, *de pestilentia*, p. 44.

[3] Raymond, *hist. de l'éléphantiasis*, etc., in 8vo., Lausanne, 1767.

[4] Büchner et Niemann, *de remediis mercurialibus spinæ ventosæ*, etc., in 4to., 1754.

[5] Desault, *dissert. sur la rage*, 1734, in 12mo.

reason that the striking similarity of the effects of mercury and the symptoms of the venereal disease, has not yet opened the eyes of physicians concerning the law of similitude? The history of no other science, perhaps, offers similar instances of obstinate blindness, than is offered by the history of medicine.

What is better still, the opponents of homœopathy themselves institute the comparison which I have pointed out. The symptomatic resemblance of the mercurial disease to syphilis, which is sometimes complete, is recognized and pointed out by them every day, and yet, they seem unable to draw from it its legitimate conclusion. Read what Professors Trousseau and Pidoux write on the subject: "bad humors, ulcerations of the mouth, tongue, pharynx, necrosis of the jaw-bones, diarrhœa, trembling, delirium, mania, acute cutaneous affections, such are the accidents which can be attributed to mercury;"[1] and, they ought to have added, to syphilis. Both mercurius and syphilis induce serious disorders upon the skin. In syphilis, etc., we have pustules, tubercles, crusts, etc. In hydrargyria, we have erythematic papulæ, vesicles, and sometimes (not very rarely) impetiginous pustules.[2] It is true between mercurial and syphilitic diseases of the skin, our authors see *very great differences;* for example: the syphilitic eruptions do not make their appearance until a few months after the venereal infection, whereas the mercurial affections are "*immediate and acute,*" which is not always true, but which would go to prove the enormous size of the doses in which the poison had been administered. Be this as it may, and although they affirm that "there is no attentive physician who is well acquainted with the pathology of cutaneous diseases, who, in the immense majority of cases, is not able to distinguish the generally evanescent forms of *mercurial cutaneous diseases* from the fixed and tenacious forms of those produced by the syphilitic virus," nevertheless, Messrs. Trousseau and Pidoux are compelled to admit that,

[1] *Traité de Therapeutique*, vol. I., p. 172.

[2] Idem, p. 173.

"in regard to the boundary between these two kinds of alterations, the diagnosis may, in some cases, be very difficult and even impossible." Hence we must conclude that, in these cases at least, the symptoms of syphilis and those of mercury which cures this disease, resemble each other perfectly.

These gentlemen, following up their comparison between the symptoms of syphilis and the effects of mercury, express themselves as follows: "Constitutional syphilis and mercury may bring about a cachexia; but the course and the forms of this malady, are, generally speaking, very marked. Mercurial cachexia, which is *generally* rapid,"—how could it be otherwise, when the mercurial poison is unceasingly administered in massive doses?—"developes itself in a few days under the influence of an *active mercurial treatment:* among the workmen who employ mercury, among miners, among patients who take for a long time small doses of mercury, the cachexia developes itself slowly, but always with its characteristic symptoms; bloating, lividity, bleeding of the gums; bloating of the face and the lower extremities; serous effusions in most cavities; habitual diarrhœa; dulness of the mental faculties, trembling. The syphilitic cachexia is not seen until after the syphilitic disease has lasted for a long time. It is always, or, at least, always seems to be the consequence of chronic organic lesions, or of acute pains, which have deprived the patient of sleep. It is accompanied with excessive emaciation of the face, and with all the symptoms which characterize marasmus."[1]

Paradoxal subtlety, or rather sophism, could scarcely be pushed any farther; for it is false, absolutely false, that mercurial and syphilitic cachexias always exhibit the characters which Trousseau and Pidoux assign to them respectively. The one, sometimes presents, indeed, acute symptoms, which the other has not. But why is this? Because the means which Allœopathic physicians employ, are very often

[1] Traité de Therapeutique, vol. I., p. 174.

more violent and more destructive than the diseases for which they are given. It will always be so, as long as we shall feel obliged to administer enormous doses of mercury to combat the syphilitic disease.

Trousseau and Pidoux, add moreover: "It has been said that the nocturnal bone-pains belong to the mercurial as well as the syphilitic disease. To this, we answer, that these bone-pains are seldom met with among the workers in mercury."[1] I confess, I have no precise information concerning this point; but Trousseau and Pidoux admit, that these pains exist *sometimes*, at least, among these workmen, since they themselves have seen them in a looking-glass tinner, who was confined in the hospital St. Antoine. Were this even the only fact of this kind, which it is not, it would authorize us to class these bone-pains among both the mercurial and syphilitic symptoms.

But what proves beyond all cavil, the similarity of mercurial and syphilitic symptoms, is the frequent error committed by physicians in mistaking them for each other. How many wretches who had been poisoned by mercury, have again been subjected to a mercurial treatment, because the disastrous effects of the poison, with which they had been saturated, were mistaken for syphilis.

Mercury having been tried, as said before, in all sorts of diseases, ever since the end of the last century, modern allœopathic physicians were unable to employ it in any new ailments. All they were able to do, was to modify its use. Indeed, they have succeeded in going much farther in the use of mercury than the most extravagant of their predecessors.

"The doses of mercurial ointment which Velpeau employed every day, in order to produce a speedy ptyalism, (in puerperal fever,) varied from one to two ounces. We have been bolder, and we have prescribed it in quantities of from three to five ounces. Paul Dubois has even used from one to one pound and a half at one dose."[1]

[1] *Loco citato.*

Will such enormities be believed some centuries hence?

The mercurial preparation which is more particularly used in homœopathy, under the name of *mercurius solubilis*, or simply *mercurius*, is the black oxyde or protoxyde of this metal. See Hahnemann's *Materia Medica Pura*, Vol. III.

Homœopathic applications.—Soluble mercury is particularly adapted to lymphatic subjects, with bad humors, debilitated in body and mind, chilly, disposed to catarrhal affections or rheumatic pains when exposed ever so little to a damp and cool air, with a sickly or nauseous breath, and sweating easily, especially at night; and lastly, *to women rather than to men.*

Here is a list of the morbid symptoms for which mercury is employed with most success:

Scrofula, syphilis, variola (in young girls); *acute erysipelas, red and round tetters: syphiliform diseases, syphilitic tubercles* in the thickness of the skin; *lepra;* ulcers with shaggy borders, a greyish bottom, and secreting an ichorous and fetid pus; *rhagades at the hands and feet; friability of the long bones*, humid *caries* of the short bones, exostoses; deformation of the nails.

Congestion of blood to the head, with flashes of heat in the face, shuddering over the rest of the body, icy coldness of the extremities; vertigo and sensation of falling or stumbling, especially on rising from one's chair after having been seated for some time, in the morning on rising from bed, during a walk in the open air, or while lying on the back; pressive headache, as if the head were strongly pressed by a cord all around, or pressed down from above downwards; throbbings, *stitches, boring pains in the head*, especially *in the left temple* or occiput; *exostosis at the cranium;* cold, viscid sweat about the head; painfulness of the whole outer head; oozing eruption at the hairy scalp; *falling of the hair. Syphilitic or scrofulous ophthalmia*, especially when the malady commences in the left eye; congestion of the vessels in the eye; *photophobia* with burning lachrymation, fiery points, muscæ volitantes, etc.; *neuralgia in the eye, with frightful pains, which proceeded from the bottom of the orbit, and sense of coldness* all around; ulcerations of the conjunctiva and cornea. Tearing in the muscles and bones of one side of the face; red and hot swelling of a whole side of the face. *Otitis*, with fetid discharges and fungous excrescences in the ear. *Caries of the nasal bones. Painful swelling of the salivary glands; greyish ulcers on the inner surface of the lips, cheeks, gums, tongue and palate; shrinking, looseness and indentations of the gums, which lays the teeth bare; nocturnal toothach; caries, looseness and falling out of the teeth; fungous swelling of the mucous membrane of the mouth; intolerable foulness of the breath; swelling of the tongue*, which is covered with a whitish, thick, *tenacious coat*, that is detached in the shape of little skins; *profuse discharge of a viscous and fetid saliva;* sweetish, sour, salt taste, or loss of taste; *caries of the palatine bones; ulcers in the pharynx;* the swallowing is rendered difficult as if the throat were obstructed by a fleshy body; *ulceration of the tonsils;* phlegmonous angina, with lancing pain that extends to the ear, and *gets worse at night.*

Nausea, with vertigo, especially after a meal; hiccough; rancid or bitter regurgitations, or tasting as if one had eaten sugar-plums; pyrosis; violent vomiting; weakness of digestion, *with constant, insatiable hunger;* aversion to food; excessive sensitiveness in the præcordial regions, epigastrium and hypochondrium; burning or cutting pain at the stomach; swelling of the liver; *hepatitis; jaundice;* hardness and swelling of the abdomen, which is painful to contact, especially in the umbilical region; incisive or contusive pains in the abdomen; sense of coldness, from the epigastrium to the throat, where it is accompanied by a sort of scraping; cutting pains after a cold; colic, followed by small mucous or frequent sanguineous stools, with tenesmus; *diarrhœic stools, especially towards evening or in the cool open air;* hard, large-sized, corrosive stools, even if not diarrhœic, grayish, greenish, bloody, excessively fetid; discharge of *ascarides* or *lumbrici.*

Constant desire to urinate day and night; burning and

smarting urine, which is emitted drop by drop; profuse urine as in diabetes, with extreme emaciation; *albuminuria;* fetid, cloudy urine, which deposits a chalky sediment; bloody urine; swelling of the urethra, in consequence of which, the stream of urine becomes thinner and twisted; inflammation of the orifice of the urethra.

Greenish gonorrhœa; chancres in the urethra, at the prepuce or at the corona glandis; *balanitis, orchitis, buboes;* sensation of coldness in the testicles, especially towards evening; erotism, with painful erections, especially in the night, and emission of a sanguinolent semen; feeble and incomplete erections; emissions without sexual desire; no thrill during an embrace; impotence. Swelling, ulceration and suppuration of the vaginal mucous membrane; *greenish leucorrhœa; chancres at the clitoris* and *labia minora; fungous ulcerations at the neck of the uterus; metritis; metrorrhagia;* suppression of the menses; *ulcerations* and swellings at the breasts.

Catarrhal affections of the air-passages, with a violent *fluent* and corrosive coryza; hoarse cough, sensation of dryness and prickings in the œsophagus; *nocturnal paroxysms of suffocation;* stitches at the heart.

Painful stiffness of the nape of the neck and of the whole neck; coldness on the back; beatings and stitches at the shoulder-blades; convulsive flexion of the trunk on the inferior extremities, with sudden and violent raising of the trunk, a double irregular movement which is repeated a hundred times in one hour; *rickets; caries of the vertebræ and sacrum;* tearing pains in the extremities; trembling of the head and extremities; *acute articular rheumatism, with red swelling of the joints,* fever, burning thirst, *fetid breath and sweat; chronic articular rheumatism,* with nodes in the joints; involuntary and sometimes strange projection of the lower extremities, forwards or sideways; *infiltration of one or more limbs,* or of the whole body; *paralysis* or *atrophy* (secondary effect) of one or more limbs.

General prostration; gaping; comatose drowsiness; fever

with shuddering, heat at the head and face, with coldness, *if uncovered ever so little;* irregular, frequent or slow, intermittent or tremulous pulse; *profuse sweat* of a *sickly or nauseous* smell, oily, and staining the linen yellow. Excessive depression of spirits; indifference to every thing or every body; apprehension of becoming crazy; imbecility; *religious monomania; mental derangement; strange neuroses; epilepsy; lethargy,* with loss of speech and of the senses, but not of consciousness, etc.

Merc. corr. and *Nitri. ac.* are the best antidotes of *Merc. sol.*

Argentum. *Metallic silver, regula argenti* of the ancient chemists.

Empirical applications.—This metal, which has been known ever since the remotest antiquity, is supposed to be without any medicinal virtues in its natural state. However, Avicenna recommended silver filings for *palpitations of the heart,* and *fetid breath,* both of which applications are justified by the pathogenesis of this agent. After having been used for a long time as an ingredient in the *electuary of hyacinth,* where it played a very obscure part, silver has disappeared from the repertory of Allœopathic drugs, and is only used by Allœopathic pharmaceutists for the purpose of covering the surface of boluses or pills with a view of disguising their taste.

But if silver is no longer used by Old School physicians, except for the ridiculous purposes above stated, some of its salts are recommended for medicinal purposes, for example, *chloride,* by Serres and Ricord, of Montpellier, *against syphilis,* and especially the *nitrate of silver,* which is so woefully abused every day.

Recommended for *dropsy* by Boerhaave, the nitrate of silver has since been used for *dyspepsia, obstinate diarrhœa, lienteria, worm affections, syphilis, whooping-cough, Saint Guy's dance,* (tarantism,) *hysteria,* and especially *epilepsy.*[1]

[1] Gmelin, appar. medic., vol. I., p. 356; Sprengel, hist. de la méd., vol. VI., p. 510; *Biblioth.* médic., vol. LI., p. 365; Mérat and De Lens, Dict. de mat. med., vol. I., p. 401, etc.

Hahnemann, who was acquainted with these facts, except those of most recent date, seems to place very little reliance in them. "The empirical reputation which the nitrate of silver enjoys in ordinary cases of epilepsy, is probably without any real foundation, and seems to be based upon the fact, that a salt of silver which contained copper, had been employed in cases of convulsions where copper was indicated; for the primary symptoms of fine silver do not by any means show that it is capable of curing the most disagreeable, and at the same time the most common form of epilepsy.[1]

"The so-called hydragogue pills of R. Boyle, and which have been so much praised by Boerhaave, are not at an adapted to their object, not only on account of the large size of the doses in which they are given, but also because silver increases the urinary secretion only during its primary action, which, in consequence of the opposite reaction of the vital force, must necessarily be followed by an opposite condition." I am sorry to be obliged to differ with Hahnemann in this instance. On the one hand, I know of cures performed by the nitrate of silver, which are so positive, that they cannot be doubted, and on the other hand, having myself cured a dropsical patient by the almost exclusive use of silver, I am obliged to admit that, if this drug is capable of curing diabetes, as Hahnemann supposes, it may also, in some cases, be able to cure dropsy.

[1] The following symptoms of silver seem to remind one somewhat of epilepsy:

"Complete dizziness on entering the room after a walk." (Hubert.)

"Before midnight, in bed, while slumbering, I was seized with a dizziness so that it seemed to me that my head was falling out of the bed; followed by a violent and convulsive starting of the body: vertigo and desire to sleep had disappeared." (Idem.)

"After dinner, during my usual siesta, I felt a violent electric shock, which first proceeded from the left, and afterwards from the right hip-joint, and disturbed my sleep. Having fallen asleep again ten minutes later, with my hands above my head, I felt another shock, much more violent, in the left arm, and proceeding from the arm-joint." (Idem.)

Besides, silver and the nitrate of silver producing effects upon the healthy organism which, probably, differ from each other, it would be wrong to draw conclusions from one of these substances, relative to the result which might be obtained by means of the other. Nevertheless, in comparing the therapeutic effects of the nitrate or chloride of silver to the symptoms of the pure metal, we will be obliged to admit that the latter agree tolerably well with the former, and even account for them in a pretty satisfactory manner.[1]

Homœopathic applications.—The most extensive pathogenesis of silver, that I know of, is that which Dr. Roth has published in the second volume of the *Bulletin de la Société de médecine homœopathique* of Paris.[2] "Until now," says Jahr, in the fourth edition of his Manual, "this agent has only been employed for *mercurial angina*, and very successfully for *chronic laryngitis*, especially in the case of lawyers,

[1] I am disposed to believe that the nitrate of silver is an antisyphilitic, and it is on this ground that I account for the fact that the cauterisation of a recent chancre with the nitrate, may sometimes have succeeded in preventing the constitutional infection of syphilis. Seventeen or eighteen years ago, a student at law, a friend of mine, was taken, after a very suspicious coïtus, with an itching at the corona glandis. Soon after, on one side of the frænulum, a small oblong vesicle, filled with a clear serum, showed itself at this spot. This young man thought he was infected with syphilis, and soon after the woman exhibited unequivocal symptoms of the disease. Before the vesicle broke, it was deeply cauterised with the nitrate of silver, and, in the place of a chancre which would undoubtedly have followed, a small wound showed itself which healed in a few days.

I ought to remark that in similar cases, which are however very rare, for the chancre-vesicle breaks easily and is not always visible, the good effects of a speedy cauterisation do not invalidate Hahnemann's doctrine of an immediate and general infection of the organism; but they go to prove that the nitrate is an *antisyphilitic.* It is said that soon after the coït the virus is absorbed; but why not the *nitrate* likewise? Both starting from the same point, pass through the same channel, meet, and neutralise each other. I will state, however, that I condemn entirely the cauterisation of the chancre, a detestable method which, by destroying the external sign, deprives us of the means of verifying the presence or absence of syphilis in the organism.

[2] This pathogenesis comprises Hahnemann's 223 symptoms, and a similar number by Dr. Hubert of Vienna.

(advocates,) preachers, and generally of persons who are obliged to speak a good deal, and for a long time in succession." However, in Beauvais' *Clinique homœopathique*, mention is made of a case of *caries*, which silver is said to have arrested. Be that as it may, according to my own observations, silver is destined to act a much more important part than that which has fallen to its lot so far.

Guided by the effects which silver has produced on myself, and which represented *syphilitic symptoms*, (such as *gonorrhœa with contusive pain in the testicles, grayish ulcers with shaggy borders, simultaneously at the prepuce and in the throat*,) I have prescribed this drug for the first time against a *yellow-greenish gonorrhœa, of an indolent character from the first, very profuse*, and of eight months' standing, for which *Cannab. Copaiv. Mercur.* (whether sol. or corr., the patient was unable to say,) had been employed for a long time and in vain. The patient was twenty-six years old, robust, active, intelligent, but had red hair, a white skin, and a very marked rheumatic diathesis. *Argentum* effected a cure in less than twelve days, and suspended for more than a year the rheumatic pains in the extremities.

This latter circumstance has decided me several times to prescribe *Argentum* for *articular rheumatism*, without swelling, and presenting, particularly at the knee, and still more at the elbow, this burning, lancing pain, which resembles a good deal the pain caused by the sting of a wasp. Let us observe moreover, that the action of *Argentum* on the muscular system and on the skin, is very similar to that of *Zincum*, after which it will indeed be found ranked. I have moreover employed argentum with success in the following cases: 1st. In two cases of *albuminuria*, of which I intend to publish afterwards an extensive account, which will be found interesting. 2d, *Seminal losses*, without erections and with atrophy of the penis, (in a man of thirty this organ was no larger than that of a child of ten years;) the primary cause of this spermatorrhœa was onanism. 3d. *Amaurosis* of the left eye, (syphilitic or mercurial, (?) rather mercurial,) which was cured in a few weeks, although the sight was already very weak, and the pupil, which was very much contracted, remained insensible at the approach of the light. 4th. *Schirrous ulceration* of the neck of the uterus.

This patient was a washer-woman of Boulogne, aged fifty years, tall, thin, emaciated, of a very irritable temperament; her father had died with a cancer at the tongue. The disease was of long standing. This woman, whose face was of a straw-color down to the lips inclusive, a characteristic symptom of the cancerous diathesis, was troubled with constant distention of the hypogastrium, which was exceedingly sensitive to contact. Every moment she felt lancing pains in this region, which she compared to pricks with a pin. There was a tension in the groins, and from time to time, crampy pains in the thighs. Her breath was fetid, *foul*, her appetite pretty good; the digestion took place without pain at the stomach; the alvine evacuations were irregular; she was often taken with a diarrhœa, or rather lienteria. The urine was pale, fetid, and profuse, especially at night. The mucous membrane of the vagina, which was considerably wrinkled by the descension of the uterus, was almost round; but the neck of the uterus, which was very much swollen, presented only, so to say, a spongy mass so deeply corroded with ulcers in different directions, that it was impossible to discover the os tincæ. The purulent, ichorous, and sometimes bloody matter which flowed from these ulcers, filled constantly the vagina, from which proceeded such a horrible stench that it would have been impossible for one to remain ten minutes in the same room with this unhappy woman, whose near death seemed to me, and indeed was, inevitable. However, she continued to live for six months, which I attribute to the action of *Argentum*. Various remedies, *conium*, *cicuta virosa*, *sepia* and *lycopodium* had been given without any effect. Argentum effected a general improvement almost instantaneously. The diarrhœa ceased and the stools became natural. The desire to urinate was diminished one half. The shooting pains in the hypogastrium diminished, so that the patient was sometimes free from them for days. A circumstance which astonished me a good deal was, that the discharge, although still purulent, lost *almost entirely*, and in *less than three days*, its foul smell. Fleshy, rose-colored granulations, of a very satisfactory appearance, showed themselves at the neck of the uterus. Her strength even returned visibly, and for two or three weeks, I flattered myself that the patient would get well. Unfortunately, this illusion was not to last long; a relapse took place. The family attributed it to a fit of anger, to which the patient was subject. The diarrhœa reappeared, and, with it, all the uterine symptoms. This time argentum had no effect. Soon the prostration was at its height. *Arsenic* was of no use. After two days spent in agony death took place; fatal, but inevitable termination of a malady against which, when it has attained this stage, medicine is of no avail; nevertheless, this partial success convinced me that, of all the medicines which I had tried, argentum was the one which had effected the most favorable change, and which, if it had been given six months sooner, might have effected a cure.

Merc. sol. is said to antidote argentum.

Kreasota. A pyrogenous product, discovered by Reichenbach, a chemist of Blausko, in Moravia.

This kind of essential oil, which was first obtained from the distillation of pyroligneous acid, afterwards from that of tar, is colorless, inflammable, a little denser than distilled water, of a burning taste, a disagreeable, exceedingly pungent smell, similar to the smell of the smoke of green wood. Water dissolves about 1–100 of its weight. When pure, this substance acts on the skin, and on the mucous membrane, like a caustic.

Kreasot owes its name (from Kreas, flesh, and Ocho, I preserve,) to the property it possesses, and which it shares with arsenic, corrosive sublimate, etc., to preserve animal matter from putrefaction. It is sufficient to dip in water in which a small quantity of kreasot has been mixed, tainted meat or fish, in order to remove at once their unpleasant odor, and impart to them the taste of smoked fish. This is accounted for by the fact that the kreasot with which they are impregnated, is contained in the smoke of the resinous woods which are used in smoking meat, and which impart to it its well known taste and flavor, and the faculty of resisting decay. This is the reason why the daily and continued use of smoked meat is hurtful to health; a sort of scurvy carries off the teeth, foul breath, costiveness, a general malaise, and a real cacochymia, are the most frequent consequences of the protracted use of such articles. It even happens that the eating of smoked meat has occasioned death. Doctor Kermes, of Weinsberg, collected, according to Mérat,[1] 135 cases of this kind of poisoning, which occurred from 1793 to 1820, and which he does not hesitate to attribute to kreasot. An acute and burning pain at the epigastrium, vomiting of sanguinolent matter, meteorism of the abdomen, violent colic with constipation, slow breathing, sinking of the pulse, and dilatation of the pupils; such had been the leading symptoms in every case.

Empirical applications.—"As soon as this drug had been introduced into therapeutics," say Messrs. Trousseau and Pidoux, "it excited a great emulation among therapeutists, and they endeavored to out-do each other in discovering new properties in the drug. Cancer, tetter, hæmorrhages, caries of the bones, scrofula, phthisis, were cured by means of kreasot. With this escort of diseases, kreasot was introduced in France towards 1829. It was a sad and deplorable infatuation, which lasted for some months; the Institute, the Académie de Médecine, were assailed with memoirs during this interval," etc.[2] That is to say, kreasot shared the fate of most other allœopathic drugs. A few successful cures were magnified into miracles, which a few reverses soon caused to be forgotten. How could it be otherwise? How could it have been possible to obtain good results from a therapeutic

[1] Dict. Univ. de Mat. Med., par Merat and de Lens, Supp. p. 20.
[2] Œuv. Cit., vol. I., p. 106.

agent, the legitimate use of which could not possibly be determined by any known means? There was assuredly some truth in what was said of the efficacy of kreasot against tetters, hæmorrhages, caries of the bones, scrofula, etc.; but this truth was indiscriminately expressed. What kind of tetters, hæmorrhages, caries, was it that kreasot cured? Nobody asked this question, and nobody could tell. The consequence was that, after having made unlucky trials with kreasot against *burns*, *ulcers*, *phlegmasiæ of the mucous membranes*, *hæmorrhages* of any kind, *phthisis*, etc., it was agreed that this substance, which however, is such a powerful and precious agent, was incapable, or nearly so, of rendering any service whatever to the healing art, and that the best use that could be made of it, was to employ it for the preservation of anatomical preparations. Now-a-days kreasot is employed only (externally) in a few hospitals of Paris, against gangrenous ulcers, bad sores, hospital-gangrene, caries of the bones. Laymen who are disposed to remember the good which a drug has done, without thinking of its failures, continue to employ kreasot against toothache and caries of the teeth. "Evidently," say Messrs. Trousseau and Pidoux, "this substance, like all those which are of a cathe-retic character, quiets, generally speaking, toothache, and keeps off caries, in the same manner as the nitrate of silver, the sulphate of copper, etc.; but it has no special properties, as might easily be seen, and latterly, kreasot is scarcely yet employed by any dentist.[1] It is very fortunate that dentists should have discontinued the external use of kreasot, which must either be of no avail, or else entail evil consequences." But let Messrs. Trousseau and Pidoux take the trouble to prove kreasot upon themselves, and they will soon find that, like mercury, it possesses a special action on the dental apparatus.

Homœopathic applications.—Dr. Wahle has rendered homœopathy a real service by his proving of kreasot. In Jahr's manual, the reader will find a synopsis of the symp-

[1] Idem, vol. I., p. 106.

toms of this agent. According to Wahle's pathogenesis, and my own observations, kreasot is best calculated to remove the following affections :—

Affections of the female sex, and more particularly of children in the cradle, of slender make, chilly, *leuco-phlegmatic*, with bad humors, and disposed to constipation.[1] General lassitude, especially in the morning, with contusive, *ulcerative*, or pinching pains in various parts of the body; yawning, drowsiness, with coldness and altered color of the skin, especially at the extremities, which seem as if mortified. *Papulous eruption*, of a bright red, and accompanied with a burning and stinging itching, especially at the arms, legs, and insteps; *syphilis neonatorum: sub-cutaneous syphilitic tubercles* (gommata);[2] *bone-pains:* painful swelling of the salivary glands, and of the lymphatic ganglions; *humid tetters*, accompanied with an intolerable itching, especially *around the mouth*, at the cheeks, eye-lids, *ears*, *elbow*, *hollow of the hands*, and insteps. Sadness and weeping in children, sometimes without stopping, but especially in the evening; *anxious sleeplessness* in the night; fever, with shuddering, which recurs every instant; bright redness of the face, thirst, small and frequent pulse; *fetid sweat: paroxysms of fainting or convulsions*, as in worm-affections; a sort of stupor.

Congestive headache, with dizziness, or stupefying, throbbing, *pressive*, especially at the forehead, temples and vertex, which is more particularly felt *in the morning on waking;* stitches, buzzing, whizzing in the head; acute pulling, which sometimes extends to the jaws and teeth; heaviness at the occiput, as if the head would fall backwards; hemicrania with a sensation of fulness, a stinging or expansive pain;

[1] In recommending kreasot in diseases of women and children, I do not mean to exclude it from the treatment of adults. Such a principle would belie my own practice. A child afflicted with *congenital syphilis* is almost always benefitted by kreasot, even if the general symptoms which I have here indicated do not exist.

[2] My colleague, Dr. Chanet, informs me that he has employed kreasot in a case of this kind with very good success, in conformity with my indications; the patient was a young woman.

painfulness of the hairy scalp; red eruption on the forehead; *falling of the hair; red and moist eyes*, or else dull and without expression; *violent ophthalmia*, with burning tears; spots and ulcers on the cornea; photophobia; dimness of sight, with dilatation or contraction of the pupil; muscæ volitantes, amaurosis; *cataract of the left eye;* redness and swelling of the eyelids; inflammatory swelling of the ear; deep prickings in the inner ear; *discharge of a purulent and fetid wax;* buzzing in the ears; hardness of hearing; complete deafness on one side; sensitiveness of the nasal bones; dry or fluent coryza; epistaxis, especially in the morning; *discharge of a fetid pus from the nostrils;* congestion and blueish redness of the face.

Accumulation of a serous or tenacious and putrid saliva in the mouth; *swollen, soft, bleeding, ulcerated gums;* drawing *toothache*, aggravated by *cold* and warm *drinks*, coming on especially in the morning or evening; *difficult teething* of children, with the ailments incidental to it, such as cough, convulsions, etc., provided the above-mentioned general conditions exist, and more particularly *when the child is constipated; caries of the teeth* in adults; *syphilitic caries of the palatine bones;* tongue covered with a thick fur which becomes detached in patches; *foul breath;* bitter taste of the food, scraping in the throat; sticky sensation in the pharynx, impeding deglutition; total loss of appetite, with burning thirst; gnawing hunger; regurgitation of a watery, sour, insipid, sweetish or bitter liquid; *nausea* and *retching* before breakfast, as during pregnancy; violent vomiting (rarely); great sensitiveness in the epigastrium; pains at the cardia; pulsations at the stomach; painful swelling of the liver; pressure, stitches or contusive pains in the liver; distention of the abdomen; *sense of coldness at the abdomen;* cutting, colicky pains, incarcerated flatulence; *constipation* or diarrhœa, watery, very fetid stools.

Scanty urine; flowing out *drop by drop, burning, smarting, cloudy*, with dark sediment; *excessive increase of the urinary secretion*, as in diabetes; watery urine with a whitish sediment and a fetid odor; *wetting the bed, in the case of children;* burning in the urethra; *swelling and excoriation of the glands;* balanitis; *recent chancres, of large size,* and *superficial,* at the corona glandis and the internal surface of the prepuce; *milky discharge from the urethra;* premature, profuse menses which last too long, preceded and followed by colicky pains similar to the pains of child-bearing, by leucorrhœa, vomiting and various other accidents; *passive metrorrhagia; corrosive leucorrhœa;* hard hearing during the menses; *milky discharge from the vagina;* excoriations between the thighs and the genital organs; painful swelling of the inguinal ganglia; *increase of the sexual desire* in the morning; pain and swelling of the sexual organs after an embrace; falling of the vagina; stitches and ulcerations at the breasts.

Hoarseness; aphonia; tickling at the larynx, trachea, and in the bronchia; dry, wheezing, *hoarse, constant, spasmodic cough,* especially in the evening, in bed, with profuse expectoration of whitish or yellowish mucus, which has sometimes a *sweetish, insipid* or *foul* taste; short breath; pains in the chest, most frequently in the region of the heart, as if bruised, or burning, or stitching; burning in the chest and throat along the œsophagus, as after having drank brandy; involuntary emission of urine when coughing; stiffness and œdematous swelling of the neck and nape of the neck; ulcerative pain in the loins; luxation-pain at the shoulders, hips, knees, feet; paralytic numbness of the superior extremities; cramps in the calves; *tetters in the bends of the knees, at the ankles and insteps; œdema of the feet;* contraction of the tendons; *fetid sweat of the feet.*

The symptoms of kreasot come on principally in the evening, at night, *in the morning, on waking, during a meal.*

In regard to kreasot, I have to observe two important facts; the first is, that the most marked effects of kreasot often only show themselves after the use of the drug is discontinued; the second is, that the symptoms which it removes, often show a tendency to reappear. It alone scarcely ever cures the *syphilitic scales or papulæ of adults.* In some of these cases, the exanthem first disappears with a speed that enchants both the physician and the patient; but soon after it reappears, and this time it resists the drug, on which account another remedy has to be resorted to. The same remark, however, applies to soluble mercury, corrosive sublimate, nitric acid, etc.

The best antidote of Kreasot, according to my experience, is metallic iron; a knowledge of this fact is not without importance, for Kreasot, when given out of place, for instance to lively, sanguine and vigorous children, makes them feel so uncomfortable that I had to consider myself fortunate to possess the means of relieving them immediately.

Arsenicum Album. See the group of which it is the *type.*

Plumbum, *lead.* This is the *molubdos* of the Greeks; the *saturnus* of the alchymists, who looked upon it as the commonest of all metals.

Lead has been employed in the arts ever since the remotest antiquity. Every body is acquainted with its physical properties. It is insipid, odorous when rubbed, fusible at 322°, and volatilizes at a white heat. Unchangeable in a dry air, it rapidly oxydizes, and then passes to the condition of a carbonate, in contact with water or damp air. Native lead, or the pure oxyde, is seldom found in a natural state. The natural compounds from which it is extracted for industrial purposes, are salts, and especially sulphurets.

Metallic lead is supposed to be without poisonous properties.[1] This opinion seems to me a serious mistake. I admit that considerable pieces of lead may be swallowed without any, or, at least, any great inconvenience, but only in compact masses, such as little balls or shot. Although the cohesion of its particles is very feeble, yet it is strong enough to prevent their absorption when swallowed. But experience has abundantly shown that absorption takes place when lead

[1] Orfila, *toxicol.* gén., vol. I., p. 639.

is introduced into the stomach in the form of an impalpable powder. The inhalation of the vapor of pure lead, not of a chemical combination in which the nature of the metal might have been altered, gives rise to the characteristic phenomena which all preparations of lead are well known to be capable of producing.[1]

This consideration is particularly interesting to a homœopathic physician, for it shows him that lead is a powerful and essentially diffusible poison, that is to say a drug which is so precious that I do not hesitate to rank it with mercury, sulphur, arsenic, lime and silex.

Empirical applications.—On account of its being thought an inert substance, metallic lead has seldom been employed in medicine. Avicenna, Amatus Lusitanus, Ambroise Paré, Johnston and Etmuller, quoted by J. F. Gmelin,[2] employed lead, it is true, but only externally, in the shape of beaten leaves, which they caused to be worn on the abdomen for their supposed anti-aphrodisiac properties, in cases of *nocturnal emissions*, or on *glandular swellings*, in order to effect their resolution. Boerhaave seems to be the first who thought of using lead internally. According to Gmelin, (loc. cit.,) he caused an impalpable powder to be prepared of it, whch he first employed as an absorbent in obstinate excoriations of the skin, but which he likewise gave for *leucorrhœa*, *dysentery*, *syphilis* and *gout*.

Passing from these uses of the metallic lead to its compounds, we shall discover in their history, through the vagueness with which all the statements of the Old School medicine are unfortunately tainted, an indication of the cases in which our dynamised lead has the best chances of succeeding.

[1] See the work of Tanquerel des Planches; *traité des maladies de plomb ou saturnines.* Paris, 1839, 2 vols., in 8vo. What is curious, is that in describing the symptoms of saturnine colic, no matter by what preparation it may have been produced, the principal symptoms contained in the pathogenesis of Hartlanb and Trinks, its authors, are mentioned.

[2] See in his *appar. medic.*, part II., the long and interesting chapter which he devotes to lead-preparations, vol. I., p. 362, etc.

The oxydes, sulphurets, chlorides, carbonates, phosphates, sulphates, sub-acetates, and more recently the tannate of lead, have been most frequently employed by the older physicians.

It cannot be doubted, that each of these preparations had its particular properties, which ought to have furnished so many special indications. But could these properties have been determined without pure experimentation? Indeed not. It was deemed sufficient to settle the *general action* of lead and of its compounds, in accordance with clinical observations, which were, for the most part, mutilated, insignificant, and doubtful. In one word, the same course was pursued with the lead-preparations that had been pursued with those of *mercury*, *iron*, etc.

United by modern therapeutists in the class of *astringents*, the saturnine preparations comprise, first, those which, on account of their insolubility, such as *minium*, *sugar of lead*, etc., are exclusively used for plasters, salves, etc.; secondly, those of a *mixed use*, (*water of Goulard*,) of which lotions, collyria, injections into the urethra, vagina, or rectum are made; third, lastly, those which, like the neutral acetate, are prescribed by a small number of practitioners, in the shape of pills or potions.

I say a *small number*, for in spite of the salts of lead having been pronounced uninjurious by Professor Fouquier, and in spite of a few authentic cures which have been effected with lead, we have to do this justice to our opponents, that they generally preserve strong and legitimate suspicions against the internal use of lead in the massive doses of the Old School.[1] They are well aware that the authorised administration of the acetate of lead, whatever Fouquier may say to the contrary, has frequently induced the frightful malady, known as lead-colic, with all its accompanying and subsequent symptoms.

[1] In the external use of lead the same reserve has not been observed. How many terrible accidents and even deaths have been caused by the water of Goulard, in consequence of repelling cutaneous diseases.

The following are the principal maladies which have been empirically cured or alleviated by lead:

Erysipelas, burns, tetters, scrofulous and syphilitic ulcers, various kinds of tumors, schirrus of the breasts,[1] *open cancer,*[2] *chronic ophthalmia, chronic coryza, ozæna, otorrhoea,*[3] *aphthæ, mercurial salivation, angina membranacea,*[4] *nervous vomiting, acute and chronic dysentery,*[5] *sporadic cholera, engorgements of the liver and spleen, with paroxysms of fever; dropsy,*[6] *gonorrhœa, leucorrhœa, orchitis, metrorrhagia,*[7] *chronic pulmonary catarrh, ulcerative phthisis* (pneumonia in the suppurative stage),[8] *neuralgia* of the head, extremities and various internal organs, such as the liver, spleen and intestines; *neurosis of the heart, hysteria, hypochondria, etc.*[9]

The good effects of lead in these diseases are accounted for by the proving of this drug; however, the empirical use of lead could not possibly lead to any great results, owing to the fact that allœopathic physicians dared not employ lead and its compounds in diseases which resembled the poisonous effects of the acetate of lead, and in which the lead preparations would have been particularly efficacious.[10]

Homœopathic applications.—Hartlanb and Trinks have published a pathogenesis of lead. Not knowing the German language, I have not been able to read this pathogenesis in the

[1] Trousseau and Pidoux, (œuv. cit., vol. I., p. 126,) relate a remarkable cure of this kind.

[2] See Nouv. bibliot. mèd., vol. IV., p. 193.

[3] Trousseau and Pidoux, œuv. cit., vol. I., p. 129.

[4] *Trans. Méd.*, vol. X., 182.

[5] Barthez. *Gaz. des hôpitaux*, déc. 1845.

[6] Etmuller, Grollius, Lieutaud, etc., quoted by Gmelin, appar., vol. I., p. 417.

[7] Aman son, *Sur l'usage des prépar. de plomb*, dans le traitem. des malvénér. (Anc. Journ. de Méd., vol. XXIV., p. 352.)

[8] Bull. des scienc. méd. de Férussac, vol. XVII., p. 369.

[9] Gmelin, loc. cit.; biblio. med., vol. L., p. 398; Morgagni, *de sedibus et causis*, etc., epist. VIII.; *Bull. des scienc. méd.* de Férussac, vol. III., p. 291, etc.

[10] It is to be observed that the internal and external forms of neuralgia, for which lead has been used with success, constitute some of the prominent symptoms of a poisoning with lead, as described by Tanquerel des Planches.

original text. Whether Jahr's synopsis is perfectly reliable, I am not able to affirm. My own observations and clinical experience have confirmed to me most of the symptoms related by Jahr. A large number of the pure effects of this metal can be collected from the cases of poisoning contained in such works as the two volumes of Tanquerel des Planches. Be this as it may, here follow the indications for the use of lead, which I think I may safely infer from my own observations.

Lead is particularly adapted to adults, males rather than females, and particularly to persons of a dry, bilious constitution, with a somewhat jaundiced complexion, irascible, hypochondriac, or disposed to religious monomania. There are acute diseases, in which it would undoubtedly be preferable to any other remedy. It might perhaps be employed with advantage (in a high potency) in saturnine colic, for the very reason that lead causes it;[1] until now I have only used it in chronic cases.

In the following affections I have employed it with particular success; *chronic inflammation of the bladder; strictures of the urethra, caused by gonorrhœa;* a sort of tenacious (mercurial) salivation, so profuse that the patient, especially in damp weather, literally inundated his pillow during sleep; *an excessively painful retraction of the testicles and penis, which seemed to re-enter the hypogastrium,* (in consequence of prolonged venereal excesses and repelled tetters); *nocturnal bone-pains, which had resisted mercury,* silver and nitric acid; several cases of pulling and pressive *chronic headache, in the forehead,* aggravated by mental labor which was almost rendered impossible, and becoming intolerable whenever the patients were in rather numerous company;[2] a case of *mental derangement* induced by syphilis, with obscure paralysis of

[1] Various dynamised substances, such as coffee, opium, cannabis, mercurius, etc., remove symptoms which had been produced by massive doses of the same drugs. Is this the case with lead? I am unable to decide this point for certain.

[2] In these cases the patients have formerly been constipated, but this condition had ceased.

the right arm, paroxysm of religious monomania, erotism without erection, periodical fever without sweat, and cramp-like retraction of the abdomen from time to time; various nervous diseases, characterised principally by wandering *pains in the* extremities, spasms in the muscles of the face, paroxysms of screams, fright without cause, and of sudden fainting, in passing from one room to another, or in entering a room full of company. In the two cases of this kind which fell under my notice, lead did not effect a cure, but a long suspension of the symptoms. In these two patients, the mind remained sound, even at the height of the paroxysms. There was a complete apyrexia, and the digestive functions took place normally, except, however, frequent paroxysms of nocturnal bulimy. It is particularly useful in *marsh intermittent*, with *quotidian or double-tertian type*, particularly when the splenic region is painful to the touch. In such a case neither china, nor arsenic, can at all be compared to lead; a trial will confirm my statement.

In some respects, lead is related to zinc, after which it will again be mentioned.

Antidotes:—*Alum.*, *Bell.*, *Hyosc.*, *Op.*, *Plect.*, *Stram.*, *Electric.* According to my experience, the best antidote is *æthusa cynap.*

Sulfuris acidum. *Sulphuric acid*, *vitriol*, etc. This powerful acid, which was discovered in the middle-ages, is found in its pure state in the neighbourhood of various volcanoes, but generally in combination with lime, baryta, alumina, iron. From the sulphate of iron it was formerly obtained for the arts. Now-a-days it is obtained in all sorts of ways, which it is needless to describe in this place.

Pure sulphuric acid is a viscid, colorless, inodorous liquid, of a specific gravity of 1.85; not very volatile at an ordinary temperature, boiling at 310°; freezing at 12° below zero, containing in this state about 20.00 water, but absorbing the dampness of the air to such a degree that, if the vial is left uncorked, the volume of the acid increases to three times its size; excessively caustic; and rapidly carbonising the organic substances with which it is brought in contact.

Empirical applications.—Formerly sulphuric acid was much used in medicine. Now-a-days it is almost abandoned by allœopathic physicians, who scarcely yet employ it, except in the preparation termed *mineral lemonade,* which is recommended as an antidote to lead-intoxication. Externally it was used in the treatment of *scrofulous, phagedenic, cancerous and venereal ulcers.* It was extensively used as a gargle for *aphthæ in the mouth, ulcerations of the gums and membranous angina,* which, among other injurious consequences, resulted in dulness and deterioration of the teeth. Even when employed externally, this agent was rarely left pure or diluted only with water. Most commonly it was incorporated in fat bodies, such a soil or lard, which it transformed into raw soap; or it was mixed in various proportions with alcohol, from which, after the mixture had grown old, a certain quantity of ether was formed. The most celebrated of these preparations were: 1. The *acid soap* of Achard, an admirable *dissolvent,* according to Macquer and Cornett,[1] who prescribed it almost exclusively for *schirrus of the breasts and calculous nephritis,* but more particularly praised by Carminati, who gave it in *obstinate intermittent fevers, visceral obstructions, dropsy, jaundice, cachexia,* provided "the fibre did not seem too irritable, and the stomach was of sufficient strength;" he used it moreover for *certain tumors of the feet.* 2. The *elixirs* of Schulz, Dippel, Mynsicht, Haller, and finally the water of Rabel. These different elixirs were almost the same, except that the relative proportions of acid and alcohol which constituted the chief ingredients, differed. All these elixirs were used internally. In the following maladies they were administered with more or less success: *intermittent, putrid, malignant, contagious fevers,* (Etmueller, Rivière), *comatose and petechial fevers, scarlatina, confluent and malignant variola,* (Sydenham), *dysentery* (Dussansay), *the plague, lepra, the*

[1] Mérat and Delens, Dict. de Mat. Med., vol. VI., p. 461.

itch and various other *cutaneous diseases; gonorrhœa,*[1] *leucorrhœa,* (Mellin), *nocturnal emissions* (Ferriar), *suppression of the menses or piles, calculous nephritis and gout,* (Dippel); *pituitous phthisis* (de Hæn and Reid); various kinds of nervous diseases, such as *epilepsy,* but particularly, according to Haller and Zimmerman, *chorea.*[2]

Lastly, according to Brult, Cramer, Roth and Brinckle, sulphuric acid, if administered as a lemonade, and for a certain period, (say about ten days,) to drunkards, has the faculty of depriving them of all taste for alcoholic beverages.[3]

For the pathogenesis, see Hahnemann, *Chronic Diseases,* vol. III.

Homœopathic applications. Where sulphuric acid was indicated homœopathically, it has removed the following symptoms:

"Tension in the eyelids, in the morning; myopia; hardness of hearing; inguinal hernia; chronic diarrhœa; profuse menses; metrorrhagia; roughness in the throat; *asthma;* swelling of the feet; cold feet."

Sulphuric acid seems also to have been employed with success in some cases of *excoriations at the skin, aphthæ* in children; chronic *ophthalmia, pyrosis, typhus-fever, hæmoptysis,* and even *pulmonary phthisis.*[4]

Two or three times I have used this drug with success against round syphilitic spots, of a bright red color, of the size of ten cent pieces, rather itching, running into each other, secreting a humor, sometimes, and generally seated at the inner and upper surface of the thighs, between the shoulders, in the face, and at the posterior surface of the forearms and hands. The subjects upon whom this acid seemed to act best, were lymphatic, ate a good deal, and were disposed to a constant looseness of the bowels, so that their evacuations were rarely in shape.

All this shows that our practical notions concerning sul-

[1] Astruc, *de morbis venereis,* cap. 12, p. 462.

[2] Gmelin, apparat. medic., t. I., p. 35, etc.

[3] Nouv. bibl. med., vol. I., p. 118.

[4] *Clinique* of Doctor Beauvais.

phuric acid, are still very limited. *Merc. corr.*, *Nitri acid.*, and *Sepia*, are the medicines, after which I have generally used it. According to Jahr, Pulsatilla antidotes it.

Stannum, *tin*, *Jupiter of the alchymists.* This metal, of a silver-white color, very soft, which is easily cut with a knife, malleable, and giving out a peculiar sound when bent, that is known in France by the name of *cri d' ètain*, (creaking of the tin,) is found in nature in the native state, but more frequently combined with sulfur or oxygen. The tin of commerce is seldom pure: it contains copper, sometimes arsenic, and almost always lead. Before it is employed in medicine, it has to be purified from all such alloy. It is fusible at 228°, and is supposed not to volatilize; but like the lead, though much less, it oxydizes in contact with damp air.

Empirical applications. "Physicians," says Hahnemann, "have never employed tin in diseases, because they did not believe that it was endowed with curative properties. Alston, was the first who gave the prescription of a domestic remedy employed by the Scotch against tænia, and which consists in a syrup to which Scotch tin is added in the shape of a powder (containing one-twentieth of alloy); after the powder a purgative is given. Since then, tin filing has been substituted. This remedy, however, does not destroy tænia; and the workers in tin are often attacked with this malady. The tin seems to stupefy it, to decrease its motions in the bowels, and therefore, only exercises a palliative effect, whence its ulterior effect is more hurtful than useful to the patient.[1]

This passage seems to be somewhat tainted with prejudice. Why should we deny incontestable facts? Every body knows that pulverized tin has very frequently cured worm-affections, and has positively freed several patients from tænia.[2] Who

[1] Chronic Maladies, vol. III.

[2] See Sprengel, history of med., vol. V.; Gmelin, apparat. med., vol. I., p. 299; bull. des sc. med. de Fér., vol. II., p. 369, etc.· In his Materia Medica Pura, vol. II., Hahnemann seems to admit the efficacy of tin against tænia; for he combats the absurd opinion which the physicians of the two last centuries entertained, namely, that tin-filings acted against

among us has not frequently seen children discharge, after taking tin, enormous quantities of ascarides or lumbrici, after which the more or less alarming nervous symptoms which seemed to be developed by these parasites, disappeared? Hahnemann's objection is that the workers in tin are frequently attacked with tænia. But what does this prove? Do gilders always find in mercury, with which their bodies are so often and so fatally saturated, a preventive against syphilis? I should say, on the contrary, that the very existence of tænia in the workers in tin, is a proof that this is an efficient remedy for this parasite. What more self-evident than that the development of worm affections ought to be favored in healthy persons by the same drug that arrests and cures them in the sick? Does not the law of similitude lead to this principle? Nevertheless, I am willing to admit that tin corresponds much more with the nervous affections caused by the presence of entozoa, than with the entozoa themselves.

Several preparations containing tin, such as the *anti-hectic liquor of Poterius* (a mixture of the oxyde of tin and of antimony,) the *magisterium jovis*, (oxyde of tin,) etc., have been recommended formerly, especially by Stahl and Fred. Hoffmann, for *pulmonary phthisis*, *hysteria*, *cancer*, *unclean*, *fistulous ulcers*, etc. But in the modern treatises of allœopathic materia medica, tin is simply classed as an *anthelmintic;* scarcely twenty lines are devoted to this agent in the work of Trousseau and Pidoux.

worms only in the ratio of their weight and roughnesses, in the following terms: "A Scotch woman," (of Leith in Scotland,) says Alston, "had a prescription against tænia, which a woman who was a wine-merchant, asked of her, and which cured this patient. Alston managed to obtain it from the daughter of the wine-merchant. Here is the prescription: Take an ounce and a half of tin, pulverise it, mix it with sugar, and take half of it on Friday before new-moon, the other half next morning, and the rest next Sunday; on Monday a purgative.

"This is not a coarse, prickly powder, but a triturated preparation. The powder contained in this prescription, by which the virtues of tin against tænia were alone known, would have been of no use, if the efficacy of the tin had depended upon the mechanical action of the points of the filings."

For the pathogenesis of this drug, we refer the reader to Hahnemann's *Chronic Diseases*, Vol. III.

Homœopathic applications.—In cases where tin was homœopathically indicated, the following symptoms have been removed by it:—

"Pressive heaviness in the forehead; bellyache during the menses; pressure and stitches in the left hypochondrium; burning pain in the hepatic region; nervous excitement; intolerable agitation."

Howsoever correct these indications are, they do not, by any means, comprise the totality of the therapeutic uses of tin. According to its pathogenesis, and certain chemical observations, we may regard the following pathological conditions as those which tin is most capable of curing, provided it is otherwise adapted to the constitution of the patient and the total character of the disease.

General weakness, which is sometimes excessive, especially in the morning and evening, with coldness of the extremities, or sensation of pungent heat, and profuse sweat when making the least movement. Extreme nervousness, as is sometimes seen in persons who have become exhausted by loss of blood, excesses, or a long-lasting sickness, with irascible disposition; misanthropy; an invincible repugnance to conversation, which is exceedingly fatiguing; disposition to spleen and suicide.[1] Attack of sudden paleness, with staring look; occasional absence of mind and dulness of ideas, *especially among children who practise onanism. Attacks of epilepsy* in the morning or evening, which sometimes come on several times in the same day. Considerable loss of flesh. Spots on the skin, round, red, yellowish, sometimes with a little blister or tubercle in the centre, pretty similar to those produced by sulphuric acid, generally with little itching. This kind of tetter is principally seen on the neck, thighs, and legs. Nocturnal restlessness; debilitating sweat in the morning; sweat in the day-time, generally in the afternoon, followed

[1] Arsenic, lead, and probably more than any other, tin, are the drugs which produce more particularly these symptoms of the emotive sphere.

by shuddering and coldness, with *thirst, periodical* febrile motion. Stupefying or contractive, or pulsative headache at the temples; *pressure with drawing* in one half of the head, (most frequently in the left half,) with constriction of the throat and desire to vomit; *painful shocks in the brain;* burning heat in one half of the head, in the eyes, face and even in the nostrils, with dulness, nausea, and desire to lie down. Redness and swelling of the eyes, as if they had been weeping; *syphilitic amaurosis;*[1] contraction, afterwards dilatation of the pupils; suppuration of the eyelids; lachrymal fistula (at the left eye;) epistaxis in the morning. Flashes of heat in the face; burning redness of one cheek only; *pale, livid, fatigued, and elongated face:* cramp-like pressure, especially during the menses, at the cheek-bone; *spasms* and *cramps of the masseter muscles:* swelling of the upper jaw; suppuration of the gums; painful swelling of one cheek; toothache after a meal or at night; sensation as if the teeth were loose and elongated; swelling of the submaxillary glands. Flow of tenacious or sour saliva; yellowish tongue; foul breath; irritation and swelling in the throat; sensation as if something sweetish and repugnant were rising in the throat; sour or bitter taste in the mouth; bitter taste of food; *insatiable hunger;* increased thirst; nausea after eating; singultus; constriction of the throat, followed by vomiting of undigested food, afterwards of a sour or bitter liquid; cutting pain round the stomach; *grasping, spasmodic pains, and accompanied with constant nausea around the umbilicus;* stitches one after the other, and sometimes excited by breathing, under the false ribs and in the hypochondria; *hypochondria;* pressure with the hand, upon the stomach or right hypochondrium, causes the pains to cease, or more frequently increases them; *vomiting of blood,* preceded by cramps and spasms of the stomach; fulness in the lower abdomen, after eating; painful distention of the whole abdomen; cutting colic, as after a cold; abundance of gas in the abdomen which shifts about with a noise; pinching round the

[1] I am in possession of a very interesting case of this kind.

umbilicus for whole days; painful distention of the inguinal region as if hernia would come on; *intestinal worms causing paroxysms of convulsions, which, in some cases, come on several times a day; tænia;* digging in the lower abdomen previous to every evacuation; stool in balls; *dung-shaped stools, fetid, with a desire for more after every evacuation; discharges of worm-shaped mucus.* Retention of urine, or frequent discharges of a watery urine; *excited sexual desire; intolerable sensation of pleasure in the genitals and in the whole body, leading to an emission of semen;*[1] profuse menses; transparent or yellowish leucorrhœa.

Stoppage of one nostril, (left); *nosebleed in the morning;* roughness in the larynx; excoriation-pains in the wind-pipe, on a level with the throat-pit; dry cough, or *with a yellowish, greenish or fetid expectoration, not excited by a titillation of the larynx, but by an irritation in the bronchia,* and *coming on in paroxysms which are sometimes excessive in the evening before midnight, and in the morning at day-break; sensation of weakness and exhaustion in the whole chest during rest as well as motion, with excessive prostration;* sensation of emptiness in the chest; *constriction as by a band, of the wind-pipe and the top of the lungs;* stitches under the left axilla, and between the shoulder-blades; *asthma* coming on after the least exercise; *ulcerative phthisis;* weakness of the nape of the neck; stitches in the back; tearings with pressure in the extremities; *partial paralysis; chorea;* eruption on the dorsal surface of the hands; *weakness in the abdominal extremities which is so great that they are unable to support the body; coldness of the knees and feet;* tension in the bends of the knees; cramps in the calves; sudden swelling around the ankles, in the evening.

[1] This singular symptom has been observed by Hahnemann. I have observed it in a virtuous young woman of 27 years, with an ardent temperament, against which she had to struggle. This poor girl had had for some weeks a red eruption on both arms, which was diminished, but not cured by Sepia. She experienced a sort of voluptuous pleasure in scratching her arms, which thence spread to the uterus and produced a real emission. Tin cured this patient completely in a short time.

The symptoms of tin show themselves principally in the morning and evening before midnight. Some of the pains to which this drug corresponds, return by paroxysms, increase slowly, and decrease in the same manner.

Pulsatilla is said to antidote tin, the same as it does sulphuric acid. The intimate relation existing between these two substances, seems sufficient to account for the fact that Pulsatilla antidotes both of them.

Mercurius corrosivus, *corrosive sublimate, deuto-chloride* or *bichloride of mercury.*—This salt which is formed of 79.09 parts of mercury, and 25.91 parts of chlorine, is white, transparent when recently prepared, opaque after it had been exposed to the air; of an astringent, biting and burning taste, soluble in water, and still more in alcohol. When heated in the open air, it spreads a whitish vapor in it which it is dangerous to inhale; when heated in a closed vessel, it suffers no change, volatilizes and crystallizes in the shape of needles on the sides of the vessel. It is obtained by the double decomposition of the deuto-sulphate of mercury and the chloride of sodium, taking care to add to the mixture a certain quantity of the binoxide of manganese, by which means the formation of calomel is prevented. It is one of our most violent poisons. The white of an egg dissolved in tepid water, is the best antidote to this agent.[1]

Empirical applications.—The corrosive sublimate was used as a drug as early as the tenth century, for it was known by Rhazes, Avicenna, and Gerber;[2] but it was only in the sixteenth century, that it was more generally used. Like other mercurial compounds, it was at first used externally only, either as a caustic or as a special modifying agent. As the latter, it formed the basis of a number of officinal prepara-

[1] Flour, or better still, fresh gluten, likewise decomposes corrosive sublimate. Rabbits, which are generally killed by five centigrammes of this poison, have taken without injury, seventy centigrammes, mixed with twelve or thirteen times their weight of dry pulverised gluten, (Mérat and de Lens, *dict. de mat. med.*, vol. IV., p. 355.)

[2] Gmelin, *App. Med.*, vol. II., p. 243.

tions, balms, pomatums, like the pomatum of Cortillo, Cirillo, etc., of aqueous or alcoholic solutions, which were used in general for *venereal or non-venereal ulcers, redness, spots, roughness and pustules in the face*, (Turquet de Mayerne,) *syphilitic ophthalmia* (Dussansay,) *venereal or phagedenic ulcerations of the nostrils, ozœna, and caries of the nasal bones* (M. Lange, Astruc, etc.,) *itch* (Rulandus,) *scald-head* (Zac. Lusitanus,) *scrofula, venereal tumors* (Hier. Rosello, Turquet de Mayerne, etc.,) *whitlow* (Pétiot,) *cancer*, especially *of the nose* or *lips*, and *more particularly the lower* (Dessault;) and lastly, for a large number of cutaneous affections, such as *lichen, impetigo, psoriasis*, etc. Next came the employment of corrosive sublimate in the shape of injections, in doses which were sometimes frightful, into the urethra or vagina, (generally for *gonorrhœa*) and even into the rectum (Fernand), which often gave rise to the most serious accidents.

The treatment of syphilis with embrocations, lotions, baths, sublimate injections, and with this poison administered even internally, constituted, so to say, as many individual methods, which were almost equally dangerous, but the origin of which belongs, with a few years' difference, to the same period. At the time when Matthiolus published his work on syphilis,[1] in the first half of the sixteenth century, the internal use of the corrosive sublimate had become pretty general.

Like other active drugs, the corrosive sublimate is scarcely ever prescribed by Allœopathic physicians, in any other than a compound form, so that it is almost impossible to tell what effect each of the ingredients which belongs to it, really exercises on the organism. Nevertheless, thanks to the *water of Van Swieten*,[2] and which, in reality, is a solution of the bichloride of mercury in distilled water, to which a little alcohol is added, and which drug had been long in use, the sublimate is still one of those drugs, the true therapeutic

[1] *Traite. de morbod gallico.* Venet. 1535.

[2] There are many receipts of this water, but the one which is most commonly used in France, is as follows: Sublimate, 40 centigrammes; distilled water, 450 grammes. (Codex.)

action of which can be most readily and positively ascertained from the records of the Old School. In the following diseases the sublimate has undoubtedly effected cures, prior to its as yet very limited use in homœopathic practice, and save, of course, the accidents which were caused by too massive doses.

1st. Venereal disease, in most of its primary or secondary forms, namely: *gonorrhœa, chancre in the urethra, at the glans or prepuce; buboes; red or copper-coloured spots on the skin; syphilitic scales, gommata, bone-pains; exostoses on the forehead, at the clavicle, elbow, femur; ulcerations of the nostrils, ozœna, caries of the nasal bones, palatine bone, inferior maxillary bone; ophthalmia; spots and ulcers of the cornea; cataract; amaurosis; deafness; asthma; spasmodic cough; hæmoptysis; phthisis; paralysis; various kinds of neuralgia and nervous diseases; epileptiform paroxysms.*[1]

2d. Non-venereal diseases: *obstinate ophthalmia,* (V. Mueller, D. Corillo, etc.,); *cataract,* (Vogler, Marke, etc.); *eruptions, pustules in the face,* (Fr. Gmelin);[2] *obstinate ulceration of the nostrils,* and *ozæna,* (Gmelin); *furfuraceous tetters,* (Ottmann); *dry itch,* (Stœrik); *humid tetters* of various kinds, (Ambr. Hosty, J. Cotton, etc.); *scrofula* and *fistulous, phagedenic ulcers,* especially at the lower extremities, (Gmelin);[3] *acute and chronic articular rheumatism, in*

[1] For facts and authorities, the reader is referred to: 1st. In the *appar. med.* by Gmelin, the excellent chapter on the sublimate, vol. II., from p. 243 to p. 313; 2d. Van Swieten, *descrip. abrég. des malad. qui règnent le plus souvent dans les armées,* etc. Paris, 1760, in 12mo.; 3d. by the same author: *Comm. in Herm. Boerhaavii aphorismos,* vol. V., p. 549, etc.; 4th. Swediaur, traité des maladies vénér. etc.

[2] A circumstance which, coupled with the indications which several authors, particularly Rapon, have furnished of merc. solubilis, has decided me to introduce the sublimate in the treatment of *variola,* which I have accordingly done.

[3] Here is the whole passage by Gmelin concerning scrofula, which it will be seen was well calculated to corroborate me in my opinion relatively to the almost *specific* nature of the corrosive sublimate in the treatment of variola: "Glandularum quoque tumores, etiam pertinaces, nisi inflammatorios, (De Horne,) ex alia longe causa natos, huic remedio obtemperare observavit B. Spielmann, (apud J. Fr. Ehrmann, l. c. p. 45,) in virgine, cui

consequence of a cold, and *gouty rheumatism, with swelling and deformation of the affected parts*;[1] *dry, obstinate cough*, and other symptoms of *tuberculous phthisis* in several children of from ten to fifteen years, of feeble constitutions;[2] lastly, *dropsy* and *paralysis*.[3]

In our time, Allœopathic physicians, many of whom, it must be admitted, do not even suspect, that the facts which I have mentioned, exist in the works of their school, scarcely employ the sublimate for any other purpose than to combat syphilis. According to them, the sublimate is, of all other mercurial preparations, (which they abuse so much,) that which is most certain in its results, and from which, salivation is least to be apprehended during the treatment. But if the sublimate has frequently cured syphilis, especially recent cases, in allœopathic doses, (and such cures cannot be denied,) how often has it, on the other hand, substituted pulmonary phthisis in the place of this latter malady.[4]

jam inde ab aliquot lustris glandulæ ab auribus usque ad claviculus sitæ induratæ intumuerant. Idem ille, œque ac Moseder, ejusdem auxilio puerum a scrophulis per omne corpus disseminatis liberavit; eamque efficaciam monstravit hic mercurius corrosivus, Ch. Hotzio (apud J. J. Zimmermann) in puero decenni post *variolas confluentes* scrophulis per totum corpus obsesso; plures ægros scrophulis affectos ejus ope sanavit Loyauté." (*Mém. de la Soc. roy. de méd. de Paris*, ann. 1777 and 1778, in 4to., etc.).

[1] See *Bibliot. Méd.*, vol. XXXIII., p. 117.

[2] See *Comment. de rebus in scient. natur. et med. gestis*, vol. XXVII., p. 92.

[3] *Bibliot. Méd.*, loc. cit.

[4] In corroboration of this fact, I will relate the following sad event. In the spring of 1837, a student at law, a friend of mine, was attacked with gonorrhœa, which was supposed to be syphilitic, and which was at first treated with *astringents*, and, these remaining fruitless, with the *pills of Dupuytren*, (opium and sublimate,) and lastly with the *water of Swieten*. At the end of two months the discharge stopped. But *at the same time* a *little dry cough* came on, which was accompanied at times with heat in the chest. Three months passed on in this way Vacation having come, my friend returned home. The cough continued, and had even become more frequent. In the first days of Sept. a slight hæmorrhage came on quite suddenly. A physician was called. My friend played on a wind-instrument, and had one of those fine bass-voices which are rarely ever possessed by persons attacked with congenital phthisis; he was ordered to quit music; but notwithstanding this rest of the respiratory organs, another hæmorrhage

Homœopathic applications.—Hahnemann's proving of corrosive sublimate is very scanty. Among the fifty symptoms which he has given us, fifteen belong to allœopathic observations, (A. Schwarz). Homœopathic physicians, who, like myself, have employed the sublimate outside of the limits of this short pathogenesis, are therefore obliged to admit, that they have used it empirically. Dr. Roth has recently published in his Materia Medica Pura, p. 526, a pathogenesis of this drug, containing five hundred and seventy-seven symptoms, which constitutes a most valuable contribution to our art, and for which I am personally obliged to him.

I must, nevertheless, remark, that this pathogenesis is still very incomplete, and that the reader will have to guard against its leading facts and the general features of the work, for these reasons.

Roth, finding that the number of symptoms obtained by pure experimentation, was so very small, has drawn largely from the works of Allœopathic toxicologists, such as Devergie, Orfila, Thénard, etc.[1] What is the consequence of this

set in, and he was bled: this was bad practice, (the patient was tall, slender, rather strong, but nervous and not by any means plethoric). Two more hæmorrhages within eight days; two more venesections. Horrible practice, an hectic fever set in, and on the 14th of September my friend died, victimised, I doubt not, by the sublimate, the poisonous effects of which were marvellously supported by his last physician.

[1] Roth might very easily have extended the list of his symptoms obtained from such sources. Here is, for example, a list which might be added to the next edition of his work, if he should think proper:

Constant anxiety of mind, (Fr. Hoffmann); vertigo, (Terras); symptoms of cerebral apoplexy, (Brambilla); loss of sight and hearing, (Ibid.); dryness of the mouth and tongue, (Loew); salivation, (Van Swieten); roughness in the throat, (Van Swieten); excessive thirst, (Loew); appearance of putrefaction of all the internal parts of the mouth, (Valleriola); nausea, deranged digestion, (Cirillo, Gardane); nausea, (Valler.); vomiting, (Colombier); violent vomiting, (Stoll, Wedel, etc.); vomiting of blood, (Stoll, Valer.); burning pain at the stomach, (Baccius); stitches at the stomach, (Valler.); horrible cutting pains in the stomach and belly, (Baccius, etc.); tenesmus, (Gardane, etc.); dysentery, (Stœrck); dropsy, (Lentin); obstinate leucorrhœa, (Gataker); miscarriage, (Brambilla); hoarseness, (Wedel); embarrassed breathing, (Terras); oppression on the chest, (Stoll); dry proceeding? Two-thirds of the symptoms related by Roth, are poisonous effects, which it is indeed useful and indispensable to be acquainted with, but which, after all, only represent very acute affections, and leave us ignorant concerning the chronic maladies to which this drug corresponds.

It is evidently owing to the fact, that we had no other knowledge of the sublimate than these general toxicological effects, even before they had been collated by Roth, that most homœopathic physicians have limited the employment of this poison to a very small number of diseases, among which, *dysentery* is undoubtedly one of the principal. This disease seems to be so inseparably connected with the sublimate that it has seemed to me that whenever I dared to propose the use of this drug in such disorders of the digestive canal as were not characterized by tenesmus and a flow of blood, my colleagues got fairly frightened. But who does not know, that whenever the sublimate is really indicated, as in *recent cases of syphilis*, and more particularly *among males*, a cure is frequently effected even by means of small allœopathic doses, without any dysenteric symptoms being developed? Of course, it has to be given under proper circumstances, otherwise, medicinal symptoms might follow. I will indicate in a few lines the general rules which experience has pointed out to me in this respect.

Corrosive sublimate is indicated in an immense majority of the cases which have been considered until now, as belonging to the sphere of soluble mercury; provided, that, with a few exceptions, CORROSIVE SUBLIMATE IS GIVEN EXCLUSIVELY IN DISEASES OF MALES, AND SOLUBLE MERCURY EXCLUSIVELY IN DISEASES OF FEMALES.[1] In observing this general principle,

cough, (Collin); violent cough, (Stœrck); spitting of blood, (Brambilla); hæmoptysis, (Stœrck, Richter, Quarin, Girtanner); slow fever, (De Horne); heat on the skin, (Gardane); sweat, (Colombier); fetid sweat, (Valleriola); cold sweat, (Wedel); clammy and cold sweat, (Stoll); hæmorrhages from the mucous membranes, (Stœrck); contraction of the extremities, (Quarin); involuntary and irregular movements of the extremities, (Id.); convulsions, (Fr. Hoffmann.)

[1] I give this as a *positive law.* It would be too long to narrate the circum-

the most beautiful results will frequently be obtained from the use of the sublimate in the following affections.

Syphilis (*chancre, gonorrhœa, buboes, ophthalmiæ, ulcerations of the cornea, cataract, amaurosis, ulcerations of the pharynx, nose, tongue*, etc., *red or copper-colored spots, pustules, impetigo, psoriasis, falling of the hair, sub-cutaneous tumors, exostosis, caries, falling off or deformation of the nails, hœmoptysis, phthisis, asthma, neuralgia, paralysis, chorea, epilepsy*, etc.); *variola* (in its natural form,)[1] some other *pustulous diseases, phlegmonous erysipelas*, in persons with *bad humors; the itch*, especially when communicated by domestic animals, such as dogs; *chronic cutaneous eruptions*, of a scaly form, a bright redness, and accompanied with a burning itching; *torpid ulcers*, with fringed borders, a grayish bottom, especially on the lower extremities; certain forms of *chronic ophthalmia*, with predominance or priority of the symptoms of the left eye; *epistaxis* in young persons of a lymphatic- sanguine temperament; *chronic ulcerations of the nostrils; fungous stomatitis and angina*, with extreme foulness of the mouth, swelling and ulceration of the gums, tongue and mucous membrane of the pharynx; *hæmatemesis*, with burning pain at the stomach; *dysentery, ascites* preceded by diarrhœa, accompanied by tenesmus and burning in the abdomen; *albuminuria, priapismus, hydrocele, induration of the testes, diabetes mellitus, seminal emissions without* erection in consequence of venereal excesses, especially of onanism; *impotence, hæmoptysis*, with a dry cough, violent dyspnœa, and burning heat in the chest; *acute articular rheumatism*, with burning thirst, frequent pulse, dry heat on the skin, or profuse and fetid sweat; *chronic articular rheumatism*, with

stances which have gradually led me to its discovery. I will mention however the following curious fact in reference to this subject:

Both the sublimate and the soluble mercury antidote sepia, which antidotes them in its turn, although imperfectly. But *this neutralisation of the sublimate by sepia, and vice versa, does not take place thoroughly except in the case of males, nor does the neutralisation of soluble mercury by sepia, and vice versa, take place thoroughly except in the case of females.*

[1] See *traité homœopathique des maladies des enfants*, p. 194.

soft or osseous tumors in the joints, false ankylosis, etc., in lymphatic subjects, after a cold, particularly at the elbows, wrists, hands, fingers, knees and feet; *gout*, where the skin is no longer red; *scrofulous caries*, *rickets*, and, in general, the chronic affections of the osseous system.

I am well aware that in most of the diseases which I have mentioned, cures have been effected with soluble mercury, *independently of the sex of the patient;* but I insist, nevertheless, that these cures would have been more speedy and striking, if the sublimate had been used instead of soluble mercury.[1]

Mercurius solubilis, *Sepia*, and *Lobelia inflata* are the principal antidotes of *Mercurius corrosivus.*

Nitri acidum; *nitric acid*, (*eau seconde*, in French, when diluted with water.) This acid, which it is impossible to render completely anhydrous, were it ever so much concentrated, is a colorless liquid, of a strong and disagreeable odor, excessively caustic, alterable by light, and, when concentrated, giving out a white vapor; boiling at 86°; and coloring organic matters yellow and destroying them. It was discovered by Raymond Lulle.

For the arts, this acid is obtained by the decomposition of the nitrate of potash by means of sulphuric acid. But before it can be used for medicinal purposes, it has to be purified, that is to say, freed from all traces of sulphuric and muriatic acid, with which it is frequently mixed. This is accomplished by treating it successively with small quantities of the nitrate of barytes and the nitrate of silver, and distilling it afterwards in a glass apparatus.

Empirical applications.—Nitric acid has but rarely been employed internally as a medicine. Surgeons used it formerly as a caustic, and some employ it as such even now, but without suspecting that its good effects, provided

[1] In some cases, however, and more particularly in the case of lymphatic boys, who have not yet attained the age of pubescence, *soluble mercury* may deserve a preference over the sublimate.

good luck helps them out, (as in the treatment of *warts, callous ulcers, dry caries* and *periostitis,*) are due to the absorption of this powerful agent. This is, however, so true, that Professor Lallemand, of Montpellier, has seen indolent periostitis speedily cured, and has cured it himself, by exciting a slight inflammation on the skin by means of nitric acid.

Fr. Hoffmann recommends nitric acid for *pernicious petechial fevers.*[1] Hull and Batemann, in England, have used it with success in *inveterate jaundice.*[2] "But, in France, it is especially Alyon," says Alibert, "who has proposed its internal use, and who has praised it as a *very powerful remedy for syphilis.* He relates a number of cases which show that this acid exercises a very powerful action on the vital forces, that it facilitates the urinary secretion, etc., and, that it combats with particular success old and *inveterate syphilitic diseases.*"[3] Several English physicians or surgeons, among others Scott, Beddoes, Geach, Hammick and Sandford, have confirmed Alyon's experience by authenticated facts. Even now a sort of lemonade is prepared of nitric acid in England and India, whose anti-syphilitic virtues are much commended. Wedekind recommends this acid for the mercurial and scorbutic foulness of the mouth. Pereira, of Bordeaux, assures us that he has used it with the best success in chronic leucorrhœa.[4]

Homœopathic applications.—Nitric acid seems to agree more particularly with individuals of a brownish complexion, a dry constitution, and especially with persons afflicted with chronic diseases, who are habitually troubled with soft stools. "It can scarcely ever be employed," says Hahnemann, "in the case of persons who are disposed to constipation." "*Chronic syphilis, ulcers, obstinate ophthalmia, general or partial atrophy, some forms of phthisis, neuralgia, chronic*

[1] Medic. ration. system., vol. IV., p. 270.

[2] See Journ. de Méd. de Leroux, vol. XVI., p. 447.

[3] Nouveaux élem. de thérapeut. etc., vol. I., p. 515.

[4] See the pathogenesis of this drug in Hahnemann's *Chronic Diseases*, vol. III.

rheumatism, diseases of the bones; and lastly, and perhaps principally, *the various affections caused by abuse of mercury;* these are the diseases for which this drug has been principally given.

According to Hahnemann, it has been used with success in the following affections:—

"Sadness, *peevish mood;* uneasiness concerning the result of one's sickness, with fear of death; excessive irritability; *quarrelsomeness* and caprice; aversion to work; vertigo when sitting or walking; vertigo which obliges one to lie down; sick headache; tearing pains in the forehead, vertex and occiput; throbbing headache; rush of blood to the head; itching of the hairy scalp; falling of the hair; paralysis of the upper eyelid; *pressure in the eyes; stitches in the eyes;* suppuration of the eyes; difficult dilatation of the pupils; *black points* which float before the eyes; stitches in the ear; swelling of the left lobule; discharge from the ear; stoppage of the ear; *hardness of hearing;* buzzing in the ears; *beating in the ear;* cracking in the ear; crusts in the right nostril; nose-bleed; disagreeable smell when breathing through the nose; *fetid smell* in the nose; pimples in the face; *pale face;* chapping of the lips; ulcerations of the vermilion border; looseness of the teeth; bleeding of the gums; heat in the throat; *smarting pain* in the throat; *bitter taste in the mouth,* even after a meal; sweetish taste in the mouth; thirst; aversion to meat; inability to digest milk; nausea after eating fat; sweat during and after a meal; sense of fulness in the stomach after eating; lassitude after dinner; acid eructations; desire to vomit; starts after drinking rapidly; stitches in the pit of the stomach; tensive pain under the false ribs; frequent pinching in the abdomen; cutting colic; stitches in the abdomen when touching it; smarting pain in the hypogastrium; swelling of the inguinal glands; inguinal hernia of children; *accumulation of wind in the belly; emission of wind* morning and evening; gurgling in the abdomen; borborygmi; *constipation;* desire to go to stool; irregular and difficult stool; *too frequent stool;*

dry stool; itching of the anus; *old piles;* difficult emission of urine; *incontinence of urine; fetid smell of the urine;* excoriation at the gland; *sycosis;* relaxation of the scrotum; want of sexual desire; want of erections; frequent nocturnal emissions; leucorrhœa.

"Suppressed sneezing; *stoppage of the nostrils;* dryness of the nose; coryza; dry stoppage of the nose; hoarseness; laryngeal phthisis; cough in the day-time; cough in the evening, after lying down; cough causing one to vomit; *asthma;* cough in working; nodous induration of the breast; atrophy of the breasts; pain in the kidneys; pain in the back; *stiff neck;* swelling of the cervical glands; stitches in the shoulders; pressive pain at the arm joint; roughness of the skin on the hands; *syphilitic tetters in the palms of the hands;* numbness of the fingers; white spots on the finger nails; itching at the thighs; *uneasiness in the legs*, in the evening; *coldness of the legs; pain in the thighs*, on rising from a chair; weak knees; *cramps* and *stiffness in the calves in walking*, after having been seated; twitching in the calves; stitches in the heel, on pressing the foot to the ground; fetid sweat of the feet; *tearing pains in the upper and lower extremities; liability to taking cold*, whence come pinching and cutting pains in the abdomen; pain in former cicatrices, during a change in the weather; acne punctata; tingling and numbness of the ends of the fingers, even when the weather is only moderately cold; itching eruption like urticaria, in the open air, even in the face; *brownish-red spots on the skin; warts;* pain in the corns and chilblains; weakness, weariness in the morning; lassitude so as to tremble; chronic lassitude and heaviness of the feet; difficulty of waking in the morning: frequent waking; restlessness in the night; waking with a start; sleep full of dreams; disturbing dreams; lascivious dreams; pains during sleep; *constant coldness;* fever, in the afternoon, coldness and heat; dry skin; night-sweat; fetid night-sweat.[1]

[1] *Chronic Diseases, loc. cit.*

The known antidotes of nitric acid are *Camph. Merc. corr.* and *Calc. carb.*

Crocus sativus. *Crocus autumnalis* of Linné; in Arab 'Zahafaran, whence safran in French, in English, saffron. Genus Crocus, family Irideæ, Class triandria monogynia.

This plant, which originally comes from the East, as its name indicates, is now cultivated in the gardens, in various parts of France. Its flower, which has the general appearance of those of all other flowers of this family, differs from them in this, that the stigma alone is odoriferous; it is these stigmata which are exclusively gathered and sold in commerce under the name of saffron.

This substance, which, in our time, is employed much more for domestic than for medicinal purposes, was very much respected by the old Greek physicians. Hippocrates recommends it in various parts of his writings, and the mountain Tmolus, in Phrygia, on whose slopes, the plant which furnishes the saffron, was cultivated, owed it a real celebrity.

As it grows old, the saffron loses its odor and appears altered; but when fresh, its emanations are said to be dangerous. "They go to the head," say Mérat and de Lens, "and it is said that persons who had exposed themselves to them, have fallen into a sort of soporous fever. Borelli, Lacoste, Koenig, Lusitanus, have seen similar effects, which even resulted in death in some persons; in other cases these emanations have caused convulsions, immoderate and sardonic laughter, etc."[1] These paroxysms of immoderate laughter, seem, indeed, to constitute one of the characteristic effects of saffron. Murray, from whom Mérat and de Lens have taken the preceding observations, relates other facts of the same kind, on the authority of Sérapion, Boerhaave, Schulz, etc.: for instance, the case of several children who were seized with an extraordinary laughing mania, from having smelled of leather bottles that had contained essence of saffron.[2]

[1] Œuv. citat., vol. II., p. 466.

[2] *Appar. Méd.*, vol. V., p. 232.

Bergius mentions a fact which goes to contradict the last-mentioned, and which completes, on this account, the series of moral effects produced by saffron. He speaks of a woman, who, whenever she took a dose of saffron, was plunged into a deep sadness.[1]

Lastly, an English physician, Alexander, who made some trials with saffron, says, that it acts without increasing the heat of the skin, and that it causes a marked depression of the pulse.

Empirical applications.—"Externally," say Mérat and de Lens, "saffron is a good resolvent; it is mixed in cataplasms to scatter *indolent tumors, ecchymoses;* it is added to anti-ophthalmic collyria, in cases of scrofulous engorgement of *the eyelids, etc.*"[3]

Internally, saffron has been used as an *antispasmodic*, for *hysteria, hypochondria,* (with a view of cheering up the patients,) for *spasms, whooping-cough, asthma,* etc. Pringle praises it as an *antiseptic*, and recommends it as such in *putrid diseases.*[4] But it is especially as an *emmenagogue*, that it has been used and abused, as is well known; witness an unfortunate woman mentioned by Rivière, who, for having taken too large a dose with a view of bringing back her courses which had been suppressed for some months, died three days after of uterine hæmorrhage.[5]

Homœopathic applications.—Abandoned almost entirely by modern allœopathy, saffron has not yet, by any means, recovered in the hands of the Homœopathic physicians, the therapeutic importance which it enjoyed in olden times, and which Cullen explicitly denies it possesses.[6] Nevertheless, it

[1] Mat. Med. e regn. vegetab. etc., vol. I., p. 58.

[2] Alexander's *experimental essays on antiseptics*, etc., p. 88.

[3] Œuv. Cit., vol. II., p. 470.

[4] Pringle, *observations sur les maladies des armeés*, etc., 2d ed., Paris, 1793, p. 24, etc.

[5] Riverii, oper. med., edit., Horstius, p. 136.

[6] According to Geoffroy, (Mat. Med., vol. III., p. 46,) the ancients venerated saffron so much that they called it *the king of vegetables, vegetable panacea, soul of the lungs*, etc. Cullen, on the contrary, who, doubtless,

has rendered some service to Homœopathic physicians, and a large number of its symptoms (see the pathogenesis of Crocus in Roth's Materia Medica pura, vol. II., p. 80,) disposes me to believe, that no remedy can replace it in many diseases of the sexual apparatus. In an actress, I have seen saffron cure speedily a *bloody leucorrhœa* of several months' standing, which the patient thought was of a syphilitic nature, although mercury had been used in various forms, but without success. But it is especially in *active hæmorrhages*, and more particularly in *metrorrhagia* and certain forms of *hysteria*, (accompanied with mental derangement, violent outbreaks of passion without any adequate cause, excessive mirth, foolish laughter, etc.,) that saffron had been employed. I am convinced that it will prove very useful in some cases of *nervous or false pregnancy*, for no other drug represents more completely the symptoms of this strange disease.

Be this as it may, I have placed saffron at the end of the analogies of mercury, with an interrogation point. Indeed, the relations existing between saffron and mercurius, are not, by any means, sufficiently striking and convincing. Nevertheless, it would not be difficult to show that these relations exist. The future will undoubtedly shed light on this point, as on many others.

Stapf regards opium as the antidote of saffron.

had only used old or falsified saffron, considered it almost an inert substance. (See his Mat. Med. translated by Bosquillon, Paris, 1790, vol. II., p. 332.)

GROUP III.

TYPE: SULPHUR.

ANALOGUES: CROTON TIGLIUM. LOBELIA INFLATA. MERCURIUS CORROSIVUS. MERCURIUS SOLUBILIS. BOVISTA. ASTERIAS. ÆTHUSA CYNAPIUM. CICUTA VIROSA. KREASOTA. RATANIA.[1]

COMMON CHARACTERISTICS.

THE arranging this group has been with me an object of particular investigations and long meditations. In order to apprehend the distinguishing features of this group, we have to lose sight, as it were, of a number of symptoms which belong to the drugs composing it, symptoms that have already been mentioned in the preceding groups; for the purpose of dwelling only upon such symptoms of the same drugs as assimilate them to their new type. It matters little to us, whether the corrosive sublimate, soluble mercury and kreasot are anti-syphilitic, whilst sulphur is not, and produce both in the healthy and sick man, effects, which would in vain be looked for in the pathogenesis of sulphur. It is sufficient for our present purpose that they should be anti-psoric like sulphur, or that they should, at any rate, have the largest number of its characteristic symptoms, (shades being of course excepted,) in order to become *analogues* of sulphur.

It is evident that the same observation is applicable to *Croton tiglium.*

Be it then well understood, that my enumeration of the characteristic symptoms which belong to the drugs of the sulphur group in common, leaves out, for the present, all

[1] I am strongly inclined to think that *Ammonium carbonicum* and *Ammonium muriaticum* will hereafter have to be added to the analogues of sulphur. (See, for these two drugs, Hahnemann's Chronic Diseases, vol. III.)

such symptoms as are not, strictly speaking, characteristic of sulphur, and which may, on this account, be classed among other groups.[1]

1st. *A sort of momentary tension of the tissues, (especially the skin and mucous membrane,) which is almost immediately after succeeded by a contrary phenomenon, whence comes—*

a. Weakness of body and mind;

b. Sickly and flaccid skin, of an altered, earthy color;

c. Sweat on making the least effort;

d. Mucous discharges of various kinds, (sub-acute catarrhs.)

2d. *Slow fever, which shows itself principally in the afternoon, and increases in the evening.*

3d. *Congestion of blood to the head, with flashes of heat in the face.*

4th. *Persistent cutaneous affections, resembling the itch more or less, and exhibiting an analogy with a certain number of cutaneous diseases, the retrocession of which, as will be seen hereafter, gives rise to internal maladies which, to judge from their outward signs, correspond to the most marked internal effects of the drugs belonging to the present group, namely:*

a. Sub-acute ophthalmias;

b. Pulmonary catarrhs;

c. Asthmatic affections;

d. Constipation, or permanent discharges of small diarrhœic stools, or alternate diarrhœa and constipation;

e. Piles;

f. Amenorrhœa or dysmenorrhœa, with chlorotic discoloration of the blood;

g. Various kinds of nervous affections;

h. Mental derangement.

A few negative features which are observable in the drugs belonging to the sulphur group, (except the anti-syphilitics,) have also a somewhat important meaning. Thus, all these

[1] All the drugs belonging to the Sulphur-group, cause: *vertigo or various kinds of pain*, or, finally, *suffocation in going up stairs.*

drugs, which act so powerfully upon the skin and the mucous membranes, but principally upon the skin—it is here that their *primary* effect takes place—seem to me to affect but very feebly the muscular apparatus and the osseous system.

Some of my readers may wonder at not finding among the sulphur group some drugs that likewise have a marked action on the skin. What has induced me to exclude them from the group of the anti-psorics is, first, that the cutaneous diseases which they occasion, are either secondary effects, or secondly, that these diseases are no more related to psora than the symptoms of these drugs are related to those of sulphur. I should have deemed it a mistake to rank *Conium maculatum* after *Æthusa* and *Cicuta virosa*, among the analogues of *Sulphur*. The action of *Conium*, which is the type of a group, although it has a great many points in common with the action of the plants of the same family, differs essentially from the action of the anti-psorics.

I will endeavor to explain myself a little more clearly by a rapid, but sufficiently thorough review of the great doctrine of psora.

"The acute and chronic diseases," says Hahnemann, "which arise from the suppression of the cutaneous symptoms, the eruption and itching, the presence of which upon the skin hushes the internal psora which is replaced by the cutaneous symptoms,—a suppression which is falsely termed *the retrocession of the itch into the interior body—are innumerable*, that is to say, as varied as the individual constitutions and the external circumstances which act upon them."

"Junker has given a succinct sketch of the pernicious consequences of repelled itch;[1] he has seen this repelled itch produce pulmonary phthisis among young and sanguine persons; among sanguine individuals, in general, hæmorrhoids, hæmorrhoidal colic and renal calculus; among individuals of a sanguine and bilious temperament, swellings of the mammary glands, stiffness of the joints and ulcers of

[1] Lud. Christ. Junker's dissert. *de damno ex scabie repulsa.* Halle, 1750.

a bad character; among stout persons, suffocative catarrh and mucous phthisis. He has likewise seen it giving rise to inflammatory fever, acute phthisis and peripneumonia. A post-mortem examination showed the lungs full of indurations and collections of pus. Indurations of another kind, osseous swellings, and ulcers, were likewise noticed by him as arising from suppressed itch. He adds, that, among phlegmatic persons, it principally causes dropsy; that the menses are delayed by such a suppression, and that, if the suppression takes place during the menstrual period, this discharge is replaced by a monthly cough, with discharge of blood from the lungs; that it sometimes drives persons who are predisposed to melancholy, to dementia, and that, if women should become pregnant at such a period, the child generally dies before it is born, that the suppression of the itch sometimes causes sterility; that, in general, it stops the secretion of milk in nurses, that it hastens the period when the menses cease to flow, and that, in women of a more advanced age, the womb goes into a state of suppuration amidst deep-seated and burning pains, which characterize this marasmus, (cancer of the womb)."[1]

Having thus declared in a manner which is rather too positive, as will be seen bye and bye; that the *acute* or *chronic* diseases resulting *from the retrocession of psora*, are innumerable, a declaration which is seconded by the observations of Junker, Hahnemann proceeds to develope his favorite notion, to wit, that *psora* comprises nine-tenths of all non-venereal chronic diseases. To prove the truth of this assertion, it strikes me, that the only reliable means was to show, that the itch had indeed been seen transformed into this number of chronic non-venereal affections. Well authenticated facts in this respect became peremptory and irrefutable arguments, which every body had to accept; but, on the other hand, I maintain that, in this matter, a single step beyond the domain of facts, must necessarily lead into the

[1] Hahnemann's *Chronic Diseases*, vol. I.

regions of fiction: let us see, therefore, whether Hahnemann has remained scrupulously true to actual observation.

It is well known, that the knowledge which this great man possessed, was immense; his memory was prodigious. He had retained in it, all that he had read, and his book-knowledge was so extensive, that all we can do after him, is to pick up a little crumb of knowledge here and there. His sketch of psoric retrocessions, and of the diseases which have resulted from them, may be called a monument of erudition. The simple enumeration of these diseases, with the authorities, forms no less than nineteen pages of the *Chronic Diseases*. These previous data show that it is absurd to consider psora, scald-head and tetters, as many Allœopathic physicians do, as affections essentially limited to the skin, and which may, without inconvenience to the general health, be treated with external means exclusively. But do they likewise show that the itch and scald-head, are solely, as Hahnemann asserts, the reflex of essentially internal and constitutional maladies? Do they likewise show that these maladies, of which the cutaneous eruption is supposed to be the outward vicarious sign, are really *innumerable*, and constitute *nine-tenths* of all chronic diseases? This is what I cannot admit.

Here follows, according to Hahnemann, a list of all the maladies which the repulsion of the itch has caused, and the names of which Hahnemann has drawn from upwards of two hundred authors.

1. Asthma.
2. Suffocative Catarrh.
3. Asthmatic oppressions.
4. Asthma, with general bloating.
5. Asthma and Dropsy.
6. Pleurisy and inflammation of the chest.
7. Stitch in the side, with cough.
8. Violent cough.
9. Spitting of blood.
10. Spitting of blood, and pulmonary phthisis.
11. Collections of pus in the chest.
12. Collections of pus in the mesentery.
13. Considerable ulcerations of several viscera.[1]
14. Alterations of the brain.
15. Hydrocephalus.
16. Ulceration of the stomach.

[1] This is very vague.

17. Sphacelus of the stomach and duodenum.
18. General œdema.
19. Ascites.
20. Hydrocele.
21. Red swelling of the whole body.
22. Jaundice.
23. Swelling of the parotid glands.
24. Swelling of the cervical glands.
25. Obscuration of sight, and presbyopia.
26. Ophthalmia.
27. Cataract.
28. Amaurosis.
29. Deafness.
30. Piles.
31. Affections of the abdomen.
32. Diabetes.
33. Retention of urine.
34. Erysipelas.
35. Acrid, ichorous discharges.
36. Ulcers.
37. Caries.
38. Osseous tumour at the knee.
39. Bone-pains.
40. Rickets of children.
41. Fever.
42. Tertian fever.
43. Quartan fever.
44. Vertigo, with complete loss of strength.
45. Epileptiform vertigo.
46. Convulsions.
47. Convulsions and Epilepsy.
48. Apoplexy.
49. Paralysis.
50. Melancholy.
51. Mental derangement.

To these fifty-one morbid conditions let us add those mentioned by Junker, namely, renal calculus, menstrual suppressions, suppression of the lochia, of the milk of nursing females, and even ulceration (cancerous?) of the womb in women of an advanced age, and we arrive at the following result: that, according to the united observations of upwards of two hundred physicians, most of whom were attached to hospitals, had a most extensive practice, and had enjoyed a vast range of observation for a long number of years, we can nevertheless legitimately attribute to *internal psora* only fifty-six different forms of disease; doubtless a large number, but not, by any means, including nine-tenths of all chronic diseases.

Among the diseases, or rather symptoms which Hahnemann enumerates as consequences of repelled itch, we do not find, for instance, *gout*, *cancer of the breasts*, *melanus*, *encephaloid tumors*, etc., etc., for this reason, that, in reality, the itch does no more change to *gout*, *cancer*, etc., than to *syphilis* or *variola*. Hahnemann has, therefore, gone too far.

But this is not all. In order to appreciate correctly the observations upon which the founder of homœopathy bases his theory of psora, it is not sufficient to mention facts; they have to be counted; for it must not be supposed that the pathological changes which have been attributed to repelled itch, have taken place uniformly in equivalent proportions. I am fully aware that numbers do not, as a general rule, deserve much confidence in medicine; nevertheless, there are cases where they are all-important. I confess that, as far as I am concerned, I feel obliged to attach a very great interest to the number of the cases which are attributed to the retrocession of the itch.

I admit with Hahnemann, (for facts cannot be denied,) that the internal psora, varying in form according to the age, sex, temperament, constitution, or idiosyncrasy of the patient, may have manifested itself under each of the above-mentioned forms, and that there may even be other unknown forms of disease belonging to the same category; but all this does not, by any means, show that these various known and unknown psoric manifestations constitute indiscriminately, and in the same degree, the *pathognomonic signs* of this obscure disease.

The determination of these pathognomonic signs, (provided they exist,) is, however, of the utmost importance, for, without it, the internal psora remains a thing of fiction. Some whose imagination has been carried away by the psora-phantom, see it all over, even where it does not exist in reality; others, on the contrary, overlook it where it really exists, and deny its existence, for the simple reason, that they cannot believe that one and the same disease can manifest itself in a hundred different forms. Let us see whether the frequency and regular recurrence of some of the phenomena which are said to be caused by repelled itch, do not entitle them to occupy the rank of the characteristic phenomena of psora. To this end let us count the facts, for, in such a business, numbers shed a real light on the question at issue.

Only one observer (Unger) has seen the retrocession of the itch followed by *erysipelas*.

Another observer, only one (Richter) has seen it cause *caries.*

In ONE CASE ONLY, it caused *cataract;* in ONE OTHER CASE, *jaundice;* in ONE CASE ONLY, *rickets;* and in ONE OTHER CASE, *bone-pains.* Now do such isolated facts deserve unlimited credence? Was the cutaneous eruption, the repulsion of which is supposed to have been followed by these diseases, really and truly the itch?[1]

We will admit, however, (because we cannot prove the contrary,) that *cataract, jaundice, rickets, caries* and *bone-pains,* may, strictly speaking, be considered as signs of the internal psora. The same will prove true with regard to *hydrocephalus, general œdema, redness of the whole body, swelling of the cervical glands, retention of urine, hydrocele, purulent collections in the mesentery, sphacelus of the stomach* and *rickets,* all which diseases have been seen once only, and sometimes twice follow the retrocession of the itch. But these are certainly not the pathognomonic signs of psora. Pursuing our statistical review, we find that the other

[1] Heaven knows what is often called itch by ancient authors, as the following case may show, to which I could easily add an hundred more: "A young woman, who was in her seventh month of pregnancy, consulted me on account of an *itch* that caused her a good deal of itching and sleepless nights, without any other trouble. I advised her to be bled, to use some cooling beverages, and to await her confinement patiently, etc. The itch resisted all these means of treatment, and the patient, anxious to get rid of her eruption, rubbed herself, by the advice of a woman, with an ointment which is kept ready-made in the shops for the purpose of driving away the itch. The itch disappeared in a few days; but in its place a hard and painful tumor, of the size of a walnut, showed itself between the labia majora, above the meatus urinarius. Consulted a second time by this lady, I had no doubt that her itch was a syphilitic disease which she had caught from her husband. I talked to him, he told me all his former adventures, and asked me to do for his wife's health all that I could possibly do," etc. (Dominique Raymond, *traité des maladies qu'il est dangereux de guérir,* p. 76.) Raymond treated his patient with mercury, and she recovered. Now, I ask any honest reader that, if Raymond had seen the repulsion of this syphilitic disease followed by *bone-pains* or *caries,* would he not have given out these diseases as consequences of repelled itch? And such an error would have been for Hahnemann an additional symptom of internal psora.

diseases have been observed the following number of times:—

Three	observers	have noticed	deafness;
Three	"	"	diabetes;
Four	"	"	amaurosis;
Five	"	"	cerebral affections;
Six	"	"	pulmonary phthisis;
Seven	"	"	paralysis;
Seven	"	"	mental derangement;
Seven	"	"	tertian fever;
Eight	"	"	convulsions;
Nine	"	"	pleuro-pneumonia;
Twelve	"	"	piles;
Nineteen	"	"	epilepsy;
Thirty-one	"	"	febris continua;
Thirty-nine	"	"	asthma, or suffocative catarrh.

This list shows that the last-named diseases constitute the most frequent manifestations of internal psora. But can it be said that these manifestations constitute its pathognomonic signs? Alas! no, for it is but too well-known that *phthisis*, *paralysis*, *epilepsy*, *piles*, *febris continua*, and *suffocative catarrh*, can exist independently of psora.

Nevertheless, it is self-evident that, if any of these diseases should manifest itself without being traceable to any particular cause, internal psora may be supposed to be the latent principle of the disease. If we consider the vague and conjectural character of the etiology of most chronic affections, it must be confessed that the supposition of an internal psora is not, by any means, without importance. In all obscure cases, it will, therefore, be advisable to have recourse to the *antipsorics*. But to which of them? To the one which is indicated by the similarity of the symptoms. This choice will sometimes seem difficult; for it is with psora as with syphilis: supposing even, (perhaps without any just cause,) that in its origin psora is *one*, it has, nevertheless, its symptomatic shades, and these shades which are already so little marked while the disease still exists on the skin, are still much more uncertain in the internal disease.

Before speaking of sulphur and its analogues, I have to point out a fact which results from the statistical review I have instituted.

If the symptoms of the drugs which constitute my group of *antipsorics*, are treated in the same manner as the symptoms of the *psoric diseases*, we obtain the following curious results:—

1st. The cutaneous symptoms of these drugs, not only correspond to the different varieties of the itch, but their most constant and truly characteristic symptoms, correspond precisely to the morbid conditions which have most frequently been developed by a retrocession of the cutaneous diseases;[1] 2d, the rare and, so to say, exceptional effects of sulphur and its analogues, corresponds to the rare and exceptional manifestations of the internal psora.

Sulphur. Simple, combustible body, or, at any rate, which has never yet been decomposed, (it is supposed to contain hydrogen,) solid, of a lemon color, insipid and inodorous, becoming electric by friction, fusible at 108° F., and crystallizing, when cooling, in the shape of semi-transparent needles. Sulphur is insoluble in water, but slightly soluble in alcohol; so that, from the first upwards, all its dilutions can be made with alcohol. This metalloid which exists extensively in nature, where it is found in its native state, in the neighborhood of volcanoes, in amorphous masses, or in the form of crystals; or in combination with hydrogen, and various metallic oxydes, (sulphurets,) or in combination with oxygen and oxydes, (sulphates,) is moreover, a constituent element of various organic substances, especially of the plants com-

[1] Is it not undeniably true that *ulcers on the skin*, *subacute ophthalmia*, *piles*, *rush of blood to the brain*, with all its consequences, (*apoplexy*, *deafness*, *paralysis of the extremities*, *epileptic vertigo*, etc.,) *febris continua*, and lastly, and more particularly, *suffocative catarrh*, *cough*, and, in general, the *mucous affections of the air-passages*, constitute, together with the *psoriform eruption*, the leading and characteristic features of the pathogenesis of *sulphur*, *lobelia inflata*, etc.?

posing the family of the Cruciferæ, of which, Baumé, Deyeux, Planche, etc., regard it as an active principle.[1]

Although sulphur acts with much less intensity than arsenic, corrosive sublimate and other poisons, it may, nevertheless, when taken in large doses, occasion death. This results beyond a doubt from Benk's experiments on dogs and cats. The following symptoms preceded death in the case of these animals: anorexia, thirst, vomiting, (only in cats,) diarrhœa; increase, followed by decrease, of the temperature of the skin; acceleration, followed by increased slowness, of the pulse; difficult breathing, marked emaciation; feebleness of the motions, prostration, slight trembling; lastly, drowsiness and convulsions. After death, all the internal organs, except the heart and bowels, were found to be remarkably pale.[2]

Sulphur seems to affect with equal intensity the carnivorous and herbivorous animals. A pound of sulphur has caused the death of a horse.[3]

The most serious accidents, death even, have befallen man, in consequence of abusing sulphur. Morgagni, for instance, relates the case of an individual, who had lost his reason, in consequence of the continued use of this drug;[4] and Olmsted, relates a case, where the continued use of large doses of sulphur, had caused a general emaciation with paralysis, ankylosis, contraction and deformity of the extremities.[5]

Empirical applications.—"Sulphur seems to have been used in veterinary medicine, previous to being employed as a remedy for the diseases of man, against which it is now used as one of the most powerful auxiliaries of the medical art.[6] From the earliest ages it has been employed as a disinfecting agent,[7] a prophylactic,[8] and in the burnt-offerings of the

[1] *Journal de Pharmac.*, vol. VIII., p. 367.

[2] *Dissert. syst. experim. de penetrat. sulph. in corpus vivum.* Tubing. 1813.

[3] *Journ. de Médec.*, de Leroux, vol. XXI., p. 70.

[4] *De sedib. et caus.*, etc., LV., c. 9.

[5] *Bullet. des sc. méd.*, Fér., vol. VII., p. 159.

[6] Mérat et Delens, op. cit., vol. VI., p. 451.

[7] Sulphurous acid could alone have been employed as a disinfecting agent.

[8] In what diseases?

ancients." Scarcely mentioned in the works of Hippocrates, it is recommended by *Dioscorides*[1] in *diseases of the chest*, against which it was employed by Plinius and Galenus, both internally and externally. Over-rated and under-rated with a like exaggeration, it has ever since remained in the Materia Medica, where its place has, however, remained very uncertain. It was successfully employed as a *sudorific*, a *tonic*, a *stimulant*, a *dissolvent*, a *deobstruent*, an *expectorant*, and a *purgative*. In the Materia Medica's of our day, sulphur remains placed among the *excitants*,[2] probably until further order.

Be this as it may, in a certain number of diseases the efficacy of sulphur was, if not generally recognized, at least established as a fact by a great many physicians, whose names are regarded as authorities. These diseases are the following:—Some acute exanthemata, particularly *measles*, of which sulphur, according to the authority of Tortual, Muhrbeck, and Hufeland, is the prophylactic;[3] *anasarca following acute exanthemata;*[4] *furfuraceous herpes*, favus, the itch;[5] *mercurial salivation*, *gastric derangement*, *colic*, *dysentery*, *intestinal worms*, *piles*, *abdominal engorgements*, *ascites;*[6] *leucorrhœa* and *amenorrhœa; cough*, *asthma*, *pulmonary phthisis;*[7] *chronic rheumatism*, *gout*, *scrofula*, *rickets*, some *forms of intermittent fever* coming on after *suppressed sweat*,[8] etc.

[1] Lib. IV., c. 73.

[2] See *traité de thérap.*, by Trousseau and Pidoux, vol. II., p. 619.

[3] Giacomini, *trait. des mat. méd.*, etc., p. 314.

[4] *Idem*, *Ibid.*

[5] "In these affections," says Giacomini, "and particularly in the itch, sulphur is, according to the opinion of all physicians, a sovereign remedy. Nobody will deny that sulphur holds this rank in the treatment of the itch." (Loc. Cit.)

[6] See *Bibliot. germ.*, vol. I., p. 93. *Nouv. bibliot. méd.*, vol. I., p. 193. *Bullet. thérap.*, 15th of Oct. 1833. J. T. Gmelin, *App. Med.*, vol. I., p. 198, etc.

[7] J. Hennius, Cardiluccius, T. Willis, F. Hoffmann, etc., cited by Gmelin, *App. Med.*, p. 1160.

[8] Mérat and Delens, *loc. cit.*

F. Hoffmann, Junker, and Rosenstein, have made this judicious remark, that sulphur not only cures the itch, but that it likewise removes the diseases occasioned by the repulsion of this disease. Hahnemann never went any farther.

Cullen, who, according to all appearances, was a great sceptic in some respects, "regards the properties which are attributed to sulphur as very uncertain;" a doctrine which seems to have revolted Alibert, who writes: "I use this drug too often and with too much success to admit the assertion of this author."[1]

Homœopathic applications.[2]—There is scarcely a disease for which sulphur has not been recommended. According to Hahnemann, it has been particularly useful in the following affections:—

Irritability; ill-humor with depression of spirits; timidity; tendency to start; tendency to weep; disconsolate in regard to every thing he does, that does not seem right to him; fixed religious ideas; *paroxysms of anxiety;* anxiety that compels him to unbutton his clothes and to go into the open air; irascible mood; *headache* and difficulty of collecting his thoughts; weak memory; frequent turns of vertigo; vertigo when sitting; heaviness of the head when stooping; vertigo on leaving the table; rush of blood to the head, with flashes of heat; headache at night; heaviness at the occiput; pulling headache as if the head would burst, every day; shooting headache; throbbing headache at the sinciput; tingling and noise in the head; cold in the head; cold spot on the head; closing of the eyelids in the morning; presbyopia; gauze before the eyes; *myopia;* pulling pain in the ears; stoppage of the ears when eating; *hard hearing;* noise in the ears; *buzzing in the ears;* dryness of the nose; stoppage of one nostril; inflammatory swelling of the tip of the nose; *discharge of blood from the nose when blowing it; nose-bleed;* pale sickly complexion; wrinkled skin of the face; heat in the face; hepatic spots on the upper lip; toothache

[1] *Nouv. élém. de thérap.*, vol. II., p. 325.

[2] Hahnemann's *chronic diseases*, vol. III.

in the evening; denudation of the teeth; swelling of the gums, with throbbing pain; sore throat, which impedes swallowing; insipid taste of the food; ravenous appetite; foul taste in the mouth, in the morning; sour taste in the mouth; aversion to fat, sweet and sour things; *canine hunger;* oppression of the chest after eating; acids, burning eructations; bitter eructations; badly-smelling eructations, at night, during sleep; regurgitation of the food and drinks; malaise before a meal; *nausea after eating;* nausea in the morning; constrictive, contractive gastralgia immediately after eating; digging at the pit of the stomach; stitch at the stomach; stitches in the left side of the abdomen, when walking; stitches in the abdomen; tearing pains in the left side of the abdomen; constrictive pain under the umbilicus; chronic pressure at the upper part of the abdomen; pressive pain in the left side of the abdomen, which extorts a cry from him, with constipation; bellyache, after drinking; the hypogastrium is painful to the touch; painfulness, in the morning, of the muscles of the abdomen, as if too short; shifting of flatulence, borborygmi; hard stool; stool every two or three days only; involuntary evacuation of fæces while urinating; falling of the rectum while straining at stool, during a difficult passage; stitches at the anus when going to stool; wetting the bed, at night; *itching at the anus;* little sexual power; *too sudden ejaculation during an embrace;* fetid sweat at the genital organs; itching and heat at the vulva; premature menses; discoloration of the menstrual blood; pressure on the genitals; itching at the vulva before the menses; headache before the menses; leucorrhœa; coryza; stoppage of the nose, roughness of the larynx; titillation in the larynx, which excites a cough; cough in the night; constant cough with fever; *blood spitting* and stitches in the side; difficulty of breathing; asthma, with wheezing and rattling in the chest, and beating of the heart; paroxysm of suffocation at night; fulness in the chest, heaviness in the chest, in the morning; weariness in the chest, from singing; stitches in the sternum; stitches through the chest, to the left shoulder-blade; heat in the chest; pressure in the sternum; itching at the nipples; pain in the loins; cracking in the sternum; pain in the back after manual labor; *pulling in the back;* tension in the nape of the neck; twitching in the arm, wrist, and finger-joints; swelling of the arms; *sweat in the palm of the hands;* trembling of the hands in executing fine work; *numbness of a few fingers;* tingling at the end of the fingers and toes; red spots on the legs, stitches in the thighs, when walking rapidly; *heaviness of the legs;* coldness about the thighs, with sweat on the legs, in the morning, in bed; weakness in the knees and arms; tingling in the calves and arms; pain in the tarsal joint, as if luxated; stiffness of the tarsal joint; sweat on the feet, uneasiness in the feet; erysipelas on the leg; *cold feet;* coldness and stiffness of the big toes; cold hands and feet; blisters on the big toes; chilblains on the feet; shocks in the extremities when sitting or lying; pains in the knee and other joints; urticaria; itching all over; *yellow spots on the body;* ecchymoses after a slight blow; sensitiveness to the air and wind; flashes of heat; numbness of the extremities, shooting pains; internal tremor; muscular twitchings; tendency to spraining joints; syncope and spasms; stooping when walking; *drowsiness in the day time;* too long night-sleep; unrefreshing sleep; desire to sleep after dinner; colic at night; *starting during sleep*, also with the whole body; sleeplessness; very light sleep; sleeplessness at night, on account of tingling in the calves and feet; *disturbing dreams;* frightful dreams, talking during sleep; hallucinations in the morning, on waking; thirst in the night; sweat day and night; night-sweat; sour night-sweat, every night; sweat in the morning; profuse sweat during work.

According to Hahnemann, *Sulphur* is the antipsoric first in rank.

"When the symptoms of the itch," says Hahnemann, "have been recognized by the physician, it will suffice to administer, without any external application, two globules of dynamized sulphur, in order to cure a child of the whole psoric disease, in two, three, or four weeks. No other remedy will be required."[1]

There is not a physician who does not know, now-a-days, what this assertion is worth. It is true, sulphur cures the itch, but almost always very slowly; so slowly, that some of Hahnemann's disciples despairing of accomplishing a cure by the internal use of the attenuations of sulphur, have resorted to the reprehensible custom of accompanying the internal use of sulphur with the external use of the sulphur-ointment. I have noticed that it is principally in sanguine and robust subjects that the itch resists with most obstinacy the exclusive and internal use of *sulphur*.

The efficacy of this drug is much more marked in the treatment of *favus;* but in any other species of scald-head it is more than doubtful. Chronic and non-venereal ulcerations of the skin are generally very speedily modified by the aid of sulphur; they change in appearance, fleshy granulations start up, and, in some cases, cicatrisation takes place with a surprising rapidity. But *sulphur* is not, as many physicians believe, the specific remedy for *scrofula*. What is supposed to be scrofula, in such a case, are simply *bad humors*, arising from bad air, bad food, or excesses of some kind; such a cacochymia is characterized by the following symptoms.

Sickly looks, pale, blanched, wan, earthy face; flaccid or wrinkled, or else fine and rose-colored skin; herpetic eruptions which are more or less distinct or have already disappeared either spontaneously or under the influence of repelling drugs; dull, but continual headache; weakness of one or more senses; slow fever, with evening exacerbations; physical and mental indolence; sweat in making the least effort; dyspnœa in working, walking, and especially in going up stairs; timid, pusillanimous, and at the same time irritable mood, etc.

This group of symptoms is indeed developed by every antipsoric in a healthy person, after its action has been allowed to continue for a time; and it is therefore cured or

[1] *Chronic Diseases*, vol. I.

at least diminished by every one of them; but these symptoms are not scrofula.

Formerly I made frequent use of sulphur against the swelling of the cervical glands, but almost always without success, except in cases where these glands were ulcerated. In such cases the pus ceased to discharge, the wound became cicatrised; and in a few months after, the disease reappeared in some other place.

In *caries* sulphur seldom effects a cure. Generally it improves the constitutional condition of the patient; but this improvement does not last unless a more suitable remedy is resorted to in season.

This drug has rendered great service in old cerebral affections, with seated pain in the forehead and diminution of the sense of hearing, and in certain forms of paralysis. The epilepsies which have been cured with sulphur, were most probably of psoric origin; I have never had an opportunity of using it in this case.

Its marked action on the rectum explains the numerous cures of piles which have been accomplished with sulphur, and likewise of the various affections which accompany them, or which break out in consequence of their suppression.

Lastly, it is especially in *chronic affections of the air-passages*, that sulphur has been found efficacious. But has it really cured *pulmonary phthisis?* If it has not cured this disease, at least its course has been retarded for several years. Sometimes, it is true, this suspension of the symptoms of phthisis, were it ever so complete for a time, for a few weeks, for instance, is only an ephemeral illusion both to the physician and the patient. There is no doubt, however, that serious affections of the air-passages have frequently been arrested by the use of sulphur; affections, which, without being tuberculous phthisis, would nevertheless have been equally fatal. I have collected several cases bearing upon this point, among others, that of a farmer of the district of Bagnoles, in Normandy, whose two brothers had both died of phthisis pulmonalis, according to the report of the physicians by whom they had been treated, and whose own case presented all the symptoms of a case of consumption of the second degree.

Sulphur is scarcely ever employed in acute cases. No drug, however, can replace it in certain abnormal phases of exanthematic fevers. "When the small pox runs an irregular course, and shows signs of being disposed to strike in; when the pustules, instead of being transparent or yellow, are greenish, pink-colored or black; when they fill themselves with blood, and a decomposition of the pus, and the development of putrid symptoms seems imminent, *sulphur* has then to be given."[1]

Camph., *Crot. tigl.*, *Puls.* and *Coff.* are the surest antidotes to *sulphur*.

Croton Tiglium. See page 84.

Lobelia Inflata, genus, *lobelia*, family campanulaceæ.

This plant grows in the United States. It is acrid and dangerous. As soon as it has entered the stomach, it causes nausea, vomiting, colic, sweat, and, it is said, a species of narcotism.[2] According to Dr. Andrew of the United States, it acts as an *emetic*, *expectorant* and *diaphoretic*. In America, it is vulgarly termed *asthma-weed*, and it is indeed in the catarrhal and spasmodic affections of the air-passages that *lobelia inflata* has been employed with most success. Dr. Cutter cured his asthma with this drug, and wrote a pamphlet on the subject.

Some English physicians have employed *lobelia* successfully against *leucorrhœa*. In France, M. Bidault de Villiers has used it only as an *emetic*.

When proved in homœopathic doses, lobelia yields a great number of symptoms which resemble those of *sulphur*. Its action on the skin, head, and mucous membranes, is more particularly analogous to that of sulphur.

[1] *Traité hom. des malad. aig. et chron. des enfants*, Paris, 1850, p. 166.

[2] *Notice sur l' emploi du lobélia inflata dans l' asthme et comme émétique*, par Bidault de Villiers, dans la *Nouv. biblioth. médic.*, vol. V., p. 226.

Jahr's Manual contains a pathogenesis of lobelia inflata, drawn from the Hygia. My own experience has furnished me the following symptoms to which lobelia seems to be particularly adapted.

Pressive headache, at the occiput, less frequently at the forehead, sometimes only on one side of the head, (left side,) increased by motion, in the evening, and especially at night; continual periodical cephalalgia, in the afternoon, increasing until midnight, every third attack being alternately more or less violent. The brain is racked by the cough, which causes an intolerable pain; vertigo in walking, especially in going up stairs; stitches at the vertex; heat and sweat about the head and face; circumscribed redness on one cheek; sense of general exhaustion, with urgent desire to remain in bed; agitated feelings, he fears lest he should have to die soon; chilly feeling; fever and ague, with more or less long-lasting shuddering towards the middle of the day, followed by sweat and heat which lasts until next morning; sensation of heat and shuddering in the day-time.

Eruption between the fingers, on the dorsa of the hands and on the fore-arms, consisting of small vesicles accompanied by a tingling itching, and resembling the itch-pustules exactly.

Mouth dry or full of tenacious mucus; bad taste in the mouth; flat taste of the food, tongue coated white; great desire for coffee; loss of appetite; aversion to every kind of food; thirst, especially during the chill; nausea; sour regurgitations; hiccough; pyrosis; desire to vomit, after drinking; constriction at the stomach; flatulence; gurgling in the left side of the abdomen; emission of fetid flatulence; distention of the abdomen which is painful to contact; constipation; frothy stools; greenish diarrhœa; increase of the urinary secretion; almost constant desire to urinate; watery or brown urine, with copious red sediment; tensive pain in the groins; pressure on the genital organs.

Titillation in the throat, causing an attack of cough at every moment; violent, racking cough, in paroxysms of long continuance, followed by profuse expectoration of ropy mucus which adheres to the pharynx. Anxious, difficult, panting breathing, with sense of constriction on the chest, sometimes on one side only; paroxysm of suffocation, with excessive anguish, and continuing sometimes the whole night; sense of rawness and soreness in the chest below the clavicle; angina pectoris, with pain extending to the shoulder and arm; painfulness of the nape of the neck and dorsal region; extreme lassitude of the legs; cramps in the calves.

This drug has not yet been much used in homœopathic practice. The striking resemblance which I observed between the *recent itch*, and the eruption which lobelia caused in one case, induced me to try it in the itch; the success answered my expectations. Afterwards I used both *Lobelia* and *Croton* for the itch, as has been stated in my *treatise on the diseases of children*. I still believe in this combination, although later experience has shown that it is not unexceptionable.

I have used *lobelia* successfully for a papulous exanthem which was evidently of psoric origin, and likewise in a desperate case of *suffocative catarrh*. The patient was an unmarried lady of about forty years; rather deaf, of a fanciful and high temper; she was pale, haggard, emaciated, subject to terrible bleedings from the left nostril. These hæmorrhages which sometimes lasted several days without interruption, caused her to faint. The bronchial affection which led me to prescribe lobelia, manifested itself with a marked intermittent character. After a chill of about an hour, the cough and dyspnœa commenced about two o'clock in the afternoon, and lasted until next morning. The pulse was rather full and frequent; the patient was troubled with profuse sweats, accompanied by a feeling of extreme malaise at night. A severe constrictive and stitching pain was felt in the whole left side of the chest, and extended all along the left arm, as far as the ends of the fingers. The cough which returned in paroxysms of long continuance, racked the head, and was accompanied with a profuse expectoration of mucus. During the paroxysms the face became red, and the sweat trickled down from it. Lastly, a very painful retention of urine, which terminated towards morning, completed this sad condition, which had not been modified in the least by such remedies as *Nux vomica* and *Digit.* This lady had never had the itch or any other disease of the skin. *Lobelia* cured her in a few days, and seemed even to have arrested the nose-bleed which had not yet returned three months after the treatment. The hearing had remained the same.

According to Jahr, *Camph.* and IPECAC. are the antidotes to *Lobelia inflata.* This drug removes very speedily several drug-symptoms, particularly the cutaneous symptoms of *Merc. corr.* and *zinc.*

Mercurius Corrosivus. See page 138.

Mercurius Solubilis. See page 105.

Lycoperdon Bovista, *puff-ball.* Genus *lycoperdon,* family *lycoperdaceæ.*

This globular fungus which, according to report, is eaten in Italy before it is ripe,[1] becomes filled, while ripening, with a blackish dust which breaks the husk that contains it, with a slight noise. According to Bulliard, this dust which causes a smarting and a more or less acute irritation if introduced into the nostrils and eyes, is very poisonous, and, if eaten in considerable quantity, might even occasion death. According to the statement of Tournefort, this dust is simply an astringent, and is used by the German barbers to arrest the bleeding in cutting the skin. Be this as it may, this fungus had never before been employed as a remedial agent: it is an interesting drug, which has some very original symptoms; hence no drug can replace it in some maladies. Its action upon the skin, the mucous membranes, the abdomen, etc., has induced me to rank it after sulphur, to which it is no doubt analogous; but, owing to certain phenomena which are peculiar to bovista, we shall find it mentioned again at the end of this volume, among the analogues of iron.[2]

[1] Paulet, *traité des champignons,* p. 446.

[2] See in Roth's *Matiére Méd. pure,* vol. II., p. 133, Paris, 1852, pathogenesis of *lycoperdon bovista.*

This drug is capable of removing the following symptoms:

Chilliness; alternate shuddering and flying heat, principally in the afternoon, with a burning thirst, especially during the shuddering; periodical attack of coldness which is not followed by febrile heat, in the morning or evening; general increase of temperature every afternoon; considerable heat all over, with thirst, the whole day. Desire to sleep, in the day time, after and even during a meal; restless sleep at night, with anxious dreams (about ghosts, serpents, etc.); *violent itching of the skin which is rather increased than diminished by scratching, especially in bed,* and felt more particularly at the front part of the hairy scalp, at the nasal wings, under the nose, at the commissure of the lips, at the chin, on the shoulders, at the inner side of the arms, on the hands, hips, at the inner side of the knees, at the bend of the knees and soles of the feet; *psoric eruptions on the hands and feet;*[1] lenticular, hard papulæ, accompanied with a burning itching at the chest and hands, aggravated by scratching.

Dulness of the intellectual faculties; absence of mind; weakness of memory; sadness; depression of spirits; gaiety; loquacity; unusual frankness concerning one's own faults; moral and physical depression towards evening. Frequent attacks of dull headache with general weakness; *distensive headache, as if there were an abscess in the brain;* violent headache towards three o'clock in the morning; which disappears gradually after the breaking out of a profuse sweat; *sensation as if the head were swelling up to an enormous size,* (this symptom generally comes on at night); *general headache, worse when lying down* or walking in the open air; dizziness in the morning, *increasing even to a loss of sense;* drawing or contusive pain, or stitches at the outer head; profuse sweat at the hairy scalp; falling off of the hair; heat, stitches or pressure in the eyes; dull eyes, without expression; dimness of sight in the morning; *illusions of sight;* objects seem nearer than they really are; *agglutination of*

[1] Bovista excited this symptom in a patient to whom I had administered the drug for a headache.

the eyelids, in the morning; itching in the ears, buzzing in the ears, weakness of hearing; *purulent and fetid otorrhœa;* stoppage of the nose, fluent coryza; crusts in the nostrils; nose-bleed in the morning; paleness of the face, in the morning; alternate paleness and redness of the face; *pustules changing to obstinate crusts under the nose, with swelling of the upper lip;* burning ulceration at the commissure of the lips; swelling of the gums; atrophy of the gums; ulceration of the gums; digging or drawing toothache, eased by warmth or exercise; *dull pain in the superior incisors, with pale and considerable swelling of the upper lip, and an occasional outbreak of profuse sweat about the head;* a sort of torpor of the tongue, and of the whole interior of the mouth, which makes one stutter; dry mouth; bitter, foul, or blood-taste in the mouth; violent hunger; thirst; vomiting of water in the morning; *painful colic, with coldness all over in the morning, on rising,* less frequently in the evening; distension of the abdomen, which is so painful externally and internally, that one dares not touch it, and has to walk bent; gurgling and borborygmi, especially in the left side; emission of fetid flatulence in the evening or morning; urging to stool *in the morning,* sometimes without result; *diarrhœa in the morning;* irregular stool; constipation; painful tenesmus; itching in the rectum, as from worms; frequent urging to urinate; cloudy urine, as if clay had been mixed up with it; smarting and stitches in the urethra; voluptuous sensation at the sexual organs of a woman; restless sleep or sleeplessness; headache with dizziness after an embrace; acrid, smarting leucorrhœa; premature menses, with discoloration of the menstrual blood; violent *pain as if bruised and weary, in the loins, lower abdomen and thighs, which prevents one from going upstairs, before, during and after the menses.*

Hoarseness in the morning, dry cough in the afternoon; constriction of the chest, short and embarrassed breathing during manual labor; stitches in the chest; anxious palpitation of the heart; *profuse and strong-smelling sweat under the shoulders.* Painful stiffness of the back; weary sensation in the articulations of the extremities; tension in the extremities, as if the tendons were too short; cramps in the calves, in the morning in bed.

I have used Bovista successfully, for a sort of red, crusty eruption on the thighs and at the bends of the knees. This eruption, which was supposed to be congenital in a youth of seventeen years, disappeared sometimes for months, without the general health appearing affected by this disappearance, and afterwards reappeared again with the hot weather; sometimes it left for a week or two, and reappeared again with the full-moon. The symptom of an enormous increase of the size of the head, led Petroz to prescribe Bovista in a case of complicated nervous derangement of the head, which Hahnemann, who had been consulted, declared incurable, on account of the great number of drugs which the patient had already swallowed under the treatment of another Homœopathic physician; the patient was cured. I have seen good effects from *bovista* in a case of *hysteria;* the patient was a lady of forty years, had all the abdominal symptoms of this drug, and was, moreover, troubled with a sort of herpetic redness at the tip of the nose, of long standing. This spot remained, but all the other symptoms disappeared very speedily.

The action of bovista is aggravated by coffee, wine, and alcoholic beverages.

Camphor antidotes this drug.

Asterias, *sea-star.* — Genus echinoderma. A decoction of asterias formerly was supposed to be *loosening.* The smoke which these animals spread when they are burnt, was regarded as a remedy *for epilepsy;* the ashes obtained from their bones were employed as a *desiccative.*

"My first notions concerning the usefulness of asterias," says Dr. Petroz, to whom we are indebted for the pathogenesis of this drug, "I derived from the fact of its being used against *epilepsy.* The celebrated Cotugno, placed some confidence in the efficacy of asterias in this disease; but this malady, the causes and seat of which are so various, will remain for a long time to come, one of those diseases against which the efforts of physicians will remain fruitless."[1]

Indeed, experience has destroyed in a great measure, the hopes which our provings, much more than dubious tradition, had induced us to build upon the curative virtues of asterias in epilepsy; but the powerful action which this medicine exercises on various organs, and principally upon the skin, constitutes it one of the most precious agents of our Materia Medica.[2]

Pathogenesis of asterias.[3]—Cerebral excitement in opposite directions; sadness, desire to weep; extraordinary mirth; desire to give one's-self up to intellectual labor, or some violent exercise; slight dulness of the mental faculties; disposed to mental labor; delicacy of the moral perceptions.

Sudden sensation of fulness in the head, as if congested; sometimes even as of a rush of blood; heat about the head; sensation of confusion in the brain; fulness of the head, whose sides seem to swell out; stitches in the right temple; passing stitches in the forehead, temples, and especially in the occiput; transitory pains in the right parietal region; pressive pains in the forehead or sinciput, which passes off towards noon; beating in the head; boring pain of short duration, above the left eye, with dimness of sight; he wakes in the night in great confusion, as if the brain were shaken by electric shocks. A sort of emptiness in the head; the consciousness is almost lost; thoughts about apoplexy; this sensation, which lasts a few minutes, is followed by fever, with a hard, quick pulse, violent beating in the right carotid; these symptoms continue until the end of the following day.

[1] Journ. de la Soc. gall. de med. homœop., vol. I., p. 502.

[2] I have had symptoms of this action on my own skin for several months, then I did not yet know that *lead* antidotes asterias.

[3] This pathogenesis has only been published in the *Journ. de la Soc. Gallicane*, and this is the reason why I republish it here, believing that this republication will be acceptable to my readers.

Vertigo in walking, with insensibility of the lower extremities. The cerebral symptoms come on in the morning, cease in the day-time, and come on again in the evening.

Heat and redness in the eyes, weary look, difficulty of bearing the light; the eyes are drawn backwards; winking of the eyelids, the free margin of which is red.

Epistaxis; sneezing and coryza, in the morning on waking.

Lightning-like stitches in the meatus auditorius; violent reports in the ears; noise in the ears as from waves; dulness of hearing in the right ear.

Transitory or permanent flush in the face; a sort of stupid, meaningless expression in the physiognomy.

Swelling of the tongue, pulling pains in the tongue; heaviness of speech, profuse flow of saliva; acute and pressing stitches in the upper teeth; thinks of biting; pressing irritation of the throat.

Loss of appetite, or else a strange and uncertain appetite; aversion to meat; dulness of taste.

Dull pain, apparently all along the œsophagus; frequent eructations; dull or constrictive pain at the præcordial region.

Shocks of dull pain in the right side of the abdomen and near the umbilicus; incarcerated wind; violent colic, with shuddering, alternating with flushes of heat in the face; alternate swelling and sinking of the abdomen during the twenty-four hours; pulling in the abdominal walls.

Constipation, with ineffectual urging to stool; diarrhœa; liquid, brown-colored stool, spirting out with force; several soft stools in the day time; heat in the rectum; hæmorrhoidal tumor; piles.

Urine frequent, clear, profuse, or else thick and slimy; heat in the urethra while the urine passes out.

Frequent erections during sleep or in the morning; twitching in the womb; sense of pressure on the inferior organs of the abdomen, which hinders walking; sensation as if the menses would appear; unusual dampness of the vagina, which affords a feeling of ease; delay of the menses, although the usual colic and other symptoms are present; these only cease on the appearance of the menses, which are more profuse than usual; excitement of the sexual instinct, every morning, in bed; violent and constant desire, with nervous agitation, and apprehension of not being able to support these painful sensations.

Stitches in the anterior and inferior portion of the chest, on the right and left of the sternum; drawing pain towards the inner portion of the chest, from before backwards, the pain starts from under the left nipple, and extends along the whole inner side of the arm, until the end of the little finger; painfulness of the whole left side of the chest, worse during exercise; pain under the sternum; sensation as if the left breast were drawn in; nightly anxiety, caused by undulating beatings in the chest; strong and frequent beating of the heart; jerking palpitations; the heart seems to have ceased beating; anxiety at the heart; itching spots; miliary or furfuraceous eruption between the breasts; swelling of the breasts as when the menses are about to appear.

Pulling pain in the back and sacrum. Uneasiness in the upper extremities; pain extending from the thumb to the shoulder-joint; numbness of the hands, with coldness of the arm; lancing pain at the left elbow; circular, red spot at the left elbow, which becomes covered with a furfuraceous, dry and friable layer; considerable itching around the nail of the left thumb.

Lassitude and great weakness of the lower extremities; pain in the left hip; burning stitches in the great trochanter and the coxo-femoral articulation of the left side; stitches at the fore part of the thigh; pain in the left knee; pain in the joints of the foot; painful pulling in the sole of the foot; gouty pain in the joint formed by the left big toe with the first metatarsal bone; redness and heat of the skin at this place; violent, very unpleasant itching at the thighs and legs, worse towards six o'clock in the evening, in the open air;

eruptions on the thighs, and insteps, consisting of small, itching vesicles, which tear easily and change to small, burning, large and superficial ulcers, lasting several days before cicatrising.

The malaise is increased by heat; great desire for cold drinks; coffee aggravates all the symptoms and excites them anew several days after they had disappeared.

The clinical observations which have already been obtained with asterias, have been related by Dr. Petroz in an interesting article, which the reader will do well to refer to.[1]

Petroz, who approves of my ranking asterias among the *anti-psorics*, has employed this drug with much success in many cases of *chronic cutaneous diseases*, old ulcers, and *cancerous affections.* Concerning the latter, Petroz observed, first, that the drug only acted well when *the left*, and not the right breast, was the seat of the disease; second, that it was not sufficient to perfect the cure. It is with asterias as with sulphur; its action in cutaneous diseases scarcely ever goes beyond the dermis. And, lastly, asterias has, like sulphur, cured *certain forms of cerebral congestion, accompanied by obstinate constipation,* and suspended *for awhile* by epileptic paroxysms.

Plumb., and particularly *Zincum*, are antidotes to asterias.

Aethusa Cynapium.— *Garden-hemlock.* — Genus Aethusa, family umbelliferæ, class pentandria digynia.

This annual plant, which grows in abandoned gardens, among ruins, on uncultivated fields, etc., has sometimes been confounded with, and eaten as chervil; whence have resulted more or less serious accidents, and even death. Not used by the older physicians, the garden-hemlock is only imperfectly known by homœopaths. We have two provings of it, one by Hartlaub and Trinks, (see Jahr's *Manual,*) and another, published in 1847, by Petroz, in the *Bulletin de la Société de médecine homœopathique.* This latter, in conjunction with several clinical observations, has enabled me to assign its

[1] *Journ. de la Soc. gallic. de méd. homœop.*, Paris, 1851, No. de Janvier.

proper place to Aethusa, which has many analogies with *Sulphur*, and many of whose symptoms resemble those of *Bovista*[1] and *Asterias*, after which I have ranked it.

Synopsis of the symptoms of Aethusa, according to Petroz.[2]

Difficulty of fixing one's attention; slowness and instability of one's ideas; absence of ideas; loss of consciousness or a sort of stupefaction as if a body had been placed between the organs of the senses and the external objects; sadness when alone; loquacious, facetious mirth; gaiety of temper; anxiety, with a sensation of weight on the chest; serious, still and whining mood; disposed to be vehement; excessive sensitiveness of feeling; these symptoms are very marked after drinking wine, and especially during a fit of intoxication.[3]

Pains in the extremities which prevent sleep; sweat on falling asleep; general coldness during sleep; rolling of the eyes, and slight convulsive motions in falling asleep; fatiguing dreams in the morning; frequent waking.

Small and frequent pulse; irregular pulse; palpitations, which react in the head; palpitations with vertigo; headache; restlessness.

Fever, especially in the morning, with shuddering; shuddering, weariness in the extremities, internal coldness, with hot and flushed face; malaise; disposition to delirium during the cold stage; sweat, after the breaking out of which the previous symptoms disappear.

Dry and burning skin; itching as from ants, in bed, especially in the evening; red spots; herpetic eruption.

Vertigo when sitting, rising, during a walk in the open

[1] Especially those of Bovista.

[2] In the first vol. of Roth's *Materia Med. Pura*, we find a pathogenesis of Æthusa, in which the symptoms of Petroz, and those of Hartlaub and Trinks, with various other symptoms from works on poisons, are put together. After a careful perusal of this combination, I have come to the conclusion that Roth had better have left Petroz's proving separate from the others, and had contented himself with merely adding his own observations.

[3] This is likewise the case with the symptoms produced by *Bovista* and *Asterias* in the emotive sphere.

air, especially in the middle of the day; sensation of tightness in the head; tightness above the root of the nose; beating in the head; pain at the vertex; pressure in the eyes; tearing pain in the eyes; the head inclines to fall backwards; these symptoms which return periodically, frequently are accompanied with paleness of the face, trembling of the jaws, pain in the præcordial region; they occur especially on waking, and are readily excited by cold; they cease during sleep, and are diminished by the emission of wind; sensation of contraction about the hairy scalp.

Stitches around the eyes; convulsions of the eyes; smarting pain in the eyes and eyelids; objects appear larger than they really are; diplopia; symptoms, such as the head-symptoms, show themselves particularly on waking and in the open air.

Stitches in the ears from within outwards; sensation of heat from the ear; deficiency of cerumen; purulent discharge from the ear; whizzing in the ears.

Pressing heat in the face; pulling, tearing pains in the face; sensation of coldness in the face and at the commissure of the lips; sweat in the face; small vesicles in the face; yellowish spots on the upper lip; twitching of the muscles around the mouth; expression of fatigue and anguish in the face.

Aphthæ in the mouth; gnawing toothache (at the lower teeth); stitching pain at the roof of the palate; sensation as if the tongue were too long; slow, embarrassed speech; redness and swelling of the curtain and the surrounding parts; impediment in the throat, even so as to cause an apprehension of suffocation; itching, scraping and redness in the throat; pains in the submaxillary glands.

Taste of cheese, onions, or salt-taste, which it is difficult to describe, before and after a meal; want of appetite, although the tongue is clean; want of appetite, only at supper; eructations tasting of the ingesta-eructations after drinking; nausea with depression of spirits; vomiting of greenish matters; vomiting, with shuddering, sweat and weakness;

cold sweat in the face; painfulness in the epigastric region; painful contraction of the stomach; digging sensation in the abdomen; beating in the abdomen; coldness in the abdomen; painfulness in the hypochondria; incompletely digested stools, some time after eating, or at night; hæmorrhoidal tumors; fluent piles; sense of dryness at the anus.

Frequent desire to urinate; pale and profuse urine, or red urine emitted with difficulty, and depositing a white sediment; cutting pain at the bladder.

Short, anxious wheezing breathing, especially when lying on the back; racking cough, especially in bed; sense of constriction in the chest, as if tied; pain in the mammary glands; swelling of the breasts.

Pulling or sense of weakness in bed.

Pain and engorgement of the axillary glands; heaviness of the arms; arthritic stiffness of the elbow-joint; swelling of the forearms and hands; cramp in the hand; digging in the fingers; contraction of the fingers.

Boring or lancing pains, or paralytic pains in the lower extremities; formication in the feet.

The symptoms of æthusa are, like those of *bovista* and *asterias*, aggravated by coffee, wine, drunkenness, cold water, and the warmth of the bed; they are diminished by a walk in the open air, and by conversation.

According to Petroz, *æthusa cynapium* has been useful in *chronic inflammation of the margin at the eyelids, pustules on the cornea, incipient amaurosis, swelling of the glands, tettery eruptions at the tip of the nose, swelling of the cervical and axillary glands, eruptions around joints, dryness of the skin, nodes of the skin, tetters which itch in the warmth, or bleed readily.*

The pathological sphere of *æthusa* is completed by the following affections, which have to be added to those above named: *nervous derangements* characterised by a *loquacious gaiety, optical illusions and hallucinations, disposition of the head to fall backwards, momentary staring of the eyes, embarrassed speech, vertigo in the middle of the day, &c., sweat on making the least exertion, dry cough and dyspnœa in the afternoon.*

Camphor probably antidotes this drug.

Cicuta Virosa—*Cicutaria* of Lamarck.—Poisonous Hemlock.[1]—A perennial plant—Genus, *Cicuta*—Family, *Umbelliferæ*—Class, *Pentandria Digynia.*

The poisonous hemlock grows on the borders of ditches, brooks and ponds, in the North and East of France. Its stem is cylindrical, fistulous, smooth, (the whole plant is likewise smooth,) striated, ramose, erect, from one to two feet in height. Its leaves are of a dark green, and, if rubbed between the fingers, exhale a nauseous and stupefying odor; they are large, with hollow petioles, many-winged, with narrow and serrated folioles. Its root is erect, tufty, and long, like the root of the parsnip, with which it has been sometimes been confounded,[2] thick, fleshy, and widening interiorly by angular turnings. When cut or crushed, a milky juice flows out, which is yellowish and of an acrid taste. This juice of the recent root, and gathered at the time when the plant is in blossom, is mixed with an equal quantity of alcohol, and forms the mother-tincture of the drug.

This hemlock is said to be the most poisonous of all umbelliferæ. Except goats, who eat it without injury,[3] it rapidly destroys all other animals by tetanus and convulsions. It is even believed that its poisonous virtues are superior to those of the *Conium maculatum.* This led Natter, and especially Bulliard, to believe that it was the cicuta that Socrates and Phocion had been condemned to drink; but the investigations of recent botanical travellers have removed all that seemed to

[1] Not the water-hemlock termed aquatica (*phellandrium aquaticum* of Linné). This grows in, but the former on the border of, water. These two plants, which are distinguished by pretty well marked botanical differences, have probably different medicinal properties. They should not be confounded under the same name. It is the poisonous hemlock, not the water-hemlock that Wepfer describes in his work, *Cicutæ aquaticæ historia.*

[2] Wepfer, *Cicuta aquat. hist.*, p. 5.

[3] Id., p. 135.

invest this supposition with the character of truth: for it has been ascertained that the *cicuta virosa* did not exist in the Peloponnesus, where the *conium maculatum*, on the contrary, abounds, especially in the neighborhood of Athens.[1]

Be this as it may, no physician had dared to prescribe the Cicuta virosa internally, prior to Hahnemann. It was only used externally *for gouty pains*, on the recommendation of Linné. On these grounds it became an ingredient of the Danish plaster of hemlock.[2]

Mayer, quoted by Roth,[3] recommends a strong decoction of galls against poisoning by hemlock.

Some homœopaths may be surprised at my having classed cicuta among the analogues of sulphur. But after having sufficiently studied the pure symptoms of the cicuta, and having perceived the natural relation and connection of these symptoms; after having noticed, as I have been able to do, 1st such derangements of the intellectual faculties, of the senses, of the muscular contractility, etc., as are occasioned by the cicuta, follow the retrocession of an old herpetic eruption, which was primarily seated in the face, and, according to the description that I have had of it, was perfectly analogous to the one that constitutes one of the primary symptoms of this drug; and 2d, after having seen all these morbid phenomena disappear one by one under the use of this drug, prescribed on no other grounds than that of the formerly existing herpes in the face, it will be admitted that *psora* and *cicuta* are not, by any means, strangers to each other. But, it may be asked, does this imply that the cicuta and the sulphur-psora are identical? Oh no, unfortunately; if this were the case, the practice of homœopathy would be much more simple than it is. But in medicine, there are no *identities;* in pathology as well as in therapeutics, we only have *analogies.* In com-

[1] Mérat and Delens, *dict. de mat. méd.*, vol. II., p. 282. It is more than probable that the Grecian conium macul. possesses much more active properties than the conium of our own climate.

[2] Hahnemann, Mat. Med., vol. II., p. 495.

[3] *Mat. Méd. Pura*, vol. II., p. 495.

paring the diseases to which sulphur, asterias, bovista, cicuta, etc., correspond, it seems to me impossible that we should not recognise a certain family resemblance between them. If I have not yet been able, like our illustrious master, to consider them as manifestations of one and the same psora, I accept them, at least, as various forms of psora, which are related to each other, and constitute varieties of the same species, distinguished from each other by the form of their cutaneous development, by the locality which they respectively prefer, and lastly, by the nature of the internal symptoms which follow the retrocession of the external eruption. In this respect, I beg leave to point out, if not a law, at least a series of facts that seem to me to merit attention. I infer from careful observation, that the organ or organs which are invaded after the suppression of the cutaneous symptoms, are generally those which are most nearly related to the original seat of the exanthem, either anatomically or functionally.

Thus, while the retrocession of the itch, to which, save their respective shades, *Sulphur*, *Croton*, *Lobelia*, *Mercurius*, *corros.* and *solub.*, correspond, and which is generally spread over the whole body, but *more particularly over* the *thoracic extremities*, gives rise to the most varied morbid phenomena, *but more particularly to pulmonary affection ;* the suppression of the eruptions to which *Bovista*, *Cicuta*, and *Æthusa* correspond, gives rise principally to *cerebral diseases*, because these eruptions are habitually situated *at the forepart of the hairy scalp, or on the face.* And lastly, the retrocession of the exanthem, which yields to *ratania*, and which, I believe, I have been the first to point out, and which is principally located *in the lumbar region*, will be found to be principally followed by *pains in the loins and uterus.*

I repeat, however, that these observations do not imply the existence of a general law; but they seem to be worthy of attention.

Hahnemann has, according to his own statement, given us simply a sketch of the action of cicuta. In Roth's Materia

Medica Pura, an extensive, though as yet incomplete pathogenesis of cicuta, will be found, (vol. II., p. 425.)

Cicuta vir., will probably be found curative in the following affections, the list of which is still rather vague and uncertain.

Chronic eruptions at the forepart of the hairy scalp, on the face and on the hands, consisting of lenticular pustules of a bright-red color, confluent, oozing, generally with a slight itching, which is only felt in the warmth, or on parts where new pustules are breaking out.

Heaviness of the head, especially in the forehead, on rising in the morning; dizziness as from intoxication, as if one had to stagger and fall forward; dull headache, with vertigo, alleviated by cold drinks and the escape of gas from the bowels; sadness; stupor; increased sensitiveness; tendency to start at every thing; starting on hearing the least noise; weakness of memory, even forgetting his own name; the patient commences a phrase, and is unable to complete it, because he forgets both what he was going to say, and had just said; illusion in regard to one's own person, imagining for instance, that one is a child; illusions of hearing, less frequently than illusions of sight; tonic and clonic spasms, with froth at the mouth, screams, vociferations, etc.; irresistible desire to stretch or to roll over the floor; complete mental derangement, changing from day to day.

Involuntary staring, redness of the eyes, photophobia, nocturnal agglutination of the lids; purulent discharge from the ear, with pain in the inner ear, as from an abscess; weakness of hearing; hæmorrhage from the ears; ulcerations in the nostrils and at the corners of the mouth.

Stuttering without any perception, trembling, or deviation of the tongue; clean and natural tongue, in spite of the existence of various serious symptoms; hiccough; watery regurgitations in the morning; *canine hunger;* pinchings and noisy borborygmi in the bowels; cutting pains after a meal; *abundant and fetid flatulence; round tumor in the left hypochondrium, not very sensitive to pressure;*[1] *constipa-*

[1] Chronic swelling of the ovary (of what kind?) in a lady of 58 years,

tion; retention of urine; frequent emission of a small quantity of watery urine.

Hoarseness: cough with itching and heat in the chest; burning pain at the nipples; swelling of the cervical muscles; *dull pain all along the vertebral column, increased by contact; trembling of the extremities, uncertainty of motion and gait.* Fever with slow pulse.

Camphor and opium antidote this poison.

Ratania, not ratanhia. — This name was given by the Peruvians, and, after them, by the Spanish physicians to the *Krameria triandra*, a bush of the genus *Krameria*, family *Polygalea*, class *tetrandria monogynia;* the name of the genus is derived from Kramer, a German botanist.

This plant, which grows abundantly in Peru and South America, was discovered in 1779, by Ruiz, who sent it to Linné. In 1808, Bourdois de Lamotte, translated in French, Ruiz's dissertation, published in 1796, on the properties of *Ratania*, and inserted in the memoirs of the *Royal Academy of Madrid.*[1] But owing to the interruption of the transatlantic navigation, the use of this plant did not spread until the year 1816, when Hurtado, an exiled Spanish physician,[2] again drew the attention of the medical world to this drug in a special memoir.

Empirical applications.—The alloeopaths have abused the ratania like all other drugs; but I am obliged at the same time to admit, that there is perhaps no plant, the properties of which have been so well indicated by chance as this.

having ceased to menstruate in consequence of a fright ever since her 30th year, of robust constitution, irritable, nervous, and excessively fanciful and odd. *Cicuta vir.* had a remarkably quieting effect for several weeks, during which period the swelling diminished considerably. *Cicuta* would perhaps have done more, if the lady who was a foreigner, had not been obliged to leave Paris and forego her treatment.

[1] Journ. de Méd. de Leroux, Corvisart and Boyer, vol. XV., p. 80.

[2] Observations sur l' efficacité de la *ratania* dans les hémorrhagies passives, (Bull. de la Soc. d' émul., et Journ. de méd. de Leroux, vol. XVI., p. 216.)

Used as an *astringent* and a *tonic*, this root sometimes arrested passive hæmorrhages (*epistaxis*, *hæmoptysis*, *metrorrhagia*, etc.) It was successfully used against *scurvy*, *mucous discharges*, such as *chronic catarrh of the bronchia*, *vagina*, *large intestines*, etc., against various forms of *incontinence of urine*, *chronic œdema of the skin*.[1] Doctor Tournel, who, no doubt, did not suspect that ratania produced abortion, had the happy idea of prescribing it as a tonic in cases of incipient miscarriage, and thus preventing this accident in delicate and nervous females who had never yet been able to go their full term.[2] Lastly, a practitioner whose high sense every body admires, and who would have been one of the first physicians of the age if he had embraced our practice, succeeded in curing with *ratania* one of the most obstinate and most painful affections, *fissure of the anus*. Trousseau and Pidoux, who mention this discovery in their *traité de thérapeutique*, accompany it with a commentary, which I cannot help reproducing here, so perfectly does it exhibit the insanity of alloeopathic theories:—

"Surely," say these authors, "if we see all surgeons, some exclusively, and others, if not exclusively, at least more than they ought to be, preoccupied with the spasmodic constriction of the sphincter, we cannot rationally be led to inject into the rectum substances which tend to increase the constriction, such as ratania."

This was, however, done by Bretonneau on the following grounds:—

"The constipation and the effort made by the fæcal ball against the sphincter, which became distended and frequently torn in consequence, being evidently, in a number of cases, the cause of the fissure, the constipation was of course the greatest obstacle to the cure.

"Now it happens that the constipation is frequently accompanied with a remarkable change in the lower portion of the rectum; immediately above the sphincter, the rectum

[1] See Bibliot. méd., vol. XVII., et Journ. de méd. de Leroux, vol. XVI.

[2] *Journ. Univ.* des sc. médic., vol. XXVIII., p. 225.

swells up into a pouch, and then contracts again on a level with the sub-vertebral angle. In this pouch the fæces accumulate, and form a ball of an enormous size, so that every time the patient goes to stool, he experiences a sort of labor-pains."

Bretonneau judged that, in order to combat these constipations, whether or not accompanied with a fissure, it was necessary to restore the reactive energies of the lower portion of the intestines, and the ratania seemed to him calculated to fulfil this object. To this end he ordered in simple constipation injections of water, mixed with the extract of ratania, and an alcoholic tincture of the same drug.

A lady was treated by him who suffered with constipation and fissure of the anus, which caused her horrible pains, and had damaged her health. He caused her to use every day an injection mixed with one-fourth of ratania, and in a short while, constipation and fissure were cured.

Other cases of constipation and fissure were treated with the same success. It was then that he tried the ratania in simple fissure without constipation, and the same success was obtained.

A very rational inference led him to the first use; afterwards facts which happened contrary to his expectations, awakened his attention; he noticed these facts, and an attentive and considerate mode of proceeding led him to a system of medication, which, according to Trousseau and Pidoux, is not, by any means, *rational*, but which effects *cures*, and this is, after all, the principal point.

This method of treatment would be rational, if the constipation were always the cause of the fissure;[1] but in many cases of fissure we have diarrhœa instead of constipation, or we have at least soft stools, so that the sphincter is not pressed against, and yet the fissure continues. We have now to inquire, how does the ratania cure fissure? We might answer: It cures, what matters it, how? And although we may admit, that, in therapeutics, this answer *seems proper*

[1] Is it rational in allœopathy to combat constipation with astringents?

and valid, the anxious reason seeks to account satisfactorily for the modus operandi of the drug in such a case of cure.[1]

A homœopathic physician accounts for such a cure quite easily; but Trousseau and Pidoux do not accept his mode of reasoning, and they are compelled to deny all truth and method, and to content themselves with this said commonplace: *This cures, because it cures.*

Symptoms of ratania:[2] *Fitful mood, gloomy and quarrelsome; deep depression of spirits when alone, it passes off in society, and is sometimes replaced by a sort of gaiety; constant disposition to irascibility of temper.* Depression of spirits and drowsiness in the day-time, especially after the evening meal. Shuddering and horripilations, with *gaping* and thirst in the evening. Fever and sleeplessness at night; frequent waking. Waking with a start, anxiety and fear; night-sweats.

Sickly skin. *Small red or white pimples which do not suppurate, especially between the shoulders and in the lumbar region, and remaining for a long time.*

Pressive headache at the forehead; rush of blood to the head and face, with heat and sense of fulness; jerking, smarting, and stitches in the head; pain in the head as if the skull would burst, especially when sitting and stooping.

Pain in the eyes as if between screws, and as if they could not be moved. Contraction and burning sensation in the eyes, especially in the evenings; inflammation of the sclerotica; sensation as of a skin before the eyes; white spot before the eye which prevents sight; myopia; jerking and shuddering of the eyes and lids; agglutination of the lids, and lachrymation in the morning.

Tearing in the ears; itching and stitches in the ears; buzzing, ringing in the ears.

[1] Vol. I., p. 108.

[2] The symptoms in italics are the result of my own observations; I have seen them *several times*, in one case on a female patient whom an allœopathic physician had drenched with *ratania*. The other symptoms are taken from Jahr, who obtained them from Hartlaub and Trinks.

Itching at the nose; smarting heat and crusts in the nostrils; frequent sneezing; nosebleed; dry coryza, with complete stoppage of the nasal secretions.

Flashes of heat in the face; tearing prosapolgia; burning vesicles on the vermilion border of the upper lip.

Dryness of the mouth, at night; flow of saliva in the mouth; *swelling of the gums, fungous softening of the gums,* which bleed easily and cause a sour taste as of blood; tearing, jerking, digging toothache, especially in the evening; burning sensation on the tongue; sore throat during empty deglutition; crampy contraction of the throat, arresting the utterance of words.

Flat taste in the morning; thirst in the evening; aversion to food and drink; eructations tasting of the food, or without any taste; violent hiccough which causes a pain in the stomach; nausea; retching, vomiting of food, especially at night; watery vomiting; *vomiting of blood-streaked mucus;* ulcerative pain at the stomach; burning, cutting, or constrictive pain at the stomach; distension of the epigastric region.

Pulling and cold feeling at the umbilical region. Distension of the abdomen; stitches, *pinchings* and motion as from a living being in the hypochondria, (especially the *left*); stitches, pinchings and contractions in the groins.

Hard stools, with urging; incomplete stools; protrusion of hæmorrhoidal tumors: fluent piles; soft, diarrhœic stools, accompanied, preceded, and followed by pains in the loins, cutting colic and burning pain at the anus. *Dry heat at the anus, with sudden stitches, which the patient compares to stabs with a penknife; dampness at the anus;* bloody diarrhœa; after the evacuation, dizziness and headache, as if the head would fly to pieces.

Pressing and frequent desire to urinate, day and night, with scanty emission. Considerable increase of the urinary secretion; pale urine. Pressure on the genital organs, followed by leucorrhœa; premature menses, too profuse and too long, with pain in the lower abdomen and loins. Metrorrhagia; miscarriage. *Delay of the menses; suppression of the menses, with swelling of the abdomen and breasts, as if she had been pregnant for several months;* this condition is accompanied by a *profuse leucorrhœa*, with *cutting colic and constant pains in the loins.*[1]

Dry cough, with tickling in the larynx, and ulcerative pain in the chest. Dyspnœa on making the least exertion; painful constriction in the sides of the chest; stitches in the chest, with suffocation, especially on going upstairs; *catarrhal cough.*

Formication and itching eruption in the dorsal region; stiffness of the nape of the neck; tearing sensation in the neck, with heaviness of the head; painful weariness in the loins and back; tensive and drawing pains from the nape of the neck to the sacrum.

Tearing in the shoulder, arms, fore-arms, and wrists; crampy contractions in the elbows and fingers. Drawing or tearing pains in the thighs, knees, legs, feet, and toes; tension and burning sensation in the thighs; jerking in the thighs, calves and feet.

Most of the ratania symptoms come on in the evening, night and morning. *They are lessened by exercise and in the open air, very much aggravated by uneasiness of mind.*

It is almost always after *Sulph.*, *Bovista* or *Sepia*, that, in uterine affections, I have obtained good effects from *Ratania.*

The antidote is unknown to me.

[1] This was removed by *Merc. sol.*

GROUP IV.

TYPE: ARSENICUM ALBUM.

There is no more powerful, no more universally applicable, and, if I may so express myself, no more complete therapeutic agent than arsenic. Its sphere of action seems to extend over every sphere of the organism. The remarks which I have offered in regard to the general action of the drugs belonging to the group *Mercurius*, of which Arsenic is likewise a member, are peculiarly applicable to it. But if, independently of its general action, we consider more particularly its special effects, it will be seen that these effects establish evident relations between this and a variety of other drugs.

Arsenic acts in a marked and almost constant manner on

1. The digestive organs.
2. The organs of the head.
3. The organs of locomotion.
4. The cutaneous organ.

Hence we have the following four series of analogues :—

1. Series.—*Affections of the Digestive Organs.*

Veratrum album.
Argentum.
Zincum.
Mercurius.
Lycopodium.
Nux vomica.
Coloquithis.
Sepia.
Copaivæ balsamum.
Alumina.
Plumbum.
Indigo.
Bryonia alba.
Sulphur.
Cina.
Lachesis.
Carbo vegetabilis.
Ferrum metallicum.
Bismuthum.
Petroleum.
Nux moschata.

2. SERIES.—*Affections of the Head.*

Belladonna.	Capsicum.
Bryonia alba.	Aconitum.
Carbo vegetabilis.	Cadron.
Opium.	Thuya.

3. SERIES.—*Affections of the Organs of Locomotion.*

Argentum.	Plumbum.
Ferrum metallicum.	Arnica.
Zincum.	Capsicum.
Opium.	

4. SERIES.—*Affections of the Skin.*

Lobelia inflata.	Sulphur.
Sepia.	Argentum.
Ferrum metallicum.	Mercurius.

The formation of these four series, and especially the relative arrangement of the drugs, have obliged me to reflect for a long time before I was able to come to any definite conclusions. The three last series are, mostly, formed of the drugs constituting the first series, but they are arranged in a different order for the reason that such and such a drug, which, by its action upon the digestive organs, occupies a rank next to arsenic, is probably remote from it in its action upon the head, extremities or skin. Leaving to the reader the task of verifying the three last series, I shall here occupy myself exclusively with a more particular description of the first series.

It will be readily perceived that the drugs of the first series are, of all the analogues of arsenic, those which come nearest to their type, either by the totality of the physiological phenomena which they produce, or by the nature of the diseases against which they have been efficacious. These diseases are especially the following:

Gastritis and gastro-enteritis, in all their shades, from epidemic cholera to simple dyspepsia; dysentery, abdominal engorgements; fever and ague, ascites; typhoid fever, chronic diarrhœa, intestinal worms, constipation, piles, periodical headache and ophthalmia; mental derangement; epi-

lepsy, especially when caused by worms; various kinds of cough accompanied by dyspnœa and paroxysms of asthma; various affections of the *genito-urinary apparatus;* various forms of *hysteria;* some acute and chronic cutaneous diseases; which are most generally accompanied by some more or less obscure disturbances of the digestive passages or the genito-urinary apparatus; *cramps in the extremities, chorea, periodical neuralgia,* especially *sciatica,* various kinds of *paraplegia* or *partial paralysis,* general or partial *emaciation.*

If Broussais had proved the arsenic, it would have confirmed him in his favorite idea, that all diseases were originally a form of gastro-enteritis. But if, with the arsenic, he had at the same time studied all the analogues of this drug, he would have been obliged to admit that, if gastro-enteritis extend through the whole organism in such a manner as to constitute a general disease, or to simulate a multitude of heterogeneous affections, it is not possessed of the unity of principle which Broussais thought it had.

But it is useless to allude to Broussais' system, which at one time made such a stir in the world. At the present day, we are as far removed from it, as if six centuries had elapsed since the death of its author. Admitting, as I do, that a derangement of the digestive functions is one of the most constant effects of arsenic and its analogues, I am far from considering this derangement as an infallible and necessary effect of their action upon the organism, or from regarding all the other symptoms in the light in which Broussais would have viewed them, as dependencies of the gastric affection.

It is very probable that my arsenic group will sooner or later be modified by homœopathic physicians, although its general arrangements may perhaps be preserved. I shall be found willing to accept any modification suggested by reason and experience.

Arsenicum album.—*Arsenious acid*—white arsenic—*Deutoxyde of arsenic.*

This compound, which has been found in a free state in

nature, but seldom and in small quantities, is generally taken from cobalt mines. It is obtained by roasting the arseniferous ore, in reverberating furnaces, with long horizontal chimneys. The arsenic oxydizes, and is changed to arsenious acid, which condenses in these chimneys, where it is collected for the purpose of being purified by new processes of sublimation, after which it is fit for use in the arts and in medicine.

Arsenious acid is a solid substance, generally in semi-transparent pieces, like glass that has lost its polish, or of a dull white on the outside, but looks like glass on the broken edge, or it is sometimes entirely opaque. If pulverized, provided not too finely, the powder looks like sugar. Its specific weight is 3.738. Semi-vitreous, it dissolves in 103 parts of water at a temperature of 15°, and in 933 parts of boiling water; if opaque and white, it dissolves in 80 parts of water at 15°, and in 7.72 parts of boiling water. The taste of arsenious acid is at first very feeble, manifests itself slowly, and becomes at last slightly acid, like the taste of sour apples, according to Devergie.[1] It is inodorous, volatilizes like metallic arsenic at a dull red heat, and, like the metal, crystallises in tetraëdric needles. When thrown on burning embers, it develops a white smoke, *having the odor of garlic.* During this process the coal becomes decomposed and sets the metallic arsenic, to which this odor appertains, free; for if, instead of throwing it on the burning embers, it is only placed in a crucible or on a red-hot metallic plate, the white smoke which rises from the plate volatilizes without being decomposed, and remains completely inodorous.

Everybody is acquainted with the deleterious properties of arsenious acid, and the innumerable crimes which have been committed with arsenic, have excited prejudices against the therapeutic use of arsenic, which are far from being extinguished. The hydrated sesqui-oxyde of iron,[2] *if administered in season*, is the antidote of arsenic. I underline these words, *if administered in season*, for the iron preparations seem to

[1] Medecine Légale, vol. III., p. 410.

[2] Or, if necessary, *the sub-carbonate of iron.*

act only *chemically*, as antidotes to arsenic, that is to say, by changing it to an insoluble arseniuret of iron; whence it follows, that, if the sesqui-oxyde is not administered until the poison has been absorbed, the use of the iron becomes insufficient, and even entirely useless. In such cases experiments upon animals, which I made six or seven years ago, and which I have been unable to repeat since, for want of a suitable apartment, have shown me that the *watery extract of opium, in massive doses*, (from five to six centigrammes for middle-sized dogs,) was the *chief and best antidote of the arsenious acid*. Unfortunately, I have not been able to confirm this observation by a single case of poisoning in man, but the fact seems, nevertheless, of interest to toxicologists.

Empirical applications.—The ancients do not seem to have known either the metallic arsenic or the arsenious acid. *Orpiment* or the yellow sulphuret of arsenic, and especially the *realgar* or the red sulphuret of arsenic, are, according to the statement of Harles,[1] the only arsenical preparations in use among the Greeks, or even the Arabs of the 10th century. Several passages in Rhazès of Avicenna, lead me to believe that the Arabs used principally, the realgar internally against *cough* and *asthma*, and orpiment externally (against the *itch*, *tetters*, and *lepra*).

After having been abandoned almost entirely for several centuries, the arsenical preparations were again used externally by Theodore and Guy de Chanliac. The former used it in the treatment of *scrofulous ulcers;* the latter, as an escharotic, to open *hydroceles*.[2] At a later period the arsenical pastes were used for *cancer;* this disease being such a frightful disorder, it was not deemed improper to combat it by the most desperate means. These preparations, although they have been of very little use, and have caused many accidents, are still used in our time. Some of them have enjoyed great celebrity, such as the paste of Rausselot, of the Friar Cosme, the powders of Justamond and Plukket,

[1] De arsenici usu in medicina, Novinberg, 1811.

[2] Gmelin, appar. medic., vol. I., p. 259.

the pomatum of Hellmund, which was purchased by the Prussian government, and which does not differ essentially from that of Friar Cosme; the anti-cancerous remedy of Davidian, that of Guy, of Chenet, etc.[1] But homœopathy has nothing to do with these poor mystifications, which are but too often invented by quacks and by interested venders.

According to Desgranges,[2] Linserbarht, better known under the name of Lentitius, and who practised medicine towards the end of the seventeenth century, was the first who employed the arsenious acid internally, at least, in intermittent fevers. But in order not to abbreviate our remarks concerning the use of arsenic in these fevers, by attaching ourselves to the chronological order, let us postpone this important subject for the present, and let us cast a rapid glance on the other diseases for which this drug was recommended.

Cancer, cutaneous diseases, scrofula, syphilis, pulmonary phthisis, asthma, angina pectoris, various forms of *periodical headache, facial neuralgia, rheumatism, chorea,* and lastly, *rage,* these were the affections which empiricism, generally, when reduced to the last extremity, dared to combat with the white oxyde of arsenic. Success, was, however, far from crowning, in every instance, these bold attempts. But some cures were effected in these cases, which is sufficiently accounted for by the pathogenesis of arsenic.

CANCER.—"For a long time past, physicians have tried to combat cancer by the internal administration of arsenical preparations. Zeller is one of the first who praised arsenious acid for such a disease. Lefebure de St. Ildephont, Ronnow, Schmalz, Adair, Desgranges, etc., assure us to have seen

[1] See Gmelin, *loc. cit.*, and Mérat and Delens, *dict. de mat. méd.*, articles *arsenic* and *arsénicaux*, vol. I.

[2] *Usage de l' arsénic dans la médecine interne*, by Dr. Desgranges, of Lyons, (Journ. génre. de méd., vol. XXX., from page 241 to 264, first part, and from 303 to 372, second part.) This memoir which Thiébault answered by common place quotations from the *annuus medicus* of Storck, is well worthy of being read. See this answer of Thiébault in the 32d vol. of the same publication, page 3, etc.

good effects from it; Dr. Minniks, of Philadelphia, says the same thing, etc.[1]

Unfortunately, these are mere assertions supported by few facts, and of a doubtful authenticity. I do not think, however, that objections have been raised against the observations of either Ronnow or Minniks.[2] Even Thiébault, who is a zealous condemner of arsenic, takes care not to mention them in his answer to Desgranges, although this one alludes to both of them in his memoir. As regards the numerous cures which Lefebure, or rather, Lefebre de St. Ildephont boasts of having made with arsenic, I confess, that they seem to me rather doubtful. Even the title of his pamphlet published in 1774, would make me suspect them: *Approved remedy* for the radical cure of the *hidden, open, or ulcerated cancer, etc.* Approved by whom? Of nobody but the author, as we learn from an official declaration of Missa, who was then royal censor.[3] Lefebre, therefore, deceived the public, and, on this account, does not deserve any confidence.

But this is not all. The method which he points out in his pamphlet, had no success whatever in the hands of his warmest partisans. Desgranges, for instance, whom Mérat and Delens mention by mistake as one of the physicians who had seen good effects from the use of arsenic in cancer, expresses himself in these terms:—"As soon as Lefebre's pamphlet was published, we tried his remedy in the hospital of Lyons on several females affected with cancer at the breasts, groins, and uterus, following his prescriptions literally; not one of these patients was benefitted in the least; all experienced anxiety in the præcordial region, spasms, pains in the stomach and bowels, and other kinds of distress, which induced us to abandon our experiments.[4] Metzger and Fodéré were not any more fortunate. But ought we to infer from these failures that arsenious acid, if administered

[1] Mérat and Delens, *loc. cit.*

[2] *Mémoire de l'académie des sciences de Stockholm*, anneé, 1778.

[3] See Ancien Journ. de Med., vol. XLIV., p. 568.

[4] Mem. Cit., p. 356.

internally, and even after Lefebre's method,[1] has never cured cancer? Such is not my opinion, for negative facts do not invalidate facts that are positive. All that can be said is, that, as a general rule, these positive facts are exceedingly scarce in the annals of empiricism.

Cutaneous diseases.—Here we have an abundance of facts, and if we had no other authorities to consult than modern allœopathic physicians, their practice, except the doses, accords so perfectly with our own, that we might almost feel tempted to regard their mode of treating cutaneous diseases internally with arsenious acid, as copied from Hahnemann; but I really believe this is not the case. For as early as 1789, Adair published the happy results which he had obtained with arsenious acid, taken internally, in *obstinate tetters.*[2] Rush, of Philadelphia, confirmed Adair's observations about the same period. Lastly, in 1806, Girdlestone, but especially Willan and Pearson, in England, had popularized this use of arsenic by a number of successful cases, and Biett was one of the first who tried it in France. Cazenave expresses himself as follows concerning the use of arsenious acid in cutaneous diseases:[3]—"It is proven now-a-days, that wonderful results are obtained with arsenious acid in the treatment of cutaneous diseases, both in the dry forms and in the chronic eczema and intertrigo. This remedy is less successful in papulous eruptions, etc., and, in general, it has almost always failed in the various forms of porrigo, acne, sycosis, etc. It may be very useful in the elephantiasis of the Greeks; to the treatment of acute exanthemata, it is not applicable, as a general rule." Homœopathy can add but little to these statements.

[1] Lefebre prescribed four grains of arsenious acid in two pounds of water, of which the patient took every day a tablespoonful mixed with milk, hence about one-sixteenth per dose, which was gradually raised to one-eighth of a grain. This was accompanied with lotions or injections into the vagina with the same solution, the use of whey, etc. (See his pamphlet.)

[2] Med. comment. of a Soc. of phys., London, 1783–1789.

[3] *Dict. de Méd.*, in 30 volumes, article Arsenic. Compare Devergie, *Bullet. de l'acad. de méd.*, Paris, 1844, vol. IX., p. 1026.

Scrofula and syphilis.—A pretty large number of well-authenticated facts testify in favor of the efficacy of arsenic in certain forms of scrofulous ulcers. The observations of Physick, of Philadelphia, of Hans Roane, of Otto, concerning this subject, made a great noise among doctors at the period when they first appeared. Those which were published by Otto in 1805, in the *Philadelphia Medical Museum*,[1] are for us homœopaths extremely characteristic. He speaks of *malignant ulcers in the face, with caries of the bones and corrosion of the upper lip.* So much for scrofula. As regards syphilis, the facts are less evident. But could it be otherwise? The prejudice which has existed for upwards of two hundred years in favor of the absolute and exclusive specificity of mercury in venereal diseases, did not allow of the introduction of another anti-syphilitic which was not mercurial; and yet it is well known that the famous anti-syphilitic decoction of Teltz enjoys even yet in England, and more particularly in India, a very extensive popularity; and the active element of this decoction is a mixture of arsenic and antimony. Cullerier, a physician of our times, has even gone so far as to substitute a fixed dose of arsenic for this mixture, and has obtained the same favorable results. "In some venereal diseases, where mercury aggravates the syphilitic ulcers, Girdlestone arrests their progress with arsenical preparations."[2] Boudin, whose writings we shall have to mention more extensively when speaking of intermittent fevers, entertains the same opinion as I do concerning the anti-syphilitic properties of arsenious acid. "Science," says this author, "has a great many facts to show, where syphilis proved rebellious against mercury, and where the decoctions of Teltz and Arnould cured the disease as if by magic. As was remarked before, the influence of these preparations is principally due to the arsenic and antimony with which they are mixed. I am disposed to think, from some cases in my own

[1] Vol. I., p. 47.

[2] Desgranges, *mem. cit.*, p. 362.

practice, that arsenic may be a very useful remedy in constitutional syphilis."[1]

Pulmonary phthisis, asthma, neuralgia, etc. Although, according to Desgranges, Hippocrates, Galenus, and the Arabs, employed arsenical preparations for *a cough with purulent expectoration,* and notwithstanding a few dubious remarks by Girdlestone and Beddoes, I do not believe that *pulmonary phthisis* has ever been cured with arsenic. But I have not by any means the same doubts concerning the cure of *angina pectoris, humid asthma, with periodical paroxysms of nocturnal suffocation and œdema of the lower extremities and face, or even ascites and general leucophlegmasia* attributed to this drug. These cures are accounted for by the provings of Arsenic.

The same is true in regard to certain cures of *phthisis meseraica, facial neuralgia, periodical cephalalgia,* (of which Fodéré relates seven cases),[2] *whooping-cough, trismus, epilepsy* and various other nervous diseases, the observations concerning which are scattered through the works of authors. *Hydrophobia* even might perhaps be included among these latter diseases, although it is generally considered incurable, for the simple reason that it is generally treated with absurd means, or at a period when it has become impossible to cure it. In this respect we read in the dictionary of Mérat and Delens: "Russel, in his work on the serpents of India, relates three experiments which he instituted, with varied success, with the pills of Tanjore, composed in a great measure of arsenious acid, on animals that had been bitten by *poisonous serpents;* he says that he has given these pills with success to fourteen persons that had been bitten by *mad dogs,* but before hydrophobia had broken out."

J. P. Ireland employed arsenious acid in massive doses, in similar cases, with uniform success; he relates five cases. In

[1] *Traité des fièvres intermittentes, rémittentes et continues,* etc., Paris, 1842, p. 266.

[2] *Recherches expérimentales sur la valeur des différents rémèdes substitués au quinquina,* etc., Paris, 1809, in 8vo.

these cases, the acid brought about vomiting or stool.[1] According to all probability, the acid, if employed in infinitesimal doses, would likewise have prevented the paroxysms of hydrophobia, and the patient would not have been disturbed with vomiting or diarrhœa. We shall have to refer again to this subject when speaking of Belladonna. It now remains for us to inquire as cursorily as may be into that property of the arsenious acid which is considered the most important by the regular physicians, and which is not even denied by such men as Störk, Didier, Peyrilhe, etc.; who look upon arsenic as a poison that can only do harm, and should, on that account, be blotted out entirely from our materia medica. I mean the *specific curative character of arsenic in fever and ague;* a question which has now been under discussion for upwards of a hundred and fifty years, and bids fair to be continued a good while longer by the orthodox members of the faculty. And yet the facts that testify to the curative character of arsenic in this disease, are almost innumerable. Indeed, from Rosinus Lentilius, whom we have mentioned already, or rather from Hadrien Stevogt[2] and Melchoir Frick[3] to Joseph Plenciz,[4] that is to say, from the end of the 17th to the end of the 18th century, arsenious acid was used in Germany all the time in intermittent fevers. The violence with which this heroic agent was assailed by its contemners, seems a guarantee for the enthusiasm with which it was defended by its friends. At the head of the former we have the celebrated Störk, who carried on this warfare with all the vehemence and bitterness which he afterwards displayed in his attacks on animal magnetism. But Keil, Bernhardt, the two Plenciz, etc., warm partisans of the arsenic, backed their arguments by thousands of cures against which the diatribes of Störk remained powerless. Even at

[1] *Loc. Cit.*, *p.* 442.

[2] *De exceptionibus, sive permissione prohibitorum et prohibitione permissiorum*, Jena, 1700.

[3] *Paradoxa de Venetis*, Ulmæ, 1711.

[4] *Acta et observata medica.*, Viennæ, 1783.

the present moment a belief in the febrifuge properties of Arsenic has remained popular in Germany.[1]

The use of arsenic in the treatment of intermittent fever was introduced in England by Fowler, in America, by Barton, in Italy, by Brera, and, in these different countries, it produced the same results which had been obtained in Germany for a century previous. But in France these decided successes were unable to conquer altogether the prejudice which this terrible name arsenic had excited among the people. Nothing short of the complete closure of the seas during the empire, was able to determine a few physicians to try arsenic as a substitute for Peruvian bark. Fodéré, Lordat, C. L. Dufour, A. Boullier, J. C. Dupont, Desgranges, etc., were the principal authors of this innovation, which, in spite of its success, excited a good deal of opposition.[2] Finally, as soon as the peace of 1815 had rendered to the French allœopaths their bark, they speedily abandoned the arsenic, which was indeed completely forgotten until recently, when one of our army-physicians tried to restore its use.

Boudin, physician-in-chief of the military hospital du Roule, is a distinguished thinker, well-informed, and in possession of that vast experience which a military physician is almost alone capable of acquiring, by studying the diseases in different countries and in different latitudes. I add that Boudin, if he was not an entire homœopath, was very near becoming one in 1842, when, in his capacity of physician-in-chief of the hospital of Marseilles, he published his *treatise on fevers*. He has read Hahnemann, quotes him two or three times, and speaks of him with respect. If he does not accept his doctrine altogether, he uses at least some of Hahnemann's proceedings. It is difficult to understand why Boudin, after having gone so far, should not have gone still farther, or should ever have endeavoured, as we shall see bye-and-bye, to retract himself.

[1] Especially in Prussia, where Prof. Schœnlein of Berlin employs this drug quite considerably.

[2] See *Journ. génér. de méd.*, vol. XLIII., p. 242.

Be this as it may, I regard Boudin's work as one of the best productions of modern allœopathy, in point of thought, originality and keenness of observation. Few works have afforded me more pleasure, and excited a higher degree of interest in my mind. This monograph is distinguished from most other monographs in this, that the details which are sometimes as new as they are ingenious, are always governed by a truly generalizing mind.

Boudin states and limits very clearly the question he desires to discuss: the *marsh-intermittent miasm*. According to him, *the type*, that is to say, the intermission, the remission, or the continuity of the febrile symptoms, does not constitute the characteristic manifestation of a particular malady, nor even of a special class of diseases. Indeed a number of very different affections may likewise assume the intermittent type, in the same manner as a number of poisons may, according to Hahnemann, whose authority our author invokes, cause a series of intermittent symptoms. We may remark here in passing, that this sound observation shows how absurd it is on the part of our opponents, to treat all intermittent fevers with one and the same drug. This is the real cause of the want of success in the treatment of intermittent fevers with Peruvian bark, and of the cachexias which are developed almost every day by the injudicious use of this drug.

In regard to marsh-intermittents, Boudin is of opinion that the phenomena of intermission, remission and continuity only express the different degrees of intensity with which the fever-miasm acts upon the organism. "If we consider attentively," says he, "the manner in which the phenomena of marsh-intermittents develop themselves, either in different latitudes, or during the change of the seasons, or lastly at different degrees of elevation above the level of the soil, we would be struck with the relation which exists uniformly and strictly between the type of the disease and the intensity of the miasm, and which is so exactly proportionate that a progression in the *quantity* of miasmatic matter, arising from the focus of the disease, carries with it a corresponding increase of *continuity* in the type of fever.

The tertian type, which prevails in the North of Europe, is replaced in warmer countries by the quotidian, remittent and even continuous type. On the other hand, as the heat increases, we see in the North of Africa a succession of types develop itself, which is analogous to the changes that take place in the type of the marsh-intermittents in proportion as we come nearer to the equator, so that the tertian winter-fevers of the North of Africa are gradually succeeded by quotidian, *remittent*, and even *continuous* fevers."[1]

This theory seems correct, and Boudin supports it by proofs which it seems difficult to gainsay. However, if it be true, as he says, that the tendency of the type to become continuous, is in exact proportion to the intensity of the miasm, how shall we account for the intermissions in cases of *febris perniciosa*, a malady which terminates fatally after the second or third paroxysm, unless it is arrested before? The violence of the paroxysms is a sure sign of the intensity of the miasm. Why then are not such fevers *continuous*, more than any other? Upon the whole, it cannot be denied, and Boudin himself will admit this, that, if the intermission of the paroxysms is not sufficient to characterize a disease, this strange and remarkable periodicity of the symptoms, does not, however, belong indiscriminately, and in the same degree, to all known maladies, no more than all drugs are equally capable of producing or arresting the intermittent disease. Would not arsenic, for instance, which is praised by Stevogt, Frick, Fowler, Pearson, Fodéré, etc., as the greatest remedy for intermittent diseases, be one of those drugs or poisons, which, if taken in feeble doses, would produce effects that are characterized by the intermittent type, more than those of any other drug? "I have seen," says Boudin, "a *quotidian* intermittent fever, for which I had to give cinchona, develope itself in the case of one of my patients, who, in the space of twelve days, had taken twenty-

[1] Loc. Cit., p. 120.

four hundredths of a grain of arsenious acid for ichthyosis. Was this a simple coincidence? I do not know; the fact, however, is, that this patient, with the exception of his cutaneous disease, enjoyed the best health, and that his fever came on at a period when no other similar disease prevailed in town."[1] This single fact proves nothing in the estimation of Boudin, and I understand the reason why. Biett, however, admits having observed similar phenomena in the hospital of St. Louis, and I have no doubt that, by ransacking authors, a number of other similar facts might easily be obtained. If I am not mistaken, Morgagni mentions one or two cases of this kind. But what would be the use of such inquiries? Boudin knows as well as I do, that all the symptoms of the marsh-intermittent fever, which he terms *limnhemic fever* or rather *affection*, from the simple *diarrhœic* to the *tetanic form*, are contained in the pathogenesis of the white oxyde of arsenic by Hahnemann and his disciples.

According to Boudin, every *limnhemic affection*, without distinction of type or development of its phenomena, arises from one and the same cause, but multiple in its unity, as we shall see bye and bye, namely, the effluvia of the marsh-vegetation. In this respect, our author believes, and I am disposed to share this belief, that it is not by the effluvia of stagnant water, nor by the emanations of decayed vegetable matter that the marsh-miasm is produced, but by the emanations arising from *living plants*. Some of these plants are already known. Such are, among others, the *chara vulgaris*, the *rizophorus*, the *calamus*, and the *anthoxanthum odoratum*, which, according to Nepples, abounds in the marshes of the Bresse, where it goes by the name of *flouve;* and lastly, according to Humboldt, the roots of the *mangrove tree*, and of the *mancanilla*, which, when not covered by water, are supposed by the inhabitants of India to be productive of fever. But how can we admit the identity of the marsh-miasm, when the fever-engendering miasms vary so much among each other? According to Boudin, the endemic

[1] See page 262.

intermittent fevers of the department of Aix in France, those of the North of Africa, of Morea, of Senegal, of the deltas of the Ganges, Nile and Mississippi, that is to say, the cholera, the plague, and the yellow fever, are forms of one and the same disease, or rather, different degrees of its intensity. "It is not only," says he, "between the ordinary endemic diseases of marshy countries, that this identity exists, and I should not think having done more than to merely lift the veil under which the truth is hidden, if I contented myself with simply pointing out the identity that exists between the intermittent, remittent, continuous and masked intermittent fevers, and the endemic diarrhœas and dysenteries of marshy regions. I have seen several times, in the North of Africa, the marsh-miasmatic diseases, not only simulate, but so faithfully express the cholera of India, that it was absolutely impossible to decide from the first, whether the disease was the real cholera or simply a *sporadic cholera fever*. In another case, which, it is true, is an isolated observation, I saw in the marshes of Navarin, in Morea, a *febris icterica perniciosa, with vomiting of black matter*, resembling tolerably well the yellow fever of the West-Indies. And in this same campaign of Greece, in 1828, I have observed among persons who had died with these severe marsh-intermittent fevers, an unusual swelling of the ganglions of the groin and neck, a symptom which greatly resembles a similar phenomenon in the disease of Constantinople and Alexandria."[1]

Independently of the symptomatic resemblance which is really remarkable in many cases, this author infers the identity of the nature of these diseases from two series of facts: 1st. From a sort of antagonism which *all* these diseases exhibit in regard to such affections as *pulmonary phthisis* and *typhus*, and which antagonism is so decided, that these different classes of diseases never co-exist in the same locality; 2d. From the fact that they are all cured by the same drug, which is *arsenious acid*.

[1] *Traité des fiévres intermittentes, rémittentes et continues des pays chauds et des contrées marécageuses*, Paris, 1842, p. 154.

Omitting this question of antagonism, however interesting it may be,[1] I hasten to admit with Boudin the efficacy of arsenious acid in all the diseases mentioned by him, or rather, I rejoice to think that he admits it with me; for I do not think that allœopathy can claim as its practice the use of arsenic in *vomiting*, *diarrhœa*, *cramps*, and other symptoms of cholera; but is this efficacy, as our author seems to think, an irrefragable proof of the identity of these diseases? To admit this identity, would imply the supposition that one and the same drug is not able to cure two apparently different diseases: an untenable hypothesis which is contradicted by thousands of facts. Upon the whole, I suppose that it is with the marsh-miasm as with psora; as I said above, it is at the same time *one and yet multiple.* But what would be of the highest interest to science in my estimation, would be to determine, by inquiries made in the different localities where marsh-intermittents are endemic, to what kind of marsh vegetation such and such a form of marsh-intermittent corresponds most generally if not specially.

As we said above, Boudin treats almost all limnhemic affec-

[1] If the antagonism which seems to exist between typhus and the marsh-intermittents, is a curious fact, though without any practical interest, this cannot be said of a similar antagonism existing between these intermittents and pulmonary phthisis. Temperate climates, or the shores of Madeira, Nice, or Italy, in general, are the regions which are generally recommended by physicians to their phthisicky patients. (See the work of Dr. Carriere: *le climat de l'Italie sous le rapport hygiénique et médical*, Paris, 1849.) The enormous mortality of consumptive patients on Malta, at Gibraltar, Corfu, and especially Naples, show that neither the warmth of the climate as is generally believed, nor the neighbourhood of the sea, as was supposed by Culler and Laënnec, can even arrest, much less cure, phthisis. Well, according to Boudin, whose assertions are based upon almost undeniable statistical facts, the marshes of Romagna, the whole of the north-west coast of Africa, the delta of the Nile, and even, despite a pretty cold temperature, the delta of the Rhine, and the marshy regions of Lancashire in England, offer all pulmonary patients an almost certain protection. (See in reference to *antagonism*, the *Annales d'hyg. publiq.*, vol. XXXIII., p. 58; vol. XXXVI., p. 5, 368; vol. XXXVIII., p. 237. *Bulletin de l'Acad. de méd.*, vol. VIII., p. 931, 936, 948; vol. IX., p. 212; vol. X., p. 1041.) The value and reason of these facts will have to be determined by experimentation.

tions, without regard to symptoms, by arsenious acid; and, in this respect, his practice is, in almost every case, perfectly conformable to the demands of homœopathy. This will be admitted by any one who has observed the various morbid manifestations of the marsh-miasm, and who, like Boudin, has studied Hahnemann's pathogenesis of arsenious acid. The physician-in-chief of the hospital of Marseilles is, therefore, knowingly a homœopath, so far at least as the treatment of limnhemic affections with arsenic is concerned; and all that seems left for settlement between him and us, seems the dose. The following passage bears upon this point: "After commencing in my experiments, with one twenty-fourth part of a grain, I gradually became convinced, together with a number of other physicians who obtained results perfectly similar to my own, that arsenious acid, if suitably prepared, preserves even at the small dose of one-hundredth part of a grain, all its medicinal energy, not only in the treatment of marsh-intermittents, but also in that of a number of other diseases. With a single dose of the one-hundredth part of a grain, I have often removed radically fevers that had been contracted in Algiers or on the Senegal, and which had resisted any kind of treatment, even the sulphate of quinine and a change of climate."[1] But this is not all. What vehicle would you think Boudin uses for the administration of his almost infinitesimal doses of arsenic? distilled water, which is used for all mineral preparations, and which is particularly adapted to the white oxyde of arsenic, which *is almost tasteless* and dissolves in this liquid? Not at all; like Hahnemann, Boudin prefers the *sugar of milk* to distilled water. It is true he allows every dose to be dissolved in water, but he directs, like Hahnemann, that the arsenic and the sugar should be previously triturated for a time. Here is his formula:

℞ Arsenious acid—one centigramme, ($\frac{1}{5}$ of a grain).

Add gradually, in small quantities:

Pulverized sugar of milk—one gramme, (20 grains).

[1] *Oper. Cit.*, p. 276.

Triturate in a glass mortar for a sufficient length of time (at least 10 minutes) to mix these substances well together, and divide the whole into 20 packages, each containing one-half a milligramme, or the $\frac{1}{100}$ of a grain of arsenious acid.

"This preparation," says the author, "is the one which I use most frequently; a package is dissolved in a spoonful of water, and the solution taken five or six hours before the time when the paroxysm is expected to set in.

"This formula is likewise applicable in obstinate cutaneous affections, and in inveterate syphilis."[1]

The following list shows that, in spite of the smallness of the doses, Boudin's results, which he obtained in 1842, were at least as satisfactory as those which had been obtained formerly with much larger doses by Fowler,[2] Fodéré, Lordat, etc.:

DISEASES.	Which had not been previously treated with any other medicine.	Resisting the bark, and cured with arsenic.	Resisting the arsenic, and cured with bark.	Resisting both bark and the arsenic.	TOTAL.
Quotidian fevers,	102	19	4	3	128
Tertian fevers,	53	11	3	0	67
Quartan fevers,	2	4	1	2	9
Quintan fevers,	1	2	0	0	3
Irregular fevers,	18	13	2	2	35
Fevers called masked,	12	8	1	1	24
Total of results,	118	57	13	8	266

[1] *Oper. Cit.*, p. 313.

[2] Of 240 fever-patients treated with his solution, Fowler cured only 171. (See his work: *Medical Reports on the effects of arsenic in the cure of agues, remitt. fevers, and period. headaches*, London, 1786.) Fodéré (*loc. cit.*) is still less fortunate than Fowler; lastly, Lordat, (*Journ. gén. de méd.*, vol. XXIII., p. 281,) accuses arsenic of leaving after the cure of the fever, a bloating of the face or even of the whole body, which has to be removed by means of the *safran de mars apéritif*, (an antidote of arsenic.)

Thus then, in 266 cases of intermittent fever, of various forms and types, the arsenious acid, administered only on the days of the paroxysms, and omitted during the apyrexia, (this was Boudin's method,) failed only in twenty-one cases, although it was only given in doses of $\frac{1}{100}$ of a grain. In these twenty-one cases, however, quinine was not more fortunate than arsenic. What is to be inferred from this fact? This truth, which homœopathic physicians should well bear in mind, that there is no *absolute specific*, and that there may even be cases of marsh intermittent which may resist both arsenic and quinine, and which the peculiar constitution, temperament, or idiosyncratic conditions of the patient may require to be treated with some other drug.

But if the arsenic is not always a specific for fevers which we know positively to have been induced by marshy effluvia, its specific character becomes still more doubtful in cases of unknown origin, existing at a distance from the focus of the marsh-epidemic, and having nothing in common with this latter disease than a small number of symptoms and the intermission of the paroxysms. Every homœopath knows that, in such a case, some fifteen or twenty drugs claim his attention as much as arsenic. Can it be, perhaps, considerations of this kind which have induced Boudin to modify his original treatment of *intermittent fevers*, and not to prescribe the arsenic until the patient has been previously vomited with a dose of ipecac, or stibium, and to give *five or six grains a day?* According to the last edition of the *traité de thérapeutique*, by Trousseau and Pidoux, Vol. I., p. 261, the present method of the physician in chief of the hospital du Roule, is as follows:—

First rule.—Commence the treatment with an emetic, (ipecacuanha one gramme; stibium one décigramme,) if the fever is accompanied with gastric symptoms, suppression or diminution of the appetite.

After the fever has been arrested, give another emetic, provided the appetite is not entirely restored; in order to allow the patient to use as soon as possible a substantial and generous diet.

Second rule.—Give arsenious acid in fractional doses, that is to say, one dose divided into several, the last dose to be given at least two hours before the time when the paroxysm is expected to come on; proportion the dose according to the character of the fever, which varies according to locality, season, and the individuality of the patient.

Give the arsenious acid according to tolerance, so as to gradually arrive at the largest possible dose, giving every *quarter of an hour* one milligramme, or only half a milligramme, (one gramme or half a gramme of the solution.)[1]

As the patient bears less of the arsenic, diminish the dose gradually, and continue the fractional mode of administration; if necessary, give the drug partially or totally by the rectum.

Take the drug both on the days of the paroxysms and during the apyrexia.

Continue it during an interval proportionate to the duration of the disease, and to its resistance to other and previously instituted modes of treatment. In a first attack of the disease, the drug should be continued at least for a week after the last paroxysm, etc.

Third rule.—Use a substantial and abundant diet, to be limited by the appetite and the digestive powers of the patient. The diet to consist principally of beef, roast mutton; a generous wine to be ordered, in quantities proportionate to the weakened state of the constitution of the patient; watery beverages to be avoided as much as possible.

All this is very different, as is seen, from Boudin's former practice. I confess I am unable to say how far his present method is superior to his former mode of treatment. Does every case of intermittent fever yield to grain doses of arsenic, even such cases as proved refractory to the $\frac{1}{100}$ part of a grain? I can scarcely believe it; or is it, according to Trousseau and Pidoux, because this mode of treatment does

[1] This shows that the sugar of milk is given up.

away with the necessity of using quinine? If this be so, is the complete abolition of the use of quinine a rational proceeding? Upon the whole, what seems to me to result most clearly from this new method of Boudin, is, first, that by means of certain accessory medicinal agents, and of certain hygienic combinations, we succeed in enabling patients to bear truly poisonous doses of arsenious acid; secondly, that this *tolerance*, all other things being equal, is proportionate to the intensity of the disease; this, however, is nothing new either to homœopaths or to the partisans of counter-stimulation. Who does not know that as many as twelve grains of the extract of opium have been given in *delirium tremens*, and as many as one hundred grains of stibium in *pneumonia?* Be this as it may, I will endeavour to account for this tolerance of the massive doses of arsenious acid in Boudin's treatment.

As we said, in speaking of the analogies of mercury, to which the arsenious acid belongs, (See page 99,) this substance is essentially depressing in its general action upon the general organism. Hence strong constitutions resist its action much better than constitutions that are naturally feeble and of a lower order of vitality, *without however being sick;* for, in such a case, the conditions of the problem might be completely changed. This is the reason why herbivorous animals, such as rabbits, chickens, etc., are readily killed by small doses of arsenic, and carnivorous animals bear, on the contrary, enormous quantities of the poison; *one ounce* of arsenic, which Reaumur gave to a bear, had no other effect on the animal than to purge it; and, in the East of France, our peasants know perfectly well that arsenic will not destroy wolves, and other dangerous or hurtful carnivorous beasts; for, it was in vain that whole pounds of arsenic were stuffed into pieces of meat, and left on the snow, along the edges of the woods, or in the midst of the thickets inhabited by these animals.

But, it may be replied, these facts simply point to a general law that has been known for a long time past. Who does not know that lions, tigers, and wolves, have a more tenacious life than horses, rabbits, and hens? It is not, therefore, to be wondered that these weaker animals are less capable than the former, of resisting the action of arsenic. I answer; if it be true that carnivorous animals resist destructive agents much better than herbivorous or granivorous animals; *there are, however, some poisons*, as we said page 55, *which are an exception to this rule, and act more powerfully on carnivorous than on herbivorous animals.* This is not an empty speculation; the nux vomica will be sufficient, hereafter, to demonstrate the truth of my remark.

If now we consider that, in all animals, and also in man, who, as respects his physical organization, is at the same time a carnivorous and herbivorous animal, the destructive action of arsenious acid, is inversely proportionate to the degree of vitality possessed by each animal; if we consider, moreover, that this vitality depends in a great measure upon the kind of diet pursued by each species and individual, we cannot fail to comprehend how Boudin's patients find in the exclusively animal diet which he prescribes for them, a sort of immunity against the excessive doses of arsenious acid used in the treatment of their diseases. Besides, ipecacuanha and stibium, (especially the former, as is well known by all homœopathic physicians,) neutralize in a measure the effects of arsenic; hence it follows, that Boudin administers the poison with one hand, and with the other the antidote. If his patients improve under this method, I have nothing to say against it, for the true medicine is that which cures. I confess, however, that, until I am further enlightened, I shall believe that Boudin was nearer the truth in 1842, than he now is.

If we will now take the trouble to reflect on what has been said, we shall obtain an explanation of a series of truths which the homœopathic applications of arsenic confirm every day. Thus:

1. Arsenic being capable of producing, in a healthy person, the general depression of the vitality, (cacochymia) which

the constant and exclusive use of a vegetable diet, (especially when consisting of herbs and watery fruits) almost always occasions, it follows, by virtue of the law of similitude, that arsenic, which is a most violent poison for individuals impoverished by a low diet, is, on the other hand, most admirably adapted to their constitutions and a majority of their maladies, if given in infinitesimal doses.[1]

2. Arsenic is essentially, and in almost every person, adapted to acute diseases, (indigestions, etc.) accidentally occasioned by the excessive use of herbacious food, (melons, strawberries, fruits in general, but more particularly watery fruits.) The diseases which arise from the abuse of vegetables, and those which are occasioned by arsenious acid, are in every respect, identical in form.

8. Lastly, arsenic seems to be, in the majority of cases, the *specific* remedy of sporadic or epidemic diseases, caused by vegetable emanations. It is to be remarked, that, in the very acute diseases which belong to this category, the *cholera*, *yellow fever*, the *febris perniciosa* and the *plague*, the patient, whatever be his constitution, seems to sink in a few hours in the lowest state of cacochymia, such as our marsh-effluvia only produce slowly, after a long lapse of time, and then only incompletely.

However, these are very general, and very vague considerations concerning the therapeutic virtues of arsenious acid. We have to study the pathogenesis of this drug, in order to obtain a knowlege of the manifold applications of which it is capable in the treatment of disease.[2]

Homœopathic applications.—The dynamised arsenious acid has been found useful in the following affections:—

Affections of persons exhausted by excesses or a bad diet,

[1] This is the reason why allœopathic physicians who have never known how to distinguish the physiological and dynamic action of drugs, class arsenic at one time among the *debilitants* and, at another time, among the *tonics*. I dare affirm that this remark embodies a general law: any drug is best adapted to a constitution which, in a normal state, is most easily affected by the poisonous action of the same drug.

[2] See the pathogenesis of arsenic in Hahnemann's *Chronic Diseases*, vol. I.

of a lymphatico-nervous constitution, irritable, disposed to sadness, to mucous discharges, to dropsy and *tetters; endemic affections which prevail among the inhabitants of low and marshy districts; cachexias occasioned by abuse of mercury, iodine*, and especially *quinine; partial or general atrophy; constitutional syphilis;* pale bloating and softening of the tissues; glandular engorgements; *paroxysms of fever, neuralgia* or *general weakness returning at fixed hours or days; paroxysms of anxiety at night, compelling one to rise from bed;* shuddering in the evening, with pandiculations and agitation; aggravation of the pains during rest; bone-pains; *aggravation of the pains, when lying on the affected parts;* pains which are felt during sleep; hypochondriac mood; compunctions of conscience, as if one had committed a bad deed; periodical paroxysms of hysteria, epilepsy, and paralysis; weakness of the memory and of the other intellectual faculties; passing excitability, followed by weakness of the senses; *mental derangement*, with tears and ominous wanderings and expressions; furious delirium; with desire to bite, as in hydrophobia; earthy, blueish, cadaverous color of the skin; burning itching, which is intolerable, and is not appeased by scratching; sanguinolent pemphigus; *malignant variola;* eruption consisting of red, rounded and burning spots; red pimples, which break and form spreading ulcers; *chronic impetigo and eczema; elephantiasis of the Greeks;* ulcers with raised and callous borders, surrounded with a red and shining areola, lardaceous or blackish bottom, and a burning pain which is eased by warmth and aggravated by cold; ichorous and fetid suppuration of the ulcers; suppression of all suppuration, with aggravation of the pain; heaviness in the forehead; headache on leaving the table; stupefying, pressive, pulsative headache; vertigo even to falling, especially in the evening, when sitting, or rather, on rising after having been sitting for a time; *excessively painful hemicrania*, in paroxysms, with viscid sweat and icy coldness of the hairy scalp, and a violent itching after every paroxysm; ulcerations at the hairy scalp; falling out of the hair and beard; swelling of the head, face and neck, sometimes enormous; *inflammation of the eyes*, with photophobia; wrenching pain in the bottom of the orbits, which is sometimes frightful; protrusion of the balls of the eyes, and profuse discharge, even in complete darkness, of corrosive tears; icy coldness at the eyes during the paroxysms of pains; contraction of the pupils; muscæ volitantes; congestion and hypertrophy of the vessels of the cornea, whence arises the phenomenon of a blackish or whitish gauze, which intercepts the visual ray; *amaurosis;* œdematous swelling; excessive dryness or continual trembling of the eyelids; noise in the ears; *otalgia;* weakness of hearing; hippocratic face; pullings and stitches in the face here and there; dull pain in the nasal bones; *red tetters on the forehead and cheeks;* acne rosacea; chapping and swelling of the lips; bleeding of the gums; dry mouth, or else filled with a viscous, bitter, sometimes bloody saliva; wrenching toothache, worse in the cold; looseness and falling out of the teeth; *foul smell from the mouth; taste as of foul flesh in the mouth and throat;* aphthæ in the mouth; tongue coated, cracked, ulcerated, brownish, blackish, tremulous: scratching in the throat between the acts of swallowing; sort of paralysis of the pharynx and œsophagus, which renders deglutition almost impossible; *gangrenous angina;* aversion to cooked food; desire for milk, fruits and coffee; *habitual difficulty of digesting vegetables and milk*, which cause acidity and flatulence; burning thirst, or rather, constant desire to nourishing the mouth and throat with a cold liquid; *periodical paroxysms of bulimy;* hiccough and *sour* or putrid eructations after every meal; nausea with flow of water from the mouth, after every meal; *indigestion caused by fruits or milk;* violent vomiting of brownish substances; *excessively acute gastritis; yellow fever; sporadic and Asiatic cholera; chronic disposition to nausea and vomiting;* subacute gastritis occasioned by a metallic body in the stomach; heaviness at the stomach; *burning pain in the stomach*, and epigastrium; *pyrosis;* distension and excessive sensitiveness of the epigastric region, with anxiety and a feeling of embarrassment in the præcordia, as if the heart would be crushed; tetters at the epigastrium; induration of the liver; *heat in the bowels;* excessive bellyache, especially on the left side; flatulence having a putrid smell; pain in the abdomen, as from a sore or burn; cold and viscous sweat on the abdomen; ulcer at the umbilicus; *ascites;* smarting stools, with violent colic; green diarrhœic stools; *lienteria; dysentery;* constipation; painful prolapsus of the rectum; *ascarides;* burning piles; swelling of the groins; paralysis of the bladder; difficulty of urinating; strangury: swelling of the genital organs; *gangrene of chimney-sweep;* momentary excitement of the sexual desire, *followed by impotence;* lascivious excitement in women; premature, pale, profuse menses, which last too long; dysmenorrhœa; amenorrhœa, with acrid discharge from the vagina.

Stoppage of the nostrils; violent coryza; dryness and burning at the larynx; blood-spitting; *paroxysms of suffocation, in the evening after lying down;* oppression on the chest when going up hill; whooping-cough; *angina pectoris;* stitches in the sternum; pressure at the sternum; pulling and tearing pains from the elbow to the axilla, at night; tearings and pullings in the hip, thigh and groin; cramps in the thighs; *sciatica;* tearing in the tibia; contusive pain in the knee-joint; itching tetters at the bend of the knee, old ulcers on the legs causing heat and stitches; weariness in the legs; varices; *spreading ulcers on the soles of the feet, and at the big toes;* smarting pain at the toes when walking.

The symptoms caused by arsenic seem to assume a nervous form the higher the attenuations with which the provings were instituted. Thence it follows that the lower attenuations of arsenic are more particularly adapted to organic affections, and especially to the very acute affections of the bowels. We know indeed from experience that the 12th dilution of arsenic was much more efficacious in cholera than the 30th; having had an attack of the cholera in 1849, I have very accurately observed the differences on my own person.

Ipecac., *veratr. alb.*, *China*, *Nux vom.*, and especially *Camph.*, are, according as such or such symptoms predominate, the best antidotes to arsenic.

Veratrum Album. *White hellebore.* Genus *veratrum*, family *Colchiacea*, class *hexandria triandria.*

This plant which grows in Europe, and especially in France, in the pastures of Auvergne, Vosges, the Jura, Alps and Pyrenees, has a tuberous, obtuse root, from one to two inches long, an erect stem, large oval lanceolate leaves, flowers in ramose, terminal tufts, of a pale-green color; fruit with three ovoid shells, containing flat, winged, numerous seeds. The mother tincture is prepared from the dry, pulverized root of the plant, and macerated in alcohol for five or six days.

Veratrum album is a violent poison. Three drachms of its root have killed a dog of middle size. Dr. Gahier, who treated dogs affected with the itch, by washing them with a decoction of this root, saw them fall immediately into a state of lethargy; they uttered plaintive and painful cries, vomited, their sides were agitated, the pulse was rapid, the eyes looked wild, as if the animals had had an epileptic fit, or had been mad.[1] When applied to the skin while recent, it acts like a caustic, and speedily occasions a burning redness and blisters; when cooked and placed upon the stomach, it causes vomiting.

Empirical applications. Almost abandoned by the Schools in consequence of its violent action on the animal economy, *veratrum album* enjoyed an immense reputation in antiquity for several centuries. In 1812, Hahnemann published a memoir on the subject of veratrum, entitled: *dissertatio historico-medica de helleborismo veterum.* This memoir contains 1st, interesting inquiries concerning the identity of the white hellebore of the Greeks and our *veratrum album;* 2d, a complete account of the *helleborismus* of the ancients, a

[1] Mérat and Delens, *op. cit.*, vol. VI., p. 858.

method of treatment which constituted, so to say, a medical doctrine by itself. This memoir, so full of facts, is not one of the most useful, at least one of the most curious documents which he has left us. The principal fact which we learn from this memoir, is the great importance which the ancients attached to veratrum.

In those times, this plant was the remedy for all desperate ailments. Patients who were supposed to be incurable, repaired in crowds to Anticyra, a city in Greece, where the veratrum treatment was more particularly pursued, and some of these patients came home again cured. "Spring," says Hahnemann, "was the season which the physicians of old deemed most favorable to evacuations by veratrum; next to spring came autumn; and, if they had to choose between summer and winter, they preferred summer for vomiting, and winter for the purgations.

"The affections for which helleborism was recommended, were asthma, cough, internal ulcers, such as pulmonary and hepatic phthisis, for example, hæmoptysis, even when the patient seemed otherwise well (they dreaded the rupture of a vein in the lungs, especially in thin persons with a narrow chest and a long neck, that is to say a phthisicky *habit*, for such subjects have almost always tubercles in the chest, a difficult respiration and a violent cough;) affections of the throat and neck; pains at the cardiac orifice in individuals that vomit with difficulty; lienteria; incipient cataract; headaches with occasional violent pains, redness of the face and distention of the vessels; lastly, hysteric suffocations."[1]

Hellebore, continues Hahnemann, was prohibited in fevers, except in some cases of quartan fever. The vomiting caused by hellebore, seemed likewise unfavorable to stout persons, or to plethoric individuals and persons subject to attacks of fainting. Persons of little nerve, no matter with what disease they were affected, were unable to bear a treatment which required much courage and energy.

The extreme violence of this treatment was the reason why

[1] Op. Cit., p. 192

it was not resorted to in the cases mentioned by Hahnemann. But these exclusions, some of which were indeed founded in reason, rested mostly upon the false inferences derived from the doctrine of contraria. Allœopathic physicians of our times would not argue that, in order to prescribe arsenic with advantage, the digestive organs must be first in good condition; this would simply be nonsense.

"The cases where hellebore was principally employed, were *long-lasting and violent diseases, without fever; mental derangements; melancholia; pains in the feet and coxo-femoral articulation of long standing; pains in the joints; incipient gout; epilepsy; spasms of the facial muscles; indolence of mind; loss of consciousness* (apoplexy); *vertigo* with gloominess of the brain; *chronic paralysis; obstinate headaches; languor; elephantiasis and other exanthemata; baldness; falling out of the beard; nightmare;* confirmed *hydrophobia;* nephritic *calculus; crudities* of long standing; *ptyalism of the pancreas; diseases of the spleen, goitre, hidden cancer*, although veratrum did not suit genuine ulcers; and lastly, an almost innumerable multitude of diseases."[1]

Notwithstanding the testimony of Ætius, Rufus, Celsius, Plinius, and others, we cannot admit that veratrum was indicated and useful in all these diseases. This drug, as administered by the doctors of Ancyra, was, upon the whole, no better than a monstrous panacea, the ravages of which were carefully hidden and the good effects exposed; which is, however, the rule with all panaceas.

Be this as it may, helleborism fell into disrepute at the period of Galenus, who contributed to its downfall by his own theories. In the middle age, it was entirely abolished; so much so that Murray does not tell us anything about veratrum, except that the Spanish hunters dipped the points of their arrows into the juice of veratrum, which rendered them so poisonous that wounds inflicted with these weapons became immediately fatal.[2] Modern physicians and botanists do not seem to know exactly what the plant was which the ancients

[1] Op. Cit., p. 198. [2] Appar. Med., vol. V., p. 145.

made use of under the name of hellebore: witness the article hellebore, in the *dictionary of the medical sciences*,[1] whose author confounds all the time our *veratrum album* with the other varieties of hellebore, which, however, differ a good deal from each other with respect to their medicinal properties.[2]

Homœopathic Applications.—Between the symptoms of hellebore and those of arsenious acid there exists the most striking analogy; so much so that these two remedies have frequently been administered in similar diseases, such as *cinchona*, *cachexia*, *gastritis and gastro-enteritis; colic*, *constipation*, *diarrhœa*, *lienteria*, *ascarides*, *dysentery*, *sporadic and epidemic cholera*, *ascites*, *periodical cephalalgia and ophthalmia; cough*, *asthma*, *whooping-cough*, *dysmenorrhœa*, *hysteria*, *chorea*, *periodical fevers and neuralgias*, *cramps in the lower extremities*, *sciatica*, *paralysis*, *emaciation*, *exanthemata* of various kinds, *weakness of the senses and intellect*, *mental derangement*, *etc*. But does this imply that arsenic and veratrum can be prescribed indifferently in these diseases? This would be an absurd supposition. It is unfortunately true that a physician may sometimes have to hesitate between these two drugs; nevertheless, if he does choose either, his choice must be based upon some rational preferences, suggested not only by symptomatic differences, such as I shall point out bye-and-bye, but principally by the constitution, temperament, and habitual mode of life of his patient.

It is almost always in the regions where maladies originate, that Providence seems to have created the means for their removal.[3] The white hellebore is neither found in valleys nor in marshy plains, but on the slopes of mountains. Analogy leads us, therefore, to think that this drug is much more appropriate to the sanguine and lively temperament of mountaineers than to the phlegmatic, *diluted* temperament,

[1] Vol. XI., p. 436.

[2] See the pathog. of verat. alb. in Roth's Mat. Med., pur., vol. II., p. 386.

[3] I have already alluded to this important point in my introduction, (page 52); I cannot sufficiently recommend it to the attention of my readers, and shall revert to it again on more than one occasion.

if I may so express myself, of the inhabitants of low and damp regions. My own experience confirms this hypothesis perfectly. In some respects, veratrum holds a middle rank between arsenic and nux vomica. Generally veratrum suits children, women, and young persons of a sanguine or nervo-sanguine temperament, gay disposition, fitful mood, and who have not been exhausted by long excesses or starvation. Among the following symptoms, those which belong, properly speaking, to veratrum, and are not produced by arsenic, will be found printed in italics.

Physical depression, *as by extreme heat;* general prostration; sinking of strength, with coldness of every part of the body; *except sometimes the face and hands; desire to lie down;* dry heat, or heat with sweat, in the evening, in bed, before midnight; burning heat of every part of the body, followed by sweat; slow and collapsed pulse; quotidian fever, every evening, or in the evening and morning; yawning; stretching; desire to sleep, *with startings, as if affrighted, which prevent sleep;* extreme brightness of the ideas, which prevent sleep; sleeplessness; comatose sleep; coma vigil; somnolence and lassitude, which oblige one to remain in bed in he morning; red and itching rash, in the warm bed; or even in the day time; psoriform eruption; extreme anxiety; *worse when standing or walking; malaise in the open air; restlessness and desire to be busy; quickness of the perceptions; gaiety; affectionate manners;* diminution of the memory and the intellectual faculties; irascibility; *still melancholy which makes one weep;* moaning, even during sleep; disturbed consciousness; ominous foreboding; *painful* recollection, especially in the morning, in bed, *of the errors or faults which one had committed in former times, and of the unpleasant events that had resulted from them;* taciturn; *timidity; paroxysms of fainting;* quiet delirium, *with cheerful countenance;* mental derangement, *with pleasant wanderings* or *frightful terrors and desire to escape;* constant dizziness; *vertigo, increased by walking;* rush of blood to the head; pain in the brain as if crushed or pressed upon; compressive headache from temple to temple, or else constrictive headache as if a cord were tied round the head; dull headache, accompanied with a sort of buzzing in the forehead; sense of coldness at the vertex, (with cold feet;) pressure at the vertex, which changes to a throbbing *during motion;* simultaneous sensations of cold and heat at the head, with sensitiveness of the hair; pressive, drawing, or throbbing hemicrania, *most frequently on the right side,* with coldness and viscid sweat on the affected part; involuntary flexion of the neck, which induces the head to incline forward, and frightful pains at the occiput on endeavoring to straighten the head again; heat in the eyes; stitch in the canthi; violent ophthalmia; *cutting pain in the eyes;* lachrymation; photophobia; severe contusive pain in the right eye-ball, which ceases on pressing the eye with the hand; dilatation or contraction of the pupils; enormous dilatation of the pupils, with momentary suspension of sight; diplopia; sparks and muscæ volitantes, especially on rising; smarting dryness of the eye-lids; *agglutination of the eye-lids by a dry gum,* after sleeping. Stitches in the ears; buzzing in the ears; noise as from a strong wind in the ears; *sensation as if an alternate current of cold and warm air were coming out of the ear;* dulness of hearing. Pressive pain at the nose; red spots and vesicles on the nose; dryness of the nostrils; dry or fluent coryza; nose-bleed; *smell in the nose as of a dung-hill.* Livid complexion; hippocratic countenance; heat and redness of the face and eyes, with *febrile shuddering* and *disposition to start;* sweat in the face *when walking;* pulling and tensive pain in the right half of the face; red rash on the right cheek; pulling and pinching in the facial muscles; contusive pain in the muscles of mastication, *when eating;* locking of the jaws; swelling of the sub-maxillary glands, with constrictive pain; pimples in the corner of the mouth, painful when touched; burning and cracking of the lips; pressive toothache, *which changes to a pulling pain while eating;* dryness and stickiness of the mouth, in the morning; dryness of the tongue and lips, in the evening; heat in the mouth, *as if one had eaten pepper;*

numbness of the palate, and dulness of taste; foul, *herby* taste, as of *dung;* sour taste in the mouth; *pungent taste like pepper-mint, in the mouth and throat,* with nausea and sensation, as if one would vomit; profuse, viscid or frothy salivation; *loss of appetite; aversion to warm food;* desire for fruit and acids; thirst in the afternoon and evening; roughness in the throat; spasmodic constriction of the throat; sense of coldness in the throat; empty, bitter, or sour eructations; nausea, with bilious taste in the mouth; nausea while eating, with hunger and pressure at the stomach, that ceases after a meal; bilious vomiting; violent vomiting, followed by extreme weakness; vomiting and diarrhœa at the same time; burning pain at the stomach; pain at the stomach, as if caused by excessive hunger; sinking at the stomach, with internal coldness, and pressure at the epigastric region. Twitching of the abdominal muscles; colic without desire for stool; flatulent colic all over the abdomen, with constipation and difficult emission of flatulence; violent and frequent emission of flatulence; cutting colic, especially in the evening and morning (about four o'clock); *the colic is aggravated by walking;* pain in the abdomen as if smashed; single stitches in the hypochondria; tension in the inguinal regions, as if hernia would protrude. Constipation as from inertia of the rectum, which is distended by the accumulated hard fæces to an abnormal size; constipation with tenesmus; involuntary liquid stool; watery stool, sometimes *without smell;* burning at the anus; blind piles. Acrid, yellow urine, which becomes turbid as soon as it is emitted; pinching in the urethra between the acts of urinating; great sensitiveness of the genital organs; sexual excitement; premature or suppressed menses; the suppression is accompanied with nausea and headache, especially in the morning.

Scraping in the larynx; spasmodic and suffocative constriction of the larynx; red and protruded eyes; dry cough, with tickling in the small bronchia; violent, constant cough, with profuse *mucous* expectoration; hollow cough, with cutting pains in the abdomen; dyspnœa; paroxysms of asthma *when walking;* painful constriction of the chest; cutting pains in the chest; constrictive and crampy pain in the left side of the chest; violent beating of the heart; stiffness or paralytic weakness of the posterior cervical muscles; pressive, drawing or laming pain the whole length of the vertebral column, *when standing or walking;* numbness of the extremities. Pain in the limbs on which one had been lying; rheumatic pain, with sense of swelling in the affected part, arms or lower limbs; sciatica; sense of lameness in the thighs; weakness and heaviness in the feet; passing swelling of the feet; cramps in the feet; burning itching at the heel; coldness in the feet, as if sprinkled with cold water; stitches in the toes; *aggravation of all the pains by motion.*

Most of the veratrum-symptoms, come on in the morning, sometimes in the afternoon, less frequently in the evening.

According to my experience, *staphysagria* is, in most cases, the antidote of veratrum.

Argentum, see page 114.

Zincum, see the group of which it is the type.

Lycopodium, see the group of which it is the type.

Nux vomica. This is the seed and not the fruit,[1] as is usually stated, of the *strychnos nux vomica*, a tree in India, of the genus *Strychnos*, family *Apocyneæ* of Jussieu, or *Strychneæ* of Candolle, class *pentandria digynia.*

The wood, bark and roots of this tree are excessively bitter, and, in the countries where the tree grows, they are employed against *intermittent fevers* and the *bites of serpents.*

[1] The fruit of this tree is a globular berry, of the size of an orange, and containing, in the midst of an aqueous pulp, 12 to 15 seeds, which are very improperly termed *vomic nuts.* According to Candolle, (*essai sur les propriétés méd. des plantes*, p. 208,) this pulp is acidulated and eatable. The contrary takes place with the fruit of the colocynth, whose pulp is poisonous, whilst the seeds are mild and harmless.

The seeds, which are the special object of this notice, are round, flat, and slightly depressed in the centre, which gives them the shape of buttons. They are of a greenish-gray color, shining, silky, inodorous, of the consistence of horn, and have an acrid and nauseous taste. On account of their felt-like texture, they cannot be pulverized; they have to be scraped to be comminuted. J. Bauhin, is the first who made them known in Europe.

The Nux vomica is a poison even more violent than arsenious acid; but there is a striking contrast between the actions of these two poisons, which we have already pointed out, (see page 213,) and which affords an interesting study. Whilst arsenic seems to extinguish life by the destruction of the vital principle, the vomic nut attains the same end, by a diametrically opposite mode of action. It would seem as though the vomic nut deranges the vital functions by exalting them, so that, upon this hypothesis, the men and animals which offer the least resistance to its deleterious action, seem to be precisely those that are endowed with the highest order of vitality. Accidental observations have fully confirmed this fact. Doctor Desportes, who was one of the first, in France, that experimented with the nux vomica, found to his great surprise, that, whilst fifteen to twenty grains of this poison were sufficient to kill a dog of middle-size almost upon the spot, three times this amount, did not affect, in the least, a goat, and that ninety-two times this amount was required to poison a hen.[1] At the present time it is well known that

[1] *Thésis de la Faculté de Paris*, 1808, No. 54. Desportes' experiments were repeated the year following by Raffeneau-Delille and Magendie with the same result. See the thesis of Raffeneau-Delille, *sur les effects du poison de Java, appelé Upas tienté, and of the vomic nut*, etc., Paris, 1809, No. 53, and the memoir which was read at the Institute on the 24th of April of the same year by Magendie. Rasori's School, it seems to me, might have drawn a great lesson from these experiments, and it is to be wondered that it did not do so. However, the results of these experiments would have often been in antagonism with the precepts of the School, for truth and error can never be made to harmonise. Be this as it may, it seems to me past all doubt that experiments on animals will be improved much better hereafter than they have been heretofore. I am well aware, and the experiments which I

the vomic nut, which acts so mildly upon animals of the ruminating and gallinaceous species, is, on the contrary, a most virulent poison for the carnivorous species, *with a tenacious vitality*, such as the wolf, fox, raven, etc., animals which are scarcely affected by arsenic, that proves such a dreadful poison to the former. Let me state, in passing, that these apparently strange facts have never yet been accounted for, and that I am, I believe, the first, who has undertaken to point out the physiological law upon which they are based.

But what merits more especially the attention of the Homœopathic physician is, that this sort of characteristic antagonism between the action of arsenic and nux vomica on animals of different, and, in some respects, opposite species, is likewise a characteristic feature of the effects which these poisons produce respectively on man. This will result from the following list of their principal contrasts, as resulting from their actually known pathogenesis.

Arsenic.	Nux vomica.
1. Symptoms principally developed on the left side.	1. Symptoms principally developed on the right side.
2. Sinking and slowness of the pulse.	2. Rising and quickness of the pulse.
3. Sinking of the general temperature of the body.	3. Rising of the general temperature of the body.
4. Aggravation of the symptoms by cold, rest and starvation.	4. Aggravation of the symptoms by heat, exercise and food.
5. Desire to eat: canine hunger.	5. Aversion to food.
6. Taste as of *foul flesh* in the mouth and throat.	6. Taste as of *foul herbs* in the mouth.
7. Aggravation of the pains by lying on the affected parts.	7. Diminution of the pains by lying on the affected parts.
8. Nervous symptoms (convulsions, etc.) coming on only after a long while, etc. etc.	8. Nervous symptoms developed almost on the spot, provided the drug had been taken in sufficiently large doses, etc.

have quoted, show, that no general conclusions with reference to man, can be drawn from the provings of poisons on animals. But, more nearly considered, the human organism will be found to be a synthetic combination of all other animal organisms, and, in its idiosyncratic dispositions, to be analogous to the individual tendencies of a variety of animals. These

Howsoever the similitude which I suppose to exist between the symptoms of arsenic and those of nux vomica, seems to be denied by these contrasts, the similitude will at once be restored so soon as the drugs are made to act upon provers of opposite temperaments and dispositions.

The antidote of large doses of nux vomica seems to be ammonia. Sauvages, at least, in his *Nosologie méthodique*, relates the case of a student of medicine, who, after swallowing an entire nut reduced to powder, cured himself perfectly by taking six drops of *volatile ammonia* every fifteen minutes. This fact is the rather interesting and reliable, for homœopathic physicians at least, that, on the one hand, the most extraordinary analogy exists between the effects of nux vomica and those of massive doses of alcohol, and that, on the other hand, liquid ammonia has been recommended for a long time past, and justly so, as an antidote to intoxication. It is also well known that alcohol is a pretty certain antidote to nux vomica.

Empirical Applications.—Allœopathic physicians having been constantly in the habit of prescribing enormous doses of this drug, have remained, on this account, unacquainted with most of its numerous and varied properties. Depending, on the one hand, upon a small number of awkwardly performed experiments on animals, and, on the other hand, upon pathological observations, which always bore upon the same facts,

inquiries into the analogies existing between man and beast, might, probably, even be pushed into the domain of the moral sphere. Many of our spiritual faculties seem indeed subordinate to the condition of the body, that is to say, to its constituent forms and principles. If, one day, we should be able to explain why the ox eats with impunity the water-hemlock which poisons the horse, whereas the horse eats without inconvenience the wild chervil and the water-parsley which destroy the ox; why several ruminating animals eat without injury the berries of mezereum, belladonna, hemlock, which are so dangerous to man; why the hog can bear enormous doses of the mineral kermes; why the pheasant digests the seeds of stramonium, the starling those of the laurocerasus, the partridge those of the ivy, the parrot the berries of the manchinella, etc.; if, I say, we should one day discover the reason of all these peculiarities, I should not be astonished if such a discovery should advance a good deal the cause of therapeutics.

they see in nux vomica nothing but an *excitant* of the spinal column, or, in the language of Rasori, an *hyposthenisans spinale.* This is one reason why many homœopathic physicians, who are not well acquainted with the old materia medica, imagine that nux, out of the school of Hahnemann, has scarcely ever been used differently from what *strychnine* is now-a-days, namely, in *paraplegia.* And yet, it is no farther back than the year 1811, when Professor Fauquier guided by the convulsive or tetanic symptoms, which he observed in animals, and reasoning, as he believed, in accordance with the doctrine of *contraria*, tried nux for the first time in a case of *paralysis of the lower extremities.*[1] From the experiments upon which Fauquier founded his practice, other inferences, might, however, be drawn. Indeed, ever since the end of the 17th century, Wepfer and Conrad Brunner, remarked, in trying nux vomica on dogs, that before these animals were seized with tetanic spasms, they had *bilious vomitings and violent alvine evacuations,*[2] and Desportes himself had observed, although in one case only, but in a very marked degree, the traces of a gastric inflammation occasioned by nux.[3] The annals of therapeutics, from 1770 to 1811, or from the period when Hufeland made his first experiments, to that when Fauquier made his, abound in facts going to prove the efficacy of nux in affections very different from paralysis.[4] Several authors have recommended it for quotidian, tertian or quartan *intermittent fevers.* Ludovico, Wedel, Buchner, Junghaus, etc., considered its efficacy against intermittent diseases equal to that of quinine. Murray, from whom I have bor-

[1] See Bull. de la Soc. de la Faculté de Médec. de Paris, vol. V., p. 219, 271, and 352.

[2] Wepfer, *Histor. cicut. aquat.*, Lugd. Bat. 1733, p. 248.

[3] *Loc. Cit.*

[4] A professor of Paris, A. L. J. Bayle, has published in the second volume of his *Bibliothèque de Thérapeutique*, (from pages 128 to 248,) a series of small memoirs, mostly translated from the German, and comprising most of the original contributions on nux vomica from the middle of the last century to our time. This precious compilation should be attentively studied by all homœopathic physicians.

rowed these names, adds, that nux vomica, has been administered with success for *cough, asthma, arthritic pains, hypochondria, hysteria, worm-epilepsy, various forms of mania, with obstinate wakefulness, dropsy, etc.*[1]

But it is especially in *dysentery*, that nux, before its use had been blindly limited to spinal affections, had acquired a well-merited reputation. "Dysentery," says Bayle, "is one of those affections in which nux vomica has been found most efficacious. Odhelvis cured several patients of this malady; Hartmann cured *nine*; Hagstrom saw good effects from this drug in several *hundred* cases of epidemic dysentery. In another epidemic, Hufeland employed it with so much success in *one hundred and forty* cases, that most were cured in two or three days." These observations, it seems to me, are sufficiently numerous to be conclusive. What, then, is the reason that alloeopathic journalists, in relating (which does not often happen) a case of diarrhœa or dysentery that had been cured with nux vomica, by some plagiarists of homœopathy, never speak of these facts in any other manner than as strange and exceptional cures? Is Bayle's work, which is an authority among them, read only by homœopaths? Perhaps. But if Bayle's work is slighted by the opponents of homœopathy, Giacomini's *traité de thérapeutique* is no less so, (not to mention Murray, who is read no longer these forty years.) Giacomini gives the following list of diseases, for which nux vomica has been used with success, in a number of well-authenticated cases: *synochal inflammations, rheumatism, gout, cardialgia, painful colic, dysentery, cholera, dropsy, plague, intermittent fevers, whooping-cough, hydrophobia, hypochondria, craziness, epilepsy, hysteria, chronic myelitis, various kinds of paralysis.*[2]

It is true, neither Giacomini, nor any of his authors, specify the peculiar conditions which are indispensable to successful treatment in the above-mentioned diseases. But these conditions can easily be inferred from the clinical observations

[1] Appar. Medic., vol. I., p. 480, etc.
[2] *Oper. Cit.*, p. 558.

with which this celebrated professor of Padua accompanies his cases, and it would not be a difficult task to derive from them such general rules relatively to the use of nux vomica as have been abundantly confirmed by the practice of homœopathic physicians.[1]

Homœopathic applications.—The vomic nut, which is such a frightful poison to beasts of prey, is, when indicated by the symptoms, peculiarly applicable to the diseases of such men as by their dry and vigorous constitutions, rigid muscles, physical and moral activity, passions, fiery, irritable, or, in case of need, tenacious disposition, exhibit a certain degree of analogy to those animals, although by their species immeasurably superior to them.

This is the reason (and daily experience confirms this truth) why the vomic nut is principally adapted to persons of a lively, choleric temperament, *with black eyes*, a brown, yellowish or very red complexion, and bilious, dry and robust constitutions. Indeed, Bayle's sixty-nine cases, and especially Fauquier's memoirs, show that these physiological conditions existed, more or less, and independently of the nature of the malady, in all cases, where the nut had effected a striking cure. I need scarcely remark that homœopathic physicians cannot deduce an absolute general rule from these cases, without falling into an error. We see it every day, how the external habits and especially the temperament of a person, are modified, and, so to say, transformed with a surprising rapidity by such or such a disease: hence a physician may have to prescribe for him such or such a drug, which had seemed incompatible with his idiosyncratic habits.

As a general rule, nux vomica is better adapted to the inhabitants of elevated, dry and warm regions, than to the inhabitants of valleys, or of cold and damp countries; all this is the opposite of arsenious acid. This is the reason why nux vomica did so well in the epidemic dysentery of 1795, in Jena, "a region," says Hufeland, "which *on account of its elevated situation*, is little disposed to this disease."[2] And it is for a

[1] See the *pathogenesis of nux* in Roth's Materia Med. Pur., vol. II., p. 446.

[2] Mém. trad. par M. Bayle, *biblio. de thérap.*, vol. II, p. 137.

similar reason that nux, according to Giacomini,[1] is such a useful agent in the clinical hospitals of Italy. And lastly, the striking similarity which exists between the effects of nux, and those of alcohol, accounts for the good effects of this drug in temporary intoxication as well as in those diseases which result from a long-continued abuse of spirits.

"Nux vomica," says Hahnemann, "is especially suitable, when the patient feels worse in the morning, than at any other time; when he wakes as early as three o'clock in the morning, and is then kept awake by a crowd of ideas, and when he does not fall asleep again until day-break, the sleep is disturbed by serious dreams, and he wakes more weary than he was on going to bed, with little desire to get up. It is likewise suitable to those who, some hours before bed-time, are unable to resist the desire of sleep, and fall asleep on a chair."[2] To this I add that heat before the chill, constipation before the diarhœa, a pungent dryness of the nasal or bronchial mucous membranes previous to the catarrhal discharge setting in, are, together with the above-mentioned physical or moral symptoms, the general indications which most frequently point to *nux vomica.*

I do not give the pathogenesis of nux, for the reason that it is generally one of the first drugs studied by a beginner, and that its pathogenesis is well known to all homœopathic physicians.

Antidotes of dynamised nux; Camph., vin., cham., and especially *lachesis.*

Colocynthis.—*Colocynth.*—Fleshy part of the peporoida of the *Cucumis colocynthis*, a creeping plant, a native of the Orient; genus, *Cucumis;* family, *cucurbitaceæ;* class, *monœcia syngenesia.*

This substance, which is of a proverbial bitterness, is one of the *drastics* of the old school. Colocynth is a poison; but less violent than is generally believed. Colombier relates that several soldiers, in order to cure an acute blen-

[1] *Loc. Cit.* [2] Hahnemann's *Mat. Med. Pura,* vol. III.

norrhagia,[1] swallowed an entire bulb in two doses, and that they accomplished their object without experiencing any untoward symptoms. I have seen an empiric administer to his patients enormous doses of an alcoholic tincture of colocynth, without causing them any other trouble than violent colic, bloody stools and a very painful tenesmus; all these symptoms seldom lasted longer than twenty-four hours. Beef broth, said this empiric, (and I can confirm his statement from experience,) is the best means to quiet the colic. Orfila, however, tells us that three drachms of pulverized colocynth introduced into the stomach of a dog, killed him in twelve hours, and that another one was killed in about the same time by means of five ounces of wine in which two drachms and a half of the poison had been mixed. In both animals the stomach and rectum were inflamed, but not the smaller intestines, through which the poison, thinks Orfila, passes too rapidly to leave a trace behind.[2] This explanation is erroneous. Colocynth acts principally on the stomach, and still more on the large intestines; these two organs constitute its legitimate sphere of action. To be convinced of this, we need but observe the effects of colocynth applied externally, a little of the recent pulp tincture or powder, to the umbilicus, for instance: these effects are exactly like the effects caused by the introduction of the poison into the digestive apparatus. Gœffroy, Hermann, and several other physicians, have attested this fact. Hermann mentions it in his *materia medica.*

Empirical applications.—It is with colocynth as with bryonia, nux vomica, etc. The enermous doses in which it has always been given by old school physicians, have disguised from them the true dynamic effects of the poison. But even, in such doses, it seems to have produced good effects in some cases of *epilepsy*, *melancholia*, *mania*, *asthma*, etc.[3] Faber,

[1] Code de médec. milit., vol. V., p. 420.

[2] *Toxicologie,* vol. II., 1st part, p. 18.

[3] Murray, *apparat. medic.*, vol. I., p. 410.

in his *traité des maladies vénériennes*,[1] recommends against *chronic gonorrhœa*, a vinous tincture, of which colocynth, saffron and cremor tartari, form the principal ingredients. It is certain that gonorrhœa has been cured with colocynth; witness Colombier, Schrœder, Hermann, etc., all of whom report cases. But what form of gonorrhœa? Further, experimentation on the healthy can alone determine this. Murray relates that his friend Dahlberg, who was physician to the Queen of Sweden, employed the colocynth with much success against *certain chronic pains of the head and neighboring parts*. We read in the *Dictionnaire univ.* de Mat. Medic., by Merat and Delens: "Colocynth had not only been employed as a drastic, but also as a vermifuge, hydragogue, emmenagogue, deobstruent; it has been used for sciatica, pains occasioned by mercury, rheumatism, gout, even rage, etc.[2]

Homœopathic applications.—Colocynth has not yet been experimented with very extensively by homœopathic physicians; its therapeutic properties are, therefore, only partially known, and have only rendered a limited, although very satisfactory use in the treatment of disease. It has been found particularly useful in the following diseases:

Anxious and concentrated mood; colds and shuddering; with heat in the face without thirst; sense of coldness at the lower extremities, especially at the knees and soles of the feet, although these parts feel warm to the hand; trembling of the extremities as after a fright or some serious disappointment; restlessness in bed, in the evening; vivid dreams during sleep; profuse night-sweat; smelling of urine, about the head, on the hands, thighs, feet; smarting itching, in the evening, in bed, only momentarily appeased by scratching, and obliging one to be in constant motion; white rash;[3] compressive headache, at the forehead or vertex; *semilateral*,

[1] Vol. II., p. 368.

[2] Vol. II., p. 481.

[3] The vomic nut likewise produces this symptom, which contrasts with the red rash of arsenic.

pressive, drawing, crampy headache, sometimes periodical, (*most frequently towards five o'clock in the afternoon;*) violent pains in the head, obliging one to leave the bed, and scattering sometimes by walking; ophthalmia; cutting pains in the eyes; prosopalgia with redness and tension of the integuments, most frequently on the left side; paleness of the face; drawing or throbbing toothache; coated tongue; bitter mouth; roughness in the throat; absence of thirst; nausea and bilious eructations, especially after eating; cramps in the throat with empty eructations; bitter vomiting; violent pressure at the stomach and præcordial region; distension of the abdomen; colic as if after a cold; cutting, constrictive pains in the bowels, obliging one to bend double and to roll over the ground; aggravation of the same pains, when sitting or lying, which are eased by violent exercise; *bilious fever, colic and bloody stools,* (*sometimes consisting of pure blood,*) in consequence of a violent contrariety, a paroxysm of anger, but especially after an *humiliation or indignation;* constipation; frothy diarrhœa, of a sour smell, consisting of a greenish substance (a bright-green like verdigris) or bloody, and, then only, accompanied by tenesmus; burning at the anus and in the rectum; *blind piles;* tenesmus of the bladder; retention of urine; profuse emission of a watery urine during the pains; rush of blood to the genitals; sexual excitement; impotence; premature and profuse menses; *miscarriage;*[1] *puerperal fever;* painful nodosities in the breasts.

Dry cough, in the evening and morning; paroxysm of asthma before midnight; drawing or bruising pains in the limbs; cramps in the hands; *rheumatic pains in the right hip, which seems limited to the united tendons of the psoas and iliac muscles;* this pain is especially felt while walking, and still more while sitting and placing the right thigh across the left; *coxalgia;* sciatica; stiffness in the knees; cramps in the calves; tearing in the soles of the feet, during rest.

Generally the symptoms of Colocynth come on in the morning, and still more in the evening before midnight. Some are

[1] I have seen one case.

aggravated by motion, most of them by rest. Contact eases the pains.

Camph., *cocc.*, *coff.*, *caust.*, *staphys.*, and *cham.*, are the well known antidotes of this drug.

Sepia, Copaivæ balsamum and **Alumina.**—See the group composed of these drugs.

Plumbum.—See page 125.

Indigo.—The product which is known in commerce under this name, is obtained by the fermentation of the leaves of several varities of *indigofera*, of the family *leguminosæ.*

The introduction of this drug into the Materia Medica, is due to Dr. Idler, of Berlin, who pretends to have used it with success in the treatment of *epilepsy.* According to his statement, among sixteen epileptic patients, five were cured without relapse, and the rest, simply relieved. Dr. Moritz Strahl, who has published several facts corroborative of Idler's statements, assures us moreover, that he obtained good effects from Indigo in the treatment of *nephritic affections*, *amenorrhœa with spasms* and *hysteria.* Andral, Bérard and Pariset, have prescribed indigo in these cases without success; other practitioners, on the contrary, among others Lenoble de Versailles, and Lesueur, affirm having seen cured with it, the one *epilepsy*, the other *St. Vitus' dance.*

Ten years ago, I gave large doses of indigo in a case of epilepsy, but without success. The truth is, indigo is no more a specific for epilepsy, than mercury, arsenic, nux vomica, etc. Moreover, I am convinced that the epilepti form diseases to which indigo corresponds, exist very seldom in practice, unless we include worm-affections.

The general action of indigo is related to the action of nux vomica, and to that of lycopodium. The following are the pure symptoms of indigo, according to Roth's pathogenesis. (See his Mat. Med. pura, vol. I., p. 293.)

Excitement of the intellectual faculties; disposition to laugh, or sombre sadness with general prostration; muscular twitchings here and there; coldness or heat all over; the pulse is generally quick or spasmodic; somnolence in the morning or towards noon; frequent waking at night; early waking, with headache; oppression of the chest and general weakness; agreeable dreams about travelling, or anxious dreams about quarrelling, etc.; pimples in the face and all over the body.

Rush of blood to the head, sometimes with palpitations of the heart and quick pulse; cephalalgia with excessive vertigo; fulness of the abdomen and emission of flatulence; pressure in the temples or around the head, as if by a band; dizziness on entering the room from the open air, or when walking; undulating sensation in the brain, with slight dimness of sight when sitting; pulsative, lancing, or tearing hemicrania, especially on the right side, sometimes with stitches at the stomach; bubbling sensation at the occiput; stitches at the left occipital protuberance, and at the same time under the shoulder-blade, and in the arm of the same side. Pressure in the eyes; stitch and itching in the canthi; twitching of the eyelids; pressing, lancing, tearing or boring pains in the ears; buzzing in the ears. Great irritation at the root of the nose; acute tearing in the right side of the nose; violent sneezing, followed by nose-bleed, especially in the evening. Flashes of heat in the face; tickling at the cheeks; red pimples, especially on the right cheek; stitch in the upper jaw; pressive pain in the parotid gland. Tearing toothache, even in the sound teeth.

Dry mouth, or flow of saliva; blisters at the tip of the tongue; sense of contraction on the sides of the tongue; constriction of the pharynx; metallic, flat or sweetish taste in the mouth; anorexia; less frequently increase of the appetite, burning at the palate, swelling of the tonsils. Eructations; acid, bitter eructations, or eructations tasting of ink; nausea; vomiting of mucus, without any violent contraction of the diaphragm, without anxiety, and without any great efforts; vomiting with diarrhœa; pressive or cutting pain at the stomach; violent cutting pain at the stomach;

cardialgia; sense of fulness and gurgling in the abdomen; nephritic colic; violent colic that wakes him after midnight, and compels him to go to stool; pain at the umbilical region; stitches in the right hypochondrium, extending to the shoulder; colic, which is followed by soft stool, and ceases after stool; several liquid stools a day; bilious diarrhœa; pressure on the bladder; frequent and urging desire to urinate, with scanty emission of a cloudy and burning urine; profuse discharge of a cloudy, slimy urine, with strong contractions of the neck of the bladder, and severe pains in the region of the bladder, only in the day-time; stitches in the urethra; itching in the urethra, at the glans penis, and at the scrotum. The sexual desire is at first very low, afterwards much excited; premature menses.

Tickling in the larynx; pain in the wind-pipe and the bronchia, as if seized with talons; profuse mucous expectorations; cough; pressure and stitches in the chest, crampy pain in the chest, (in the open air). Stitch in the breast, (left,) ceasing after rubbing, but felt again either above or below this place; tensive pain in the region of the heart; palpitation when walking rapidly.

Boils at the neck; pulling stitches in the rhomboideus muscle, (left side). Lancinating shocks and dull stitches in the lumbar region; weakness or lassitude in the extremities; throbbing pain in the joints; itching and blotches on the dorsum of the hands; acute pain, swelling and sense of contraction in the tendons at the sole of the left foot.

Two or three times I have employed indigo with great success in *worm fevers*. The children were from ten to twelve years old, lymphatic, apathetic, peevish, and ate a good deal. The symptoms which these cases presented, were the following:—chilliness, catarrhal cough, coming on in paroxysms of long duration, in the evening; whitish and moist tongue; sour and foul breath; large but soft abdomen; small diarrhœic stools, like a grayish pap, of a sour smell, two or three stools in the twenty-four hours; ascarides in the rectum, which even crawled out during sleep. I have used indigo successfully in a case of semi-liquid diarrhœa, without colic, (from three to four stools a day, which came on, especially after exercise,) in the case of a stout old man, who was frequently given to excesses of eating. This drug has likewise been of service in my hands in chronic catarrh of the bladder, and, in company with *plumbum* and *sepia*, in a case of stricture of the urethra, which had remained after an old gonorrhœa.

Camphor antidotes indigo.

Bryonia alba. See the group of which this drug is the type.

Sulphur. See page 161.

Cina. *Semen contra*, abbreviated from *Semen contra vermes, seeds against worms.*

This substance, which contains half developed blossoms, scales belonging to the calyx, small rolled-up leaves, parts of branches, heterogeneous vegetable remains, and, lastly, various foreign bodies, such as sand, small shells, etc., seems to come from two species of artemisia, (which, is not exactly known,) cultivated in the East, some say in Mongolia, others in Persia, etc. Be this as it may, the semen contra, which Russian caravans import from Western Asia, and which we generally obtain in Europe by the Baltic Sea, has been, for a long time past, employed by European physicians, as a *vermifuge.*

Bouillon-Legrange has extracted from semen contra, an essential oil of a pale lemon-color, an acrid and bitter taste, having somewhat the odor of mint, and which he says contains all the active properties of our drug.[1] Indeed, a few drops of this oil, when applied to the navel, have been found sufficient to purge the bowels, and cause the expulsion of lumbrici.

[1] *Journ. de Pharm.*, vol. VII., p. 542.

The large doses which are sometimes given of this drug, have caused death in more than one case. More frequently its want of success was owing to its not being given for the right disease. Nothing can be more erroneous, as is well known, than the anthelmintic theory of the allœopaths. Instead of considering the worms as effects of the disease, they are treated as the cause thereof, and it is believed, that the disease will disappear of itself, as soon as the worms are killed. "The truth is," says Hahnemann, "that, when these worms exist in large numbers in the bowels, their presence is always caused by some morbid state of the system, some psora which is developing itself in the system, and which has to be cured, otherwise the worms will continue to reappear in spite of the semen contra, so that the expulsion of the worms proves useless, and a treatment which is so inconsistent and irrational, causes the death of the child after long and unnecessary tortures."[1] To attribute the worms *to the development of psora*, is, undoubtedly, a hazardous theory in many cases; but it is a fact that the presence of worms in the bowels, is always accompanied by some intestinal affection of a changeable nature, which may have to be treated with various drugs, and that the worms do not disappear until this malady has been cured. I admit that *cina* frequently corresponds to this affection of the bowels, and this is the reason why it has frequently cured worms, even when given in massive doses, without being any more a vermifuge, on this account, than *arsenic*, *lycopodium*, etc. But allœopathic practice does not heed such logic. In Trousseau and Pidoux, *traité de Matière Médicale*, for instance, in the chapter on *anthelminthics*, we find Mercurius, arsenic, antimony, tin, Corsical moss, semen contra, etc., mentioned in beautiful confusion as *vermifuge drugs*, the choice of which is left to the good pleasure of the reader, without any further indications.

"Semen contra has also been recommended as a remedy te strengthen the stomach, dissolve visceral engorgements,

[1] Mat. Med. Pura, vol. III.

quiet spasms, combat dyspepsia, various nervous diseases, etc.; now-a-days its use in these diseases has been abandoned."[1]

This drug has been found particularly useful in the following affections:—

Capricious mood; crying and *weeping of children, when merely touched;* anxiety which is worse in the open air; *quotidian intermittent fevers, with bulimy and vomiting; coldness unto shaking,* even near the fire; paroxysms in the morning on waking, or more frequently in the evening; heat about the head, and sometimes on the hands; *sickly looks;* yawning and drowsiness in the day-time; *anxious sleep;* painful dreams, *grating of the teeth and starting during sleep;* delirium; *partial or general convulsions; tetanic or epileptiform paroxysms,* but most frequently *without complete loss of consciousness.* Pressive headache from above downwards, or compression from temple to temple, sometimes less when stooping; *headache, alternating with a dull, pressive pain in the lower abdomen;* dizziness and cries, (in children,) in the morning on waking; shining or dull eyes; *dilatation,* less frequently *contraction* of the pupils; *amblyopia;* formication in the eyelids; *formication and itching in the nostrils, obliging the children to scratch their noses all the time, and bore with their fingers in the nose until it bleeds; frequent nose-bleed,* in the morning, and especially *in the evening; coryza;* purulent discharge from the nostrils; face pale, fatigued, *bloated, with bluish rings around the lips;* pressive or pulling, sometimes periodical pains at the malar bones; itching of the cheeks; toothache, caused by inhaling cool air; sickly, sourish or foul breath; the tongue is generally clean and moist, or white without coating; dryness in the mouth and throat; eructations in the morning; deficient appetite; *bulimy;* sinking at the stomach, with shuddering; thirst, hiccough; *regurgitation of a sour or bitter liquid after a meal; vomiting, with violent efforts,* of ropy *phlegm, and even of ascarides;* pressure at the pit of the stomach, which

[1] Mérat and Delens, *loc. cit.*, vol. VI., p. 303. See the pathogenesis of Cina in Hahnemann's Mat. Med. Pura, vol. III.

hinders breathing; *large, distended abdomen, sensitiveness to contact, especially in the umbilical region; twisting around the umbilicus; constant pinching, either in the umbilical region, or in the left hypochondrium; colic,* (in consequence of a cold by the feet,) *with urging to stool, and desire to void the bladder,* followed by a *soft, whitish stool like tape; worm fever; whitish, sour-smelling,* diarrhœic stools; white, frothy urine in a large quantity, and becoming cloudy shortly after emission. *Voluptuous formication at the genital organs, in children of both sexes, inducing them to commit onanism; menses accompanied with cutting colic and labor-like pains;* pulsations at the hypogastrium, before or after the menses, directly above the mons veneris; redness at the vulva; *acrid, greenish leucorrhœa,* and even discharge of blood *in little girls.*

Tickling in the larynx and wind-pipe, obliging one to cough; hoarse hacking cough in the evening; cough, preceded by a sort of eclampsia, during which, the child raises himself suddenly, with a staring look and a stiff body, as if an epileptic fit were approaching; moaning in consequence of the paroxysms of cough; attack of asthma, while standing erect; *whooping-cough* in children with bad humors or worms; cough with profuse expectoration of a thick phlegm (in children or women); oppression of the chest; stitch under the sternum and in the sides of the chest; crampy constriction of the left side of the chest.

Distress and weariness in the back as after standing too long, increased by motion, and not diminished by pressing with the hand; stitches with pressure, here and there, in every part of the body; crampy tearings in the arms and hands; trembling and weakness of the hands; laming, pulling or crampy pains in the lower limbs; crampy extension of the legs and toes.

Camphor antidotes the semen contra.

Lachesis.—A number of symptoms establishes undoubted analogies between this drug and arsenic. Its general action, however, is still more analogous to that of *Belladonna*, and more especially to that of *Agaricus muscarius*, after which, I have deemed proper to place my remarks concerning *lachesis*.

Carbo vegetabilis, *vegetable charcoal.*—"In former times, charcoal was supposed by physicians to be without any medicinal properties; some kinds of charcoal, such as the charcoal made of linden-wood, were used by empirics in their powders, for instance, in the powders for epilepsy, without, however, being able to assign any reasons for the efficacy which these powders were supposed to possess. It was not until Lowitz announced the chemical property of which charcoal is possessed, to destroy the odor of putrefying bodies, and to guard liquids from corruption, that physicians commenced to use it as a local application. They ordered persons who had a bad smell from the mouth, to rinse it with pulverized charcoal, and they applied the same substance to old ulcers, and, with it, suppressed instantaneously, the unpleasant smell which emanated from them. If taken internally, in doses of several drachms, it removed the foul smell of the stools in the fall-dysenteries. But this was not a dynamic application of the charcoal affecting the vital principle itself. The mouth, which had been sweetened with charcoal, remained sweet only for some hours, and the foul odor reappeared soon after. The ulcer, likewise, did not become altered in its nature, and the foul emanations returned. This was likewise the case in regard to the putrid smell of the dysenteric discharges. Pulverized charcoal can only produce chemical effects. It may be swallowed in pretty large quantities, without affecting the organism in health."[1]

I confess that I do not find it easy to draw the line of demarcation between the *chemical* and the *dynamic* action of charcoal. I am not even fully convinced that such a distinction, as is drawn by Hahnemann, exists, with regard to charcoal. It is evident, however, that charcoal, when simply

[1] Chronic Diseases, vol. III.

reduced to a powder, cannot be absorbed with the same facility as dynamized charcoal. This shows that pulverized charcoal acts scarcely otherwise than locally, but it remains nevertheless unproven 1st that its more penetrating action, when absorbed into the organism, is different from its external action on tissues with which it is simply brought in contact; 2d that no absorption whatsoever, takes place, unless the charcoal is communicated in the Hahnemannean fashion.

It is well known that, following the example of Dr. Belloc, many allœopaths now-a-days cure gastric affections with more or less success, by means of pulverized charcoal.[1] The question here is not now, whether Belloc has borrowed this practice from homœopathy. The fact is, that the charcoal of poplar, (there does not seem to be any reason why this kind of wood should be preferred to any other) has effected cures without any previous dynamisation. Belloc found that 1st pulverized charcoal of poplar, in doses of from 10 to 12 grammes, generally produced frequent and copious stools, without being, strictly speaking, diarrhœic; 2d that it was useful in *gastralgia* with constipation, or in *chronic gastritis*, accompanied with foul eructations, and occasional diarrhœa. In the latter case especially, charcoal is most apt to effect good results, and this circumstance alone induces me to believe in the correctness of Belloc's observations, which prove, contrary to the opinions of Hahnemann, that the non-dynamized charcoal is capable of producing dynamic results.[2]

But how is it that Belloc contented himself with such a trifling sketch of the medicinal properties of charcoal, whereas, so many important inductions are suggested by the pathogenesis of this drug ?[3]

The following morbid conditions are more particularly cured by charcoal.

Anxiety; ill-humor; irritable mood; one feels so unhappy

[1] *Bullet. de l'académie de médec.*, Paris, 1850, vol. XV., p. 280, etc.

[2] It will be seen hereafter that the same is true with regard to lycopodium.

[3] See the pathogenesis of charcoal in Hahnemann's *Chronic Diseases*, vol. II.

that one desires to die; constant restlessness, with trembling; spasmodic mirthfulness; tendency to start; beating in the body, here and there; partial convulsions; extreme prostration, even unto fainting; desire to sleep in the morning, afternoon, and early in the evening; sleeplessness at night, with internal restlessness; waking with a start; *fear of ghosts at night;* disposition to take cold; general coldness; shuddering and horripilations in the afternoon or evening, or even at night, followed by flashes of heat; frequent hot flashes; intermittent fever, with burning heat at the extremities; sweat at night and in the morning; itching of the skin; nettle-rash; foul and readily-bleeding ulcers; *emaciation;* congestion of blood to the head; heaviness of the head; liability to taking cold in the head; pressive headache, especially above the eyes, in the temples, and at the occiput; headache after the nausea; nocturnal headache; crampy tension in the brain; sharp drawing pain in the scalp, especially at the forehead and occiput; pain in the eyes from straining them; heat in the eyes; pressive pain in the eyes; nightly agglutination of the eye-lids; buzzing in the ears; purulent discharge from the ears; *deficiency of ear-wax;* otalgia in the evening; itching in the nostrils; profuse coryza, with hoarseness; *frequent and prolonged nose-bleed, especially at night, and in the morning, after stooping or after straining at stool;* paleness of the face; drawing, pulling, burning pains in the bones of the face; tetters in the face; swelling of the parotid glands; cracking of the lips; constrictive or gnawing toothache, caused by something warm or cold taken into the mouth; looseness of the teeth; bleeding of the gums; dryness of the mouth, or flow of water in the mouth; foul breath; *bitter mouth;* salt taste in the mouth; scraping in the throat; secretion of a quantity of phlegm in the throat; deficient or excessive appetite and thirst; long-continued aversion to meat; desire for salt food, or food sweetened with sugar; eructations; *bitter eructations;* rising of the fat that one had been eating; rising of food, especially of fat food; sour eructations, especially after eating; heaviness of the stomach after eating; sweat when eating; pressure at the pit of the stomach, as if the heart would be crushed; constant nausea.

Stitches under the ribs; stitches in the spleen; lancinating and tensive pain in the liver; contusive pain in the hypochondria; sensibility of the epigastrium when touching it; *unceasing emission of flatulence by the rectum;* colic excited by the motion of a carriage; constipation; slimy stools of light color; insufficient stools; itching at the anus; piles; bleeding from the anus at every stool; diminution of the urinary secretion; frequent urging to urinate; wetting the bed; dark urine; smarting pain when urinating; pressure in the testicles; *extraordinary rush of voluptuous thoughts; frequent emissions; onanism during sleep;* too sudden ejaculation during an embrace; soreness, itching, or burning at the genital organs, *even in little girls;* swelling of the genital organs; profuse and premature menses; *scanty and pale menses;* vomiting during the menses; leucorrhœa previous to the menses; milky, *yellowish, greenish* discharge from the vagina; *excoriations at the vulva;* inflammation of the breasts.

Long-lasting hoarseness; hoarseness in the morning; cough with expectoration of yellowish or greenish phlegm; *oppression when walking;* stitches or smarting pains in the chest; hydrothorax; brownish spots on the chest.

Stiff neck; pulling pain in the back; *pain in the left side of the hypogastrium, as after having raised too heavy a weight;* numbness of the extremities; weariness in the limbs, especially in the morning after rising; luxation-pain in the joints; pain in the elbow when closing the hand; heat in the hands; uneasiness in the lower limbs; numbness of the knee; tetter at the knee; cramps in the calves; constant insensibility of the feet; sweat at the feet; redness and swelling at the toes with lancing pain.

Long continued aversion to fat food and milk-diet, is one of the most characteristic symptoms that indicate vegetable charcoal. But this drug is principally adapted to the sub-acute forms of *gastro-colitis*, and I am disposed to think that it is abused in *epidemic cholera*, for which some homœopaths consider it a *specific remedy*.[1] As an *antiseptic*, like arsenic, but in different conditions, charcoal is capable of rendering the most distinguished services in cases where it is indicated. I have seen it cure radically, and in a few days, a little girl of seven years, who, *for upwards of six months*, had been affected with the following symptoms: excessive *irascibility;* yellowish complexion, with slight redness of the cheeks, during her paroxysms of ill-humor; emaciation, especially of the upper half of the body; heaviness of the head; cough with oppression when walking; distension of the abdomen; constipation; itching at the anus; itching at the vulva, with *acrid leucorrhœa*, (cause or effect of onanism?) Charcoal, as well as semen-contra, has been used several times with success, for vaginal discharges of little children. The powerful action of this drug on the sexual organs fits it, in certain cases for combatting an excessive excitement of the sexual organs, redness and excoriations at the vulva, nocturnal emissions with erections, lascivious fancies and involuntary onanism, as I have had many opportunities of witnessing.

"Arsenic, camphor, and crude coffee have been recommended (according to Hahnemann) as antidotes to charcoal; but nitric ether seems preferable." According to my own experience, *metallic iron* is still preferable to nitric ether.

Ferrum metallicum. See the group of which this drug is the type.

Bismuthum—*Oxyde of Bismuth.*

This drug is very little known by homœopathic physicians. Its pathogenesis, of which Hahnemann has published a few symptoms in his Mat. Med. Pur., Vol. I., is almost wholly to make, and has been very little used by allœopathic physicians. I believe Hahnemann is mistaken, when he speaks of the

[1] If such a specific remedy existed, it would certainly be *arsenic* much rather than vegetable charcoal.

praises which Odier, Carminati and Bonnat, have lavished on the *oxyde of bismuth;* it is the sub-nitrate of bismuth, (*calx bismuthi alba,*) that was used by these physicians. I suppose, however, that the greatest analogy exists between the effects of these two drugs; my opinions in this respect, are based upon the most conclusive evidence.

The sub-nitrate of bismuth seems to have been used with most success against the following diseases.

Cerebral congestion; megrim (even when existing independently of a gastric affection;) *febrile delirium,* (in acute diseases;) *tetanus; epilepsy; intermittent fevers; acute gastritis,* (after blood-letting,) with fever, redness of the tongue, vomiting and acute pain at the stomach; *cardialgia,* with excessive irritability of the stomach; *cardialgia,* caused by the abuse of spices; *spasms and cramps at the stomach; intestinal worms, obstinate dysentery, Asiatic cholera; crampy pains in the loins and at the pubis during the menses; inflammation of the womb; painful amenorrhœa; urethritis; venereal blennorrhœa,* (very probably of a *sycosic* nature); *rush of blood to the chest; pneumonia; arthritis.*[1]

This dry enumeration of affections which seems so different from each other, does certainly not imply any exact indication of the therapeutic properties of bismuth. But after a careful study of this drug, it will no doubt be found that, among its symptoms, there exist indications for every one of the above-mentioned affections.

To judge from my own experience, the oxyde of bismuth is particularly adapted to slender and irritable children, to nervous women, and more particularly to persons that have been debilitated by emotions or long-lasting diseases; thin, exceedingly excitable, and disposed to mucous discharges without fever.

In the last edition of their *traité de thérapeutique,* Trousseau and Pidoux have laid down rules concerning the use of the sub-nitrate of bismuth, which I deem very proper, and which, as I know from experience, can be applied to the

[1] See Giacomini, *traité de thérapeutique,* p. 479.

oxyde of bismuth as well as to the nitrate. "The sub-nitrate, say they, is adapted to persons suffering with slow digestion, nidorous eructations, and a tendency to slow diarrhœa. When the eructations are sour, or the flatulence is strictly inodorous, the drug is scarcely ever of any use.

"It is indicated in the chronic non-febrile vomiting following an acute gastritis, or indigestion, or the ingestion into the stomach of a violent irritating drug, and in the gastralgias with which this condition is so often complicated. It is particularly useful in acute gastritis, etc." This is vague, and much less correct than that which precedes or follows:

"But when the gastralgia is accompanied with habitual constipation, without vomiting, or with vomiting of insipid or sour ropy phlegm, etc., etc., the sub-nitrate of bismuth is of little use."[1]

In general:

Absence of fever, nidorous eructations, mucous or brownish, foul-smelling vomitings, small, serous, intermittent diarrhœic stools, or papescent stools, of a light color and a foul odor, *preceded by crampy pains at the stomach and pinching in the stomach;* these are the gastric symptoms which indicate more particularly the oxyde of bismuth.

When, among infants at the breast, these symptoms characterise a state of difficult and painful teething, the oxyde of bismuth is best calculated to arrest them.

I have used the oxyde of bismuth with success, 1st, for a wearing, nightly cough, (in a hysteric lady, whose strange and odd manners almost amounted to craziness); 2d, in a case of *sub-acute cystitis,* (after *plumbum,*) accompanied with violent crampy pains at the bladder, which came on in irregular paroxysms; 3d, in several cases of dysmenorrhœa in hysteric females; 4th, and lastly, with brilliant success in a case of *phlegmasia alba dolens.* The left lower extremity was the principal seat of the disease. This fact, coupled with another almost similar fact, communicated to me by Petroz, and the characteristic action of bismuth on the genito-urinary

[1] *Oper. Cit.,* vol. II., p. 724.

apparatus, have decided me more especially to number this drug among the analogues of *thuya occident.* among which it will be found.

Bismuth is antidoted by camphor, and especially by colchicum.

Petroleum, *oleum petræ, oleum gabianum,* petrol, petroleum. Bituminous substance of a reddish-yellow color, an oily consistence, and a penetrating and tenacious odor.

Petroleum is found in France, England, Italy, and is almost abandoned now-a-days by allœopathic physicians. Formerly it was employed for *toothache, chilblains,* and even worms, (in the shape of frictions on the abdomen;) internally, as a *tonic* and *anti-spasmodic,* from which we do not learn much.[1]

According to Hahnemann,[2] petroleum has been principally useful in affections characterised by the following symptoms:

Anxiety; tendency to start; sur-excitation of the nerves; deficient memory; dizziness; *vertigo;* headache in consequence of chagrin; oppressive, lancinating headache; beatings in the occiput; eruptions on the head and nape of the neck; crusts on the hairy scalp; falling off of the hair; gauze before the eyes; presbyopia; myopia; dryness of the inner ear; deafness, (after acidum nitricum.) *Various kinds of noise in the ears;* yellow color of the face; swelling of the sub-maxillary glands; white-coated tongue; bad breath; foul and sticky taste in the mouth; aversion to cooked and warm food; aversion to meat; canine hunger; noisy eructations; *desire to vomit;* sea-sickness; loss of appetite; swelling and painfulness to contact, of the epigastrium; cutting colic in the bowels; ingüinal hernia; *hard stool;* frequent stool in the day time; diarrhœa; incontinence of urine; wetting the bed; stricture of the urethra; burning in the urethra; *itching* and dampness of the *scrotum;* frequent emissions; discharge

[1] Gmelin, *apparat. medec.*, vol. I., p. 153.

[2] See the pathogenesis of petroleum in Hahnemann's *Chronic Diseases*, vol. III.

of prostatic fluid; dryness of the nose; coryza; hoarseness; cough in the evening, after going to bed; dry cough at night; suffocative cough at night, without expectoration; stitches in the side of the chest; palpitations of the heart; tetter on the chest; *pain in the loins* which does not allow him to remain standing; pain in the back; tetter at the nape of the neck; rhagades in the hands; brown spots at the wrists; chapping of the hands and fingers, in winter; arthritic stiffness of the finger-joints; tetter at the knee; stitches in the knee; cold feet; swelling of the feet; corns; obstinate ulcerations at the toes; pulling pains in the head, forehead, temples and molar teeth; *numbness of the extremities;* cracking and stiffness in the joints; aversion to open air; pain in the chilblains; proud flesh in ulcers; vivid dreams; difficulty of waking in the morning; heat at night; fever in the evening, first a chill, afterwards heat in the face, cold feet, even at night.

A few empirical observations have induced me to employ petroleum in dysentery, together with ipecacuanha; this seems to have done very well.[1]

According to Hahnemann, Camphor is the antidote of Petrol.

Nux moschata; *nutmeg*, fruit of the *myristra moschata*, (*aromatica* or *officinalis* of some botanists.) Genus *Myristica*, ranked by Jussieu among the Laurineæ, but which has since been separated from this family, and has been made the type of another one, the *myristicæ*.

The nutmeg tree attains a height of from twenty-seven to thirty feet, with whorled branches, oval, entire and alternate leaves. It is a native of the Moluccæ, where it grows still in large numbers, especially on the islands of Banda and Amboine, whence it has been transplanted to Barbadoes, Mascareigue, île de France, to the Antilles, to Cayenne, etc. What is peculiar to this tree is this, that, in hot countries, it requires for its full development, a fresh, moist and covered soil. The Dutch, who, for several centuries past, have had

[1] *Treatise on the diseases of children*, Paris, 1850, p. 323.

the exclusive monopoly of this spice, take care to cultivate it in the shade of tall and bushy trees: *the Canarium commune* was, and probably still is, the tree with which they sheltered their plantations. Now, if we keep in mind this wonderful arrangement of nature to bring together, in the same region of country, the causes of diseases and the most appropriate agents to neutralise them, it is difficult to overlook the fact, that the peculiar conditions required for the growth of nutmeg, do not imply some striking indications of its use in disease.

The fruit of this tree, with which we have more particularly to do, is a piriform or slightly ovoid drupe, somewhat depressed at both extremities, of the thickness of a hen's egg, and marked with a longitudinal furrow. It has, 1st, an outer envelope or shell of a rosy white, fleshy, fibrous, about four lines in thickness, and splitting, when ripe, into two incomplete valves; 2d, a second envelope, or tunic, a sort of cup, which completely surrounds the nut at its base, where it adheres to and penetrates the seed, and then divides into flat, branching, jagged, unequal bands, which creep over and plough the whole surface of the nut in every direction. It is this part of the plant which is the most aromatic of any, bright-red when fresh, but turning yellow when drying, which commonly goes under the name of *mace;* 3d, lastly, the seed, or nut, properly speaking, with a thin, fragile, smooth, brown shell, striated externally by the furrows of the mace, and containing a kernel of a woody consistence, and slightly grooved at the centre when dry, ovoid, like the entire nut, of a grayish color, with a slight purple tinge, a hot taste and a strong aromatic and well-known smell; this is the nutmeg used in the shops and in medicine.

This substance which has, for a long time, enjoyed great celebrity in the culinary art, is consumed in enormous quantities, in the tropical and temperate regions, and so far as I know, has never been regularly proved upon the healthy organism. All that we know, in this respect is, that the pigeons, according to Rumphius,[1] eat it with impunity, as does likewise the bird of paradise, which however, according to Forster,[2] is sometimes intoxicated and killed by the nut.

The ill effects of nutmeg on man have been noted by a number of observers. Rumphius, Lobel, Schmidt, Cullen, Ainslie, etc., have seen it produce various nervous derangements, especially a sort of intoxication, vertigo, delirium, stupor, insensibility, oppression of the chest, and even cerebral apoplexy; according to Ferrein,[3] these and other results are common in India and in other countries where nutmeg is consumed in quantity. Several authors even look upon the emanations of the nutmeg-tree as poisonous, and assure us that it is dangerous to repose in its shade.

Empirical applications.—Nutmeg is one of the favorite remedies of Hindoo physicians. They give it especially in *adynamic fevers*, in *long-lasting maladies of the bowels*, and in *humid asthma*.[4] According to Murray, it is especially suitable for *spasmodic vomiting*, *weakness of the stomach and bowels*, *incarcerated flatulence*, *apyretic diarrhœa*, and *dysentery*.[5] "In Europe," says Mérat and Delens, "nutmeg is seldom prescribed alone; it is combined with other aromatics, and is only prescribed as a tonic, when the digestive organs are weak, in certain chronic forms of diarrhœa, or as a cordial in order to reanimate a depressed circulation, and sometimes for the purpose of stimulating certain functions, such as the uterine functions, in such diseases as chlorosis, or the muscular energy, as in paralysis; it is also administered in hypochondria, with spasmodic vomiting, after certain forms of dysentery, in atonic gout."[6] Nutmeg has also, (with what success I know not,) been masticated for the cure of *paralysis of the tongue*, and of *the cough of pregnant females*, and F. Hoffman and Cullen,[7] have recommended it in *intermittent fever*, but combined with alum.

[1] Quoted by Murray, *appar. medic.*, vol. VI., p. 138.

[2] *Observat. during a voyage round the world*, p. 171.

[3] Mat. Med., vol. II.

[4] Ainslie, *Mat. Med.*, vol. I., p. 201.

[5] *Loc. Cit.*

[6] Dict. de Mat. Med., vol. IV., p. 536.

[7] *Treatment of the Mat. Med.*, Vol. II., p. 201.

Homœopathic applications.—We are indebted to Helbig, for the only pathogenesis of nutmeg that I am acquainted with. A synopsis of it, containing all the characteristic symptoms of this drug, is contained in Jahr's Manual. Some of these symptoms which, in their general expression, remind one of the symptoms of arsenic, correspond very clearly to various affections which prevail in warm climates, especially in such regions as produce the nutmeg-tree; such affections may arise from a cold which is contracted by reposing, when in perspiration, in such cool and damp places as are found in parts where this tree grows habitually. Among these symptoms we have the following:

Diarrhœa as after a cold; great sensitiveness to cool air, with dryness of the skin which is not disposed to perspire; toothache worse in the cool air, and eased by warm water; drawing pains in the extremities and joints, as after a cold; rheumatic condition, as is caused by cooling off too soon when in perspiration, with pain in the nape of the neck and in all the bones; extreme sensitiveness of the whole body; ephemeral, wandering pains, which cease for a while, and then come on again, etc.

Most of the symptoms of *Nux moschata*, are like those of arsenic, aggravated by rest, by cold and darkness, and, on the contrary, diminished by motion, the light of day and heat.

Nutmeg has been used by Homœopathic physicians very nearly for the same affections that it was formerly used empirically, namely, for *adynamic fevers*, *rheumatisms* caused by the suppression of sweat, and especially for retrocession of the gout, when the gouty pains had left the extremity and had attacked some internal organ, especially the stomach.

It is said, I know not with how much reason, that nutmeg is particularly adapted to affections of women and children. I have given *Nux moschata* successfully, to old and to middle-aged men (affected with the gout.) Upon the whole, I do not believe that this drug will ever be of much use in the diseases incident to our climate. According to Helbig, caroway is the antidote of this drug.

GROUP V.

TYPE: PULSATILLA.

ANALOGUES: SILICEA, GRAPHITES, CALCAREA CARBONICA, PHOSPHORUS, HEPAR SULPHURIS CALCAREUM.[1]

COMMON CHARACTERISTICS.

THE drugs which make up this group, act principally on the vascular apparatus. All the symptoms which they have in common, seem to depend upon a small number of primordial phenomena (such as *impeded respiration*, *engorgement of the air-passages*, *tumultuous* or *irregular beating of the heart*, etc.) all of which indicate a disturbed condition of the vascular sphere; hence we have,

Throbbings here and there, isochronous with the pulse.

Blackness and diminished fluidity of the blood.

Swelling of the veins and capillary engorgement, constituting a sort of ill-conditioned plethora.

Diminution of the vital heat and action.

Congestion of blood to the head, and engorgement of its sinuses.

Sensation of heaviness and fulness in the brain.

Pain of the same kind, accompanied sometimes with apoplectic shocks, either in the centre of the brain, or, which is more frequent, in the right side.

Vertigo and cloudiness as in complete apoplexy, especially when the atmospheric pressure is below the ordinary standard, as is the case at the approach of storms, on the summit of mountains, and more generally on elevated regions.

[1] *Ferr. muriat.*, *Cham. vulg.* and *Gadus* will very probably, one day, be added to the analogues of Pulsatilla; but, at all events, Chamomilla will always remain the type of a group, on account of its possessing several symptoms which appertain neither to pulsatilla nor its analogues.

Paroxysms of comatose somnolence, as in asphyxia (by charcoal, for instance,) after a meal (which increases the frequency of the pulse,) in the afternoon or evening.

Dulness of the senses.

Swelling of the eyes and lachrymal glands; lachrymation.

Stickiness and bilious bitterness of the mouth and throat, with swelling of the salivary glands, salivation (at the commencement of the action of the drugs,) frequently loss of thirst, and in some cases aversion to liquid food, as if one had an instinctive dread to increase the excessive fulness of the vessels.

Aversion to fat food, and especially to real fat.

Fulness at the stomach and in the whole abdomen, which is doubtless owing to the venous engorgement of the liver, of the portal system, pancreas, etc.

Nausea, rancid eructations, watery and bilious vomiting.

Suppression of the biliary secretion, hence: constipation, colorless clay-colored stools; stools consisting of undigested food; or (as I believe, a secondary and ulterior effect:) excessive secretion of bile, and especially of intestinal mucus; hence result:

Soft stools, and a passive diarrhœa, without colic, which seems to ease the patient rather than to weaken him, and continues for an indefinite period.[1]

Venous or catarrhal engorgement of the genito-urinary apparatus.

Sort of numbness, torpor of the genital organs, with absence of erections and pleasurable sensation (especially among women,) during an embrace, or else permanent sexual excitement.[2]

Heaviness of the uterus.

Delay of the menses in spite of evident symptoms of a flow

[1] As in phthisicky patients, for instance.

[2] Probably owing to the compression of the cerebellum by the blood which flows to it in excessive quantity and remains there, as is the case in certain forms of asphyxia; this is perhaps the cause of the sexual excitement with which phthisicky persons are so often troubled.

of blood towards the uterus; the menstrual blood is black, coagulated, impoverished, and the menses are generally either too early or too late.

Discharge of blood from the vagina between the menses.

Passive metrorrhagia.

Milky leucorrhœa.

Fluent coryza preceded by stoppage of the nose, and generally by irritation in the throat.

Angina, with puffing up of the pharyngeal or tracheal mucous membrane.

Loose cough preceded by dyspnœa, pains and oppression at the chest.

Pains in the chest as from an abscess.

Obstinate catarrh, which terminates in some cases in suppuration; hæmoptysis; ulceration of the lungs.

Heaviness of all the extremities.

Pain in the extremities as from an abscess.

Wandering pains, generally distensive; pains which cut short the breathing.

Blueish redness of some parts, but without increase of the temperature of these parts.

Varices.

Petechiæ.

Red papulous blotches on the skin (especially on the sides of the head, in the face, on the neck, chest.)

Infiltration of the feet.

Abscess (whitlow) at the extremities.

Night-mare.

One is obliged to lie with the head much higher than the rest of the body.

Pains which manifest themselves principally in the parts upon which one is not lying, but aggravated breaking out of these pains, in shifting one's position, in the parts upon which one had been lying, etc.

Pulsatilla and its analogues will be found in several other groups, especially in the one which has ipecacuanha for its type.

Hepar sulphuris, which terminates the series of the analogues of pulsatilla, is the drug which is farthest removed from the sphere of action of pulsatilla. The symptoms of hepar seem to partake of the character of its two constituent elements, sulphur and lime. This is the reason why it is an antipsoric, although I have not mentioned it among the group *sulphur ;* it holds an intermediate rank between the sulphur and pulsatilla group.

CORRESPONDING DISEASES.

Affections of men and women of a plethoric and at the same time feeble constitution, (the plethoric condition prevailing first;) organic diseases of the heart, arteries or veins, (aneurisms, varices, etc.;) passive congestions with swelling, without any increase of heat in the affected parts; cutaneous abscesses; diseases of the air-passages; acute or chronic catarrh; pulmonary engorgement; pneumonia; abscess in the lungs; tuberculous phthisis; Cerebral apoplexy, (especially on the right side,) with numbness, convulsions or paralysis of the extremities of the opposite side; vertigo; headache; periodical headache, especially when the paroxysm takes place immediately before or after, or during the menstrual period; ophthalmia; cataract; amaurosis, (especially of the right eye;) varicose condition of the veins of the cornea and sclerotica; epiphora; lachrymal fistula; indigestion from eating meat or fat; bilious, petechial, purple and miliary fever; typhus; typhoid fever; chronic constipation; lienteria; diarrhœa without colic; nightly diarrhœa; prolapsus of the rectum; piles; cystitis; catarrh of the bladder; stricture of the urethra; pains in the loins; swelling of the right testicle; metritis; various affections of pregnant women; amenorrhœa; dysmenorrhœa; passive hæmorrhages from the womb; leucorrhœa, (thin or milky;) impotence; sterility; cancer of the breast; measles, rash (on the chest;) wandering erysipelas; red tetters in the face (acne rosacea;) tetters on the sides of the head, (with falling of the hair;) adipose cysts; rheumatism, (especially at the neck, shoulders, at the small of the back, in the hips and knees;) wandering gout; ulcers (at the extremities;) panaritia; warts; various kinds of intellectual derangements.

Pulsatilla, *anemone;* small herbaceous plant of the genus *anemone*, family *ranunculaceæ*, class polyandria polygynia.

This plant grows in most countries of central Europe, on arid and bare hills, or in sandy woods. It is recognised by its leafless stems, which are about three inches high, furnished with an indented sheath under the flowers. These are terminal, large, composed of five petals, which are straight, hairy on the outside, without chalice, and enclosing in the midst of stamina and numerous pistils, seeds which are surmounted by a long silky extremity.

Pulsatilla is usually considered identical with the anemone of the meadows. Some botanists, however, protest against such a confusion, and Mr. Spark, among others, goes so far as to make two different genera of these two plants.[1] This seems to me superfluous ; for, the only difference which exists between pulsatilla and the other variety, is this, that, in the former, the petals, instead of being straight, are bent back at their tops. The medicinal properties of these two plants seem to be the same, except what difference may be derived from the localities where they grow.

The leaves of the recent pulsatilla, its stem and root have an acrid, burning and nauseous taste. Its juice draws blisters, to the extent, it is said, of causing gangrene, if allowed to remain in contact with the part for a sufficient length of time ; but these properties are, in a great measure, lost by desiccation, and ruminating animals, such as sheep and goats, eat the dry pulsatilla, if mixed with other herbs, without aversion or inconvenience.

We are indebted to Stœrck, for a knowledge, if not of the physiological effects, at least, some of the therapeutic properties of pulsatilla.[2]

Empirical applications. — Stœrck employed pulsatilla, especially, in chronic affection of the eyes (*cataract, amaurosis, spots on the cornea*). Among his twenty cases, the most remarkable, is that of a young girl, who had been afflicted with amaurosis of both eyes since her infancy, and whose sight he restored in two months. He prescribed pulsatilla in two different forms, namely, an extract inter-

[1] *Dict. univers. d'hist. natur.* article *anemone.*

[2] See *libell. de usu pulsat. nigricantis medico,* Vindeb. 1771, in 8vo. Stœrck used for his experiments the anemone of the meadows, which is very common in the neighborhood of Vienna, where the pulsatilla on the contrary, is scarce.

nally, and a dry powder externally, which was blown into the eye. This process of insufflation, at first caused an acute pain, and a profuse flow of tears; after which, the pains which had existed previous to the lachrymation, diminished as soon as it commenced, and finally disappeared with it.

It seems to me that Stœrck did not properly appreciate the action of pulsatilla in the diseases of the genito-urinary apparatus. According to him, this drug had *anti-syphilitic properties*, and he ascribes to them the cures of syphilitic conditions, which he says, were effected with pulsatilla, such as *ulcers at the pudendum*, *at the tongue* and *in the throat; nocturnal arterial pains*, (one of the most characteristic symptoms of pulsatilla,) *caries of bones*, and lastly, *condylomata*. All this may be, but were all these various morbid conditions really syphilitic? this is not shown conclusively by the Vienna physician. Most of Stœrck's cures are accounted for by the physiological action of pulsatilla. No homœopath will wonder that he should have cured with the extract of pulsatilla: 1st, *a foul ulcer at the foot, with serpiginous tetters at the neck and shoulder;* 2d, *a paralysis of the right arm*, of five years standing; 3d, *a paralysis of the thighs;* 4th, *a white swelling at the knees;* 5th, lastly, *melancholia*.

Murray,[1] mentions the physicians who repeated Stœrck's experiments with more or less success. Bergius tried pulsatilla without success in a case of amaurosis, which is not astonishing.[2] Bonnet was more fortunate. With pulsatilla he cured *tetters*, which had resisted all other means of treatment.[3] In 1808, Dr. J. de Raum, published several cases, showing the good effects of pulsatilla in *asthma* and *whooping-cough*,[4] against which diseases we Homœopaths frequently employ it, in accordance with the principle *similia similibus*.

In our time, pulsatilla has been totally abandoned by

[1] *Appar. Medic.*, vol. III., p. 99, etc.

[2] *Mat. Medic.*, p. 491.

[3] Ancien *Journ. de Medec.*, vol. LVIII., p. 476.

[4] *Même collection*, vol. XVI., p. 604.

Allœopathic physicians, who, for the most part, do not even seem to know that any of their predecessors has ever made use of this drug. Trousseau and Pidoux do not even mention it in their *traité de thérapeutique.*[1]

Homœopathic applications.—"Pulsatilla will be found the more useful, the more the physical symptoms to which this plant is most adapted, are accompanied by a disturbed condition of the feelings, a tendency to silent grief, or to a sad and resigned mood, especially if, during health, the patient was of a benevolent and mild disposition, (even inconsistent and frivolous). It is, therefore, particularly suitable to lymphatic temperaments, and not very suitable to men of decision and rapid action, even when disposed to be benevolent.

"A favorable indication is, when the patient complains of chilliness every now and then, with absence of thirst.

"Pulsatilla suits females with delaying menses, or when it takes them a long time to fall asleep in the evening, or when they feel worse in the evening. It is a good remedy for ailments arising from the use of pork."[2]

To this I add, that the general action of pulsatilla seems to correspond to the immediate or consecutive effects of fat food, not as it is generally understood, but of real *fat ;* in the same way as arsenic corresponds to the consequences arising from the abuse of raw food, and nux vomica to the effects of rich viands and strong spirits ; I say, moreover, that pulsatilla is particularly suitable to persons who, by the relative predominance of the adipose tissue in their constitution, by the whiteness of their flesh, the roundness of their forms, the mildness of their disposition, and their fitful mood, exhibit all the marked features of the female sex; that this drug is particularly indicated when the moral and physical symptoms of the disease are very changeable, that is to say, when there are

[1] See the pathogenesis of Pulsatilla in Hahnemann's Mat. Med. Pur., vol. III., of the numerous provings left to us by Hahnemann, that of pulsatilla seems to be the one to which he has contributed himself more than to any other; it is one of the most interesting and most characteristic provings of his Mat. Med.

[2] *Loc. Cit.*

frequent alternations of sadness and mild gaiety, of redness and paleness of the face, of shuddering and heat, of dryness and moisture of the skin, and, finally, when the pains frequently shift without any apparent cause.[1]

Pulsatilla has been tried for almost every disease, but principally for diseases characterized by the following affections:—

Symptoms caused by the abuse and improper use of *sulphur*, mercury, cinchona or *chamomilla*, (especially sulphur-springs;) sadness; disposition to *cry* or laugh without any apparent cause; aversion to any kind of work; lassitude *with heaviness* of the whole body; uneasiness concerning one's health or business; *want of decision;* disposition to be afraid (of ghosts,) in the evening or at night; *anxiety*, with apprehension of near death; *anxiety, in the evening in bed, as if threatened by an attack of apoplexy; anxiety with beating at the heart* and trembling of the extremities; here and there *painful arterial pulsations, perceptible to contact; prominent veins*, on the hands for instance, *even without heat of the skin; varices;* heat and redness of the cheeks, very frequently *of the right cheek only*, followed by coldness and paleness; paroxysms of fainting setting in with sudden heat, profuse sweat in the face, obscuration of sight as by a cloud and trembling of the extremities; internal pains here and there, as *from some abscess;* pains *which cut off the breath, although they are seated in other parts than the air passages; wandering* pains, with swelling of the affected parts; blueish redness of certain parts, without increase of heat, and even with coldness; *chilblains; chilliness;* fever, generally with coldness followed by dry heat, or chills alternating with the heat at short intervals, especially at *sunset*, or in the afternoon; *loss of thirst during the chill*, and thirst only during the heat, and then only when it is very considerable, or the thirst is only felt during the sweaty stage; disposition to sweat on making the least effort; sweat, in some cases, on

[1] Every physician knows that not one of these indications is to be taken in an absolute sense.

one side of the body only, generally *the right side; somnolence*, which is sometimes irresistible, either in the evening or afternoon: *restless sleep at night*, with *dry heat;* frequent waking; disagreeable, frightful dreams; insomnia, with strange and confused ideas crowding upon one; *pains which manifest themselves principally on the side on which one is not lying, and quieted sometimes by lying on the affected side;* comatose sleep with loud dreaming; profuse and sometimes fetid sweat during sleep; *smarting itching not appeased by scratching*, especially on the chest, (above the sternal region,) on the sides of the neck, and in the face; *red papulous blotches; measles; wandering erysipelas;* eruption in consequence of an indigestion from grease, *especially pork; alternating symptoms*, most frequently aggravated *by a sitting posture*, sometimes by a recumbent posture, less frequently by gentle exercise, but almost always by passing from a cool air into the warm air of the room.

Vertigo recurring in paroxysms in the afternoon, especially *in the evening*, less frequently in the morning, *when sitting, stooping, raising one's eyes*, or even when *walking: oppressive*, tensive, *throbbing* headache, with *sense of fulness* in the head as from an indigestion, or a sensation of emptiness as after a night's watching or as after an excess at table; *single acute shocks in the right half of the brain;* stitches *proceeding from the occiput* and passing through the whole head; *nocturnal headache with nausea;* throbbing and pulling headache, *which is alleviated by pressure with the hand;* small pustules on the hairy scalp, filled with pus; bloating of the eyes; itching in the eyes; *congestion of the vessels of the sclerotica; ophthalmia;* deep-seated pains in the orbits; *cloudiness of sight; cataract; amaurosis; photophobia; flickering of flames before the eyes, especially in the open air;* rush of blood towards the organs of hearing: buzzing in the ears; *acute otorrhœa; stoppage of the ears;* sense of tension in the face; abscess at the root of the nose; swelling of the salivary glands; toothache, with sense of fulness in the gums, which manifests itself especially in the afternoon or evening, generally aggravated by *warm drinks* and alleviated by cold water, although the reverse likewise takes place, but much less frequently; *coated tongue, without the sensation of taste;* foul, herby taste, *or taste of spoiled flesh, rancid grease or pus* in the mouth, in the morning; bitter taste in the mouth *after eating; aversion to butter* or milk; all kinds of food seem *bitter* or too salt; *tenacious mucus coating the inner mouth and throat as with a fur; want of appetite; loss of thirst;* nausea and desire to vomit, *as if one had drank oil:* nausea, with profuse salivation and headache; hiccough after eating; aversion to tobacco-smoke; eructation after having eaten pastry, *tasting of rancid grease or old tallow; vomiting, with violent straining, of a sour, greenish phlegm burning the pharynx like fire, in the evening after eating and going to bed;* heaviness at the stomach; *beatings in the epigastrium, which are isochronous with the pulse;* bellyache, when walking; flatulent colic after eating, especially in the evening; pain as from an abscess, under the false ribs, extending to the sacrum; pinching, griping, bellyache, *as if diarrhœa would set in;* bellyache *after stool; typhoid fever:* frequent soft stools mixed with mucus; *bilious diarrhœa* (especially at night;) *diarrhœa without any pain; stools consisting of whitish substances;*[1] constipation; *blind or fluent piles;* acute sensitiveness to contacto ver the whole hypogastric region; pressure and stitches in the vesical region as if wind were incarcerated there; *tenesmus of the bladder;* discharge of watery urine; stricture of the urethra; brown urine, with gelatinous or brick-dust sediment; *mucous discharge from the urethra and swelling of the right testicle;* itching at the prepuce and scrotum; *sexual excitement,* morning and evening; tensive drawing pains in the uterine and lumbar regions, resembling labor-pains; *delay of the menses; suppression of the menses by a fright;* premature menses; insufficient menses *which flow only in the day time;* difficult menses, although profuse, with blackish

[1] All the drugs belonging to the pulsatilla group, have alternately an excessive secretion and a deficiency of bile in the duodenum, which causes white, clay-colored stools.

and coagulated blood; *spasmodic pains in the lower abdomen, nausea, stricture at the throat, flow of water in the mouth, cloudiness, desire for stool; numbness of the abdominal extremities during the menses;* stitches in the chest during the menses; *milky leucorrhœa.*

Coryza with loss of smell, or a bad smell in the nose; purulent discharge *from the right nostril;* nosebleed during the coryza; *catarrhal angina,* with headache, moist and burning skin, and absence of thirst; *acute bronchitis; cough especially in the evening and at night, with profuse expectoration; cough when one is extended in bed, and disappearing in a sitting posture; engorgement of the lungs; rusty sputa; pneumonia; hæmoptysis;* constriction at the base of the chest; purulent expectoration with hectic fever; paroxysm of suffocation, especially while lying down; *rush of blood to the heart,* with paroxysms of anguish; *swelling of the breasts as if the milk were setting in; acute rheumatism,* with or without swelling *at the nape of the neck, at the right side of the neck and at the right shoulder;* stitches between the shoulders; painful stiffness in the back; painful lameness at the sacrum, aggravated by motion; rheumatism with sensation of heaviness at the right shoulder; *paralysis of the right arm;* luxation-pain in the hip, especially when the menses delay; *painful lameness of the lower extremities; weakness of the knees which causes one to stagger,* even without vertigo; *swelling around the ancles;* ulcers at the instep; boring in the heels; pain at the soles of the feet, apparently in the periosteum, with insensibility of the soft parts.

Many practitioners make a wrong use of pulsatilla in *amenorrhœa* and *dysmenorrhœa.* They seem to imagine that pulsatilla is indicated whenever these symptoms exist in any disease, and they prescribe it accordingly. What is still worse, is the practice of undertaking to combat a disease, which breaks out shortly, before the menstrual period, by hastening the appearance of the menses by means of pulsatilla. Pulsatilla is only suitable in amenorrhœa when there is an evident tendency of the blood to the uterus, and in dysmenorrhœa when the little blood which flows out, is black and coagulated.

Chamomilla, sulphur, coffee and the vomic nut, are the principal antidotes of pulsatilla. But when the improper use of this drug affects the air-passages, *calcarea phosphorata* seems, according to my experience, to be the most suitable antidote.

Silicea.—*Silicea, oxyde of silicium, decarbonized white pebble.*—Although in some of the older treatises on Materia Medica, mention is made of silica and its compounds, under the vague denomination of *terræ siliceæ*, yet there is such a complete absence of all allœopathic documents relative to the use of this drug, that we may safely consider it as a new element in the practice of medicine, due to our peculiar art. Indeed, of what use could have been a mineral to allœopathic physicians, that *seems inert* in the form in which it exists in nature? I say, *seems inert*, for I am not sure that a finely pulverized pebble, if introduced into the alimentary canal, is without any effect whatsoever. This experiment might not be attended with any important result, but it has yet to be made.

Rapou, in his *History of Homœopathy*, calls Sepia the "*pulsatilla of chronic diseases;*" it is silicea which should be considered in this light. There are few drugs that are as intimately related to each other as pulsatilla and silicea.

I have even been tempted to suppose that silicea might be a constituent portion of the active elements of pulsatilla, a supposition which will not appear unfounded if we consider that pulsatilla and all the other varities of anemone, are fond of *sandy bottom*, and may, on this account, readily incorporate the leading principle of the soil in their own constitution. But I admit that this is a very bold hypothesis, which is not even based upon facts furnished by a chemical analysis of the plant.[1]

[1] Pulsatilla has been analysed several times, especially by Vauquelin and Schwartz, but these chemists have contented themselves with the immediate results of their analysis, neglecting the discovery of the real constituents of

Be this as it may, if we compare attentively, and symptom by symptom, the pure effects of silex to those of pulsatilla, we are struck with their resemblance to each other, which is sometimes complete. But it is in the clinical results obtained with these drugs, that their perfect analogy is most strikingly evidenced.

Silicea corresponds to the chronic form of such diseases as pulsatilla cures when acute: rush of blood to the head, more particularly in the right temple, and at the vertex; headache every day; photophobia; lachrymation; loss of taste; aversion to fat food, with rancid or oily taste in the mouth; catarrhal affections of the air-passages; lateral swelling of the nape of the neck, right side; rheumatic pain at the right shoulder, in the back and sacrum; numbness of the limbs; pain as from chilblains or whitlows; suppression of the menses with beating of the heart; swelling of the lower abdomen, etc. The symptoms of silicea differ, however, from those of pulsatilla in this, that they are more constant, more deep-seated, and last longer. For instance, the mucous secretions caused by pulsatilla, become easily purulent under the action of silicea. Silicea exhibits likewise, two series of phenomena, which, at different degrees and in different forms, belong to most other powerful drugs: these are, first, a sort of internal

the plant. A white, crystalline, insipid, inflammable substance which they termed *anemonine*, was considered by them the active principle of the plant, and engaged their particular attention. Does anemonine contain silica? I do not know.

It would be interesting to inquire whether white burgundy, that has a *bouquet of flint*, and which the vine-dressers of the Côte d'or drink every morning in order *to remove the phlegm*, does not contain silica. I am not, by any means, convinced of the efficacy of this white wine in removing a disease which the peasants of Burgundy term "*pituite*," (phlegm); but what I am, on the contrary, convinced of, is that this wine causes the disease. Any other wine, it may be objected, will cause the same effect. This may be. Nevertheless it is positive that the chemical properties of drugs depend, to a certain extent, upon the chemical composition of the soil in which they grow. Who will assert that these properties do not, in part at least, result from the salts of lime and others inherent in the various soils, and naturally dynamised by the process of assimilating growth?

sinking, accompanied with a sort of canine hunger, a desire to restore one's strength by eating, etc., and secondly, nervous crises, of a more or less strange character, and apparently connected with this sense of exhaustion. It has seemed to me, at least, that this coincidence between a craving for food and the nervous derangements was, in all purely nervous affections, one of the most reliable indications for silicea. And I have likewise observed that all nervous affections in which this drug exists with the best chances of success, are such as are either roused again or aggravated when, by some accidental circumstance, by caprice or by the requirements of a system, patients were condemned to excessive abstinence from food.

These, together with the thirst and the predominance of the symptoms in the morning on waking, or rather in the afternoon or evening, are the principal differences between silicea and pulsatilla. But, in their general action upon the vascular system, these two drugs either act alike, or, at any rate, similarly. It might be said, however, that silicea affects the capillary system more specifically than does pulsatilla.

Another observation which I regret having limited to a few experiments only, has led me to believe that the effects of silicea are the more strikingly analogous to those of pulsatilla, the lower the dilutions with which the provings were instituted.

According to Hahnemann, (see his *Chronic Diseases*, Vol. III.,) silicea is principally indicated by the following symptoms. A comparison of the pure effects of pulsatilla to those of silicea, goes to show that pulsatilla is indicated by the same morbid conditions:

Tendency to anger; *ill-humor;* aversion to work; excessive excitability; chagrined and irritated on the least provocation; discouraged; agitated; want of memory; *malaise while reading and writing; inability to think;* dizziness; sort of intoxication in the evening; vertigo, obliging one to hold on to something; heat in the head; headache on getting heated; *headache from the nape of the neck to the vertex*, hindering sleep; *headache every day;* tearing in the forehead, with heat in the morning; heaviness in the forehead from noon till evening; pulling pain in the head; pain in the head, as if it would burst; pulsative headache; megrim; tearings and stitches in the eyes and facial bones; *sweat about the head in the evening; humid and itching crusts* on the head; tuberculous elevations on the scalp; *falling out of the hairs; presbyopia;* photophobia; *blindness by the light of day;* cataract; *black spots floating before the eyes;* a sort of gray veil before the eyes; *amaurosis;* sparks before the eyes; weakness of the eyes; the letters look blurred, when reading at candle-light; sudden paroxysms of blindness; one has to use spectacles to read and write; lachrymal fistula; *lachrymation in the open air;* tearing in the eyes: *agglutination of the lids in the morning;* redness of the eyes, with pain in the canthi; inflamed eyes; noise in the ears; *hardness of hearing;* boring pain in the ears; stitches in the ears from within outwards; eruption of pimples on the nose; redness at the tip of the nose; eruption of pimples in the nose; *painful sensation of dryness in the nose;* stoppage of both nostrils; loss of smell; *nose-bleed;* cracking of the skin of the face; heat in the face; osseous swelling on the lower jaw; pulling and stitch in the lower jaw, at night; stiffness in the neck, preventing one from closing the jaws; ulceration at the vermilion border of the lower lip; tetter on the chin; swelling of the sub-maxillary glands; digging and stitch in the teeth; boring pain in the teeth; tearing pain in the teeth and cheek, night and day; shocks in the teeth when sucking at them with the tongue; tearing toothache which strikes to the ear when eating; bleeding of the gums; dryness in the mouth; *smarting at the tongue; loss of taste;* mucus in the mouth, constantly; *bitter-mouth,* in the morning; eructations; eructations which are sour or taste as of rancid grease; eructations which taste of the food one had eaten; nausea in the morning; *constant nausea and vomiting;* nausea after every heating exercise; nausea after eating; vomiting after drinking; nausea every morning, with pain in the head and eyes when turning them; inability to digest meat; *desire to vomit with shuddering; a good deal of thirst,* he loathes every thing he eats; aversion to boiled things; *aversion to meat;* the child refuses the breast and vomits as soon as it takes it; *heaviness at the stomach;* heaviness at the stomach after drinking rapidly; *pain at the pit of the stomach when pressing upon it; tightness in the pit of the stomach; pain at the stomach*, after eating; *it had existed for years;* fulness after eating; hardness and swelling in the hepatic region; hardness and swelling of the abdomen on the right side and in the middle, above the navel, with hardness when touching it; tension and hardness of the abdomen in children; swelling of the lower abdomen; heat in the lower abdomen; borborygmi in the abdomen when stirring with the body; *shifting of flatulence;* difficult emission of flatulence; painful inguinal hernia; pinchings in the abdomen; cutting pains in the abdomen; *cutting in the hypogastrium without diarrhœa;* colic from constipation; belly-ache, with diarrhœa; worm-fever in scrofulous children; several fæcal stools a day; constipation; indolence of the bowels; retention of stools, with frequent unsuccessful urgings; itching at the anus; frequent urination; *wetting the bed at night;* no sexual desire and weakness of the sexual organs; frequent involuntary attacks of lascivious ideas; excessive sexual desire; itching at the prepuce; *profuse menses;* menstrual suppression of several months' standing; too early and too scanty menses; discharge of blood from the uterus during the period of nursing; acrid, excoriating leucorrhœa; *leucorrhœa when urinating;* leucorrhœa with cutting colic in the umbilical region; *itching at the vulva.*

Suppressed sneezing; *excessive or too frequent sneezing; stoppage of the nose for years;* dry stoppage of the nose; frequent coryza; coryza, after which a chronic stuffing of the nose ceases; *hoarseness;* asthma during rest; *asthma during work;* asthma during a rapid walk; loud breathing when walking rapidly; loss of breath when lying on the back; loss of breath when stooping; loss of breath when running, coughing; *cough, with purulent expectoration; cough*, with mucous expectoration; suffocative cough at night; *oppres-*

sion of the chest; oppression of the chest when coughing or sneezing; beating in the sternum; stitches from the chest to the back; stitches under the left ribs; pain in the loins; spasmodic pulling in the sacrum, which obliges one to lie down and does not allow one to rise again; stitches in the back; tearing in the back; lameness at the trunk; stitch in the loins, when sitting or lying; contusive pain between the shoulder-blades; weakness in the sacrum, back and nape of the neck; glandular swellings at the nape of the neck; painful numbness in the arm on which one is lying; heaviness at the arm; inability to hold the arm raised a long time; weakness and trembling of the arm, after performing some slight manual labor; pulling pain in the arm; rheumatism in the arms; warts on the arm; incipient paralysis at the fore-arm; the hand drops the object which it seizes; stitches in the wrist-joint, at night, extending along the arm; formication in the fingers; pains in the finger-joints in pressing upon them; *stiffness and want of strength in the fingers;* whitlow; pulling and stiffness in the legs; pressure in the muscles of the thigh; swelling of the knee; pulling pains in the legs; numbness of the calves; numbness of the feet, in the evening; cramps in the calves, in the evening, after working; stitch in the ankle when pressing the foot to the ground; *cold feet; sweaty feet;* suppression of the sweat on the feet, and cold feet; fetid smell of the feet; swelling of the feet; voluptuous and furious itching when slightly scratching a little spot on the sole of the foot; hard and painful cutaneous tubercles on the sole of the foot; corns; stitches in the corns; ulceration at the big toe, with stinging pain; vascular excitement and thirst after drinking a little wine; tendency to spraining joints; sweat during a slow walk; *tendency to taking cold* when uncovering the feet; foul smell of the ulcers; itching all over the body, on the legs, with ill look; itching ulcer on the thigh and at the ankle; carbuncle; stitches in every joint, at night; twitchings in the limbs, day and night; epilepsy; rheumatism in the arms and legs; numbness in the extremities; weakness in the extremities, in the evening; painful feeling of weariness in the extremities, in the evening; nervous debility; general prostration; tendency to faint away when remaining lying on one side; drowsiness, in the afternoon; frequent yawning; one remains awake late, in the evening, in bed; slight sleep at night; many dreams and frequent waking; *a good many dreams every night; disturbing dreams;* snorting during sleep; startings during sleep; talking during sleep; night-sweats; frightful visions at night; dryness of the nose, at night; frequent shuddering every day; profuse and sour night-sweat.

Until recently, silicea has been principally used in chronic diseases; but there are also many acute maladies where it is sometimes indicated. I use silicea as often and as successfully as any other drug. In the following affections I have used it with marked benefit: 1st. *Measles*, when first breaking out, *with thirst*, pressive headache and dizziness *in the morning*. 2d. *Cerebral apoplexy*, with loss of consciousness, preceded (for three or four days) by a stupefying headache, *deep-seated stitches in the right parietal region*, and dull, *heavy and crampy pains in the arms*, and followed by an almost complete paralysis of the motor and sentient nerves of the left arm and left lower limb, in a young woman of short stature, *very fat*, blond hair, white and rose-colored skin, a lively and irascible temperament, and *mother of* four children, *the youngest of whom she was yet nursing*. I was called to this patient on the morning after the paralytic stroke, and silicea removed in two days all the symptoms, including the headache, which still existed. 3d. *Metrorrhagia* of six weeks standing, in the case of a *fat* and robust woman, of a brown complexion. This woman, who was a washer-woman at Grenille, and whom I saw only three or four times at my office, attributed her sickness to her constantly standing in cold water. *Silicea* arrested the hæmorrhage almost immediately, and effected such an improvement in one week, that I scarcely knew her again the second week; she did not take any other medicine. 4th. *Sterility*, with descension of the uterus, anteversion and slight induration of the neck of the uterus, scanty and painful menses, which come every month some seven or eight days sooner; *pulsative* pain in the right ovarian region, incapacitating her from standing; unpleasant heat on the skin of the hypogastric region, whilst the feet and knees feel icy-cold, especially at night; *complete absence of the thrill during an embrace, without, however, experiencing any aversion to sexual intercourse,* in a very brown complexioned but thin lady. I may feel disposed to publish this case *in extenso,* some time or other. Silicea, which was administered for three months without an interruption, but in various dilutions, produced a regular, progressive amelioration, which never ceased *until the moment when the patient became pregnant.*[1] 5th. *Miscarriage.* A young woman, of blond hair, lively, easily impressed, who had been married for some ten months, was in the eighth month of pregnancy. For some days past she had felt a dullness about the head, and a dull pain at the lumbar region. After a somewhat long walk, and a little unpleasant excitement, she was suddenly seized with violent pains in the loins, which soon increased to real labor-pains. The uterine contractions could be felt distinctly; a little rose-colored blood appeared at the vulva. *Silicea* arrested the symptoms immediately, and the lady went her full term. 6th. *Constant pressive headache* from above downwards, (over the whole head,) *with intermittent itching at the vulva,* without any other apparent symptoms, in the case of a lady of forty years, blond hair, apathetic, *very fat,* and rosy complexion. 7th. *Chronic affections of the heart.*

As a general rule, and contrary to the opinion which a number of homœopathic physicians seem to entertain, silicea is particularly suitable to lymphatico-sanguine individuals, rather than to persons who are simply *lymphatic* or *cachectic.* A remarkable contrast exists in this respect between *sepia* and its two analogues. I have observed in several instances,

[1] She had been married for two years, and had already been under homœopathic treatment the previous year, but without deriving any perceptible benefit from it.

that sepia, copaïva or alumina produced bad effects on persons to whose temperament silicea was especially adapted, and who had, indeed, been cured by silicea. Nevertheless there are certain chronic maladies which it may be proper to treat alternately with *Silicea*, *Sepia* and *Alumina;* but such a combination never suits persons of a sanguine, or a sanguine-nervous, temperament. The use of sepia, like arsenic or mercurius, always presupposes a condition of *hyposthenia*, if I may so express myself, in the affections for which it is prescribed; the reverse is generally the case with the remedies of the group *Palsatilla.*

Sulphur antidotes silicea, as it does pulsatilla; but hepar sulphuris corresponds much more completely to the symptoms of silicea.

raphites—*Plumbago*, *Percarburet of Iron;* now-a-days, it is considered as pure, or almost pure carbon, that is to say, carbon with which atoms of native iron are mixed, but not combined in the minutest proportions. "The first idea of making use of this substance as a drug (see Hahnemann's Chronic Diseases, Vol. II.) is due to Doctor Weinhold, who was led to it during his voyage in Italy, by the workmen in a looking-glass factory, who employed it externally for tetters. He imitated them, and described the results which he obtained. From this period, and perhaps even before the publication of Weinhold's memoir,[1] Ruggieri employed Graphites internally and externally, in the cases for which it is recommended by the German physician. Some time after, in 1812, Hufeland related, in the third report of the Polyclinical Institute of Berlin, the case of a lady of forty-one years, who was cured by the internal and external use of Graphites of an *acne rosacea*, which had defied all the means of treatment that had been employed until then. In 1817 and '18, the same author published several other cases of the same kind."

As regards French allœopathic physicians, I am not aware

[1] Graphites considered as a remedy for tetters, (in German,) Leipsic, 1809, 2d edit., Meissen, 1812.

that any of them, except Doctor Marc, have ever employed Graphites. Marc[1] published several cases tending to confirm the experience of Weinhold, Ruggieri, and Hufeland concerning the efficacy of this drug in various cutaneous affections. But, according to Hahnemann's judicious remark, it is a mistake to suppose that the use of Graphites is limited to the treatment of a few kinds of tetters.[2]

The more one studies the pathogenesis of graphites, the more one must feel convinced of the many points of contact it has with pulsatilla and (perhaps more particularly) with silicea. Graphites, for instance, has the following symptoms in common with pulsatilla and silicea:

Anxious, changeable, wavering mood; aversion to work; vertigo with cloudiness; sort of intoxication in the morning; sense of fulness or emptiness in the head; drowsiness in the day-time; single, acute, deep shocks in the right half of the brain; flickering before the eyes; suspension of the visual power; photophobia; lachrymation in the air; foul smell in the nostrils; prurulent coryza; wandering heat in the face; red, papulous eruptions, or resembling flea-bites, in the face and over the whole body; bitter taste in the mouth; aversion to liquid food; thirst (less frequently); nausea in the morning; rancid eructations; aversion to fat food; pressure and beating in the epigastrium; soft, thin, tape-shaped, incomplete and frequent stools; pain in the abdomen after stool; swelling of the lower abdomen; piles; tenesmus of the bladder, followed by flow of watery urine; amenorrhœa and dysmenorrhœa, watery leucorrhœa, swelling of the right testicle; itching and swelling of the right half of the scrotum; sexual excitement; no thrill during an embrace; impotence; catarrhal engorgement of the air-passages; palpitation of the heart; arterial throbbings here and there; pains as from deep-seated abscesses; swelling of the veins; wandering pains; pains in the parts upon which one is not lying; weak-

[1] *Bibliothèque Médicale*, vol. XLV., p. 109.

[2] See the pathogenesis of Graphites in Hahnemann's *Chronic Diseases*, vol. II., p. 230.

ness in the extremities, with heaviness in the affected parts; hemiplegia; rheumatism at the nape of the neck, with swelling of the right side of the neck; painful lameness at the scrotum; swelling of the feet; sweat at night, having the odor of urine; drowsiness in the day-time; sleep is disturbed by dreams, etc. These affections seem to be the same for the three drugs; the reader will have to decide for himself, agreeably to the totality of the symptomatic indications, which of them requires a preference in a given case.

I doubt not that graphites can be usefully employed both in acute and chronic affections. I have never used it in measles, but I believe that in certain cases of measles graphites may be found more efficacious than any other drug.

"When chronic constipation, and a delay of the menstrual show of several days, are prominent symptoms, Graphites is often required."

According to Hahnemann, arsenic and nux vomica are its antidotes.

Calcarea carbonica—*Carbonate of Lime.*

It is quite natural that the almost complete insolubility of this salt was an obstacle to its being used as a drug by the older physicians. Nevertheless several substances, such as chalk, egg-shells, oyster-shells, or the concretions which are known by the name of *crabs'-eyes*, are, in reality, mere varieties of the carbonate of lime, and have formerly enjoyed a certain celebrity in therapeutics. This is not the place to inquire into the real or supposed merits of these substances as remedial agents; moreover, they were scarcely ever prescribed without being combined with other drugs, so that it would be impossible to determine their genuine effects upon the organism. But there is one calcareous preparation which might, in some respects, be considered a substitute for our Calcarea carbonica, and the uses and effects of which are pretty well known; I mean *lime-water*. I do not pretend to say that lime-water and the carbonate of lime are identical in their action; but, if Hahnemann considered the acetate and carbonate of lime so nearly alike that he deemed it proper to range their symptoms side by side in a common pathogenesis,[1] we may certainly be allowed to believe that the difference between the action of lime-water and of carbonate of lime cannot be very great. What justifies this hypothesis is the fact, that, when lime-water remains exposed to the air for a while, a pellicle of sub-carbonate of lime is very speedily formed by the absorption of the carbonic acid. It is, therefore, interesting to us homœopaths to inquire how far the empirical applications of this drug coincide with the pathogenesis of the carbonate.

Lime-water seems to have been employed in medicine from the remotest antiquity. Hippocrates mentions it in several of his works, especially in the second book on epidemics, 5th section, and lauds it for several diseases, especially *lepra.* Fabricius d' Aquapendente recommended it for *encysted dropsy.* According to Gmelin,[2] Monro prescribed it internally and externally for *scaldhead;* Bell for *soft* and *suppurating warts*, and in general for *humid chronic exanthems*;[3] Girtenner for *old gonorrhœa;* Jæger for *ulcerated whitlows;* Morton,[4] Boerhaave,[5] and Graham[6] considered lime-water as one of the best remedies for *scrofulous or scorbutic ulcerations of the mouth, the genital organs and extremities.* These physicians used lime-water, as they expressed it, as a *desiccative*, an *astringent*, *a dissolvent*, and an *antiseptic* (doubtless, because they had remarked that it arrested the fetid smell of ulcers, which is, indeed, one of its effects *in some cases*). Hence they recommended it in *chronic diarrhœa*, *ulcerated cancer*, *gangrene*, etc. In many cases, according to Gmelin,[7] phlegm (or probably the chronic catarrh of the air-passages) has been known to yield to the prolonged use of this drug: a

[1] The symptoms of the acetate are marked with asterisks.

[2] *Appar. Med.*, vol. I., p. 11, etc.

[3] See symptoms, 1475, and foll. of calc. carb.

[4] *Opera Medica*, edit. of Geneva, p. 148.

[5] Elem. chem., vol. II., p. 316.

[6] Med. observ. by a societ. of phys., London, 8 vol., vol. I., p. 286.

[7] *Loc. Cit.*, p. 13.

statement which was afterwards confirmed by Monginot, who maintained that lime-water had been of great use to him in whooping-cough.[1] Lime-water has, lastly, been praised in *rheumatic* and *arthritic* affections, in *worm* and *intermittent fevers.*

It is to be remarked, that the warmest advocates of lime-water, notwithstanding all the good effects which they said it had in the above-named affections, were all agreed on the following points: 1st, that it was only suitable in the chronic forms of these affections; 2d, that it was counter-indicated by inflammatory fever, or by acute inflammation of some important organ; 3d, that it had unpleasant effects on individuals of a dry constitution and disposed to spasms; 4th, lastly, that it was able to do mischief at the commencement of dysentery, or when there was a sanguineous congestion of the head or kidneys.[2] Most of these counter-indications evidently reposed only on allœopathic prejudices. If an improperly administered dose of lime-water produced, in a single case, spasms, fever, congestion of the head or kidneys, (and such a thing might and must have happened,) it was supposed deleterious in all cases where such symptoms existed.

Now-a-days, lime-water has lost its former charm, and is scarcely used for any other purpose than to transform uric acid calculi into soluble urate of lime, an iatro-chemical proceeding, the success of which I dare not warrant. A few physicians, however, among whom I should mention Dr. Bretonneau, have tried to improve, in their practice, some of the traditional uses of lime-water. Bretonneau uses it in *chronic diarrhœa,* especially when ulcerations of the lesser intestines, and especially of the rectum, may be suspected.

This is a short synopsis of the history of lime-water, which is, I dare say, little known to allœopathic physicians, but which, no doubt, suggested to Hahnemann the idea of proving the oyster-shell for the purpose of determining the

[1] Journ. génér. de méd., Vol. XLIV., p. 290.

[2] Gmelin, *loc. cit.*, p. 23.

pure effects of lime, which may be found recorded in the first volume of his Chronic Diseases.

Calcarea is frequently, but contrary to rule, employed empirically, in chronic diseases, even by homœopathic physicians, in the hope of modifying, they know not how, an old or congenital diathesis. A few successes do not justify such a mode of proceeding, which I must reject. I know that the carbonate of lime, phosphorus, phosphoric acid, and all other substances which enter largely into the composition of the human body, exercise a deep and pervasive action on the organism; but this is, it strikes me, an additional reason why it should not be administered at random.

As a general rule, lime, when it is indicated by the symptoms, suits blond and fat children, of a peevish and whining mood, having a certain appearance of vigor, or in whom the process of ossification takes place with difficulty; fat youths; adults of both sexes, with fair complexions, blue eyes, disposed to sub-acute catarrhal affections and chronic rheumatism; women with white skins, mild or listless dispositions, whose menstruation is generally too early and profuse, and who, after a meal, or during a walk in a somewhat cool air, are attacked with heat in the face and redness at the tip of the nose; lastly, aged persons of both sexes, with dry, southern constitutions, yellowish complexions, having been troubled with tetters formerly, and being subject to attacks of peevishness, neuralgia or gout. It is especially in affections characterised by one or more of the following symptoms, that the carbonate of lime has been found efficacious:

Depression of spirits; peevishness, or weeping without any apparent cause; *tendency to start;* apprehension of near death; excessive sensitiveness; egotism; laziness; indifference for every thing; fatigue after walking ever so little; *great sensitiveness to the cold;* sweat after the least effort; dryness and roughness of the skin; furfuraceous tetters; *warts* on the extremities, and even in the face; papulous red spots on different parts of the body; *lipomata; anxiety* and shuddering towards evening; *drowsiness early in the evening;*

frequent waking at night; sleeplessness; restlessness in bed; disturbing dreams; paroxysms of epilepsy in the night; tertian fever in the afternoon or evening, with heat before the chill. The head feels generally dull, as if a board were pressing against the forehead, with difficulty of thinking; *vertigo in ascending an eminence; deep and sudden pain in the right half of the brain when stooping;* dizziness and trembling in the morning, after leaving the bed; heaviness and pressure at the forehead, obliging him to close his eyes; headache, caused by the least mental exercise; boring pain at the forehead; *pulsative* headache at the occiput; beating in the centre of the brain; hammering headache after a walk in the open air; flashes of heat about the head; headache and noise in the head, with heat about the cheeks; *icy coldness at the right side of the head; sweat about the head, in the evening; falling out of the hair;* itching of the eyes; *swelling of the eyes; congestion of the vessels of the eye;* stitches in the eyes: *deep-seated pain, proceeding from the bottom of the right orbit, as if the ball of the eye would be crushed from behind forward; photophobia;* lachrymation in the morning, in the open air; lachrymal fistula; obscuration of sight after eating or when reading; hemiopia; muscæ volitantes, or a sort of opaque gauze before the eyes; sensation as if electrical sparks started out of the eyes, (even in darkness;) *agglutination of the eyelids* during the night, and still more *during the morning slumber;* stitches in the ears; discharge of pus from the ears; cracking in the ear when swallowing; *beatings in the ears;* ringing in the ears; buzzing in the ears; noise in the ears, with hardness of hearing; noise in the ears, ending in a report; *dulness of hearing; pains at the nose;* stoppage of the nostrils by a yellow and fetid pus; bleeding of the nose; foul smell from the nose; smell of manure in the nose; pain in the face; itching and eruption in the face; freckles; itching, and itching pimples in the beard; eruption around the mouth; pain in the submaxillary glands; toothache after a cold drink; pulling and stinging toothache, day and night, excited again or aggravated by cold or warmth; digging and smarting in the teeth; *difficult teething of children;* painful swelling of the gums; ready bleeding of the gums; *dryness of the tongue,* night or morning, on waking; ranula; accumulation of mucus in the mouth and throat; *bitter mouth, in the morning; want of appetite; loss of appetite, with constant thirst;* aversion to warm food, especially warm meat; urging hunger in the morning; hunger shortly after having eaten; insatiable hunger; heat of the skin after eating; rush of blood to the head and face, sometimes with palpitation of the heart, after eating; eructations after eating; bitter eructations; sour eructations immediately after taking milk; heaviness of the stomach, before breakfast, and after eating; heaviness at the pit of the stomach, (with thirst,) at night; spasms of the stomach; pinching, lancing or cutting pain at the pit of the stomach; sensitiveness of the epigastric region, which does not allow one to wear tight clothes; swelling of the epigastric region, with pressive pain; tension in both hypochondria; pressive, lancing pain in the abdomen, without diarrhœa; cutting pain in the upper part of the abdomen; cutting colic in the lower abdomen, in the afternoon, with vomiting of the food that had been taken a few hours previously; coldness in the lower abdomen; *swelling and hardness of the lower abdomen; shifting of flatulence;* constipation; scanty and hard stools; *soft, thin and frequent stools; stools consisting of undigested food; chronic diarrhœa without bellyache;* stools white as clay; involuntary discharge of liquid stool; protrusion of the piles, with burning pain, when going to stool; *violent, fetid diarrhœa, at night or towards morning, with prolapsus of the rectum, enormous pressure on the anus and the genitals, which are swollen, constant and painful erections, excessive anguish;*[1] prostration and painful weariness after stool; *itching and ascarides in the*

[1] In the case of a man of sixty-six years, of a dry and nervous constitution, afflicted with tetters and the gout, Calcarea arrested these alarming symptoms very soon.

rectum; tenesmus of the bladder, or, rather, frequent emission of urine; discharge of blood from the urethra; blood urine; lascivious fancies; deficiency of sexual desire; weakness of the genital organs; *absence of thrill during an embrace;* stitches and burning in the male genital organs during the ejaculation of the semen; pressive pain in the vagina; pressure on the uterus; *symptoms of miscarriage;* stitches at the uterine orifice; itching at the vulva; varices on the labia majora; *uterine hæmorrhage; premature and profuse menses;* cutting colic during the menses; *acrid leucorrhœa previous to the menses.*

Stuffing in the nose, especially in the morning; excessive coryza; *chronic coryza; purulent coryza;* hoarseness; excessive phlegm on the chest; cough in the evening, in bed; *cough all night,* during sleep; cough in the morning; *dry cough;* yellow and fetid sputa; heaviness at the stomach when coughing; oppression on the chest; loss of breath when stooping; *stitches in the side of the chest during motion;* heat in the chest; *palpitation of the heart at night; stitches in the region of the heart;* formication in the pectoral muscles; swelling of the breasts; *stiffness of the nape of the neck; swelling of the cervical glands;* pain in the loins; liability to attacks of lumbago, either by making an effort, or by exposure to a draught of air; pressive pain in the right arm; rheumatic pain in the arms, at night; *weariness in the arms;* paralytic weakness of the hands; swelling of the hands; *sweat on the hands;* arthritic nodes on the hands and feet; numbness of the fingers, even in warmth; heaviness of the extremities, and particularly of the feet; spasms in the nates; stitches in the thighs; *varices at the thighs;* numbness of the legs when sitting; stiffness of the legs; cramps in the legs; ulcers at the legs; stitches and tearing in the knee; pulling in the knees; swelling of the (right) knee; heat at the sole of the foot; swelling of the soles of the feet; cold feet in the evening; *sweaty feet;* numb feet in the evening; sensitiveness of the big toes; *stitches in the corns.*

The Calcarea-pains are most generally felt while lying in bed, or while sitting; they are felt in the parts upon which the body had been lying for a time.

In some respects, there exists a sort of negative relation between the symptoms of Mercurius solubilis, or rather between those of nitric acid and the symptoms of Calcarea. This contrast has struck me several times, and it is the more remarkable for this reason, that nitric acid is one of the best antidotes of calcarea.

Phosphorus.—A simple body which was discovered in 1673, by Brandt, an alchymist of Hamburgh, and shortly after by Kunkel, in Saxony, and by Robert Bayle, in England.

Phosphorus is a solid substance, colorless, transparent, flexible, luminous in the dark, exhaling an odor *sui generis* which has been compared to that of garlic. Fusible at 43 degrees of the centigrade thermometer, it is very volatile, and has such a strong affinity for oxygen that, when exposed to the open air, it burns in any temperature, disengaging a white smoke of phosphoric acid, which shines in the dark. It is insoluble in water, but tolerably soluble in alcohol, ether, fat and volatile oils. Phosphorus, which exists in large quantities in nature combined with oxygen and lime, is never found in a free state. It is extracted from urine, and still more generally from the bones of animals, the solid portion of which consists, as is well known, for the most part, of phosphate of lime.

Empirical Applications.—As soon as phosphorus had been discovered, attempts were made to use it as a drug. Kunkel made it into his so-called *luminous pills*, which he used for various chronic diseases, and some years after, Kramer, physician to the Elector of Saxony, pretended having cured with phosphorus, as by enchantment, several cases of *dementia, epilepsy* and *malignant fevers.*

Bayle has collected in the second volume of his *bibliothèque de thérapeutique* a very considerable number of cases successfully treated with phosphorus in Germany and France, but especially in the former country, from the time of Kramer to that of Lœbenstein-Lebel, or from 1738 to 1815. The principal cases,—there are not less than a hundred in all, in this learned compilation—are taken from the reports of Mentz, Morgenstern, P. J. Hartmann, Bœnnekenius, Weickard, Conrad, Alphonse Leroy, Jacquemin, Hufeland, Coindet, Odier, Lobstein, Frank, Crell, Midy, Poilroux, Pilger and Lœbenstein-Lebel.[1]

The following diseases were treated by these practitioners:

1st. Twenty-five cases of *continuous fever* (of the kind generally termed typhoid, putrid, ataxic, adynamic, etc.); the principal symptoms being; increase of temperature, more or less accelerated pulse, delirium, coma, various nervous symptoms, petechial, miliary or purple eruptions, (almost always on the chest and neck,) restlessness or prostration, foul odor of the excretions frequently; and lastly, in most cases, at the period when the use of phosphorus was decided upon: precursory signs of approaching death, such as, feeble, imperceptible pulse, cold extremities, loss of sensibility and cessation of the action of the senses.

2d. Six cases of *bilious fever*.

3d. Three cases of *tertian intermittent*, having been unsuccessfully treated with cinchona and other remedies.

4th. Six cases of *general œdema* following putrid fevers, with excessive prostration, coldness of the extremities, small pulse, interruption of the sensual perceptions, etc.

5th. A case of *measles* of a suspicious nature, with disappearance of exanthem, (which the phosphorus brought out again,) dyspnœa, anxiety in the præcordia, etc.

6th. Two cases of pneumonia (left lung) accompanied with ataxic symptoms.

7th. Two cases of very *serious pleurisy*, the symptoms of which unfortunately are described incompletely.

8th. A case of *croupy disease*.

9th. A case of chronic *ophthalmia*.

[1] Lœbenstein-Lebel, *recherches et observations sur le phosphore*, Strasburgh 1815.

10th. A case of *chronic rheumatism* of the legs, (described incompletely).

11th. Two cases of *cerebral apoplexy*, one of them accompanied by convulsions of the right arm and right lower extremity, and the other case having been several times aggravated by bleeding.

12th. Two cases of *hydrocephalus*.

13th. Two cases of *periodical headache;* in one case the attacks came on almost every ten days, in a nervous and delicate female whose menstruation was irregular; the other case was of a gouty nature.

14th. A sort of *catalepsy* coming on after confinement, and which ceased after the breaking out of miliaria.

15th. Two cases of *convulsions*, incompletely described.

16th. Two cases of *epilepsy*.

17th. One case of *mania*.

18th. Five cases of *paralysis*, among which two cases came on after an attack of gout.

19th. A well marked case of *gutta serena*, the cure of which cannot be attributed to any other agency than that of phosphorus.

20th. A case of *amenorrhœa*.

21st. An obstinate case of *cardialgia*.

22d. A case of *asthenia senilis*, in a man of eighty years, who used other medicines at the same time.

23d. Three cases of *gout*, with swelling of the joints and typhus, the cure being accompanied with profuse sweat and emission of urine.

24th. A case of chronic-*lead poisoning*.

25th. A case of *chlorosis*.

The following cases were not cured, but a temporary relief, which was sometimes most extraordinary, was experienced under the administration of phosphorus: Two cases of *purple* and *petechial typhus;* a case without any particular name (by Alphonse Leroy,) with evident symptoms of agony, and the fatal termination of which was kept off for a fortnight; a case of *bilious fever;* a case of *paralysis;* a case of *anasarca;* and one case of *ascites.*

The other cases, related by Bayle, were treated with phosphoric acid; we shall recur to them in time and season.

There is no doubt that the cases which were unsuccessfully treated by these physicians, are much more numerous than the cures. This, however, only shows that phosphorus is, no more than any other drug, a panacea for all diseases, and that it cures only such cases as correspond to its remedial virtues. Let allœopathic physicians study Bayle's cases as I have done, pen in hand, draw up a list of the symptoms of these cases, compare these symptoms with the pure effects of phosphorus on the healthy organism, and they will soon learn why phosphorus cured in some and failed in other cases. Unfortunately such a comparison could not have been instituted before the drug had been experimented with, and this is the reason why phosphorus, in spite of the cures it had effected, has fallen into disuse among allœopathic physicians to such a degree that it is not even mentioned in their modern treatises of therapeutics.

Bayle, who is not a homœopath, (which I am at a loss to comprehend, after having read his treatise,) sums up the therapeutic action of phosphorus as well as could be expected of an observer who is not accustomed to the Hahnemannian mode of investigation. He says: "Phosphorus is indicated, 1st, in every disease where death has become imminent in consequence of the deep-seated injury inflicted upon the vital forces, without the structure of the organs being much altered. We see this state of things in all severe continuous fevers, when they have attained their last stage, be they caused by some miasm, such as typhus, plague, etc., or by a spontaneous alteration of the blood, as in the so-called adynamic or putrid fevers. In such cases, phosphorus reanimates the vitality, furnishes nature the means of effectually resisting the disease, and eliminating, by the natural excretory outlets of the system, the material causes of the disease. Phosphorus is indicated, 2d, in all acute exanthemata when the eruption had disappeared quite suddenly, with aggravation of the symptoms, (measles, variola, scarlatina, miliaria, erysipelas, low fevers, with exanthem;)[1] 3d, in malignant pustule, when the low fever has reached its acme, and the strength seems on the point of becoming extinct; 4th, in gout and chronic rheumatism, which nature relieves or cures by profuse sweat or urine; 5th, in all morbid conditions, where it is proper to excite these secretions, and, at the same time, to stimulate the vitality in a speedy and energetic manner."[2]

Homœopathic applications.—I infer from the clinical observations of homœopathic physicians, and from mine in particular, that phosphorus, when it is indicated by the symptoms of the disease, is principally suitable to adults of both sexes and to old men (much rather than to children) of a lymphatico-sanguine, sanguine-nervous temperament, fair complexion, sensitive disposition, lively and quick perceptions, inclined to corpulence, or else thin and slender, with a narrow chest, and what is generally termed, a phthisicky habit. Here follows a list of the symptoms, a majority of which is taken from Hahnemann, against which phosphorus has been used with the best effect:—

Sadness; *weeping;* or involuntary laughter; want of decision; indifference for one's own family; aversion to society, in general; tendency to start; irascible disposition; timidity; *aversion to work;* paroxysms of anxiety, with *embarrassed respiration;* bitter eructations, and heat in the hands; anxiety, especially in the evening, with palpitation of the heart, and trembling of the extremities; *pulsations in*

[1] Bayle's remark, which is often founded so far as measles, purple-rash, miliaria, pétechiæ, and some forms of erysipelas are concerned, is much less applicable to variola and scarlatina. As a general rule, phosphorus is only useful in retrocessions of exanthemata when ataxic symptoms and derangements in the region of the heart and the air-passages spring up in consequence of these retrocessions.

[2] *Loc. Cit.*, p. 124. (See the pathogenesis of Phosphorus in Hahnemann's Chronic Diseases, vol. III.)

different parts of the body; vertigo of various kinds; stupefying headache; rush of blood to the head; *headache in the morning;* pulsations in the brain; sudden shock in the brain, (when stooping,) stitches in the side of the head, externally; itching about the head; *falling off of the hair;* heat and smarting in the outer canthi of the eyes; inflammation of the eyes, with heat and pressive pain; lachrymation in the open air; photophobia; dimness of sight; hemeralopia; *myopia;* every object looks as of a grayish color; cataract; glaucoma; *black spots hovering before the eyes;* difficulty of opening the lids; nightly agglutination of the lids; *beatings in the ears; buzzing in the ears;* difficulty of hearing the human voice; *nose-bleed;* bad smell from the nose; want of smell; earthy complexion; redness and heat of the cheeks; tearing in both jaws, at night; toothache in the morning, when eating; lancing toothache every night, until two o'clock; bitterness of the mouth; excoriation in the inner mouth; mucus in the mouth; *dryness in the throat,* day and night; *a good deal of phlegm, in the morning;* slimy taste in the mouth; cheesy taste in the mouth; loss of taste; *eructations;* spasmodic eructations; sour eructations; *absence of thirst;* thirst in the middle of the day; nausea in the morning; obstinate or periodical hiccough; hunger after eating; nausea after eating; canine hunger; nausea after having eaten sour things; burning in the hands after eating; laziness and drowsiness after eating; *heaviness at the stomach after eating,* with vomiting of the ingesta; sort of tightness of the cardia, causing a rising of the food that had just been swallowed; sensitiveness of the pit of the stomach; formication in the pit of the stomach; *rancid regurgitations;* difficulty of digesting milk; *flatulence* after dinner; bellyache in the morning, in bed; *borborygmi, gurgling in the abdomen; inguinal hernia;* violent urging before stool; tearing in the abdomen, with violent urging to stool; *discharge of blood during stool; diarrhœa of phthisicky patients;* discharge of pieces of tænia; itching at the anus; *internal and external piles;* discharge of mucus from the anus; tension in the urethra; smarting in the urethra when urinating; hot urine; burning twitching in the urethra; erection in the evening; *excessive desire for an embrace;* too rapid ejaculation of the semen; *frequent emissions; stitches in the vagina, extending to the uterus;* too profuse and watery menses; *megrim at the period of the menses;* leucorrhœa.

Stuffing of the nose; fatiguing dryness in the nose; constant discharge of mucus from the nose; smarting in the throat; mucous sputa; *tickling in the throat,* which excites a cough; chronic cough; cough excited by laughter; cough, with vomiting; *cough, with pain in the chest and hoarseness;* cough during the night, with stitches in the larynx; difficulty of breathing; noisy respiration; pressure on the chest; chronic stitches in the side; smarting pain in the chest; pain in the left side of the chest, when resting upon it; *palpitation of the heart when sitting;* palpitation of the heart during the least movement; spasms of the pectoral muscles; swelling of the breasts, (especially the left;) contusive pain in the back; *stiffness of the nape of the neck;* swelling of the neck; pain in the arm when raising it; tearing stitches in the arms and shoulder-blades; heat in the hands, *with swelling of the veins;* trembling of the hands; pulsative pain in the buttocks; spasms in the glutei muscles; stitch in the hip striking to the chest; pulling pain in the knees; twitchings in the calves; exostosis at the tibia; cold feet at night; smarting pains at the soles of the feet when walking; shocks in the feet, in the day time and at night before falling asleep; rheumatism in the extremities; numbness of the ends of the fingers and toes; round, *papulous,* yellow spots on the chest and lower abdomen; brown spots on the body; drowsiness in the day time; drowsiness in the morning; *difficulty of falling asleep, in the evening;* sleep full of dreams; frightful dreams; cold in bed, every evening; *dry heat, without thirst, in the evening, in bed;* transitory heat; *sweat in the morning.*

Sulphur, chamomilla, carbo veg. and viola, are most generally employed with phosphorus, at least in chest affections.

I do not believe that the antidotes which Jahr points out in his Manual, *Camph. Coff. Nux vom.* and *wine*, will prove of much avail. *Chamom.* may, perhaps, neutralise the action of phosphorus with tolerable speed.

Hepar sulphuris calcareum, *sulphuret of lime.*—This compound exists in nature; but the homœopathic preparation is obtained artificially, by calcinating in closed vessels equal parts of purified flowers of sulphur, and finely pulverised oyster-shells.

The therapeutic history of this substance is very short. At first it was only used externally against the *itch, rheumatism, gout, goître and scrofulous swellings.* C. L. Hoffmann and Stoll, among others, recommended it very strongly for the two last named affections.[1] In 1794, Hahnemann, who is quoted by Gmelin, proposed to use it internally to arrest *mercurial salivation.* A few years after this, it was tried for *asthma* and *pulmonary phthisis.* This was one of the happiest applications that could have been made of this drug. I believe that this idea is due to Dr. Busch, of Strasburgh. In the first period of the disease, Busch prescribed the extract of aconite, and hepar sulphuris in the subsequent periods. He states that by means of this empirical proceeding, he has effected several cures of confirmed pulmonary phthisis.[2] Professor Bang, of Copenhagen, pretends having arrested by the same means an incipient *pulmonary phthisis*, (which is very vague.)[3] In our time, Dr. Harel de Tancrel, pretends curing pulmonary phthisis by means of a mixture of extract of aconite and hepar sulphuris. Such assertions are only imperfectly justified by the physiological action of hepar. There

[1] Gmelin, *appar. medic.*, vol. I., p. 164.

[2] Recherch. sur la nature et le traitem. de la phthisie pulm., par J. J. Busch, in 8vo., 1800.

[3] *Bullet. des sc. méd.* de Férussac, vol. I., p. 213.

are some forms of phthisis the symptoms of which correspond to hepar, and which may, therefore, be cured by means of this drug; but in other forms of this disease, hepar would be out of place and might do harm. Experience shows this every day.[1]

According to Hahnemann, hepar has been used with success in the following morbid conditions:

Dissatisfaction with one's self and others; unpleasant recollections; dreamy, atrabilious mood, *a sort of ferocious spleen, as though one could murder a man in cold blood,* (even in persons who are generally of a benevolent and merry disposition);[2] boring pain at the root of the nose, every morning, from seven o'clock until noon; smarting pain above the eye, every evening; stitches in the eyes; photophobia; discharge of fetid pus from the ear; erysipelas of the face, with prickling tension; dryness of the throat; scraping in the throat, with difficulty of talking, but not of swallowing; canine hunger; eruptions; paroxysms of nausea, with coldness and paleness; swelling and pressure at the epigastric region; frequent stomach-ache; constrictive pain in the lower abdomen; stitches in the left side of the abdomen; shifting of flatulence; difficult emission of flatulence, in the morning; emission of urine during sleep, at night; mucous discharge from the urethra; deficient sexual desire; absence of erections; feeble erections during an embrace; *discharge of prostatic fluid while urinating after hard stool;* considerable delay of the menses; leucorrhœa and excoriations of the vulva; cough; violent cough, in the evening, in bed; spasmodic constriction of the chest, after talking; cancerous ulcer at the breast, with a lancinating, burning pain, and an odor as of old cheese; tearing pain in the arm; pulling in the back, between the shoulders; fetid sweat in the axillæ; cyst at the point of the

[1] See the pathogenesis of this drug in Hahnemann's *Chronic Diseases,* vol. II., p. 283.

[2] These symptoms are not mentioned by Hahnemann; but I have seen them yield so often under the action of *hepar,* that I look upon them as characteristic effects of this drug.

elbow; numbness of the fingers; pulling pains in the extremities, especially in the morning, on waking; weakness and trembling after smoking; yawning; liability to sweating, in the day-time; transitory heat, with sweat.

Hepar is frequently indicated in the diseases of children. It is antidoted by silicea, chamomilla, and especially by belladonna.

GROUP VI.

TYPE: SEPIÆ SUCCUS.
ANALOGUES: COPAIVÆ BALSAMUM. ALUMINA.

We have seen these three drugs figure on a previous occasion among the analogues of arsenic, to which they seem indeed related by their generally depressing action, their mode of affecting the digestive apparatus, and, to a certain extent, all the mucous membranes, the nervous system and the cutaneous envelope. But their peculiar action upon the organs of generation, has decided me to unite them into a special group. The resemblance which they bear to each other, is clearly evidenced by their pathogenetic effects, and still more by the clinical verification of their curative virtues; this assertion will appear the more correct, the more frequently alumina is made use of by our practitioners.[1]

COMMON CHARACTERISTICS.

Excessive excitability of the whole nervous system.

Weakness of the intellectual, and excitation of the sentient powers.

Hysteric derangement of the cerebral functions, as though the mind were deranged, (especially under the action of alumina.)

Paroxysms of weeping, sobbing, and of spasms.

Indifference, misanthropy, loathing of life, and, at the same time, *extreme fear of death.*

Tendency to start, to be uneasy, and particularly *to feel vexed.*

[1] Further on, the reader will find a pathogenesis of the balsamum copaivæ, which, although still very incomplete, is, however, much more complete than Hahnemann's proving, which is, however, included among the symptoms of the former.

All the symptoms are aggravated by chagrin and contrarieties.[1]

Extreme sensitiveness to cold and dampness.

Fever in the morning, with coldness; smallness, depression, and sometimes slowness of the pulse.

Flashes of heat in the face, followed, in some cases, by a passing sweat, during or after a meal, a discussion, or after the least disagreeable excitement.

Red, itching and oozing spots, flat or papulous here and there.

Restless sleep at night, full of frightful or lascivious dreams frequent or too early waking, with inability to fall asleep again.

Hysteric headache, pulsative, boring; *beatings in the occiput; pain at the root of the hairs; falling out of the hairs* and eyebrows; coldness at the head.

Buzzing and whizzing in the ears; *extreme sensitiveness of hearing.*

Pressure at the eyes, ophthalmia, *with agglutination of the eyelids* by dry gum or pus; contraction of the pupils; dimness of sight; *great sensitiveness of the eyes to light.*

Tetter at the tip of the nose; bad smell in the nose; *excited sense of smell.*

Paleness and sickly looks; tension at the cheeks; *red tettery spots on the cheeks or chin.*

Cracked lips; drawing toothache; *caries of the teeth;* sense of coldness in the incisor teeth; *sensation as if the teeth were too long*, which renders chewing painful; *looseness of the teeth*, with ulcerative pain at their roots.

Bad smell from the mouth; putrid breath, or breath having

[1] Every practitioner knows that intensely unpleasant emotions react very unfavorably upon the powers of the sexual sphere, which exalt to the highest degree the receptivity of the soul. I have seen a gonorrhœa which I had fancied cured for a week past, break out afresh with great violence in consequence of a paroxysm of anger. But it is especially in uterine diseases that we frequently see aggravations or morbid paroxysms caused by violent emotions.

a penetrating odor, *sui generis; dryness of the mouth; flow of saliva;* coated tongue in the morning; sour taste in the mouth.

Acute angina; swelling and ulceration of the tonsils; *secretion in the mouth and throat of phlegm, which it is difficult to spit up.*

Changeable, irregular appetite; sense of emptiness and pressure as from a stone, at the stomach; nausea; *sour eructations;* difficulty of digesting milk and various kinds of vegetables; paroxysms of spasmodic vomiting, with violent straining, and threatening suffocation; swelling and sensitiveness of the epigastrium.

Pressure and heaviness in the abdomen; distension of the abdomen as if it would burst; borborygmi; *emission of fetid flatulence; tearing and cutting colic; swelling of the lower abdomen.*

Several stools a day; diarrhœa, causing a good deal of prostration; violent diarrhœa, with cholera symptoms; ascarides, crawling out of the rectum; incomplete stools; scanty stools, like sheep's dung; *serous or purulent discharge from the anus between stools stitches in the rectum;* blind or fluent piles; *burning pain and stitches at the anus.*

Constant pressure on the bladder, with pain in the loins, frequently unsuccessful urging to urinate; catarrh of the bladder; spasms of the bladder; smarting pain and stitches in the urethra; gonorrhœa; large and superficial ulcerations (false chancres) *at the glans and prepuce; swelling of the inguinal glands; swelling and induration of a testicle* (generally the left,) *heat and swelling at the scrotum; profuse sweat at the perineum.*

Constant excitement of the sexual instinct; desire, with impotence; too speedy ejaculation of the semen; absence of thrill during an embrace.

Pressure on the uterus; spasmodic contractions of the uterus; heat in the vulva and vagina; stitches in the vagina extending to the os tincæ, and even to the interior of the womb; excoriation at the neck of the uterus; leucorrhœa before and after the menses; and sometimes in the place of them; *gonorrhœa from the urethra or vagina* (in women;) *red papulous tetters at the vulva* (speciall y in the case of alumina,) *and causing a very unpleasant burning itching.*

Premature, pale, not very copious menses accompanied by several hysteric symptoms, or also suppression of the menses.

Sensation of exhaustion and restlessness, depriving her of sleep, after an embrace.

Coryza; hoarseness with constrictive and excoriative pain at the larynx; cough morning and evening; or continual, dry cough, or *cough with profuse expectoration of whitish, greenish or blood-streaked purulent mucus;* stitches at the base of the chest, on the right side, in both sides of the chest; *palpitation of the heart;* irregular and intermittent beating of the heart.

Rheumatic pains *at the nape of the neck, back, sacrum; stitches between* the shoulders and shoulder-blades; sweat and tetters in the axillæ; tensive and tearing pain *in the hips and thighs; swelling of the knee;* swelling of the feet and legs.

Uneasiness in the extremities; contusive pain in the extremities; tendency of the limbs to go to sleep; *partial* paralysis; twitching in the extremities; cold feet and hands.

The pains are eased by motion, aggravated by cold, rest, and by lying on the affected parts; general emaciation; most of the symptoms are worse at night and in the morning.

Several homœopaths having supposed that there exists a resemblance between sepia and pulsatilla, at least in the general action of these drugs, I have deemed it advisable to contrast the differences existing between the general action of the drugs of this and the former group, in the following arrangement:

General Symptoms of the Pulsatilla Group.	General Symptoms of the Sepia Group.
1. Symptoms which seem, all of them, to proceed from the heart and lungs.	1. Symptoms which seem, all of them, to proceed from the lower abdomen, and more particularly from the genital organs.

2. Engorgement of all the blood-vessels, especially the veins, (varices, etc.)	2. Depression of the pulse, a sort of eruption of the vascular apparatus.
3. Congestive headache, sometimes followed by hemiplegia.	3. Hysteric headache; partial paralysis.
4. Numbness of the nerves; dulness of the senses; sort of plethora.	4. Excited nerves; excessive nervous sensitiveness: loss of flesh.
5. Engorgement of the parenchyma; slow mucous discharges, (diarrhœa, etc.) which do not cause exhaustion.	5. Mucous discharges, without marked congestion; painful diarrhœa, and causing much prostration.
6. Derangement of the digestive passages which is never very acute, and seems to proceed from a sort of inertia.	6. Gastric and intestinal symptoms which are sometimes so acute that they resemble sporadic cholera or a case of poisoning by arsenic.
7. Dysmenorrhœa, with black and coagulated blood, showing at the same time a tendency to plethora, and a vicious state of the blood, etc. etc.	7. Dysmenorrhœa, with rose-colored, pale, impoverished, discolored blood, etc. etc.

CORRESPONDING DISEASES.

Nervous headache. — Ophthalmia. — Coryza. — Dyspepsia. — Dysentery. — Diarrhœa.—Sporadic cholera.—Ascarides.—Intestinal spasms.—Ascites. —Nephritis.—Dysuria.—Cystitis.—Catarrh of the bladder.—Gonorrhœa, (not syphilitic.)—Hardness of the testicles.—Buboes, (not syphilitic.)—Metritis. — Metrorrhagia. — Precursory symptoms or consequences of miscarriage, (in hysteric females.) — Dysmenorrhœa. — Leucorrhœa. — Hysteria.—Nymphomania.—Acne rosacea.—Erythema, (sometimes very obstinate, at the vulva, tip of the nose, etc.)—Angina.—Pulmonary catarrh, etc.

Sepia. The sepiæ are molluscæ of the seas, with heads and feet, without any outer shells, of variable sizes, and provided with pouches that contain a blackish-brown liquid with which they disturb the water for the purpose of escaping from an enemy or catching prey.

This liquid has for a long time past been confounded with Chinese ink; we owe a knowledge of its remedial properties to Hahnemann, (see *Chronic Diseases*, vol. III.)

The flesh of these animals, which is said to pass for a delicacy in Greece, and in some parts of Italy, is not much esteemed in France; it is generally tough and indigestible.

The flesh of some varieties exhales a marked odor of musk, which few persons find agreeable. The fact that this flesh is endowed with medicinal properties, is an additional reason, why its use as an article of diet should be relinquished.

Empirical applications. According to Mérat and Delens, Hippocrates prescribed sepia in the diseases of women. He regarded it as an *astringent*,[1] contrary to the opinion of Plinius, who looked upon it as a *diuretic* and *purgative*. I confess I have never seen the passage where Hippocrates speaks of the astringent properties of sepia; but I have read in his works[2] that he recommended a broth made of Pulpe or *Calemar*, (varieties of sepia,) 1st, to recently confined women who had retained their placenta; 2d, to those whose lochiæ did not appear or remained suppressed. According to this, it would seem that Hippocrates believed the flesh of sepia possessed of the same properties which are ascribed to the liquid in the pouch. What is still more remarkable is, that several physicians among the ancients, such as Dioscorides, Soranus, Plinius and Marcellus, used either the flesh, the eggs, or even the only bone which constitutes the skeleton of this animal, for *leucorrhœa, gonorrhœa, catarrh of the bladder, gravel, spasms of the bladder, baldness, freckles, and certain kinds of tetters*, in other words for the very diseases for which we employ the *juice of sepia* in our own practice.[3] I need scarcely say, that this drug has been out of use for centuries.

Sepia, if indicated by the symptoms, is principally suitable to young people of both sexes, or, rather, to persons between the age of pubescence and the critical period of life; of delicate constitutions, with fine, white skins, or skins having a rosy tinge; blond or red hair; nervous or lymphatico-nervous temperaments; exceedingly excitable, and anxious for emotions; and lastly, and particularly such as are disposed to

[1] *Dict. univ. de mat. méd.*, vol. VI., p. 329.

[2] Complete works of Hipp., translated by Littré, Paris, 1853, vol. VIII., p. 105, 119, etc. *Treatise of female diseases*, book I.

[3] See *Suite* de la mat. méd. de Geoffroy, vol. I., p. 137, and foll.

sexual excitement, or have been exhausted by sexual excesses. It is particularly indicated by one or more of the following symptoms:

Restlessness obliging one to change one's place or position all the time; *anxiety and prostration, as after deep emotions;* paroxysms of discouragement, weeping, sobbing; extreme uneasiness concerning one's health, even in persons who, when in good health, would not hesitate to brave the greatest dangers, and death itself without fear; excessive excitability of all the senses; aversion to one's habitual occupations; indifference for one's family; momentary paroxysms of vertigo, with loss of consciousness; weak memory; inability to attend to mental labor; *boring headache,* with *coldness of the external head;* headache with nausea and vomiting; heaviness of the head; lancinating and pulsative headache, *especially at the occiput;* tendency of the head to fall backwards; *rush of blood to the head,* when stooping; the headache is worse when leaning or lying on the affected part of the head; itching of the hairy scalp; red, vesicular eruption, with ulcerative pain at the back part of the head; *falling off of the hair;* itching in the ears; *buzzing in the ears;* otalgia; formication in the eyes, especially at candle-light; *purulent ophthalmia; presbyopia; gauze before the eyes;* black points and fiery zigzag before the eyes; amaurosis with contraction of the pupils; dry crusts at the free margin of the lids, in the morning; *red obstinate tetter at the tip of the nose;* frequent flashes of heat in the face; yellow complexion; itching in the face; erysipelatous bloating of a whole side of the face, proceeding from a carious tooth; *caries of the teeth;* lancinating toothache in the evening or at night, worse in the cold; the teeth feel elongated, and as if they would start out of their sockets; *dry and cracked lips;* swelling and bleeding of the gums; smarting of the gums; *dry mouth and throat;* profuse flow of salt saliva; strong breath; white-coated tongue; smarting at the tip of the tongue; constric-

[1] A flow of saliva, and dryness of the mouth, or, at any rate, of the throat, may very well exist together; I have seen this in a number of cases.

tion of the pharynx; phlegm in the morning; canine hunger; aversion to food; *aversion to meat and milk; acidity in the mouth after eating; sour eructations;* eructations tasting of the food; pressive pain at the pit of the stomach, even before breakfast; stitches at the stomach; twisting pain at the stomach, followed by a profuse flow of saliva in the mouth; beatings at the pit of the stomach, increasing in proportion as one eats more; cramps at the stomach, with spasms in the chest; *stomach-ache,* with heat at the face and head, scraping in the throat, and hacking cough after eating; *sense of emptiness in the stomach;* boring in the hypochondria; *digging, pressure and cutting pains in the hypogastrium;* pressure in the lower abdomen, ascending to the stomach; sensation as if some hard body had lodged in the lower abdomen; swelling of the abdomen; sense of emptiness in the abdomen; coldness at the abdomen;[1] *ascites;* noisy borborygmi; a good deal of wind in the bowels, especially after eating; cutting pains, brought on again by motion; ineffectual urging to stool; delaying stool; *stool which is too soft; exhausting diarrhœa;*[2] violent diarrhœa, with spasmodic pains in the bowels, especially at night; incomplete stool; stool like *sheep's dung;* heat in the rectum; formication and stitches in the rectum; spasms of the rectum; *falling of the rectum during stool;* discharge of mucus, blood or even pus from the anus; pressure on the bladder; *spasms of the bladder; tenesmus of the bladder;* dark urine; smarting in the urethra when urinating; *gonorrhœa; painful swelling of the testicles,* (especially the left;) *superficial ulcerations at the glans and prepuce;* sweat at the genital organs; red and oozing tetter at the genital organs; *pressure on the womb; spasms of the womb;* penetrating stitches in the vagina; *leucorrhœa, gonorrhœa, from the urethra* and *vagina* of the

[1] Pulsatilla and several of its analogues have the opposite symptom (unpleasant heat) at the skin of the abdomen, and especially the hypogastrium.

[2] The contrary is the case with the diarrhœa caused by Pulsatilla, which often does *not exhaust* and is not accompanied with pain.

female; *engorgement of the inguinal glands; pale, not very profuse*, and too early menses; *active metrorrhagia; superficial ulcerations at the neck of the uterus; sexual excitement in either sex; weakness of the genital organs.*

Fatiguing dryness of the nose; *stuffing;* fluent coryza; hoarseness, which sometimes comes on suddenly; cough, morning and evening, with white and salt sputa; yellowish sputa, which it is difficult to raise; fetid sputa; blood-streaked sputa; oppression of the chest when walking, ascending an eminence, or in the evening, in bed; pressure on the sternum; pain in the chest during motion; smarting pain in the chest; *stitches at the base of the chest*, on the right side; *stitches in the left side* of the chest; stitches in the side when breathing or coughing; irregular and intermittent beating of the heart, especially after eating; pain in the loins; pressive pain at the sacrum; beating in the sacrum; frequent backache; itching eruptions at the back; shuddering in the back; tearings and cramps in the back; stiffness of the back; *stiffness of the nape of the neck;* sweat in the axillæ; moist tetters in the left axillæ; lassitude in the arms; stiffness in the arms; *pullings in the arm*, which obliges one to let it hang down; heat in the palms of the hands; cold sweat at the hands; deformity of the finger-nails; tearing stitch proceeding from the superior skin of the pelvis round the groin, to the front part of the thigh; paralysis of the lower limbs; lancing shocks in the thighs, which oblige one to raise the leg; rheumatic pain and swelling at the knee; stitches in the legs; painful pullings in the legs and the big toe; *cold legs and feet;* cramps in the calves; swelling of the legs and feet; twitching of the feet during sleep, in the day-time; stitches in the instep; heat and formication in the feet; sweaty feet; suppression of the sweat of the feet; numbness of the arms and legs, especially during manual labor; stiffness of the wrists, knee and tarsal joints; ulcers at the joints of the fingers and toes; restlessness and beating in all the limbs; burning pains in different parts of the body; *paroxysms of passing heat;* heat excited by anger or a lively conversation; profuse sweat during the least motion; *deficiency of natural temperature;* sensitiveness to the open air; *tendency to taking cold;* aggravation of all the pains by cold, especially a damp cold, and still more by the contact of cold water; *brownish spots on the chest*, abdomen and back; *shocks and twitchings in the extremities, in the day-time;* frequent stretching; aversion to exercise; fatigue when making the least effort; fatigue even to trembling; drowsiness in the day-time, or early in the evening; reveries during sleep; disturbing or frightful dreams; frequent waking at night; aggravation of several symptoms at night; *slow pulse.*

Is sepia, which, by the totality of its symptoms, corresponds to corrosive sublimate in man, and soluble mercury in woman, like these two agents, an *anti-syphilitic?* This question deserves to be examined, though I am disposed to doubt the anti-syphilitic virtues of this drug.

It is undoubtedly true that certain kinds of infectious gonorrhœa can be, and have been, cured with sepia in a number of cases. But I do not believe that these kinds of gonorrhœa belong to the syphilitic class, and, if left to themselves, would taint the whole organism, and develop the venereal chancre, buboes, gommata, exostosis, caries, necrosis, and all the other forms of secondary syphilis.

Not that I believe that the gonorrhœa which yields to sepia, must *necessarily* be a local disease only. Any one who has observed with becoming care the development of this class of diseases from their commencement, must have noticed symptoms of constitutional disturbance, which show themselves as soon as the infectious disease has been contracted, and are sometimes abundantly accounted for by the relations of locality and sympathy that frequently exist between the apparent seat of the disease, namely, the urethra and vagina, and various important organs, such as the testicles, bladder, kidneys, uterus and its appendages, the cerebellum, larynx, etc.,[1] without mentioning the accidents which frequently

[1] Every body knows that there is an intimate relation existing between the organs of generation and the vocal organs. We can hardly explain this

result from the material transfer of the gonorrhœal matter, whether venereal or non-venereal, from the urethra to the nostrils, lips, and particularly to the eyes, I am not at all surprised even now at what my teachers, and I with them, used to term a *metastasis* of blennorrhagia. The urethral or vaginal discharge which yields to sepia, is, so to say, the most marked symptom of a disease *sui generis*, which, if not as penetratingly pervasive as syphilis, is at least capable of tainting the whole organism. Nevertheless I confess that the genito-urinary apparatus seems to me to constitute most generally the elective sphere of this disease, even in cases (which, by the by, are much more frequent than is commonly supposed,) when it is not caused by infectious contact, but develops itself spontaneously. In such cases, a discharge from the urethra or vagina is not, necessarily, the first perceptible symptom of the disease, no more than the chancre at the glans, clitoris, or in the urethra, is necessarily the first perceptible symptom of syphilis. But whatever be the apparent seat of the sepia disease, it may safely be affirmed (I know this from experience) that it implies *in every case* certain apparent or latent, organic or functional disorders of the genital apparatus. As regards the secondary effects of this disease, even the most serious, I cannot persuade myself to rank them in the same category with syphilis, although the symptoms may sometimes seem to exhibit a confused image of this disease, sepia does not, by any means, exercise upon the human organism, the deep action of mercury, arsenic, lead, nitric or sulphuric acid, etc., or, in one word, of the truly anti-syphilitic agents. Sepia alone has never cured, and will never cure, syphilitic papulæ or scales, syphilitic caries, or even a recent chancre. I maintain, moreover, contrary to some homœopaths, that sepia has never arrested pulmonary phthisis. The forms of phthisis which sepia is said to have cured, like those which are supposed to have

anatomically, but what matters it? It is, therefore, not to be wondered that the diseases of these respective parts react upon the non-affected organs. This takes place in a most marked manner in syphilis, hysteria, etc.

been cured with the balsam of copaiva, were doubtless some chronic catarrh, but without tubercles or organic lesions, or at most some superficial ulcerations of the mucous membrane of the larynx, trachea or bronchi.

Be this as it may, and notwithstanding the fact that sepia is powerless both in constitutional and recent syphilis, it is nevertheless true that it constitutes a capital remedy in gonorrhœa, which, even when not venereal, proves so often the despair of both homœopathic and allœopathic physicians. It is therefore desirable that the shade to which sepia corresponds in this disease, should be correctly and unmistakeably determined. This would at the same time facilitate and elucidate the other cases where this remedy is to be applied. Unfortunately, a most distressing vagueness still prevails in this branch of our therapeutics, which is principally owing to the fact that the term gonorrhœa comprises a multitude of exceedingly varied diseases, every one of which requires a particular treatment.

There are *primary* and *secondary* gonorrhœas. By primary gonorrhœa I mean a discharge which marks the beginning of a disease, the nature of which is still unknown, and of which the gonorrhœa is sometimes the only symptom.[1] By secondary gonorrhœa, I mean a discharge which develops itself subsequently to all other morbid conditions, such as various kinds of tetters, rheumatic, gouty pains, and other symptoms which constitute the characteristics of the disease of which the gonorrhœa is only an evanescent symptom. The treatment of this latter kind of gonorrhœa, is necessarily subordinate to the totality of the symptoms. Primary gonorrhœa may be syphilitic, sycosic, or lastly non-venereal. But, even if non-venereal, this does not show that the discharge must always be of the same kind, and yield to the same remedy. The fact that different remedies have often to be given, renders the treatment of this kind of gonorrhœa frequently so very difficult.

[1] This symptom is always of a complex nature, and requires to be analysed.

However, if the physician should have become convinced that the gonorrhœal discharge is not only a primary disease, but belongs neither to the class of syphilitic, nor sycosic diseases, one great difficulty in the way of a successful treatment will have been removed. But how is he going to obtain this conviction?

1. So far as I know, the inoculation after Ricord's fashion,[1] is the only means of establishing the syphilitic character of a gonorrhœa. I do not know how far this is reliable. The syphilitic character of the disease being once established, some remedy of the group *Mercury* will have to be selected, which is most appropriate to the age, sex and constitution of the patient.

2. Here is what Hahnemann tells us relatively to sycosic discharges: "In these kinds of gonorrhœa, the discharge generally resembles, from the commencement, thick pus; the emission of urine causes little pain, but the body of the penis is swollen and hard; glandular nodes are seen on the dorsum of this organ, and it is very painful to contact."[2] *Thuya* and its analogues are suited to this kind of discharge.

The non-syphilitic or non-sycosic nature of the gonorrhœa being settled, we have then to determine to what shade of gonorrhœa *sepia* corresponds. This shade is recognised by the following symptoms:

Such general conditions of age and temperament as have been indicated, page 301; *absence of fever and of every other symptom which indicates inflammation;* complete inertia of the genital organs for some days previous to the appearance of the discharge; coldness of the genital organs, or disposition to get cold; general nervous excitement, which is almost always accompanied by sleeplessness, less frequently by loss of appetite: formication, voluptuous titillation, and occasion-

[1] See J. Hunter's *treatise of the venereal disease*, with additions by Ricord, Paris, 1851.

[2] Chronic Diseases, vol. I.

[3] Sepia is no more an anti-sycosic than it is an anti-syphilitic; I believe all homœopaths are agreed on this point.

ally acute stitches in the urethra or vagina; frequent urging to urinate, with dark urine, which becomes cloudy shortly after it is passed; discharge of mucus which gradually becomes milky, and lastly slightly *greenish;* it increases from the first to the tenth day, then decreases spontaneously from the fifteenth, but may continue for months and even years; nocturnal erections which are either painful or not painful, and are, in some cases, accompanied *by sexual* excitement.[1]

It has to be remarked that sepia, which is essentially depressing in its general action, has little chance of succeeding in simple gonorrhœa, if the patient is of a strong constitution, sanguine, and disposed to acute inflammations, and if the disease presents, as we said above, truly inflammatory symptoms. Sepia is likewise indicated in any of the various metastatic diseases resulting from this primary discharge, such as swelling of the testicles, hydrocele, hydrarthrosis, ophthalmia, angina, etc.; in all such affections, it does the same good as in the original discharge.

Acetic acid, aconite and nitric ether, have been pointed out as the antidotes of sepia; but I know from positive experience, that the true antidotes of sepia are the corrosive sublimate *in the case of man,* and soluble mercury *in the case of woman.*

Copaivæ balsamum, *balsam of copaiva.*—A species of turpentine or oleaginous rosin obtained from the *copaibera officinalis,* a tree belonging to the family of *leguminosæ,* which is frequently found in Brazil, where it is known under the name of *copaïba* or *copaïva.*

[1] I admit that these symptoms are vague; but, in the present state of our science, it seems impossible to furnish more precise indications. A simple, non-venereal gonorrhœa may likewise be successfully treated with *Petroselinum,* (an empirical remedy, of which no proving yet exists,) when the discharge is, from the first, *rose-colored,* and accompanied by acute pains and constant erections, without desire; *Cannabis,* when the discharge is from the first greenish and profuse; *Pulsatilla,* and still more *Silicea,* when it is an *indolent,* serous, mucous or even purulent discharge, but *without erections.* Moreover, *Merc. corr.* and *sol., Kreasot., Thuy., Plat.,* etc., are useful in gonorrhœa, even if neither syphilitic nor sycosic.

At the time it flows out of the tree, the balsam of copaiva is of an oily consistence, almost colorless, of an aromatic odor, of a heating, acrid and long-remaining taste; as it grows older, it assumes a yellower tinge, becomes thicker, and loses some of its odor. Such a large quantity is consumed of it that it is exported from Brazil in casks of from one hundred to one hundred and fifty pounds.

Empirical applications. This balsam has been employed in medicine for at least two centuries past. The writings of F. Hoffman, Pringle, Fuller, Valcareugh, Monro, Simmons, Pisan, Jacquier and Swediaur, testify to this fact. It is recommended for *blennorrhagia* and *affections of the chest, accompanied with profuse expectoration*, by Tournefort, Ferrein, Geoffroy and Cullen. Schwilgué and Alibert do not mention it in their systems of materia medica. Some modern physicians of high repute fancy, on this account, that they were the first who made use of this drug, and they have even gone so far as to dispute about the priority of this discovery; an unheard-of fact, and which alone would suffice to prove the inconceivable ignorance of most allœopathic physicians in medical matters.

With his wonted conscientiousness, Murray[1] collects the opinions of his predecessors and cotemporaries concerning the medicinal properties of the balsam of copaiva. At first it was used externally, on wounds, and as an antiseptic in the treatment of sores and atonic ulcers, the cicatrisation of which it hastened. Afterwards it was, undoubtedly by analogy, received as an internal agent, for the treatment of all such affections as were reputed to be characterized by processes of ulceration, such as *pulmonary phthisis*. But its use in this affection is condemned by Pringle, Rosenstein, Tissot, Fothergill and Quarin; they accuse it of augmenting the fever, the inflammation, and the obstruction of the lungs around the ulcerated portions. According to others, with Fuller at their head, it was possessed of extraordinary healing virtues in these very cases. Fuller says that it cleanses

[1] *Appar. medic.*, vol. IV., p. 47 and foll.

the air-passages,[1] strengthens the tone of the lungs, dissolves tubercles, and stops the most dangerous kinds of cough, even phthisis when far advanced. Fr. Hoffmann recommends its use in *ulcerations of the lungs*, *kidneys*, *bladder* and *prostate gland*, provided it is directly used.[2] Valcarengh, relying upon his own experience, and upon that of Rega and Sommers, likewise admits the efficacy of copaiva in ulceration of the lungs ; but only when employed in small doses, and for a long time in succession.[3] Monro[4] thinks that it is very useful in phthisis, when there is a state of weakness and looseness. Gessner recommends it for the same disease, but only in persons of thin blood, a lymphatic constitution, and whose nerves are not too sensitive. And lastly, Simmons,[5] Lentin, and several other practitioners of the 18th century, give opinions concerning the antiphthisical properties of copaiva, which are not very different from the opinions expressed a little while before.[6]

The other quotations made by Murray, refer to the use of copaiva in gonorrhœa. Murray condemns its use in the inflammatory period. Theden did not prescribe it until the discharge had become almost serous. Swediaur[7] praises the massive doses of this drug, from 50 to 100 drops of which he caused his patients to swallow every twenty-four hours. J.

[1] *Pharm. extemp.*, p. 275.
[2] *Obs. phys. chim.*, p. 24.
[3] *Spect. pract. de præcipuis febribus*, p. 173.
[4] Dis. in the Brit. Milit. Hosp., p. 129.
[5] *On the treatment of consumption*, p. 36, 39.
[6] The opposite opinions of authors, says Bayle, concerning the efficacy of copaïva in phthisis, are easily accounted for. It is well known, on the one hand, that this drug is frequently useful in pulmonary catarrh, and, on the other, that it was impossible formerly to distinguish these two diseases. It is therefore probable that those who praise copaïva in phthisis, had only to combat pulmonary catarrhs, whereas the opponents of copaïva had to deal with genuine phthisis, (*Bibl. de Thérap.*, vol. I., p. 435.) Let us add that not all bronchial catarrhs are cured with the balsam of copaïva, so that, even if we define these affections exactly alike and in the commonly received manner, the most contradictory results may nevertheless yet be arrived at.
[7] *Traité des maladies vénériennes*, Paris, 1817.

Hunter[1] observes that the discharge is frequently suspended only during the use of the drug, and reappears as soon as the medicine is discontinued, whence he infers that the copaiva has to be continued for five or six days after the apparent cure of the discharge, etc.

Murray relates finally, although he does not seem to place much credence in his own statements, that, beside blennorrhœa, pulmonary catarrhs, phthisis, and sores, (by external applications,) copaiva has cured *leucorrhœa*, *pains in the loins*, *calculi*, *dysuria*, *colic*, *diarrhœa*, *dropsy*,[2] and *paralysis*. My present knowledge of the action of copaiva, induces me to think these cures very probable.[3]

Agreeably to the spirit of modern allœopathic practice, almost every thing that has been said recently with reference to copaïva, is intended to defend its use in massive doses. But without examining this gross mode of treatment, which

[1] *Traité de la maladie vénérienne*, avec des additions par Ricord, Paris, 1851, p. 194.

[2] In the *Nouvelles de la république des lettres et des arts*, a remarkable cure of dropsy by the balsam of copaïva may be found related, No. 33, p. 73.

[3] Besides Murray's work, all other publications concerning copaïva, contain very little that is interesting, or that is not contained in the former work. The most familiar of these works are in chronological order: 1. *Un mémoire sur le traitement de la blennorrhagie par le baume da copahu á haute dose*, by Dr. Ansiaux, chief surgeon of the civil hospitals of Liége, published in 1816. 2. *Un mémoire sur l'emploi du baume de copahu á haute dose, dans la gonorrhoé et l'engorgement consécutif des testicules*, by M. T. Ribes, published in 1822 in the *Revue Médicale*, vol. IX., p. 10 and foll. 3. *Un mémoire sur l'emploi du baume de copahu dans la blennorrhagie, le catarrhe de la vessie et l'engorgement consecutif des testicules*, by Delpech, also in the *Revue Médicale*, vol. VII., p. 403; 4. *Des recherches sur l'emploi du baume de copahu administré en lavement*, by Velpeau, professor in the university of Paris, 1824. 5. *Des observations de catarrhe pulmonaire guéris par le baume de copahu*, by Dr. Laroche, published in 1826 in the North American and Surgical Journal, and translated into French in the *Journal universel des sciences médicales*, vol. XLVI., p. 365. 6. Lastly, *several cases of orchitis, leucorrhœa*, etc., published in various medical journals. All these cases have been related by Bayle in his bibliothèque de thérapeutique, vol. I., partly in substance, partly literally.

the organists alone can possibly justify, let us examine the facts which we cannot reject as doubtful.[1]

Auriana, who, however, scarcely ever used copaïva alone, treated with it acute gonorrhœa exclusively. In most cases he used *Chopart's potion.* Of twenty-six patients he cured twenty-four. In one the drug effected nothing, and in another it caused a serious aggravation. Do not these two exceptions show that copaïva is not, as Ribes believes, a specific remedy for all cases of gonorrhœa?

Ribes' memoir is, however, much more interesting than that of Auriana. With copaïva alone, Ribes cured various diseases which had developed themselves in consequence of the suppression of the blennorrhœa, namely: *various engorgements of the testicles, a swelling of the cavernous bodies resembling priapism, several recent catarrhs of the bladder;* several cases of *nephritis;* two cases of *hydrarthrosis of the knee,* two cases of *headache,* two of *ophthalmia,* one case of *subacute laryngitis,* a case of profuse *mucous expectoration.*

Delpech, independently of a number of cases of gonorrhœa, like Ribes, treated successfully with copaïva *several catarrhs of the bladder,* and several subsequent *swellings of the testicles.* Delpech terminates his memoir by a curious observation, but which I do not think founded, namely, that copaïva has very little, or no effect in cases of women.

The only interesting fact contained in Velpeau's memoir, is taken from Bretonneau. This is the case of a young woman who, after her confinement, was seized with a *large abscess* in the iliac fossa and in front of the pelvis; this abscess had opened into the bladder and discharged by the urethra. The pus from this abscess, combined with the quantities of mucus which came in increased quantities from the bladder, and which nothing could stop, flowed so profusely, that the patient came near sinking under it. The discharge was speedily

[1] Patients have been given as many as 30 grammes of copaiva in 24 hours, sometimes with success, but also to their great ruin, as I know from observation. May not the prostration which is caused by these enormous doses, have favored the natural action of the drug?

stopped by injections, consisting of two drachms of copaïva, and a small quantity of a decoction of *cinchona*. But is the cure attributable to the cinchona or the copaiva? As regards the gonorrhœa, Velpeau has shown, contrary to the statement of Delpech, that copaïva cures it as easily in females as in males; according to this author, it is his peculiar mode of administering the copaïva, that is the cause of his success.

Laroche cured *seven* cases of chronic bronchial catarrh with copaïva. They are interesting; but they lack, like most other cases of allœopathic observation, the precision of details in the statement of the symptoms, which would justify the use of such or such a drug. After reading these seven cases, I am unable to say for what variety of pulmonary catarrh copaiva is the specific remedy.

The cases of *leucorrhœa* which Degaëz, Castel, Lacombe, Armstrong, Larrey, etc.,[1] have cured by means of copaïva, prove at least one thing, namely, that it is not, as Cullen supposed,[2] and as Trousseau and Pidoux still seem to believe,[3] by the immediate contact of the medicinal molecules with the diseased parts that copaïva heals certain *phlegmasiæ* of the mucous membranes.

From the accidental observations of Old School physicians, we may infer a small number of the physiological effects of copaïva. According to the language of these physicians, these effects, which are unavoidable consequences of the daily abuse of this drug, constitute its unpleasant results, not its dangers, for copaiva is never supposed to be dangerous.

"The *miliary* and *erythematous exanthem*," say Trousseau and Pidoux, "the *swelling of the testicle*, phenomena which are sometimes remarked during the administration of copaïva, are not to be considered in the least as counter-indicating causes of copaïva.[4]" In another passage, the same authors

[1] See *Biblioth. Méd.*, vol. XXXV., p. 202 and foll.

[2] Mat. Méd., vol. II. This is one of the gross errors with which Cullen's works abound.

[3] *Traité de Thérapeutique*, vol. II., p. 601

[4] *Traité de thérapeutique*, vol. II., p. 105.

admit that, independently "*of various vesicular eruptions*, copaïva frequently *causes obstinate headaches*." But how do Trousseau and Pidoux, after such confessions, explain to themselves the cures of swollen testicles, and of *headache*, which are attributed to copaïva?

Fred. Hoffmann, Pringle, Fuller, Monro, J. Hunter, Chopart, Swediaur, etc., have seen copaiva produce *nausea*, even *vomiting*, and frequently *colic* and *diarrhœa*.[1]

According to Mérat and Delens, the balsam of copaiva does not always act only against the disease for which it is administered. Generally it *purges*, when given in large doses of one or two drachms; then it may even cause *vomiting*, especially if the dose is still larger, in which case it may occasion a real *gastritis*, or *enteritis*, with evacuations upwards and downwards, etc. At other times, it causes an *inflammation of the urinary passages* and the adjoining parts. It has been KNOWN *to cause urethritis*, *retention of urine*, *phlegmasia of the bladder*, *prostate gland*, *anus*, *rectum*, etc. IT IS REMARKABLE THAT THIS DRUG SHOULD BE ADVISED BY SOME AUTHORS FOR NEARLY THE SAME DISEASES THAT OTHERS HAVE KNOWN IT TO CAUSE.[2] Is there a single drug to which this remark does not apply?

If the alloeopathic physicians would watch their patients with the same attention that the practice of homœopathy requires, they would not be slow to find out that the balsam of copaiva, besides the therapeutic virtues which they accord to it, and the unpleasant results which they attribute to the over-doses, or to the untimely action of the drug, produces a variety of symptoms, of which they have never kept any account. The following pathogenesis is a proof of this:

This pathogenesis is the result of two different experiments, instituted at periods of two years' interval. The first experiment took place in 1847. These provings were instituted on myself and on seven or eight persons besides, of both sexes. Each experiment lasted several weeks; the drug

[1] Murray, *App. Medic.*, (*loc. cit.*)

[2] *Dict. univ. de mat. méd.*, Paris, 1830, vol. II., p. 419.

was taken in drop doses of the sixth dilution by myself and some of my co-provers, a dose every morning and evening; the others took it more irregularly. Unfortunately most of these persons lived in the country; they were tolerably sensible to medicinal action, but did not know how to observe properly and correctly the effects of a drug, and still less, how to describe them. Howsoever short the following list of symptoms may seem, it is not without much patient labor that I have succeeded in perfecting it.

Pathogenesis of the Balsam of Copaiva.

1—*Depression*, with anxious sadness.

In the morning, immediately after waking, deep sadness, which passes off during a walk, but returns in the evening.

Excessive sensitiveness of the whole nervous system, so that the least noise makes one start, and angry.

Attack of weeping, in a young girl, on hearing the sounds of a piano.

5—In the afternoon, periodical attacks of sadness and tears, with cold extremities and flashes of heat in the face.

Uneasiness on account of one's health.

Quarrelsome, irascible, gloomy, intractable mood for a week, with vascular excitement, heat about the heart and trembling of the limbs, on meeting with the least contrariety.

Absurd recriminations concerning trifling things that had happened a long while ago.

Misanthropy.

10—Insurmountable *aversion* to one's usual occupations.

Complete inability to perform any manual labor; the head feels empty, and the ideas are confused; a dull pain is felt at the forehead, when trying to struggle against this inability.

Deficient memory; this makes one impatient, and plunges one into a gloomy depression of spirits.

Loathing of life, and, at the same time, *fear of death.*

Passing attacks of vertigo when sitting, working, walking, but especially when *standing immoveable.*

15—Attack of vertigo when riding on horseback, in the morning, although he was talking at the time, and going a pace.

Headache in the morning.

Every step he takes jars the head, this ceases in half an hour.

Pulsative, deep-seated stitches at the occiput.

Dull pain at the occiput.

20—Lancinating pressure, proceeding from the right occipital protuberance.

Stitches at the left occipital protuberance, with occasional shocks in the whole head, only in the morning.

Hemicrania, (on the left side,) with boring pain, sense of coldness in the affected part, weeping and constant moaning, for three days, in a young man of twenty-two years, disposed to hypochondria.[1]

Pressure at the forehead.

Heaviness of the head, and especially of the occipital region, which is instinctively pressed against the collar of the coat; this affords relief.

25—Pulsative stitches at the top of the head, not synchronous with the pulse.

Headache with nausea, (*Spielmann*).

Stitches in the temples and behind the ears.

Tearing pain in the temporal regions, especially in the left, alleviated by gentle pressure with the hand.

Contusive pain at the right temple, evening and night, and which becomes intolerable when leaning on the pillow.

30—Sudden stitches in both temples, when washing one's face with cool water in the morning.

Sensitiveness of the hairy scalp, and even of the hair.

Small, red, slightly-itching pimples at the upper part of the forehead and hairy scalp, above the ears and at the occiput.

Falling of the hairs, after the first doses.

Formication in the canthi of the eyes, in the evening.

[1] This symptom was so violent that I had to give the patient, who had only taken three doses of copaiva in all, *mercury* to relieve him.

35—Redness of the left eye.

Passing obscuration of sight.

Black points hovering before the eyes.

Upon alternately closing the right and left eye, the same objects look much paler when seen with the left, than when seen with the right eye.

40—Contraction of the pupils.

Sensitiveness of the eyes to the light.

Involuntary contraction of the orbicularis muscle of the eyes, in the morning.

Spasm at the right upper lid, recurring several times in the day-time, and accompanied by a slight pressive pain at the eyes.

Agglutination of the lids, in the morning.

45—Stitches, for a whole night, in the left ear, causing one to cry out (at the end of three days); some days after this, a little purulent matter is discharged from the meatus.

Buzzing in the ears.

Humming in the ears.

Formication in the ears.

Small furfuraceous tetter at the concha of the left ear, with burning pain, only when touched.

50—Excessive sensitiveness of hearing, especially when sharp sounds are perceived; the report of a pistol caused a disagreeable and even painful sensation; this unpleasantness did not arise from the detonation of the powder, but from the shock of the ball against the metallic disk at which it was fired.

Paleness and sickly look of the face.

Bloating of the face.

Heat in the face, in the morning, on waking.

Itching of the cheeks, here and there, in the eye-brows and at the chin.

55—Small white miliary vesicles, on a red ground, at the left wing and at the tip of the nose.

Yellowish spots, of the size of a dime, of irregular shapes, and slightly itching, on the right cheek, morning and evening.

Passing tearings in the left cheek.

Red, humid tetter (after eight days,) at the upper lip, which is swollen and painful when touched.

Sensitiveness without any appreciable swelling at the parotid glands, but contusive pain and perceptible swelling at the submaxillary glands.

60—*The teeth are on edge.*

Sensation as if the teeth were longer.

Gnawing and throbbing pain in a carious tooth, worse when drawing in cool air, or when touching it by some cool drink.

Sense of coldness in the teeth.

An unpleasant odor seems to come out of the teeth.

65—The teeth seem less firm, and to start out of the sockets.

Dryness of the mouth, especially at night and in the morning.

Flow of saliva in the the evening, at night, and in the morning.

Every now and then a sudden and profuse flow of a sweetish saliva.

Foul breath in the morning.

70—*The tongue is covered with a whitish coating, greenish at the base.*

Redness, with smarting, on the sides and at the tip of the tongue.

Excoriative pain at the gums, palate and pharynx.

Tenacious phlegm in the mouth and throat, which is constantly reproduced.

Sensation as of a foreign body in the pharynx.

75—*Swelling of both tonsils,* (especially of the right.)

Troublesome pressure in the pharynx.

Constriction of the throat.

Bitter taste in the mouth.

Thirst and diminished appetite.

80—Excessive hunger, (the first two days,) then loss of appetite.

Hunger in the evening, (contrary to his habit,) when on the point of going to bed.

Sort of fainting at the stomach, without any real appetite.

Every article of food seems too salt.

Rush of blood to the head and face, when eating or *after a meal.*

85—Hiccough after eating.

Eructations after eating.

Violent cutting pains, followed by two diarrhœic stools, immediately after taking a cup of coffee with milk (as usual.)

Eructations tasting of the ingesta.

Sour eructations.

90—Foul eructations.

Flashes of heat in the face, heat and sweat in the palms of the hands, with anxiety and general malaise, after eating.

Beating at the pit of the stomach, followed by beating of the heart, and cloudiness on leaving the table after eating.

Pressure at the pit of the stomach, even before breakfast.

Burning pain at the stomach.

95—Nausea in the morning.

Desire to vomit, (*Hahnemann.*)

Vomiting, (*Fred. Hoffmann, Swediaur, Monro,* etc.)

Stitches at the stomach, every now and then, as if in paroxysms.

Spasms of the stomach.

100—Pressive pain in the region of the spleen, which becomes pulsative from time to time.

The whole epigastric region is tensive and painful to contact.

Sense of burning in the abdomen, (*Hahnemann.*)

Stitches in the hypochondria.

Noisy borborygmi.

105—Pinching in the abdomen.

Tearings in the abdomen, preceded by pullings in the femoral bones, (*Hahnemann.*)

Swelling of the lower abdomen.

Pressure in the lower abdomen, as from a stone.

Discharge of fetid flatulence in the morning, in bed, and after rising.

110—Beatings in the lower abdomen.

Pressure on the rectum, causing a constant urging to stool.

Coldness at the abdomen.

Several soft stools every day, especially in the morning, followed by general prostration.

Diarrhœa in the morning.

115—Violent diarrhœa in one night, (fifteen evacuations in ten hours,) with spasms at the stomach; coldness of the extremities and cramps in the calves.

White, diarrhœic stools, generally in the morning, with coldness and drawing tearings in the abdomen, obliging one to bend double, (*Hahnemann.*)

Involuntary stools, (*Hahnemann.*)

Diarrhœa, (Monro, Fred. Hoffman and others.)

Whitish, fæcal stools, of a sour smell, *with discharge of ascarides.*

120—Stools which are at first dry and in shape, and terminate in diarrhœa.

Stools like sheep's-dung.

Insufficient stools.

No stool for five days.

125—Piles, (*Montegre.*)

Fluent piles.

Stitches in the rectum.

Spasms of the rectum.

Burning itching at the anus.

130—Constant oozing, from the anus, of a serous or even purulent liquid.

Pressure on the bladder.

Dull pain at the bladder.

Tenesmus of the bladder, (*Ansiaux.*)

Frequent unsuccessful urging to urinate.

135—*Constant unsuccessful urging to urinate, (Hahnemann.)*

The urine is discharged drop by drop, (*Hahnemann.*)

Unpleasant itching at the tip of the glans.

Itching, smarting and burning sensation in the urethra before and after urinating, (*Hahnemann.*)

Excoriative pain at the orifice of the urethra, (*Hahnemann.*)

140—*Inflammation and swelling of the orifice of the urethra which remains open*, with a throbbing pain in the whole length of the penis, (*Hahnemann.*)

Absence of erections the first days.

Violent erections on the following days, (night and morning,) with or without thoughts of the other sex.

Constant and permanent sexual excitement, (during the whole time of the proving.)

Violent desire for an embrace, with absence of erection.

145—*Mucous discharge from the urethra.*

Yellow, purulent discharge from the urethra, (Hahnemann.)

Profuse milky discharge, for three days, and which stops of itself, although the use of the drug is continued.

Dull, heavy pain in the testicles.

Swelling of one of the testicles (left) which is very sensitive to contact.

150—Heat at the skin of the scrotum.

Boil at the pubis.

Superficial excoriation at the glans and prepuce.

Redness and slight dampness between the scrotum and thigh.

The inguinal glands are painful to contact.

155—(Not very considerable) swelling of the inguinal ganglions.

Constant pressure on the uterus, as if prolapsus would set in.

Pulling pains in the suspensory ligaments of the uterus.

Deep stitches in the vagina and neck of the womb.

Spasms of the uterus.

160—Beatings in the right ovarian region, when standing.

Milky *leucorrhœa*.

Acrid leucorrhœa, which causes excoriations at the vulva.

A leucorrhœa of long standing disappears during the use of the drug.

Heat and red spots at the vulva.

165—Itching at the vulva.

The menses are too early by three days.

The menses are too early by seven days.

The menses are too early by ten days.

The menses appear on the regular day, but they are pale and much less profuse than usual.

170—During the menses she is sad in the morning, depressed, has pains in the loins, and is very nervous.

During the menses, tightness at the larynx, hoarseness in the morning, dry cough morning and night.

Stomach-ache during the menses.

During the menses, rheumatic pain (as from some great fatigue) in the left hip and knee, and uterine spasms.

Cold feet and knees during the menses.

175—Leucorrhœa after the menses.

The menses reappear after they had ceased for several days.

Sleeplessness and restlessness, all night, after an embrace.

Metrorrhagia, (Hahnemann.)

Stuffing of the nose for two days, only in the morning.

180—Frequent sneezing.

Fluent coryza with headache, pressive pain at the root of the nose, and itching in the eyes.

Dryness and roughness in the larynx.

Excoriative pain in the larynx.

185—*Hoarseness* especially in the morning, with excoriative pain in the larynx when talking.

The voice, although not much altered, loses its compass during the whole time of the proving; the lower notes are the same, but the higher notes cause an excoriative pain which finally prevents one from bringing them out.

Cough excited by tickling in the larynx, trachea and bronchia.

Dry cough morning and evening.

Rough cough, with difficult expectoration of greenish mucus.

190—Cough with profuse whitish expectoration, sometimes saltish, sometimes flat and nauseous.

Heat in the chest.

Stitches in the right side of the chest.

Acute stitches in the left axilla, penetrating into the chest.

Sense of fulness at the chest, which frequently obliges one to sigh.

195—Difficulty at the chest, with labored breathing, while working in a stooping position, (digging).

Pressure at the sternum.

Palpitation of the heart during work.

Beating of the heart, (*Hahnemann*).

Palpitation of the heart, (*Spielmann*).

200—Stitches between the two shoulders, cutting off the respiration.

Rheumatic pain at the nape of the neck and left side of the neck.

Dull pain, like spasms, in the lumbar region.

Stiffness in the back, disappearing when walking.

Burning pain in the dorsal spine.

205—Red spots, slightly itching, in the sternal region and right axilla.

The axillary glands are sensitive to contact.

Stitches in the left shoulder-blade.

Pullings in both shoulder-blades.

Luxation-pain in the right shoulder-blade.

210—Acute pain in the left shoulder-joint.

Numbness of the arm, on which one is lying, at night.

Red, itching spot on the left arm.

Pulling in the fore-arms.

Stiffness in the fingers.

215—Cold hands.

Trembling of the hands.

Crampy pains in both hips, worse in the right.

Contusive pain in the right hip, when lying on it.

Contusive pain in the right thigh, when walking and when touching it.

Dull pain in the knees.

220—Cracking in the knees, when stretching the leg.

Numbness of the legs, when sitting.

Pain as if sprained, in the feet, very troublesome when first commencing to walk, and which the walking causes to disappear.

Swelling of the left foot.

Swelling of both feet.

225—*Icy-coldness of the feet*, from morning till noon.

Twitching of the limbs, during rest.

Intolerable uneasiness in the lower limbs.

Pulling in all the muscles, especially in the evening and at night.

Trembling of the extremities.

230—Pulsations here and there.

Slowness of the pulse, (*Giacomini.*)

Excessive sensitiveness to damp and cold.

Quotidian fever; cold and shuddering before noon, followed by a general heat and thirst for cold water, (*Hahnemann.*)

Hæmorrhage, (*Monro.*)

235—Urticaria, (*Hahnemann.*)

Eruption of a number of red blotches all over the body, but especially in the face, (*Montège.*)

Paroxysms of spasms and other hysteric symptoms.

Epileptiform attacks, (in a boy of eighteen years, who had prostrated his mind and body by onanism,) decrease gradually, and finally cease altogether.

Drowsiness in the day time.

240—Restless sleep at night.

Coldness of the feet, knees and thighs, at night.

Frightful or *lascivious dreams*.

Frequent waking.
Wakes early, and is unable to fall asleep again.
245—Sour-smelling sweat at night.
Profuse and inodorous sweat in the morning.

For some years past I have used copaiva freely in my practice. I use it for the same conditions that indicate sepia, and I am as yet unable to point out the least difference between the therapeutic properties of these two drugs. A circumstance worthy of remark is this, that they have both the same antidotes. I know from various trials, that *corrosive sublimate in the male,* and *soluble mercury in the female,* neutralise the action of copaiva almost on the spot, the same as they do that of sepia.

Alumina. A basic salt, which Guyton Morveau was the first to disengage from alum, and which chemists, after the example of Sir H. Davy, consider as the oxyde of a metal, (aluminium,) the existence of which is not yet generally admitted. Alumina, which has been confounded for a long time past with lime and silica, is like these, a constituent of clay, schist, etc., and is, therefore, found all over in nature. When isolated, and sufficiently dry, it forms a white, fine powder, very soft to the touch, adhering to the tongue, insoluble in water, infusible and without taste. And yet, it seems to me, beyond doubt, that even in this form, without being comminuted by the process of dynamisation, alumina is possessed of medicinal properties. The alumina which is found in dry and anhydrous earths, says Mialhe, is insoluble in water, and therefore inactive; but the dissolving action of the gastric juice, which is acid, imparts to it very marked astringent properties.[1]

Empirical applications.—Bojean, of Chambéry,[2] has shown the presence of alumina in the flesh of a hare that had induced symptoms of poisoning. What were these symptoms? Vomit-

[1] *Essai sur l'art de formuler,* p. 95.

[2] *Comptes rendus hebdomadaires de l'Academie des Sciences,* vol. XVII., p. 134

ing, cramps at the stomach, colic and diarrhœa; for which symptoms alumina has been employed by some modern allœopathic physicians with success. Professor Ticinus of Dresden, affirms that this drug has always helped him out in every case of *obstinate or light dysentery*, in adults as well as children, but especially in children.[1] Drs. Weese and Seiler, although less explicit, express themselves nearly in the same way.[2] Upon the whole, however, allœopathic experience concerning the use of alumina, is limited to these few observations.

Homœopathic applications. — Alumina is to sepia what silicea is to pulsatilla; it is indeed the sepia of chronic diseases. A most complete pathogenesis of this drug is contained in the 1st Vol. of Hahnemann's *Chronic Diseases*, who has doubtless contributed to it greatly.

The peculiar adaptation of alumina to the treatment of chronic diseases, did not escape Hahnemann's keenly observing genius. Hence, among the symptoms which best indicate the use of this drug, he points out: *disposition to eructations, for years; disposition to colds in the head, of very long standing*, etc. "I do not know of any drug whose action is more durable than that of alumina. I have often derived the greatest advantages from the use of this drug in the case of aged females, against diseases that had been apparently seated in the sexual system, but whose primary symptoms had disappeared with the complete cessation of the menstrual periods. Generally they were cases of dyspepsia, with rush of blood to the face after eating, tettery redness at the tip of the nose and on the knee, sour eructations, vomiting, accompanied with suffocation, and returning every now and then with such violence, that the life of the patient seemed placed in jeopardy, when these paroxysms took place, which was generally the case in the evening or at night, the vomiting was soon accompanied by cutting pains, spasms in the abdomen, cramps in the lower extremities, and a violent diarrhœa, as if the patient had been attacked by cholera. In the case of a

[1] *Nouv. journ. de med.*, vol. IV., p. 300.

[2] *Bull. des scienc. med.* de Férussac, vol. I., p. 364.

lady, whom several homœopathic physicians had treated for years without any success, alumina frequently produced a surprisingly speedy improvement, if not a cure. The vomiting, spasms of the stomach, etc., were arrested for good by the first doses, but the herpetic eruption which the patient had had for upwards of twenty-five years at the tip of the nose, on the cheeks and chin, remained. The blueish redness of these parts which did not itch at all, gradually decreased, but did not entirely disappear.[1]

I have likewise cured with alumina, various kinds of *angina* or *laryngitis*, chronic gonorrhœa which had lasted for years, *chronic hardness of the testicles* coming on subsequently to gonorrhœa, various kinds of *obstinate leucorrhœa*, and lastly spots at the vulva and in the vagina, of a burning redness, prominent like papulæ, *with violent itching*.

This drug is one of those the use of which requires a good deal of discretion. It is hurtful when given improperly, as it is advantageous and efficacious in cases where it is indicated.

I have seen a few doses of alumina excite and maintain, for two months in succession, a tearing cough, every turn of cough being accompanied by involuntary emission of urine, which reduced the patient to despair. Bryonia which is pointed out as an antidote in such cases, did not seem to do any good. As a general rule, alumina does not suit persons of a lively and sanguine disposition. This feature is possessed in common by every drug belonging to the *sepia* group.

I should like to know the true antidote of alumina. Hahnemann, after the example of Bute, mentions bryonia, and, in accordance with the suggestions of other provers, chamomilla and ipecacuanha. I do not believe that these indications repose upon facts. Each of these drugs may, according to circumstances, be able to combat a few of the symptoms of alumina, but not one of them, it seems to me, is sufficient to neutralize the action of alumina in its totality.

[1] I have never succeeded in effecting a cure of this kind, nor do I believe that other practitioners have been more successful.

GROUP VII.

TYPE: CAUSTICUM.

ANALOGUES: COCCULUS. COFFEA CRUDA. CORALLIA RUBRA. NUX VOMICA. STAPHISAGRIA. ARSENICUM ALBUM.[1]

Two of these drugs, *Arsenicum album* and *Nux vomica*, have already been described in the *arsenic-group*. But no one will be astonished on seeing these two polychrests again mentioned in the *causticum* group. All that is required, in order to justify their position in this group, is to bear in mind that it is only when used at a high potency, say the one hundredth, that they become true analogues of causticum; at this potency their physiological action remains unaltered, but the primary symptoms of the drug are less permanent, and give room more speedily to the manifestation of the secondary effects. I will illustrate my idea by a single example. When experimented with at the twelfth, or at a lower dilution, arsenic causes diarrhœa very generally, whereas the hundredth dilution produces almost always constipation. I know that constipation is one of the ordinary symptoms of arsenic, as it is one of the common effects of *nux vom.*, *causticum*, *coral. rubr.*, etc., but it is nevertheless true that this symptom manifests itself the more tardily the lower the attenuation which had been administered, so that, provided the poison is administered in sufficiently massive doses, death even may take place before the constipation developes itself. These considerations, if suitably dwelt upon and applied, explain my

[1] It is more than probable that tea is one of the analogues of Causticum, of which I have published a pathogenesis in the *Journ. de la Soc. gall. de méd. hom.*, vol. II., p. 233. But not having made as yet any use of it in practice, I have not deemed myself authorised to add this drug as one of the members of this group.

reasons why it is only in reference to the higher attenuation of *arsenic* and *nux vom.*, that I desire to establish their analogy with *causticum.* It will be seen, at the same time, that arsenic closes the causticum-group. This is intended to show that the analogy between these two drugs is of the most remote kind.

COMMON CHARACTERISTICS.[1]

Two series of successive and opposite phenomena; the former of short duration, consisting in a sort of universal exaltation of all the functions; the latter which succeed the former more or less rapidly, consist in a general depression of the vital forces, and constitute the real and permanent action of the drugs of this group.[2]

[1] The primary symptoms are in Roman; the secondary ones in italics.

[2] This antagonism of symptoms or effects is a rule in regard to every other drug. It would be a great progress in homœopathy, if we knew exactly the primary and secondary effects of every drug; our opinions in reference to this point have been recorded in the introduction page 38. Symptom **1321** of *Causticum* has this curious remark attached to it by Hahnemann: "The primary symptoms of Causticum seem to develope themselves more slowly than those of the other antipsorics." I can scarcely believe, however, that this remark should come from Hahnemann himself. I do not understand its meaning; it seems to me even that it is erroneous and absurd. It would seem that the author of this remark had made up his mind beforehand not to regard certain effects of *Causticum* as primary; or does he simply mean that all the effects of Causticum, whether primary or secondary, develop themselves slowly? This cannot be, and I protest against this doctrine, for there is not perhaps any drug that acts with more promptitude than *Causticum.* I am inclined to think that Hahnemann often mistook for curative effects certain ephemeral phenomena which were simply primary effects of the drug. To mention only a few moral symptoms, I will quote: for *Causticum*:—**49.** *Mirthfulness*, sometimes, and soon after *ill-humor*,—**51.** *For the first twelve hours, cheerfulness, ready comprehension and generation of ideas*, etc.; and at the end of twenty-one hours, *anxiety, peevishness*, etc. (How can this antagonism be looked upon as a curative effect?)—**53.** *Mirthfulness, cheerfulness, satisfaction with one's-self, loquacity.*—**54.** Disposition to talk and work. *For Cocculus*:—**555.** *Joyfulness, contentment, hilarity, he becomes playful and is disposed to jest* (at the end of six hours.)—**556.** Hilarity, self-contentment.—**557.** *Irresistible inclinations to hum a tune, sing; a sort of delirium,* (a better expression would

A sort of foolish and talkative gaiety; passing excitement of the mind and feeling; satisfied with one's self and every thing else; *sadness even unto loathing of life; irascibility; vehemence; inability to perform any mental labor; deficient memory; complete absence of all imagination; want of feeling, sometimes amounting to revolting hardness of heart*, etc.

Increase of the frequency, and particularly of the fulness of the pulse, and of the temperature of the body; disposition to perspire; *depression and weakness of the pulse, general coldness, icy coldness*, or sometimes a *dry, pungent heat at the extremities, excessive sensitiveness to the open air.*

Sleeplessness, with restlessness and an excessive flow of ideas; sleeplessness, especially during the first half of the night,[1] *yawning, stretching, constant drowsiness, with waking as in affright, irresistible desire to sleep in the morning.*

Slight moisture on the skin; *dryness of the skin; stinging or burning itching all over the body, but particularly at the hairy scalp, at the dorsum of the nose, neck, chest, between the shoulders, at the buttocks, thighs, calves, around the ankles, in the palms of the hands and at the soles of the feet; eruptions which are at first moist, vesicular or pustulous, and which most frequently change to red and dry tetter.*

A sort of intoxication, *vertigo with nausea, as in sea-sickness;*[2] *headache in the morning; pressive headache at the forehead and occiput; pressure mingled with acute stitches, in the temples; hemicrania; acute neuralgic pains in one*

have been *intoxication;* but in what way is this a curative effect?) For *nux vomica:*—**2.** *Intoxication.*—**1299.** He is scarcely able to control his senses, so rapidly do the ideas crowd upon his mind, etc.—**1300.** A very lucid perception of one's own impressions, exquisite feeling of right and wrong, etc. For *Staphisagria:*—**536.** Changeable mood; at first cheerful, etc.—**537.** He is in good spirits and likes to talk.—**538.** Good humor, cheerfulness, inclination to talk, self-contentment. And lastly for *arsenic:*—**69.** Good humor, and fond of talking.—**70.** Tendency to be cheerful and busy.—**71.** *For the first minutes*, composed and cheerful, but, after the lapse of half an hour, he feels anxious, etc.

[1] The reverse is the case with opium; sleeplessness is its permanent effect.

[2] The nauseous vertigo of Staphisagria is much more permanent and deep-seated than the similar effect produced by the other drugs of this group, except perhaps *arsenic.*

side of the head; headache as if the hair would be pulled out; falling out of the hair.

Shining and moist eyes; dilatation of the pupils; *itching of the eyes; redness of the eyes; ophthalmia* (acute and chronic, and, in this case, with secretion of gum that dries rapidly); *contraction of the pupils; black, shining spots floating before the eyes; white cloud before the eyes; photophobia.*

Excessive sensitiveness of hearing, (any kind of noise is unpleasant to the ear.)

Caries of the teeth: gnawing toothache, which is aggravated by cold drinks, with cold in one of the cheeks; painful neuralgia in one or the other jaw.

Flow of saliva, especially after supper, and the first part of the night; *intolerable dryness of the mouth and throat at night; absence of mind; gnawing hunger; burning and scraping eructations, causing a dry cough; pyrosis; spasmodic gastralgia.*

Copious emission of flatulence; *incarcerated flatulence; constrictive pain in the lower abdomen;* sudden and violent diarrhœa, but short-lasting; *dry, frequent, but insufficient stools; alternate constipation and diarrhœa; piles; acute stitches at the anus and in the rectum; itching or rather burning at the anus, even without diarrhœa.*

Scanty, red and watery urine, with brick-dust sediment; *profuse watery urine.*

Sexual excitement, generally of short duration; *absence of all sexual desire; impotence; discharge of prostatic fluid during stool;* premature menses; *delaying, pale and watery menses; leucorrhœa; dryness and stitches in the vagina.*

Coryza, first fluent, afterwards *dry; dry crusts in the nostrils; hoarseness; scraping and excoriative pain in the larynx and trachea; cough with mucous expectoration, becoming dry, afterwards; dry, spasmodic cough, in paroxysms, with short and panting breathing after a meal, in the evening, middle of the night, or in the morning; nocturnal asthma.*

[1] This symptom belongs more especially to *Cocculus* and *Staphis.;* but all the drugs of this group, even coffee, attack powerfully the bulbs of the hair, and cause them to fall out.

Pressure on the sternum; acute stitches, as with very fine needles, in the sides of the chest, or in the region of the heart.

Stiff neck; pulling in the back; painful neuralgia in the trunk or limbs; pains mingled with pressure or sharp stitches, or resembling stitches with burning needles, which are felt along the length of the extremities, in the tract of the nerves, seldom increased by pressure, and in some cases (which is especially true for arsenic and staphisagria) *as if seated in the periosteum of the long bones; trembling of the extremities and even of the head; cramps in the calves; contusive pain in the parts which, though only for a short time, have been exposed to cold and draughts of air.*

It is only by a deep study of the physiological action of the drugs constituting the group *Causticum* that the various shades of symptoms which indicate particular agents, can be correctly determined and perceived. In spite of this, it is sometimes next to impossible, to arrive at such a determination. In such cases, however, it is generally of little importance, whether we give the preference to one or the other of such drugs. I am persuaded, for example, that in many cases where *causticum* should be given, *coffea cruda* will very nearly effect the same results, and vice versa.

Several of these drugs seem to strengthen each other's action in such a manner that, if given at short intervals from each other, they produce an aggravation rather than a modification of the symptoms. This is the case with *caust.*, *coccul.* and *coff.* This consideration which is entirely founded on experience, raises a very delicate question, which it is certainly worth while to look into.

Suppose a person who had been disturbed by taking *causticum*, should go to consult a homœopathic physician, without telling him anything about the cause of his indisposition. If the physician be acquainted with his materia medica, and be otherwise a man of judgment, he will prescribe *causticum* or *coff.* Well, if he prescribes *causticum*, it will aggravate the symptoms, this is evident. But *coff.*, which is chosen in apparent homœopathicity to the symptoms, will likewise produce an aggravation. Nevertheless, the selection of *coffea* for a train of symptoms that indicates causticum, would show skill and judgment, for there are no two remedies whose symptoms are as nearly alike as those of coffea and causticum. Is not the law of similarity applicable to this case? At any rate, I feel unable to account for this fact upon any other grounds than by assuming an *identity of principle* in the physiological action of *coffea* and *causticum*. Happily this similarity of the symptoms and this identity of action exist only between a small number of drugs. I recollect a case of *gastralgia*, accompanied with nauseous vertigo, where *cocculus*, which seemed to be clearly indicated by the symptoms, produced an aggravation of the pains. *Staphisagria* effected a rapid cure. Was it as an antidote to cocculus, or as a remedy for the morbid affection? I am unable to decide. But I can affirm positively that this disease had lasted for several months, and that it only yielded to the *antidote* of the drug, to the symptoms of which the original disease corresponded. Was there then an identity of action in this case between *cocculus* and *staphisagria?*

CORRESPONDING DISEASES.

Nervous apoplexy.—Hypochondria.—Megrim.—Alopecia.—Tetters of the hairy scalp, (very different from favus.)—Acute and chronic ophthalmia. —Prosopalgia.—Toothache.—Caries of the teeth.—Gastralgia.—Sea-sickness.—Typhoid fever, (intercurrent malady.)—Intestinal spasms, (especially of the rectum.)—Piles.—Impotence.—Amenorrhœa.—Dysmenorrhœa.—Leucorrhœa.—Coryza.—Hoarseness.—Nervous cough.—Endemic whooping-cough. — Asthma. — False croup. — Neuralgia. — Paralysis. — Chorea.—Variola and varioloid.—Dry tetters, etc.

Causticum, according to Hahnemann, *the active principle of quick-lime.*

This substance which owes its introduction into the Materia Medica, to the author of homœopathy, had not only never been employed, before him, as a drug, but was even unknown to chemists. It is obtained by distilling a mixture of quick-lime, bisulphate of potash and water. That which, after the operation, remains in the retort, is, of course, a mixture of the neutral sulphate of lime and sulphate of potash; but as regards the product of the distillation, which is nothing else than a concentrated solution of *causticum*, we are entirely ignorant concerning the constituent elements of this substance, (Hahnemann, at any rate, has not apprised us what they are, and, probably, did not know.) All that we know of this liquid is, that it is colorless and clear like distilled water, that it smells like ley, causes a smarting on the tongue, a pungent heat in the throat, congeals, like water, at a low temperature, favors to a great degree the putrefaction of animal matter suspended in it, does not redden vegetable blues, as other acids do; and that sulphuric acid is not detected in it by means of the chloride of baryum, nor lime by means of the oxalate of ammonia.

Be this as it may, *causticum* which, together with the caloric, is spontaneously disengaged from the moistened quicklime, and is no longer present in hydrated lime, possesses therapeutic properties very different from those with which the Hahnemann causticum is endowed: this is one of the most valuable drugs known to me. Its action is well defined, characteristic; and although the provings of this drug seem to have been instituted with high potencies, yet the symptoms are pretty clearly marked and easily studied and remembered. Causticum is one of our most frequently used drugs.[1]

According to Hahnemann, the following symptoms have been principally cured with causticum:

"Hypochondriac depression of spirits; melancholy; saddening thoughts at night, and weeping in the day time; anxiety; mistrust in the future; despair; tendency to start; disposition to anger, chagrin, ill-humor; vertigo; dull pressure in the brain; stitches in the head; stitches in the temples; stitches at the top of the head; lachrymation; ophthalmia; *suppuration of the eyes;* incipient amaurosis; black spots hovering before the eyes; buzzing in the ears; eruption at the tip of the nose; old warts on the nose or in the eye-brows; painful teeth, starting out of their sockets; old suppuration of a spot in the gums; *dental fistula;* mucous

[1] See its pathogenesis in Hahnemann's *Chronic Diseases*, vol. II.

affections of the throat and velum palati; phlegm in the throat; aversion to sweet things; malaise resembling a state of fainting; vomiting of a sourish liquid; heaviness at the stomach after eating bread; pressure and griping in the stomach; *spasmodic gastralgia;* stitches in the pit of the stomach; pressure at the epigastrium; pressure in the whole lower abdomen, after eating; large abdomen of children; swelling of the lower abdomen; shifting of flatulence, with chronic constipation; light-colored and white stools; cutting pain in the rectum and at stool; discharge of blood during stool; itching at the anus; protrusion of the piles; fistula ani; urging to urinate, with thirst; *involuntary discharge of urine day and night; involuntary discharge of urine during cough, when sneezing, walking; frequent emissions;* deficient erections; *aversion to an embrace in females: delaying menses;* scanty menses; excoriations between the thighs; *discharge from the vagina; stoppage of both nostrils;* constant stuffing of the nose; *chronic hoarseness; barking cough;* inability to spit up the phlegm in the throat; *asthma; stitches in the region of the heart;* painful stiffness of the back, especially when rising from a chair; stiffness of the neck and loins; pulling and tearing in the shoulder-blades; goïtre-shaped swelling of the cervical glands; rheumatism in the arms; eruption on the arms; pressive pain under the elbows; sense of fulness in the hands, when grasping any thing; stitch in the fingers, striking to the elbows; pains in the soles of the feet, ankles and big toes, when walking; *cold feet; swelling of the feet;* pain in the varices; vacillating gait of a child that is in the habit of stumbling forward; restlessness in the body; palpitation of the heart; *weakness, even unto trembling;* disturbing dreams; disposition to feel cold; night-sweat."

This picture of symptoms is doubtless drawn by the hand of a master, and there is scarcely a drug, the effects of which Hahnemann has more happily condensed in a similar synoptical arrangement. Nevertheless, I beg leave to add to this synopsis an interesting observation from my own practice; it is this: "*Causticum frequently proves wonderfully efficacious in the treatment of small-pox.*"

"In my treatise of the diseases of children, I have stated that *Merc. corr.*, in conjunction with *causticum*, is a most powerful remedy for *variola*. Prescribe, for instance, as soon as the first pocks break out, or in the course of the second or third periods, if we should not have been called sooner, 8 globules of *causticum* 30, in four ounces of water, and give two table-spoonfuls in the morning, at three or four hours' intervals; and 8 globules of Merc. corr., in the same quantity of water, and to be taken at the same dose and interval; and in the vast majority of the cases, the exanthem and all the accompanying symptoms, will, under the influence of these two drugs, be found to disappear as by enchantment."

Several physicians, among whom I have the privilege of mentioning my friend, Dr. Delavallade, have tried this treatment to their highest satisfaction. The cutaneous action of *corrosive sublimate* is somewhat analogous to that of *causticum*, but these two actions, so far from neutralising, strengthen each other. Before giving these two drugs together, I had given them separately in small-pox, and I did not resort to the former method of using them conjointly, until I had become perfectly satisfied, first, that either of these drugs extinguished the small-pox exanthem from its commencement with a surprising rapidity; secondly, that they neutralised each other no more than did causticum and coffee, or causticum and cocculus; bryonia and ipecacuanha, etc., etc.[1]

[1] Independently of the general action which *causticum* has on the nervous system, eyes, throat, the digestive canal and the extremities, the following cutaneous symptoms of this drug, have induced me above all to try it in variola:—**351.** *Burning blisters in the face discharging an acrid liquid which forms crusts when drying.*—**1337.** Itching all over;—**1338.** Itching all over at night, with dry heat.—**1340.** Itching here and there, especially on the head and in the face.—**1341.** Prickling itching of the skin.—**1342.** Prickling itching, obliging one to scratch, on the back, in the axillæ, on the arms, thighs, and especially on the backs of the fingers.—**1345.** Heat wherever she touches herself.—**1346.** Itching all over, with redness and numerous

Laurocerasus is, in most cases, the antidote of *causticum.*

Cocculus, *cocculus indicus.* Fruit of the *cocculus suberosus,* a climbing bush, which grows in India, where it goes by the names of *loctan, lobtang, saura, tuba flava,* etc., and which constitutes one of the species of the genus cocculus, family menispermeæ.

The Indians esteem the root of this bush very highly. They term it *root for all diseases.* They use it *for loss of appetite, colic, diarrhœa,* etc. Allœopathic physicians sometimes use the *colombo*-root, which is another species of cocculus, but never the fruit of the *cocculus suberosus,* which Hahnemann has been the first to introduce as a drug, after having studied its medicinal properties by pure experimentation.

The violence of its action upon animals is, probably, the reason why its introduction into the materia medica has been so long delayed. Orfila states, that dogs into whose stomachs three or four grains of the pulverized drug had been introduced, and whose œsophagi were afterwards tied, to prevent vomiting, died in half an hour, in the midst of frightful convulsions, *without any traces of inflammation being seen in their stomachs on opening them after death.*[1] Such experiments do not prove much, as a general rule, I admit, and it seems to me even, that such horrible cruelties might be dispensed with as not advancing the cause of true science;

vesicles: *the itching continues even after scratching.*—**1347.** Pimples all over, with *gnawing itching,* and smarting after scratching.—**1394.** *A species of varioloid in a child at the breast.*—**1350.** *Large vesicles* on the chest and back, with oppression on the chest, and cold, followed by heat and sweat.—**1451.** *Large painful vesicles,* on the left side of the chest and back, with *much febrile heat, sweat and anxiety,* etc. I knew that coffea had been used in varioloid with success. To me there seemed to be such a striking analogy between the effects of causticum and those of coffea, that it did not seem as though I risked any thing if I tried causticum instead of coffea. The action of causticum in varioloid is more clearly defined than that of coffea; but it is evidently similar.

[1] *Traité de toxicologie,* vol. II., second part, p. 22.

nevertheless, the experiment which I have just quoted, seems to establish a very remarkable fact.

The ligature of the œsophagus causes the death of a dog only five or six days after the operation had been made. Hence, if death take place half an hour after the introduction of cocculus into the stomach, it must be this poison that caused it. But we are told that the stomach presents no visible signs of inflammation or disorganization, and yet we know, on the other hand, that it is upon the stomach that cocculus exercises a specific action. We have, therefore, to conclude that it is the nervous system that is specifically affected by cocculus. This opinion is confirmed by daily experience.

Cocculus, which, as regards the totality of its symptoms, has its natural place after *causticum*, affects moreover the brain in a more marked manner than do any of the other drugs of this group, and in this respect, is vaguely analogous to *aconite*, among the analogues of which it will again be found mentioned. But it is principally in the diseases which resemble those to which *causticum* corresponds, and, frequently even in certain stages of such diseases, that cocculus is particularly useful.[1]

Cocculus is principally indicated by the following symptoms:—

Sadness; *irascibility;* anxiety; *tendency to start, especially at night;* trembling of all the extremities; paroxysm of fainting and convulsions; shuddering, in the afternoon or evening, with or without any perceptible coldness; restlessness, with anguish at night; startings when falling asleep; restless sleep; frightful dreams; irresistible desire to sleep in the morning; *itching of every part of the body;* miliary eruption; itching, particularly in warmth; red spots on the neck and chest; *paroxysms of vertigo with nausea;* cloudiness after eating or drinking; pressive headache, especially in the forehead; hemicrania, with or without nausea; pulsative,

[1] See the pathogenesis of Cocculus in Hahnemann's Mat. Med. Pura, vol. II.

pulling, lancing headache, especially in the evening; trembling of the head; pressive pain in the eyes; stitches in the eyes; dryness of the lids; black spots and muscæ volitantes before the eyes; optical hallucinations; various kinds of noise in the ears; swelling of the nose; dry nostrils; *crampy pain in the temporal and masseter muscles; acute stitches in the cheeks;* passing heat at the cheeks, *with cold feet and legs;* swelling of the salivary glands; acute stitches in the teeth, especially in those that are carious; sensation as if the incisors were longer and would start out of their sockets; painful swelling of the gums; *dry mouth and throat;* heat at the curtain; contusive pain at the base of the tongue, which feels swollen; profuse flow of saliva in the mouth; heat and scraping in the throat; *painful deglutition;* sensation, when swallowing, as if the food were too salt or had too much pepper; sort of constriction of the pharynx, impeding the breathing, and exciting a cough; metallic, brassy, or sour taste in the mouth; thirst, (which is generally middling); eructations, which taste bitter or of the food; *burning eructations,* which are sometimes suppressed; nausea, with profuse flow of saliva in the mouth, especially after supper; nausea after eating or drinking; *violent nausea during a ride in a carriage;* drowsiness, caused by the cold; *spasms at the stomach;* pressive, lancing or crampy pains at the stomach; stitches, or contusive pains in the hypochondria; contractive, pinching or burning pains in the abdomen; acute colicky pains; flatulent colic; distention of the abdomen; *sudden attack of diarrhœa; hard and knotty stools; itching in the rectum;* constrictive pain at the anus; *frequent and copious emission of urine;* itching at the scrotum; contusive pain at the testicles; *great desire for an embrace; excitability, afterwards relaxation of the sexual organs;* premature or *delaying, pale, watery* or suppressed *menses.*

Irritation and dryness of the larynx, which does not allow one to read in a loud tone of voice, and excites a cough; difficult expectoration of mucus, which is secreted in small quantities; *dry cough,* coming on in parcxysms in the evening and at night, *sometimes after having ceased for some days; dry, fatiguing cough, owing to the dyspnœa that accompanies it;* constriction at the base of the chest, which hinders breathing; paroxysms of acute stitches in the inner chest, in the region of the heart, sternum, and in the axillæ; pressure and *stitches* at the nape of the neck and at the shoulder-blades; *luxation-pain in the dorsal vertebræ and at the sacrum;* painful cracking of the cervical vertebræ in shaking the head; paroxysmal stitches in the soft parts of the shoulders, arms and fore-arms, especially during rest; stitches at the elbows; *paralytic pain* at the arms and fore-arms, sometimes coming on suddenly; twitching of the arms; sweat in the palms of the hands; cold sweat at times on one, at others on the other hand; numbness of the hands; contractions, pullings, boring or drawing pains in the fingers; stinging itching at the ends and palmar surface of the fingers; pinching in the buttocks; *contusive* or *lancing pains* in the *thighs;* pimples on the thighs; cracking in the knees; cramps in the calves; *coldness* and swelling of the *feet;* pulling pains in the toes.

Cocculus is especially suitable to women and nervous children of a lively turn of mind, and who are disposed to being troubled with imaginary fears. It is often used (especially in gastralgia, nervous cough, toothache, etc., together with causticum and coffee. Like these two agents, it antidotes the effects of chamomilla. It aggravates the effects of *causticum* and *coffea,* for the simple reason that its action is analogous to that of these agents. Staphisagria, on the contrary, which belongs to the same group, and seems to act upon the organism much more like cocculus than can be said of any of the other drugs, nevertheless, neutralises this agent, as I can affirm from experience.

Nux vomica. See page 227.

Coffea cruda, *raw coffee.* Seed of the *coffea Arabica,* a bush of the family rubiaceæ; the Arabs name it *quahouëh* or *cahouë.*

The history of coffee is very generally known. It comes originally from the East, where it has been known from time immemorial, and was imported in France in the year 1664. Hahnemann's treatise on the "*effects of coffee*," has been so universally read, that I can dispense with the trouble of going into extensive details in reference to this subject.

Allœopathic and even homœopathic physicians have accused Hahnemann of exaggeration in drawing a picture of the pernicious effects of coffee. As far as I am concerned, I am entirely of Hahnemann's opinion, that the daily use of coffee is one of the commonest causes of a number of chronic affections, and more particularly of a variety of nervous derangements, which it is so very difficult to cure. Hence it is that I look upon coffee as one of the most valuable agents of our art.

I am inclined to think, from a number of trials which I have made, that there is very little, if any, essential difference between the effects of raw and roasted coffee. It is certain, however, that the raw coffee, after having been rendered more diffusible by the process of comminution adopted by Hahnemann, acts much more promptly, and more pervasively, than any infusion of roasted coffee. This is so true, that in our provings with the crude coffee, the secondary effects, which always constitute the true and permanent effects of the drug, develope themselves so rapidly that we might almost feel tempted to take them for symptoms of the primary action of the drug.[1]

Empirical Applications.—Some Allœopathic physicians, (generally they only notice the primary or immediate action of a drug) have discovered that, among the effects of coffee, *its anaphrodisiac properties* are particularly striking. It does indeed possess such an effect on the sexual organs, but this is not its primary, but its secondary effect. But coffee is very seldom used in allœopathic practice, except as an antidote to belladonna and opium. G. Musgrave, J. Pringle, and some

[1] The same remark applies to the *Cannabis indica* which, when dynamised, never produces the good-humored craziness of the *haschich*.

other authors, recommend it as a remedy for *true asthma*, when characterized by periodical nocturnal paroxysms. Professor Grindel, of Dorpat, in Russia, says that he has used it with success in certain forms of *intermittent fever*, which is a very vague statement;[1] Dr. Arnati, in a pamphlet published at Naples, in 1823, praises an infusion of crude coffee, and the vapor of roast coffee in *chronic ophthalmia*.

It is worthy of remark, that the dynamised coffee, as I can affirm from long experience, prevents or neutralizes in many persons, the secondary effects of roast coffee. This would seem confirmatory of the *idiopathic* method of treatment. In some, *stramonium*, or *tabacum* had to be resorted to in the place of the coffee-globules, to antidote the effects of strong coffee. This might have been owing to a variety of physiological or other circumstances, which I am unable to account for. This idiopathic property is not, however, by any means an exclusive property of coffee, for I have had many opportunities of convincing myself that the dynamisations of opium, belladonna, cannabis, cinchona, lead, mercurius, etc., are possessed, in many cases, of antidotal virtues against the secondary effects of massive doses of the crude drug.

Homœopathic applications.—According to Hahnemann's own observations, as well as according to my own experience, coffee produces the following symptoms, which it is, therefore, capable of curing.

Primary symptoms:—More or less agreeable exaltation of the vital action; increase of heat, especially in the upper part of the body; slight increase and fullness of the pulse, which, however, remains soft, without ever assuming a feverish state; exaltation of all the intellectual and moral faculties, increasing to the degree of enthusiasm; the memory is more tenacious; increased facility of conception; liveliness of spirits; expansive tenderness; contentment with one's

[1] In the Eastern parts of France, I have often seen peasants use coffee without milk to cut off a paroxysm of fever, frequently with success; they were pretty severe marsh-intermittents.

self, and every thing else; forgetfulness of one's grief; crowd of ideas; desire to communicate one's ideas and emotions; talkativeness, witty remarks, puns, foolish gaiety; absence of sleep; fantastic visions (this symptom occurs rarely, I have experienced it twice); animated eyes and countenance; slight tension in the eyes; circumscribed redness of the cheeks, which does not lose itself gradually, but terminates abruptly like a spot; uniform rose-color of the face (in persons having a white skin, and who are habitually pale); warm moisture on the forehead, and in the palms of the hands; wild sweat all over; agreeable taste of nuts or almonds in the mouth; smokers have an increased desire for tobacco; suspension of the appetite and thirst; the digestion takes place more rapidly; greater facility of stool; soft stool shortly after a meal; profuse and clear urine; the sexual appetite is easily excited, with orgasm (although transitory); premature menses; the lungs are more completely and more readily dilated; ease and rapidity of the bodily movements; muscular mobility; exaggerated gestures; slight trembling of the extremities; swelling of the veins on the backs of the hands; cold feet.

Secondary symptoms.—A sort of relaxation of all the faculties of the organism; disagreeable sensation of life; excessive moral and physical sensitiveness, which renders all the sensations, as it were, painful; dullness of the mental faculties; stoppage of one's thoughts; weak memory; complete absence of imagination; sombre, gloomy, irascible mood; quarrelsome; irresolute; timid; fitful; hard-hearted; indifferent; apathetic; disposed to weeping; nervous in every part of the organism; loathing of life; aversion to exercise; chilliness; depression, and almost complete collapse of the pulse; constant yawning; stretching; desire to lie down; desire to sleep, at every moment of the day; inability to go to sleep; a sort of slumber in the place of sleep; startings, waking one at the moment when one is on the point of going to sleep; light, unrefreshing sleep, full of frightful or painful dreams; frequent waking; waking with a start;

panic fright at night, on hearing the least noise; anxious beating of the heart at night; illusions of hearing, which wake or frighten one; thirst at night; pungent heat of the skin, followed by profuse sweat; irresistible desire to sleep in the morning; sadness on waking; unhealthy skin, sensitiveness to cool air, and easily becoming sore; pricking itching, which ceases sometimes, but not always, by scratching; small vesicles here and there, with red areolæ all around; vertigo with cloudiness, and sometimes with nausea; stupifying headache; headache in the morning, with pressure in the forehead and occiput, which does not allow one to attend to mental labor, and increases on making the least effort towards it; constrictive headache, as if the head were tied by a band which passes over the forehead, and compresses the sides of the head; hemicrania; violent megrim;[1] slight pres-

[1] In reference to the headache to which coffee-drinkers are subject, and which, therefore, belongs to the symptoms of coffee, Hahnemann expresses himself as follows:

"This megrim must not be confounded with that which comes on in consequence of particular causes, such as a chagrin, an overloading of the stomach, a cold, and which generally disappears again at a certain hour of the day. The nervous headache of which I speak, comes on in the morning shortly after waking, and increases little by little. The pain becomes intolerable, and sometimes burning; the integuments of the head are very sensitive, and hurt when touched ever so slightly. Body and mind seem excessively sensitive. The patients look exhausted, they retire to lonely and dark places, and they close their eyes in order to avoid the light of day, and they remain seated in an arm-chair, or stretched upon a bed. The least noise or motion excites the pain. They avoid talking or being talked to, or hearing others talk. The body is colder than usual, although no chills are experienced; the hands and feet especially are very cold. They loathe every thing, especially food and drink, on account of a continual sickness at the stomach. If the attack is very violent, a vomiting of mucus takes place, which, however, does not diminish the headache. There are no alvine discharges. This kind of megrim scarcely ever ceases before evening. If the paroxysm is less violent, a little strong coffee, which was the first cause of such a headache, will produce a palliation of the pain, but the disposition to relapses becomes so much greater. The attacks come on irregularly, every fortnight, or every few weeks, without any apparent cause, and quite suddenly, so much so that the patient often does not feel a single unpleasant symptom the evening preceding the attack. Such a headache has never been seen by me except in real coffee-drinkers."

sure in the temples, with rapid stitches, which are felt at times in the right, at others (and more frequently) in the left side, they do not penetrate deeply, but are sometimes so acute that they extort cries from the patient; similar stitches in the occipital protuberances; involuntary twitching of the head, as in delirium tremens; formicating itching of the hairy scalp; *falling off of the hair;* itching in the eyes; pressure at the eyes; *redness of the eyes; acute ophthalmia; chronic ophthalmia* (especially in children) with an eruption of the face; lameness and sinking of the upper eye-lids, which does not allow one to open the eyes, and excessive photopobia; congested condition of the vessels of the cornea; blisters and ulcers on the cornea; dimness of sight which prevents one from reading or writing at candle-light, and sometimes even by day-light; diplopia to such a degree that objects can only be seen by closing one eye; *whizzing in the ears;* stitch in the ears; weakness of hearing; small red pimples around the wings of the nose; flashes of heat in the face; yellowish, livid complexion, with languid look and blueish lips; acute tearing pains in the cheeks; generally in one only; eruption in the face resembling varioloid; erysipelas of the face; chronic ulcers in the face; painful neuralgia in the lower jaw; *tooth-ache, especially at night,* with redness and rheumatic catarrh in one cheek; painful pullings in various parts of the body, sometimes in one side of the face, at other times in one or the other extremity; caries of the teeth, especially the incisors; painful teething of children; *excessive dryness of the mouth and throat, especially at night; flow of saliva, in bed;* excoriations, with burning pain on the edges of the tongue;

(See Hahnemann's memoir on coffee, forming the concluding part of his Organon in the Paris edition of 1845, page 308, note.)

This species of hemicrania is much less frequent in countries where coffee is drank with more moderation than it is in Germany. I have cured it in the case of a young man, simply by stopping the use of coffee. Although this kind of headache is a real coffee-disease, yet we may avail ourselves of all such indications, and similar ones in the case of other drug-diseases, each of which is, strictly speaking, perfectly distinct, for the purpose of curing analogous affections. There are, therefore, various kinds of hemicrania, which yield to coffee, as we know from experience.

loss of taste; tobacco-smoke, which in general is pleasant during the primary action of coffee, is no longer so during the secondary action, and seems even to have an unpleasant smell, like that of burning wool; sensation of excessive hunger, which ceases after eating a few mouthfulls; loss of appetite; moderate thirst, generally; phlegm in the pharynx; excruciating pain in the pharynx during empty deglutition; eructations immediately after a meal; *burning eructations; sour eructations; violent spasmodic eructations, with rising of the ingesta; heartburn* in the evening; sour vomiting; spasmodic gastralgia; *burning pains at the cardia; tension of the epigastric region, with sensitiveness to the touch,* which does not allow one to wear tight clothes; acute and sudden colic at night; *lienteria; dry, knotty, insufficient stools; constant alternations of constipation and diarrhœa;* painful retention of flatulence; acute stitches in the rectum and anus, making him cry out; blind piles; *spasmodic contraction of the sphincter; burning itching at the anus; scanty, dark, and sometimes burning urine;* copious and frequent emissions of a clear urine; stitches in the urethra, between the acts of urinating; *excited sexual instinct, with deficient erections, and even complete impotence; total loss of sexual desire and power;* emissions without *erection; delaying menses, accompanied with acute colic—of a pale color, watery and scanty;* suppression of the menses; metrorrhagia alternating with amenorrhea; *unceasing; acrid leucorrhœa,* and sometimes coming on in the place of the menses, which have either ceased, or have become very scanty; *aversion to sexual intercourse in women; it is painful;* the breasts are relaxed and flaccid.

Dryness and excoriative pain in the larynx; extinction of the voice after talking for a time or reading loud; *sensation of rawness in the windpipe;* dry barking cough, with constant tickling in the larynx; violent and dry cough, that wakes one in the middle of the night, comes on again in the morning on waking, and attacks one in the day time in short and not frequent paroxysms; *spasmodic cough, like whooping-*

cough, with this difference, that the spasms of the glottis are principally experienced during the inspirations, not the expirations; violent cough, with ropy expectoration, especially in the morning; *constriction of the chest; asthma at night;* stitches in the chest and region of the heart; itching eruptions between the breasts; stitches in the sternum; chronic ulcers in the breasts, (in nurses who make an inordinate use of coffee with or without cream;) stitches in the extremities here and there; vacillating gait, (in children;) tearings in the nape of the neck, *back*, sacral region, *in the flesh and cellular tissue rather than in the bones, in the parts between the articulations rather than in the articulations themselves;* rheumatic pain at the insertions of the muscles; *trembling of the hands;* stitches in the ends of the fingers; *heat in the palms of the hands, with coldness of the backs of the hands;* stiffness in the lower extremities; *itching eruption at the knees and calves;* unpleasant itching of the soles of the feet; *cold feet.*

If indicated, coffee is particularly suitable to women and children, or, as an intercurrent remedy, to male adults. Its action is less durable than that of causticum, but these two remedies are so nearly alike, that coffee probably does not possess a single symptom which is not likewise possessed by causticum. It must not be supposed that, because a drug is said, rightly or wrongly, to act only for a short period, it is, on this account, inefficacious in chronic diseases. With coffee and opium, the action of which is likewise supposed to be of short duration, I have succeeded in curing, in less than two months, a case of neuralgia of the head,[1] which had baffled all the resources of Old School practice.

[1] The patient was a student at law, and had been suffering for three years past. The symptoms were as follows: constant, pressive pain in the forehead, mingled with acute stitches; yellow complexion, gloomy, senile look; dry stool without constipation; tolerably fair sleep, but full of disagreeable dreams; his feet were usually cold, and his inability to study was so complete that he had made up his mind to renounce a profession for which he had expressed a fondness since his boyhood.

Tabacum is generally, and for all persons, the most speedily effective antidote of *coffea cruda.*

Staphysagria, *stave's-acre.—Perennial* plant of the genus *Delphiniæ*, family Ranunculaceæ, section of the helleboraceæ, class polyandria trigynia. It grows in the south of France, in Italy, Greece, etc.

The seeds are the only portion of this plant used in medicine. Formerly they were used for the destruction of the lice of children, on which account this plant was termed by some of the older botanists *pedicularia*, (lice-bane.) In some diseases it was also given to chew as a *sialagogue*. This must have been sometimes unpleasant and even dangerous, for these seeds have not only a bitter, pungent and burning taste, but are likewise poisonous. Murray informs us that Hillefeld gave a dog five scruples of this drug, and that the animal was soon after seized with nausea, vomiting, and a convulsive trembling, after which it ceased to bark, as if the larynx had lost the faculty of uttering sounds, and finally it fainted away and died soon after.

Empirical applications.—They are few. Dioscorides recommended the chewing stave's-acre for *toothache*, which, indeed, may have succeeded in some cases. But Schulz, desirous of curing himself of a toothache with which he was afflicted, aggravated it to such an extent by chewing these seeds, that it almost made him crazy. Not all toothaches are alike.[1]

Now-a-days staphysagria is abandoned and scarcely known by Old School physicians. In some countries it is only used for the purpose of intoxicating fish.[2]

Homœopathic applications.—Hahnemann, who ranked causticum among the anti-psorics, on account, doubtless, of the long action which he attributed to this agent, has omitted

[1] Murray, *apparat. medic.*, vol. III., p. 36.

[2] Cocculus, as is well known, is used for similar purposes, a peculiarity that becomes doubly interesting on account of the great analogy existing between these two drugs. For the pathogenesis of Staphysagria we refer the reader to Roth's Mat. Medic. Pura, vol. III., p. 78.

staves-acre among this list. However, I am satisfied that the action of staves-acre is much more thorough and lasting than that of causticum. This is the reason why I believe staves-acre much more suitable in chronic than in acute affections, although it is likewise useful in some acute diseases, such as *sea-sickness* and others that will be mentioned bye-and-bye. *Staphisagria* is principally efficacious in diseases that are characterized by one or more of the following symptoms:

Hypochondria of long standing, with taciturn disposition, constant uneasiness concerning one's health, anxious imagination, weak memory, disposition to suicide, occasional glimpses of a cheerful humor, queer notions which even exposed him to the suspicion of being thought crazy; imaginary fears, but which one endeavors to keep secret; *extreme sensitiveness of feeling; deficiency of animal heat, which compels one to wear winter clothes in summer;* heat in the palms of the hands, after a meal; disposition to sweat breaking out on the forehead; shuddering in the day-time; *shuddering in the back, with absence of thirst, in the evening in bed;* yawning and stretching; sleepiness after eating, or *in the afternoon; slumber in the day-time, with waking as if in affright;* difficulty of falling asleep before midnight; starts on falling asleep, which wake one; *light sleep;* cold at night which hinders sleep or even wakes one; *frequent night-mare;* long sleep in the morning, even after waking several times; *burning itching of various parts of the body; old miliary eruptions;* small red tubercles, finally changing to vesicles that break and discharge for a long time; *long-lasting vertigo, and accompanied by continual nausea, as in sea-sickness;*[1] *vertigo which*

[1] From this symptom which I experienced several times on myself, I inferred that Staphysagria might perhaps be an excellent remedy for sea-sickness. I prepared 100 doses of the drug, three drops of the 6th dil. to each, and had them given to 100 persons going some to England, others to America. Unfortunately, in spite of my prayers, I have only been made acquainted with the results, in a small number of cases. Of 20 persons, 7 who had already taken cocculus and arsenic without success, found in stavesacre a perfect preventive against a disease which had proved unconquerable until then; 8 were strikingly relieved, did not vomit, for instance,

ceases on rapidly turning round on one's heel, after *waltzing*, for instance, (in other words,) performing the kind of movement that causes the species of vertigo which is cured by staves-acre;[1] *headache in the morning;* constrictive, pressive or boring headache in the forehead; acute stitches in the temples; *itching at the hairy scalp as from red-hot needles;* burning itching at the occiput; red, moist and very obstinate eruption at the hairy scalp; *profuse falling off of the hairs;* hollow eyes, without lustre, *half closed, as if one had not slept long enough; smarting in the internal canthi;* redness of the whites of the eyes; pricking in the eyes, as when one is sleepy; *painful ophthalmia:* contraction of the pupils; small, black shining spots passing before the eyes from time to time, and rapidly;[2] pressure on the upper lid on opening the eyes; *chronic inflammation of the margin of the lids;* winking; dry gum at the commissure of the lids, all the time; stitches in the ears; dry crusts in the nose; *old prosopalgia*, on one side of the face; *neuralgia of the lower jaw;* disposition of the lower jaw to be sprained; *blackness and caries of the teeth; gnawing toothache, with swelling of the cheek; violent pain in the hollow teeth, when eating*, and especially when *drinking any thing cold;* excoriative pain at the tongue which makes tobacco-smoke sting; sense of rawness at the pharynx, rendering speech and deglutition painful; *nausea in the morning*, accompanied with stitches in the chest, (in the tract of the œsophagus;) *scraping eructations, and pro-*

which they had always done previously: on 5 the drug had no effect. I have found that—1. Staves acre had no effect except when taken before vomiting had set in, at the moment when the dizziness and the nausea commenced; 2. That it always helped nervous persons, not over-fat, and disposed to sadness.

Some of my patients, but very few, have found relief, in sea-sickness, from *causticum* and *coffea cruda.*

[1] This observation, which comes from myself, agrees with Hahnemann's symptom in the pathogenesis of Staphysagria: vertigo when sitting, as if things were turning round, *decreasing by walking in a circle*, (C. A. Cubitz,) Mat. Med., vol. III.

[2] *Caust., Cocc.* and *Coff.* also have this symptom: sensation as if one saw fleas jumping about.

voking a dry cough, after eating; pressure and tension at the stomach, hindering breathing; digging pain at the stomach; *old gastralgia,* caused either by coffee, or by the oriental custom of swallowing the tobacco-smoke;[1] tension in the hypochondria; *incarceration of flatulence in the lower abdomen; constrictive pain in the lower abdomen;* prickings in the lower abdomen; the abdomen is not very sensitive to contact or pressure; sweat at the abdomen, at night; *frequent, but dry and insufficient stools; frequent urging to stool, with constipation as from inertia of the rectum; slight diarrhœa, alternating with constipation; pain at the anus, as if excoriated; scanty urine, of a deep yellow or reddish color, with brick-dust sediment in either case;* discharge of prostatic fluid at stool; no sexual desire; *relaxation of the penis;* dull, contusive pain in the testicles; *impotence,* having lasted for years; *chronic amenorrhœa,* with general debility.

Chronic dryness of the nostrils, dry coryza, or secretion of thick mucus in the nasal fossæ, after an intense, fluent coryza of short duration; hoarseness, with excoriative pain at the larynx, not allowing one either to talk or read aloud; *dry cough after eating; chronic dry cough, which is sometimes very violent,* especially in the evening, in bed, or in the morning after rising, with pain in the chest as if raw; acute stitches in the chest; pressure at the sternum, especially when sitting; constriction of the chest which hinders respiration; *inordinate beating of the heart,* after every emotion or every effort; miliary eruption on the chest; general lameness and weariness; stiffness of the nape of the neck, back and articulations of the extremities; *pressive pain in the periosteum of every bone, which is not altered, either by motion or rest, nor increased by pressure;* deep stitches here and there, *contusive pain* in the flesh, when exposed ever so little to the cold.

Of all known drugs, *staphysagria* is probably the best remedy for the nausea of pregnant females.

[1] I have cured patients who had this habit, with staves-acre.

Camphor is said to antidote staphysagria; but it is only incompletely that it neutralises the effects of this drug.

Corallia rubra, *red coral.*—A species of cortical polypus of the genus *isis* of Linné, or *corallium* of Lamarck.

This substance, which has disappeared from allœopathic pharmacies for a long time past, and which is not even mentioned in Gmelin's *apparatus medicaminum*, is a compound, or rather, a mixture of carbonate of lime, oxyde of iron, gelatine, and perhaps, other elements that have escaped the eye of the chemist.

Empirical applications.—"Coral," say Mérat and Delens, "has been lauded by Schrœder, Ettmueller, Rivière and a number of other physicians, as endowed with strengthening properties, such as precious stones were formerly supposed to be possessed with; it was likewise considered as a tonic, astringent, sudorific, diuretic, and particularly as an absorbent; this last-mentioned property is easily accounted for by the calcareous nature of coral. It was administered in the shape of a powder, ground, sifted, and generally in the shape of round tablets, under the name of *prepared coral*, for *diarrhœa, dysentery, hæmorrhages*, (especially *hæmoptysis*, according to Dioscorides, and for *uterine hæmorrhage*, for which Bourgeois, who is quoted by Fourcroy, gave it with success,) *epilepsy, leucorrhœa, blennorrhagia.* Externally it was used as a desiccative and cicatrising agent applied to old ulcers, in certain salves, etc."[1] This passage, which contains pretty much the whole history of coral as a drug, sufficiently shows, that allœopathic physicians have never had any definite notions concerning the medicinal properties of this agent.

Homœopathic applications.—Stapf has given us a very incomplete pathogenesis of the coral in his *Archives*, which may be found translated in Jahr's Manual. In Paris, it is scarcely used by any but Dr. Petroz. In the provings which I made with this drug upon my own person, some years ago, I elicited a few exceedingly characteristic symptoms, which

[1] *Dict. univ. de mat. méd*, article Isis, vol. III., p. 663.

induced me to prescribe it, sometimes with striking success, for *nervous cough, asthma Millari, endemic whooping-cough,* and for certain forms of *gastralgia.* I believe, that the action of *corallia* is very similar to that of *causticum, coffea,* etc. However, I should be unable to determine the exact symptomatic indications of coral as preferable to *causticum* or *coffea.* I have seen *corallia* succeed in cases where *coffea* had failed, and vice versa. But in such cases of failure there was never any aggravation; the drugs simply exhibited no effects whatever. In a case of gastralgia, I used with tolerable success, and alternately, *Coff., Staphys.,* and *Coral.*

Arsenicum album. See page 193.

GROUP VIII.

TYPE: IPECACUANHA.

ANALOGUES: PULSATILLA, NUX VOMICA, BRYONIA ALBA, IODIUM, CHAMOMILLA VULGARIS, PHOSPHORUS, ANTIMONIUM CRUDUM, SILICEA, ARSENICUM ALBUM, SPONGIA TOSTA, ZINCUM, IGNATIA, FILIX MAS, TARTARUS EMETICUS.[1]

VOMITING, upon which, Old School physicians have founded an absurd and barbarous system of medication still in vogue, consists essentially in an anti-peristaltic movement of the stomach, which is generally accompanied with more or less violent spasms of this viscus, in consequence of which, the food which had been swallowed, or the gastric juices contained in the stomach, are diverted from their natural channel, and compelled to return by the œsophagus and mouth. This phenomenon may be produced by almost any drug, when given in sufficiently large doses, or even by any indigestible substance, even though it should not be exactly medicinal. But the medicinal agents, which, even when given in small doses, produce vomiting as a permanent and positive result of their action, are much less numerous than it would seem. This is the characteristic property of the drugs of this group. I will endeavor to show that most of the symptoms which these drugs have in common, depend upon the faculty which they possess, of exciting vomiting by

[1] Perhaps we might add to the analogues of *Ipecacuanha: Paris quadrifolia*, if it were only better known, *Dulcamara*, *Belladonna*, *Chelidonium majus*, and even *Cannabis indica*, which affects the head, throat and air-passages similarly to *Ipecac.;* lastly, *Natrum mur.*, *Stannum* and *Sambucus nigra;* however, they had better remain in the groups to which I have assigned them respectively, and where a description of their medicinal properties and uses may be found.

their primary action upon the stomach, independently of the mode in which they are introduced into the system.

It is evident that one of the first results of drug-vomiting, or of a prolonged nausea, excited by artificial means, must be a rush of the blood and all the vital fluids from the stomach to the upper half of the body; that is to say, to the chest, throat, head, which may give rise to the following symptoms:—

Engorgements of the lungs.

Deranged condition of the circulation, and the functions of the heart.

Swelling of the mucous membrane of the throat and air-passages.

Swelling of the breasts, salivary glands, tonsils, cervical ganglia, and all the soft parts of this region.

Flow of saliva and buccal mucus.

Bloating and redness of the face.

Congestive headache.

General clogging of the venous and lymphatic systems, which may result in hæmorrhages, swelling of the glands, etc.

If the anti-peristaltic movement should extend throughout the whole intestinal canal, another series of symptoms developes itself; besides abdominal pains of more or less intensity, we then have:

Frequent and unsuccessful urging to stool, that is to say, tenesmus with constipation, or, in consequence of the above-mentioned states of congestion, a sanguine exudation in the rectum, and a painful discharge of blood from the anus, which, on account of its fluid nature, is enabled to escape in spite of the restraining action of the tenesmus.[1]

All these, however, are only the primary effects of our

[1] Although these last mentioned symptoms, which constitute such marked effects of *Puls.*, *Silic.*, *Nux vom.* etc., are not mentioned among the symptoms of *Ipec.* in Hahnemann's Mat. Med. Pur., I have found, in my own experience, that they belong equally as much to this drug, only the tenesmus of *Ipec.*, like all its primary symptoms, is of short duration; the diarrhœa that comes after it, and which sometimes lasts a long while, is a secondary effect.

drugs; let us now proceed to an examination of their secondary effects.[1]

After the vomiting (which continues for a longer or shorter period, according to the nature of the drug and the constitution of the patient) stops, an opposite effect takes place; the peristaltic movement of the stomach, and generally of the bowels, succeeds the former anti-peristaltic movement of these organs. But the intensity with which this reaction develops itself, is just as abnormal a phenomenon as the vomiting itself. The symptoms which characterise this reaction, will appear just as violent and intense as those that characterised the primary action of the drug; such symptoms, for instance, are: diarrhœa, sinking at the stomach, bulimy, impoverished quality of the blood, dwindling of the breasts and other glands; emptiness of the head, neuralgia, weakness of the senses, etc.

This shows that the drugs which constitute the *Ipecac.*, or, indeed, any other group, can be given for apparently opposite states of disease, hypertrophy or atrophy of glands, plethora or marasmus, etc.

Among the analogues of *ipecac.*, there are some that seem to occasion at one and the same time an anti-peristaltic movement of the stomach and an abnormal intensity of the peristaltic movement of the bowels, so as to occasion at the same time vomiting and diarrhœa. Supposing now that, by virtue of a physiological law which seems to be invariably true, these two abnormal conditions are succeeded by their opposites, what must be the necessary consequence of such a change? Sinking at the stomach; paroxysms of canine hunger, accompanied with constipation; antagonistic pheno-

[1] These symptoms, at least so far as Pulsatilla is concerned, are not regarded by Hahnemann as secondary symptoms of the drug, but as *reactions of the organism.* As I have said before, this distinction seems to be purely speculative, and without any practical value. It is immaterial whether we attribute effects which uniformly manifest themselves after the exhibition of a drug, to the secondary action of this agent, or to the reaction of the organism.

mena, which, beside a deep and general derangement of the health, and an universal emaciation, result in *hypertrophy of the abdominal glands*, (liver, spleen, mesenteric glands, etc.;) *intermittent fevers*, that never fail to make their appearance; *ascites*, etc., etc.; to all of which diseases, arsenic, as is well known, corresponds more exactly than any other drug, for, of all the analogues of *ipecac.*, it is the one that produces in the most signal manner these antagonistic effects on the digestive canal.[1]

CORRESPONDING DISEASES.

Hydrocephalus.—Periodical headache.—Dyspepsia.—Gastric derangements.—Indigestions.—Bilious fevers.—Intermittent fevers.—Diarrhœa.—Dysentery.—Peritonitis.—Puerperal fever.—Angina.—Croup.—Asthma.—Whooping-cough.—Bronchial catarrh.—Pneumonia.—Pleurisy.—Hydrarthrosis.—Hypertrophy and atrophy of the glands.—Goître.—Scrophula, etc.

Ipecacuanha.—*Radix Braziliensis*, root of the *cephælis ipecacuanha, ringed or officinal ipecacuanha.*—The plant from which we derive this celebrated root, belongs to the family of the rubiaceæ, and the pentandria monogynia of Linné. It is found in large quantities in Brazil, in the provinces of Pernambuco, Bahia, Rio de Janeiro, Mariana, etc. But the exportation of this root from Brazil is so considerable, and it is consumed in such immense quantities in that empire itself, that the crop in the neighborhood of Rio is actually failing, and the root has to be gathered in the interior provinces.

The root of the *cephœlis ipecac*, as sold in trade, is from two to three inches long, about the thickness of a goose-quill, flexible, and furnished with a line of irregularly shaped, rugose, and closely-joined rings. The root consists of a thick, hard, brittle bark, of a grayish color externally, and whitish internally; and secondly, of a much whiter, flexible, and almost wooden core. This root has not a very marked

[1] This remark, of course, does not include the diseases to which the various analogues of *ipecac.* respectively correspond, when viewed independently of the relations they hold to *ipec.* as their type.

odor, but the taste of its cortical portion is acrid, bitter, and nauseous.

Empirical applications.—For a long time past *ipecacuanha* had been used in Brazil as a remedy for *dysentery*, when Pison and Musgrave furnished the first description of it, and informed European physicians of its medicinal properties. But it was not until some 30 or 35 years after this period, towards the end of the seventeenth century, that the use of *ipecac.* became more general, owing to the recommendations of the Dutch physician, John Helvetius, who resided in Paris, and is the grandfather of the celebrated author of the book, *De l'esprit.* Since then, ipecacuanha was made the subject of a number of memoirs, theses, dissertations, etc.; in spite of which, and notwithstanding the very correct but neglected description of Pison and Musgrave, the plant which furnished this root was not yet exactly known, even as late as the end of the eighteenth century, and even later. It was successively attributed to several distinct plants, especially to a species of the genus *Paris*, then to a species of the genus *lonicera*, and lastly to a plant of the genus *viola*, which is found in Brazil, the root of which is indeed an emetic, and which Linné, in his *Mantissa*, termed *viola ipecacuanha*, which name is given by Murray to the *officinal ipecacuanha*. All such historical details, however, are of no sort of practical importance, and such of our readers, as desire more extensive information in reference to these matters, are referred to Sprengel's *history of medicine*, or to Murray's *apparatus medicaminum*, or finally, to Mérat and Delens' *Dictionnaire de Matière Médicale.*

According to Trousseau and Pidoux, the most interesting experiments with ipecacuanha, are those that have been made by Dr. Bretonneau. (The experiments of Hahnemann and his disciples, are, of course, ignored by these gentlemen.) "This practitioner (see their *Traité de Thérapeutique*, Vol. I., p. 602,) discovered that the powder of ipecac., when applied to the skin, which had been deprived of its epidermis, excited

[1] *Historia naturalis brasiliensis*, Amsterdam, 1698.

a most violent local inflammation; that a small pinch of this powder, when blown into the eye of a dog, caused such an intense phlegmasia of this organ, that the corner sometimes became perforated. He showed, by these experiments, that the ipecac. is capable of producing a local irritation, and he inferred from this fact that it excites vomiting and purging in consequence of the inflammation which is produced by this agent in the mucous membrane of the stomach and bowels." These experiments are certainly not uninteresting; but are they as important as Trousseau and Pidoux seem to believe? I think not. They simply prove that what is true of a number of other drugs, is likewise true of ipecacuhana, namely, that when applied to the cutis, or a mucous membrane, this root causes a local irritation. But does this faculty of causing a local irritation, imply that ipecacuanha cannot be absorbed, especially when it is given in small, extremely comminuted doses, or that it is not possessed of therapeutical properties of a much greater importance than the power to irritate the skin? Bretonneau never intended to prove any such a thing. It is true, to alloeopathic physicians, *ipecacuanha* is an emetic, nothing else, and all the experiments which they perform with this drug, are simply intended to find out the manner in which the vomiting is provoked.

Nevertheless, Trousseau and Pidoux themselves have to admit that, in some cases, ipecac. possesses other properties besides that of causing vomiting. After having mentioned and praised unreservedly its good effects in *dysentery*, they add:—"In simple diarrhœa accompanied with saburral symptoms, etc., ipecacuanha stops the disease almost immediately."[1] How is this, I ask? Is it by determining an *inflammation of the gastro-intestinal mucous membrane?* But what becomes of this inflammation, *if the symptoms cease almost immediately?* An explanation of this kind seems absurd.

Trousseau and Pidoux continue:—"Ipecac. exhibits a remarkable action on the respiratory apparatus. We knew

[1] *Oper. Cit.*, vol. I., p. 608.

two apothecaries in Tours and St. Germain who were seized with paroxysms of asthma every time the flask which contained the powdered ipecac. was opened in their shops. In the *Transactions Philosophiques Abrégées*, Vol. II., p. 69, a similar fact is related. The pathological laws which we developed in speaking of the method of substitution, explain to a certain extent, the good effects of ipecacuanha in nervous, and in moist asthma; but whatever explanation be offered, the fact has to be admitted." This is a frank and explicit concession to the principle of similarity; ipecac. causes and cures *nervous and humid asthma;* homœopathy is nothing more than a generalization of this fact, embracing all other diseases. As regards the pretended laws of this *method of substitution*, this is not the place to discuss them; but every body now-a-days knows that this method of substitution is simply a fanciful theory put in the place of the only true interpretation of the facts upon which this pretended theory is based, an interpretation which is embodied in the doctrine of homœopathy, and which no practitioner who desires to escape the charge of ignorance, is permitted to remain unacquainted with.

But it is not only in the method of substitution that error, nonsense and contradictions abound, when the effects of ipecac. are attempted to be explained. Mérat and Delens express themselves in this wise:—

"The *incisive* action (I confess I do not well understand the meaning of this term), is quite evident, and it is most frequently depended upon by modern practitioners. Thus, it is prescribed in small or broken doses, for bronchial derangements, for an excess of mucus in the lungs, flaccid condition of the pulmonary parenchyma, serous inflammation of the lungs, etc. *It procures a more profuse and easier expectoration, by increasing the exhalation of the pulmonary mucous membranes, in cases where it is deficient, and distinguishes it by its tonic action, whenever the expectoration is too profuse.*"[1]

[1] *Oper. Cit.*, vol. III., p. 646.

It seems then that ipecac. acts two opposite parts, that it is alternately *incisive* when the expectoration has to be rendered more profuse, and *tonic* when the expectoration has to be diminished. The reason of this antagonism is not inquired into. Is it possible that learned authors should thus content themselves with empty words, without perceiving the inanity of their theories ? Be this as it may, the positive and undeniable facts upon which these fanciful doctrines are based, are still less reconcilable to the principle of local inflammation established by Bretonneau. The truth is, that until this moment, science has been unable to explain or to deny the effects of ipecac. any more than those of a number of other heroic agents. Its uses have been altogether empirical. It has been given with more or less success for *diarrhœa, dysentery, leucorrhœa, acute angina, inveterate catarrhs of old people, laryngitis, whooping-cough, intermittent fever, and even puerperal fever.*[1] "Experience shows," say Trousseau and Pidoux, "that almost all the dangerous symptoms which occur during confinement, yield to ipecac.; we mention this, not on the strength of books, but of what we have seen and done. For five years past we have constantly attended at the hôtel dieu, sixty women in confinement; we have never failed to give every woman, who had been recently confined, a dose of ipecac.; no matter with what derangement she might have been affected, and we can affirm that we have never seen the least trouble arise from this practice; on the contrary, in most cases, we have either effected a cure or a perceptible improvement."[2] Homœopathic physicians will not fail to appreciate the vagueness or extreme explicitness of these statements which, be it said in passing, do not harmonize with any known allœopathic doctrine. I have mentioned them here for the purpose of substantiating in the eyes

[1] Concerning the use of ipec. in this last named disease, read the cases collected by Doublet, in the hôtel-dieu of Paris in 1782, and contained in vol. LVIII. and LIX. of the ancient *Journal de médecine.*

[2] *Oper. Cit.*, vol. I., p. 607.

of homœopathic practitioners, some of the real and most important properties of this drug.

Homœopathic applications.—Hahnemann's pathogenesis of ipecac. (see his Mat. Med. pur. Vol. II.) comprises only 233 symptoms, including those which have been furnished by his disciples; this seems a small number, considering the importance of the drug, but I am inclined to believe that this list contains all the characteristic effects of this powerful agent.

"This drug," says Hahnemann, in his Mat. Med. Vol. II., "acts only for a short while, massive doses for a few days, small doses only a couple of hours." But, if this action be of short duration, it is, on the other hand, speedy, intense and well-marked. The throat, stomach, salivary glands, thyroid body, abdominal glands, pancreas, liver, spleen, the mucous follicles of the larynx, trachea and bronchia; and, lastly, the heart and head seem to be affected by the drug, at once and at the same period. Hence, I infer that ipecac. corresponds naturally to acute affections of short duration, but running a rapid course, and capable, on this account, of reaching in a short period a high degree of intensity, such as *croup* and *pneumonia.* We shall refer to this again bye-and-bye. I infer, moreover, from this rapidity of action, that ipecac. is particularly suitable for various affections of children, in whom the pathological and physiological phenomena develop themselves much more rapidly than in adults. Indeed, it is in the diseases of women and children, and of young male adults with fair complexions, and a lively and plethoric disposition, such as must have developed itself out of a similar disposition in infancy, that ipecac. has exhibited the most successful curative effects.

I have used it with good effect in constrictive and contusive headaches, seated in the left parietal region, coming on every day, at 11 o'clock in the morning, increasing progressively, until the pain became intolerable, then decreasing again in the same manner, and ceasing so completely, about two in the afternoon, that the patients only preserved a remembrance of their sufferings, and were perfectly able to resume their usual avocations.

Ipecac. evidently corresponds to various forms of dyspepsia, nausea, idiopathic vomiting, or vomiting caused by fat pork or fat in general, or such a condition of the stomach as was formerly termed saburral, and lastly to certain kinds of acute diarrhœa. But Hahnemann does not admit the efficacy of this drug in dysentery. Here are his remarks in reference to this subject: "Originally ipecac. was brought to Europe as a remedy for fall-dysentery. It is now more than one hundred and thirty years since it was recommended by Leibnitz for dysentery, and since it has been falsely used in this disease, in accordance with the very false conclusion that, because it cures certain kinds of diarrhœa, it must, therefore, be able to cure dysentery, which, however, is the contrary of liquid and excessive diarrhœic discharges. Physicians begin to perceive their error, for experience has shown them in thousands of cases, that it is not by any means suitable for dysentery. So many unfortunate experiments, which have destroyed the lives of a number of patients, might have been avoided, if the specific effects of ipecac. had first been ascertained by experimentations upon the healthy organism, which would have revealed the diseases which this drug is capable of curing by virtue of a similarity of the symptoms. It would have been seen that ipecac. is capable of diminishing the bloody discharges and some of the abdominal pains in dysentery, but that it is not capable of arresting any of the essential symptoms of this affection, for the simple reason that it is not endowed with the faculty of producing similar ones in a healthy person."[1] It is true, tenesmus, which is one of the characteristic symptoms of dysentery, is not among the list of symptoms furnished by Hahnemann and his disciples; but it is not the less true that this drug has more than once stopped the tenesmus, if not in the real fall-dysentery, at least in certain kinds of diarrhœa. But do not symptoms 38, 39, 40, 42, 45, 46, 47, 48, 49, 50, 53, 59, 60, 61 and 62 of Hahnemann's pathogenesis point to

[1] *Loc. Cit.*

dysentery? It is these symptoms, and a few empirical reminiscences that have induced me, contrary to Hahnemann's opinion, to prescribe ipecac. in dysentery, and, indeed, with success. I ought to state, however, that I never succeeded with ipecac. except when used in alternation with *Petroleum;* hence the mode of treatment in dysentery which I have pointed out in my *traité des maladies des enfants.*

"On the other hand," continues Hahnemann, "the symptoms of ipecac. show that, as it is capable of arresting vomiting, which it likewise produces, so it is also capable of exercising specific curative effects in hæmorrhage, in spasmodic asthma characterized by paroxysms, in suffocative spasms and some kinds of tetanus, provided, however, that all the other symptoms correspond." And, lastly, certain quotidian intermittents, with absence of thirst during the heat, and nocturnal paroxysms, cannot, according to Hahnemann, be cured as effectually with any medicine as with ipecac.

Let us briefly mention the value of this drug in croup and pneumonia.

In almost all cases of croup, where allœopathic physicians have substituted ipecac. and stibium to their horrible blood-letting, they have not had any cause to regret the change. But the success which they obtained by this violent method of treatment, which was sometimes dangerous and yet powerless, in consequence of the excessive size of the doses and the improper use of the drug, was not owing, as they supposed, to the vomiting, but to such symptoms as Nos. 70, 71, 72, 73, 74, 78, 79, 80, 81, 104, 109, 110 and 111 of Hahnemann's pathogenesis, all of which point to croup, and to the powerful and specifically characteristic action that ipecac. has on the mucous membrane of the pharynx, larynx, trachea, and, probably, of the bronchial tubes. In some cases, I have seen *ipecac.* arrest the following symptoms with such a marked rapidity that I cannot help believing it capable of producing similar symptoms, if not in full-grown persons, at any rate in healthy children:

Rapid bloating of the mucous membrane of the pharynx, and very probably also of the larynx and trachea.

Secretion, on the inflamed surface of this membrane, of a thick, plastic, whitish, mother-of-pearl humor, looking at first like small white or grayish points, either on the tonsils, or on the pillars of the palate, or even in the pharynx.

If we unite these symptoms to those mentioned before, we shall have as complete an image of croup as possible.

The cures of croup, which have been and are being effected with the attenuations of *ipecac.*, or of *ipecac.* and *bryonia*, given in alternation, agreeably to my method, are indeed quite numerous, and become more so from day to day.[1] But does this mean that other drugs, besides *ipecac.* and *bryon.* may not be useful in croup?

It would be absurd to suppose any such a thing. I know that croup has often been cured with *Bell.*, *Stibium*, *Spong. tost.*, *Hep. Sulph.*, and even *Acon.*, which latter drug is far from possessing the specific action on the air-passages, that *Ipec.* and its analogues can boast of. But what are we to infer from this? In the first place, nothing shows that the cases, where the former drugs were successful, *Ipec.* and *Bryon.* would not have effected a more rapid and decisive cure. In the second place, I admit, that all the analogues of *Ipecac.*, are capable of producing, each in its own degree, not only the general symptoms of croup, but even the pseudo-membranous exudation which constitutes the pathognomonic sign of croup, and that they must, therefore, be capable of curing this disease. I go still farther: I admit that cases may occur where a peculiar idiosyncrasy, or an exceptional

[1] *Croup*, which scarcely ever varies in its symptoms, is, like *scarlatina*, *variola*, and other affections of this kind, one of those *essential* diseases, for which it is perfectly proper to endeavor to discover a *specific mode of treatment*. For the mode of treatment which I propose, and which now enjoys a certain degree of popularity, I refer the reader—1st, to my *treatise on the diseases of children*, p. 365; 2d, to my *answer to a note of Dr. Peschier* in the *Journ. de la Soc. gall. de méd. homœop.*, vol. I., p. 195; 3d, to two cases reported by Dr. Turrell of Toulon in the same Journal, vol. II., pages 492 and 496, and being part of a remarkable essay, entitled *Etudes cliniques*.

development of the symptoms, its sub-acute form, etc., may require *Pulsat.*, *Silic.*, *Spong.*, *Hepar.*, etc., in preference to *Ipec. or Bryon.* But I maintain that these cases are rare, and that, as a general rule, *Ipec.* and *Bryon.*, constitute the specific remedies for croup.

It is not necessary, however, by any means, that an inflammation of the larynx, and more particularly of the air-passages, should be accompanied with plastic exudation, giving rise to the formation of a false membrane, in order that *Ipecac.* should be the appropriate remedy. I might corroborate this assertion with numerous facts. *Ipecac.* is almost the only remedy that is indicated in all cases of very acute inflammation of the throat, wind-pipe, bronchia, and even the parenchyma of the lungs, no *matter what the cause of the inflammation may have been*, when the patient is from six months to ten years old, with blond hair, of a sanguine and lively disposition, and if it is more particularly at night that the disease reaches its acme or first breaks out. Under such circumstances, I have seen *pulmonary engorgements*, and even *genuine pneumonia*, yield to ipecac., especially one case of the latter disease, in a child of ten months, which came on in consequence of the repercussion of a scarlatina-exanthem, and for which, *Belladonna* was given without effect.

As an intercurrent remedy, I have used *Ipec.* with marked success in *goïtre.*

I believe, although I am unable to prove it, that *veratrum album*, is the surest antidote to *Ipecac.*

Pulsatilla.—See page 260.

Silicea.—See page 268.

Nux vomica.—See page 227.

Arsenicum.—See page 193.

Bryonia.—See the group of which it is the type.

Spongia marina tosta, *spongia officinalis, burnt sponge.*

Formerly, sponge was ranked among the zoophytes; but at present it is classed among the polypi, although the animal that inhabits it, is unknown, and seems only to consist in a sort of a thin jelly, which, when dry, leaves scarcely a trace of its existence.

For medicinal purposes, sponge is first cut in small pieces, and then roasted like coffee, until it has a brown color, and can be pulverized without much difficulty. "Sponge,[1] when changed to a black coal, as it is often found in the shops, appears to be without any strength, whereas, sponge that is only roasted to a brown color, preserves much of its odor, and imparts all its powerful properties to alcohol. When the tincture is poured into water, this liquid assumes a milky aspect; but it retains a good portion of it in solution. Sponge is said to contain iodium." It is precisely because an excessive degree of torrefaction decomposes the salts of iodine contained in sponge, that most of its medicinal properties are destroyed. It has to be observed, that iodium is not, by any means, the only medicinal ingredient of sponge; if this were the case, iodium and spongia would produce the same symptoms, which is not the case. But independently of the iodides of potassa, chemists have discovered in spongia officinalis, a fat oil, a large quantity of carbonate and phosphate of lime, muriate of soda, sulphur, alumina, silica, magnesia, and more recently, bromine.[2] The physiological effects of sponge, doubtless, result from the combined, or, at any rate, the simultaneous action of these various substances. The probability is, that in the production of these effects, the chlorides which are decomposed by the roasting, namely; chlorine, bromine, and more particu-

[1] See Hahnemann's Mat. Med. Pur., vol. II., p. 284.

[2] If chlorine and bromine are not, side by side with Spongia, found ranged among the analogues of *Ipecac.*, it is because I was not in possession of a sufficient number of precise facts concerning the medicinal properties of these drugs, and I considered it, on this account, proper to avoid classifying them; but there is no doubt that they belong to the present group as natural constituents.

larly iodine, are principally concerned. But, howsoever much these hypotheses may be founded, they can only be of minor interest to the homœopathic physician. Rejecting medicinal compounds under whatever form they are used, and placing very little confidence in the results of chemical analyses, which are but too often of a conjectural nature, homœopathy considers every product of nature as an homogeneous and unitary whole, and uses it as such in the treatment of diseases.

Roast sponge, which has been banished for a long time past from the Allœopathic Materia Medica, as an *illusory and ridiculous drug*,[1] was, nevertheless, and very properly considered a specific remedy for goître, for several centuries. Arnold de Villeneuve, appears to be the first who conceived the idea of using it for this disease ; this was in the thirteenth century. But I do not believe, that this precious drug has been used for any other purpose, nor do I admit that iodium is a substitute for it in all cases, although this agent has completely superseded spongia in the practice of allœopathic physicians.[2]

It is more particularly in diseases characterised by one or more of the following symptoms, that Spongia has been found efficacious :—

Moral and *physical debility;* tendency to start; *paroxysms of anguish;* sense of weariness in the upper portion of the body, and of numbness in the lower portion; alternate sadness and mirthfulness; *fever with shuddering in the back and coldness all over, followed by dry heat or accompanied with sweat;* drowsiness in the day time ; sleep full of dreams and fantastic visions, which sometimes continue after waking; *frequent waking with a start;* itching of the skin, as if sweat would break out; red spots; rush of blood to the head; vertigo, as if one would fall sideways or backwards; pressive headache, *at the top of the head*, at the occiput or temples; stitch in the temples; pressive pain in the forehead from

[1] *Dict. des sc. méd.*, article *Eponge.*

[2] See the pathogenesis of Spongia in *Hahnemann's Mat. Med. Pura*, vol. II.

within outwards; fullness of the head, with heat, which is perceived by the hand, and sometimes *sudden flow of saliva;* semi-lateral headache; sensitiveness and itching of the hairy scalp; stitches in the eyes; redness and burning of the eyes; lachrymation; heaviness and nightly agglutination of the lids; myopia; constrictive otalgia; retention and thickening of the nasal mucus; *nose-bleed;* pale face, with sunken eyes and anxiety in the features; crampy pain in the articulations of the jaw; blisters at the edges of the tongue, and on the inner surface of the cheeks; *stitches in the throat; pricking sensation above the throat-pit;* induration of the sub-maxillary glands and of the *thyroid body; sickness at the stomach;* sense of sickness and faintness at the stomach, as if one had drank a quantity of warm water; sour regurgitations; vomiting; contractive pains at the stomach; *pinching in the abdomen;* cutting colic after a meal; crampy pains at the groins; swelling of the inguinal glands; diarrhœic stools, with tenesmus; hard stools; formication in the rectum; smarting at the anus; increase of the urinary secretion; urine with a white, yellow or grayish sediment; crampy pain in the testicles; *induration of the testicles; premature and profuse menses.*[1]

Great dryness of the larynx, with short and barking cough, embarrassed breathing, as if the larynx and trachea were narrower; pain at the larynx when touching it; hoarseness, dry, hollow, wheezing cough, worse in the evening, excited by a sense of tickling and burning in the larynx and trachea; crampy pains in the whole chest; *stitches resembling pleuritic stitches in both sides of the chest;* vascular excitement in the chest on performing the least movement, with dyspnœa, anxiety, nausea and weakness, as if one would faint; anxious pain in the region of the heart; *crampy pain in the cervical muscles;* stitches in the shoulder-blades; wrenching pains at the shoulder-joint; boring pain at the elbow; *drawing stitches in the fore-arms and hands;* swelling of the

[1] The profuse and premature menses of spongia, as well as the uterine hæmorrhages caused by *Ipecac.*, are probably *primary* effects of these drugs,

hands; numbness at the end of the fingers; twitching of the glutei muscles; acute stitches in the thighs, above the knees and in the feet; stiffness of the lower extremities.

Roast sponge, which acts for several weeks, is, like iodium, or, rather, much more than iodium, a specific for goïtre. It is necessary for me to observe, that this term specific, in the sense in which I use it in this instance, is justified by Hahnemann. He says in the second volume of his Materia Medica, art. Spongia: "The particular swelling of the thyroid body to which the name of goïtre is given, and which is peculiar to the inhabitants of low valleys and of the adjoining plains, depends upon a conjuncture of circumstances, which, although mostly unknown to us, yet seem to remain pretty much the same, and, for this reason, constitute a disease which remains essentially the same, and against which a drug which has once effected a cure, ought to show itself efficacious, it would seem, in every case." Experience does not justify these conclusions. Some goïtres resist any attenuation of Spongia. I have frequently been obliged to have recourse to ipecac., iodium, bromine, in the treatment of goïtre, after having vainly tried *spongia*. As a general rule, this agent is only suitable in the second stage of *croup*. But I do not hesitate to place it in the first rank in the treatment of acute and chronic affections of the serous membranes, (*pleurisy*, *pericarditis*, *peritonitis*, etc.,) with or without effusion; my opinion concerning this subject is based upon a few facts only, but they are decisive to my mind.

Camphor is said to antidote Spongia.

Iodium. This is a simple body, a metalloïd, the name of which is derived from the Greek word *Ioeidès*, violet-colored, and has been given to it on account of the beautiful color it assumes when volatilised.

The iodium of the shops consists of laminæ, or scales of a blueish-gray color, specific gravity 4,946, fusible and volatile, almost insoluble in water, but soluble in nine times their weight of alcohol, at a temperature of 35 degrees, and still more soluble in ether. The odor of iodium is similar to that of dilute liquid chlorine, or rather to the odor of the chloride of sulphur. Its taste is acrid, penetrating, persistent, and very unpleasant. It was first discovered in 1813, by Courtois, in the mother-ley of the saline ashes of the kelp, and only seems to exist in saline combinations. In this form it has been found, 1st, in a number of algæ and weeds which are very abundant on our coasts; 2d, in some sweet-water plants; 3d, in the saline marshes on the borders of the Mediterranean; 4th, in sea-sponges, in various species of polypi and molluscæ; 5th, in some silver ores; 6th, and lastly, in a considerable number of mineral-waters that are indebted to iodium for a portion of their properties, especially the waters of Cauterets, Saint Sauveur, Plombières, Hambourg, Aix-en-Savoie, Castel-nuova-d'Asti, Montechia, etc. Almost as soon as iodium had been discovered, it was introduced into the Materia Medica by Coindet, of Geneva; the therapeutic powers of the sponge were attributed to it alone.

Empirical applications.—Iodium was from the first considered the specific remedy for *goïtre*, and with the exception of the accidents it caused, it maintained this reputation tolerably well. Although the scrofulous nature of goïtre was not, by any means, proven, yet iodium and its compounds were used as specific remedies for all sorts of scrofulous diseases. These drugs were successively lauded and prescribed, but with variable success, and sometimes without any, for *strumous tumors*, with or without ulcerations on the neck, breasts, in the axillæ or groins; for *meningitis* and *tuberculous phthisis*, *mesenteric phthisis*, *ulcerations of the mucous membranes;* also for affections that were not, properly speaking, of a scrofulous nature, such as *passive dropsy*, *encysted ovarian tumors*, *hydrocele*, *hydrothorax*, *dropsy of the bursæ mucosæ or of the articular and tendinous bursæ*, *amenorrhœa*, *leucorrhœa*, *nervous diseases*, (always depending upon accident;) and lastly, for tertiary syphilis, such as *tubercles of the cellular tissue*, known by the name of gommata, *bone-pains*, *periostoses*, *exostoses*, *caries*, etc. It is true, that in these latter cases, it is the hydriodate of potash, not iodium, that is given to patients, so that it would be difficult to determine to which of the constituents of this compound the good effects which it is said to produce, should be attributed.

Be this as it may, I have no hesitation in saying that Iodium is very much abused by allœopathic physicians in their every day practice. All honest and enlightened practitioners will admit this. The ill effects of large doses of iodium, administered without reason, and out of all rule, are so numerous on the very records of the allœopathic school, that they almost suffice to constitute a complete pathogenesis of the drug. Among these effects we distinguish the following:

General irritability, (John).

Restlessness, (Zink).

Trembling of the limbs, (Zink and Matthey).

Tendency to convulsive motions, (Dessaignes).

Sleeplessness, (Coindet, Wallace).

Frequency of the pulse, (Zink).

Feverish excitement of the pulse, (Mérat and Delens).

Small, tense and concentrated pulse, (Zink).

Extreme heat on the skin, (Zink).

Pungent heat on the skin, (Trousseau and Pidoux).

Sweat, (Trousseau and Pidoux).

Various acute exanthems, erythema, urticaria, prurigo, acne, eczema, (Trousseau and Pidoux).

Fainting, loss of strength, emaciation, (Coindet).

Dwindling of the breasts, (Hufeland and others).

Headache, (Coindet, John).

Sort of intoxication, (Lugol).

Frontal headache, with stitches in the eyes and ears, and transitory dizziness, (Lugol).

Headache with vertigo, (Dessaignes and Montcourrier).

Cerebral congestion, (Lugol).

Pains in the whole length of the nose, as far as the forehead, (Wallace).

Trembling and oscillating motion in the eyes, (John).

Considerable discharge from the nostrils, (Wallace).

Violent coryza, with lachrymation and frontal headache. (Trousseau and Pidoux).

Flow of saliva, (Wallace).

Sticky mouth, (Zink).

Anorexia, (Wallace).

Abnormal increase of appetite, (Wallace, Coindet and others).

Looseness of the teeth, (Schmidt).

Constant desire to spit, (Carro).

Burning in the pharynx, with dryness and stiffness of the tongue, (Matthey).

Intense thirst, (Zink).

Burning from the pharynx to the epigastrium, (Dessaignes and Montcourrier).

Irritation of the throat and air-passages, (Joerg).

Saburral irritation in the primæ viæ, (Gendrin).

Nausea, (Dessaignes and Montcourrier).

Vomiting, (the same).

Vomiting of liquid and yellowish matters, (Orfila).

Burning heat and acute pain at the epigastrium, (Orfila).

Tearing pain at the stomach, (Dessaignes).

Unsuccessful straining to vomit, (Dessaignes).

Various derangements of the digestive canal, (Trousseau and Pidoux).

Violent colic, (Chevalier).

Constipation, (Wallace, etc.).

Constipation, with increase of appetite, (Wallace, Trousseau and Pidoux).

Diarrhœa, (Wallace).

Profuse diarrrhœa, (Wallace).

Increased urine, (Trousseau and Pidoux).

Violent and constant erections, (Zink).

Increase of the menses, (Guersant, Mérat and Delens).

Uterine hæmorrhage, (Schmidt, Bréra).

Uteritis, (Trousseau and Pidoux).

Miscarriage, (Magendie).

Sterility, (Zink).
Atrophy of the testes, (Mojsisovitz).
Dry and frequent cough, (Coindet).
Dyspnœa, (Coindet, etc.)
Blood-spitting, (Mojsisovitz).
Acute pleurisy, (Wallace).
Nervous phthisis, (John).
Palpitations, (Coindet, Zink, etc.).
Swelling of the legs, (Matthey).
Atrophy of the lymphatic ganglions, (Guersant)[1]

It is worthy of remark that allœopathic physicians have very often, and successfully, prescribed iodine for the very derangements which they describe in their works as the injurious effects of iodine to be avoided and guarded against in practice. Although *iodine* produces salivation, for instance, it is nevertheless recommended as one of the best remedies for *mercurial salivation*. It is capable of causing *emaciation*, according to universal testimony; nevertheless Doctor Lebert[2] affirms in his *Recherches sur les maladies scrofuleuses*, that he has cured with it *marasmus*. It causes *dyspnœa*, *cough*, *spitting of blood*, *nervous consumption*, and yet a number of practitioners assure us that they have employed it with success in these various affections. Such cures are not effected in accordance with allœopathic principles, and, it seems to me, ought to startle old-school physicians. But, thanks to Trousseau and Pidoux, the *method of substitution* explains these anomalies, and saves the credit of allœopathic wisdom.

Iodine, like spongia, appears to exercise a powerful action on the serous membranes. This, at least, seems to result from a multitude of cases of *ascites*, *serous articular tumors*, etc., that have been cured empirically with iodine. But does

[1] Hahnemann's pathogenesis of this drug is, in a great measure, composed of the poisonous effects of this drug, as observed by Kunliz, Gairdner, Richter, Perrot, Kolley, Græfe, Voigt, Massalien, Neumann, Henning, Jœrg, Formey, Schneider, Rust, Baup, Suttinger, Muhrbeck, Gœden, Rœchling, Vogel, Wolf and others.

[2] *Traité pratique des maladies scrofuleuses et tuberculeuses*, Paris, 1849, p. 97 and the following.

this prove the efficacy which Doctor Laffore, (of Agen,) ascribes to iodine against *tubercular meningitis*, seven cases of which he pretends to have cured with iodine? When invited to repeat his experiments at the Hospital of Children, in Paris, (*hôpital des Enfants*), Laffore failed to conquer this incurable malady. It is, therefore, more than probable that his assertions were based upon errors of diagnosis. But, although I look upon tubercular meningitis as a disease for which we do not possess, as yet, any remedy, I am, nevertheless, willing to admit that in some cases of hydrocephalus, whether of recent origin or of long standing, but not tuberculous, iodine may, like spongia, render eminent services. All this is, however, mere conjecture, for I am not aware that the curative virtues of iodine in this disease have ever been verified by experience.

Homœopathic applications.—According to Hahnemann, in Vol. II. of his Chronic Diseases, iodine is particularly indicated by the following symptoms:—

"Dizziness in the morning; beatings in the head; smarting in the eyes; buzzing in the ears; hardness of hearing; coated tongue; salivation; taste of soap in the mouth; sour eructations, with burning; *heart-burn*, after eating heavy food; *canine hunger;* nausea; *shifting of flatulence;* meteorism; constipation; wetting the bed; delay of the menses; cough; old morning-cough; difficulty of breathing; external swelling of the neck; lassitude of the arms in the morning, in bed; numbness of the fingers; distortion of bones; dryness of the skin; night-sweat." In this short list of symptoms, Hahnemann has evidently given us only the most important secondary symptoms of iodine, without mentioning the primary symptoms which are evidently exceedingly similar to those of ipecac.

I have tried iodine, but with very doubtful success, for the unpleasant consequences of weaning, on the supposition that the secretion of milk is diminished by iodine. The antidote of this agent is unknown to me.

Zincum.—See the group of which it is the type.

Chamomilla vulgaris.—See the group of which it is the type.

Ignatia amara, *St. Ignatius' bean.*—This is the seed of the *strychnos ignatii*, a climbing bush of the genus *strychnos*, which, like the *strychnos nux vomica*, grows on the Philippine Islands, and in India, where it goes by the name of *papreta.* It is known that the name of *St. Ignatius' bean*, was given to this seed, by Father Camelli, in honor of the founder of the order of the Jesuits. The fruit of the *strychnos Ignatii*, which is of the size of a small melon, or a large pear, is ovoïd, smooth, and contains from fifteen to twenty seeds, which are of an irregular shape, angular, hard, of the size of olives, of a pale-brown color, and striated on the outside, inodorous, but very bitter.

The action of this drug is less violent than that of nux vomica, but, nevertheless, very powerful, at least, on carnivorous animals, for from fifty to sixty centigrammes of the pulverised, that is to say, scraped bean suffice to kill a middle-sized dog in a few hours; the animal expires in convulsions.[1] In spite, however, of the nervous symptoms which this drug likewise causes in man, it seems to me, nevertheless, that, like ipecac., iodine, sponge, etc., it acts principally upon the stomach, throat, salivary glands, etc. Murray, who has inserted in his work, all the observations and clinical experiments, with *Ignatia*, known up to his time, expresses himself as follows: *Ignatia apud homines facile vomitum ciet alvumque movet;* imo exempla sunt *spasmorum et convulsionum, risus involuntarii, angustiæ pectoris, vertiginis, sudorum frigidorum inde et apud homines natorum, vel exteriori eorum natura, vel juste majori dosi.*[2] Professor Jœrg's, of Leipsic, observations go to strengthen Murray's opinions. "Eleven members of the society who had convened for the purpose of instituting such experiments, swallowed, at different periods, from nine to ninety drops of the tincture of

[1] Orfila, *toxicologie*, vol. II., 1st part, p. 328.

[2] *Apparat. Medic.*, vol. VI., p. 29.

Ignatia; four other persons took this drug in the form of a powder, from half a grain to four grains, ground together with equal parts of sugar of milk, and stirred in from one to two ounces of water. The action on the glands was evident, and the salivary secretion was at first increased; there was nausea, heaviness and pains at the stomach; afterwards colic, borborygmi, constipation and diarrhœa. These primary effects were followed by headache, vertigo, dull and heavy pains in the eyes, which became inflamed; lastly, prostration, a very marked drowsiness and general apathy set in. These secondary symptoms were sometimes succeeded by a marked acceleration of the pulse, considerable oppression, a sense of formication and smarting in the urethra."[1] It will be seen, that in these experiments of Professor Jœrg, although made with enormous doses, there were neither spasms nor tetanic stiffness. From his experiments, Jœrg drew the very logical conclusion, that the St. Ignatius' bean may prove useful in *weakness of the stomach and bowels, accompanied by chronic induration of the mesenteric glands,* and for *atony of the eyes* or *weakness of the eyes,* provided the patients are not too nervous. Jœrg, in order to be consistent in his deductions, ought to have said, that ignatia, which he had seen cause dyspnœa, formication and smarting in the urethra, must possess a certain amount of curative power in bronchial and urinary affections; but Jœrg's deductions were necessarily made at random, for the reason that he was not acquainted with the law of "*similia similibus.*"[2]

Empirical applications.—The inhabitants of India esteem the St. Ignatius' bean very highly, and use it for a multitude of diseases, particularly for *cholera morbus,* I know not with what success. In Europe, where it was introduced by Portuguese missionaries from the Philippine Islands, allœopathic physicians first used it in the diseases indicated by Jœrg, *in intermittent fevers,* that would not yield to cinchona, in

[1] *Bull. des sc. méd.* de Férussac, vol. XXV., p. 100.
[2] See the pathogenesis of Ignatia in Hahnemann's Mat. Med. Pur., vol. II.

neuralgia and *epilepsy*, brought on by violent emotions, such as fear, etc.; but at present it is almost abandoned.

Homœopathic applications.—According to Hahnemann, the principal difference between the action of *ignatia*, and that of *nux vomica*, consists in their different manner of affecting the mind. "Whatever analogy may seem to exist between the effects of ignatia and nux vomica, it will, nevertheless, be found that these two drugs are essentially different from each other, for the moral condition to which one is suitable, is essentially different from the moral condition to which the other seems to correspond. The St. Ignatius' bean does not by any means suit persons or affections characterized by anger, vehemence, a violent disposition; on the contrary, it is required, when sudden changes from mirth to tears, etc., prevail.[1] Ignatia is principally indicated by the following symptoms:—

Great *fitfulness of temper;* gaiety; sadness; quarrelsome mood; alternate paroxysms of boldness and *timidity;* sadness occasioned by chagrin, such as unhappy love; *fixed ideas;* spasmodic laughter; fainting fit; convulsions; tetanus; shuddering with thirst, *followed by heat without thirst;* partial chill, changing from one part of the body to another; spasmodic yawning; restless sleep, full of dreams, sometimes very light, at times very deep; moaning during sleep; *constant desire to change one's position in bed; painful sensitiveness to cool air;* aggravation of the symptoms by coffee, tobacco, alcoholic drinks. Itching of the skin, eased by scratching; sensation on the skin as if sweat would set in; urticaria; *sweat during rest, at night or in the morning;* sense of fulness in the head, with cloudiness; vertigo and staggering as if drunk; pressive headache at the root of the nose, at the forehead, and sometimes at the occiput, diminished by lying down, or less frequently on rising from a recumbent position; hemicrania, with nausea; digging, pulling, crampy headache, changing to facial or dental neuralgia; falling off of the hair; redness of the eyes, with dimness of sight; flow

[1] *Loc. Cit.*

of tears; swelling of the Meibomian glands; dilatation of the pupils; swelling of the upper lid; agglutination of the lids; heat and redness of the outer ear; swelling of the parotid glands; formication in the nostrils; nose-bleed; fluent, afterwards dry coryza; *sweat in the face;* pale face; redness of one cheek; *spasmodic twitching of the facial muscles;* contraction of the masseter muscles; chapped lips; small stinging ulcers on the inner surface of the lips; loose teeth; *swelling of the submaxillary glands;* dry mouth, or else constantly filled with a watery, acid or frothy saliva; smarting at the tip of the tongue; extreme sensitiveness of the inner mouth; stinging at the curtain; coated tongue; *redness and stinging in the throat,* ceasing sometimes during deglutition; *inflammation of the tonsils;* aversion to warm food, to meat, milk, and tobacco, although he was in the habit of smoking; flat, doughy taste in the mouth; bitter taste of drink and food; desire for or (less frequently) aversion to *fruit and acids;* loss of appetite, or else a good deal of appetite, which ceases as soon as one begins to eat; rising of food or of a bitter liquid; nausea; sickness at the stomach with anxiety, without one being able to vomit; vomiting of bile; desire to vomit, which sometimes ceases while eating; distress at the stomach caused by food; crampy stitches at the stomach; sensitiveness of the epigastric region to contact; at three in the morning vomiting of the food which one had eaten at supper; anxious fulness of the abdomen after eating; sense of burning, coldness, turning or pinching in the bowels; flatulent colic, especially at night; sensation in the lower abdomen as if a cathartic commenced to act; pressure on the anus and the left inguinal region, as if hernia would protrude: mucus or bloody diarrhœa; *frequent unsuccessful urging to stool; large-sized stool which it is difficult to get out,* sometimes of *a whitish color;* involuntary contractions of the anus, sometimes occurring periodically; stitches at the anus which extend high up in the rectum; dull pain in the rectum, as if distended by gas; itching swelling of the border of the anus; itching at the perinæum, especially when walking; pressure on the bladder; frequent emission of urine; profuse, watery urine; *scanty, dark-colored and acrid urine;* griping, drawing, pressive pains at the root of the penis, coming on in sudden shocks; painful pressure in the testicles; *sexual desire with impotence;* loss of sexual desire; sweat and swelling of the scrotum; expulsive, bearing-down pressure on the uterus, as in labor; premature menses; scanty discharge of black and badly-smelling blood during the menses; acrid and corrosive leucorrhœa.

Itching at the larynx causing a dry and frequent cough; *constrictive sensation (without tickling), and sometimes coming on quite suddenly, above the throat pit, and which compels one irresistibly to cough; constant hacking cough in the evening, in bed; dry and hollow cough, in the morning on waking;* cough which does not arrest the tickling that causes it; constriction of the chest; *dyspnœa at night;* asthma; difficult expectoration of a yellow mucus, smelling and tasting like old catarrhal mucus; want of breath during a walk, and cough as soon as one stands still; pressure at the sternum, after eating; stitches in the chest, especially on the left side; palpitation and stitches in the region of the heart; painful nodes at the neck; stiff neck; pulling pain or painful stitches in the shoulder-blades and back; contusive or pressive pain at the sacrum, in the morning, even when lying on the back; wrenching pain in the deltoid muscle; luxation pain in the shoulder-joint; intolerable *pains in the long bones and articulations of the side on which one had not lain; paralytic numbness of the extremities;* itching at the hands; *tepid sweat in the palms of the hands;* fetid sweat at the hands, in the evening; *spasms of the fingers;* luxation-pain in the hips; violent contusive pain at the posterior surface of the thigh; stiffness and cracking in the knees; heat at the knees; cramps in the calves; pulling at the insteps; *cold hands and feet, up to the knees; numbness of the feet, legs, and sometimes of the whole lower limbs;* stinging heat of the feet, which are sensitive to the pressure of the shoes; burning pain in the corns.

Although the *bean of St. Ignatius* is very seldom superior to *ipecac.* at the commencement of *metro-peritonitis*, nevertheless, it is a valuable auxiliary in some cases, of this kind, especially when uterine spasms are present, or convulsive symptoms become imminent. *Ignatius* deserves a place side by side with *chamomilla* in the spasmodic diseases of parturient females and new-born children. As regards its efficacy in genuine epilepsy, it is more than doubtful. "A first attack of epilepsy," says Hahnemann, "brought on by some disagreeable emotion, and which assumes a threatening aspect on account of the length of time it lasts, and the frequent recurrence of the paroxysms, is almost always, and generally permanently, cured by a single small dose of ignatia, as I can testify by my own experience. But in chronic epilepsy ignatia affords no permanent relief, no more than it is capable of doing any thing of the kind in other chronic diseases."[1] Hahnemann adds, that unless the delay should be dangerous, the morning is the best time to give ignatia, which he thinks produces too much restlessness, if it is taken at the moment of going to bed. In regard to nux vomica, Hahnemann recommends the opposite course, and directs that it be taken at night, before retiring.

The symptoms of *ignatia* manifest themselves more particularly in the morning and evening, but more particularly in the morning, like those of nux vomica, they are generally aggravated by contact, motion, the open air and artificial warmth.

Cham., *Puls.*, *Coff.*, etc., are said to antidote this drug.

Phosphorus. See page 285.

Filix mas, *Polypodium filix mas* of Linné, *male fern.*

The root of this plant, which was looked upon by Ætius as an agent endowed with a specific power to excite the genito-urinary apparatus, or even to produce miscarriage, is mostly employed as an *anthelmintic* by modern physicians. But a

[1] Mat. Med., vol. II., pathog. of Ignatia.

few provings and various clinical experiments induce me to think, that filix mas possesses far different properties besides its anthelmintic virtues. The manner in which it affects the stomach, throat, air-passages, is so very much like the mode of action of ipecac., that I have felt authorised to range it among the analogues of this latter drug. Filix mas has done me good service in a case of violent dyspnœa without cough, with stitches in the region of the heart and obscure symptoms of pericarditis. The patient was a young lady of a lymphatico-nervous temperament, and very much weakened by a long sickness. Her symptoms were: amenorrhœa, frequent attacks of fainting, a general coldness, paroxysms of clammy sweat in the face, anorexia, constipation, perceptible bloating of the præcordial region, which was painfully sensitive to the least contact; no palpitation, but dull, distant sounds of the heart, remarkably feeble and slow (from 50 to 52 beats a minute.) After having given several medicines without success, filix mas produced a rapid and marked improvement. Since then I have used it with the same success for an almost similar case. The patient was likewise a female, and visited my dispensary. I am now engaged in proving this drug, and shall publish my list of symptoms as soon as it is completed.

Antimonium crudum,—*crude antimony.* This drug is undoubtedly related to ipecac., but still more to Lycop., to whose group the reader is referred.

Tartarus emeticus,—*antimonial tartrate of potash, tartar emetic.* This salt is not found in nature, and was first prepared by Mynsicht, a chemist of Hamburgh, since which time it has acquired an extraordinary celebrity as a medicinal agent. It exists in commerce in the shape of small octoedral or tetraedral crystals, which, when exposed to the air, shoot out in the form of flowers, and thereby lose their transparency and part of their weight. They dissolve in fourteen parts of cold, and a much smaller quantity of boiling water. It is a poison that, though less violent than was supposed previous to the experiments instituted by Rasori, has nevertheless destroyed a number of lives. The extract of opium in large doses is its best antidote.

Empirical applications.—For the two centuries that tartar emetic has been employed as a drug, it has been prescribed for almost any disease. The following are the diseases which have been most successfully treated with this agent: *certain affections of the head, gastric derangements, bilious fevers, engorgements of abdominal viscera, ascites, metro-peritonitis, acute angina, croup,*[1] *whooping-cough, asthma, shifting rheumatism,* and lastly, and more particularly, *acute pneumonia, pleuro-pneumonia,* and acute articular rheumatism.[2]

Homœopathic applications.—Many of the symptoms in Stapf's pathogenesis of tartar emetic, which Jahr has republished in his Manual, are evidently strikingly similar to those of ipecac. Stibium has not yet, however, acquired in our practice that importance which allœopathic physicians, especially the partisans of Rasori, attribute to it. I have used it as yet very seldom. In the following cases I have prescribed it with more or less success: 1st, the case of a lady who was in the fifth month of pregnancy, of good constitution, with

[1] Kœhler, quoted by Gmelin, relates a case (see appar. med., vol. I., p. 211,) where the patient was unable to swallow, and where a cure was effected by injecting a solution of tartar-emetic into a vein.

[2] See Gmelin, *loc. cit.* and Giacomini's *traité* de mat. méd., p. 257, etc., the chapter entitled, on *Vascular-arterial hyposthenisants.* Although very remarkable in some respects, and very learned, yet this chapter is based upon a fundamental error. Tartar-emetic being one of the corner-stones of Rasori's system, Giacomini heaps facts upon facts to prove the *contra-stimulating* agency of this drug. Unfortunately the author does not succeed, in spite of the greatest efforts, in reconciling contradictory facts, some of which are taken from physiology, others from the domain of pathology. This, however, is a radical fault of Rasori's system. His partisans will not see the difference between the physiological and therapeutic action of drugs. Tartar-emetic depresses, moderates, *contra-stimulates* the pulse in pneumonia; this is proved by incontestable facts; but that tartar-emetic affects in the same manner the circulation of a man in good health, Giacomini makes vain efforts to prove; witness Magendie's experiments who saw the lungs of animals that had been poisoned with tartar-emetic, engorged with blood, as if hepatised; witness likewise Stapf's pathogenesis of this drug.

the following symptoms: febrile motion after every meal, with pungent heat in the face, dampness in the palms of the hands, anxiety during the paroxysms which lasted two or three hours, mouth slightly bitter, not much appetite, no thirst, constipation; 2d, after *bryonia* and *causticum*, in two or three cases of dyspepsia of long standing, in adults; 3d, in a case of articular rheumatism, the symptoms of which have escaped my memory.

According to Stapf, *Cocculus*, *Ipec.* and *Puls.* antidote the effects of small doses.

GROUP IX.

TYPE: BRYONIA ALBA.

ANALOGUES: ALLIUM SATIVUM. LYCOPODIUM CLAVATUM. DIGITALIS PURPUREA. NUX VOMICA. COLOCYNTHIS. IGNATIA AMARA.[1]

ALL the drugs, composing this group, act with much power upon carnivorous animals, whereas graminivorous or herbivorous animals are scarcely affected by them at all.[2] This is a fact full of meaning. I do not hesitate to infer from it that these drugs may safely be struck from the list of those that are required for the diseases of horses, ruminating animals and the gallinaceous tribes, and that they will have to be reserved for the diseases of carnivorous domestic animals. The fact which I have pointed out, is, however, as important to a physician as it is to a veterinary surgeon. The symptoms which Bryonia and its analogues generally produce, independently of those which are peculiar to each and respectively differ from those of any other co-members of its group, resemble such symptoms, as are caused by habitual or accidental overeating, or by the exclusive and excessive use of animal food, without excepting even the shades of difference arising from the constitutional idiosyncrasies of the patients. These drugs must, therefore, principally suit persons that are disposed to

[1] Hereafter *Indigo*, *Oleum animale* and *rhododendron chrysanthum*, will probably be added to the analogues of Bryonia.

[2] This remark applies, at any rate, to all those among these drugs that have been tried on animals. Garlick has not been regularly experimented with, that I know. It is exceedingly unpleasant to *cats* who eat it, even when boiled, with an extreme aversion. I should like to see lycopodium tried in the same way, although it is probable that this drug is less adapted than any of the other analogues of *Bryonia*, to the constitution and diseases of enormous meat-eaters.

commit excesses at table, have strong constitutions,[1] dark, rather than fair complexions, with firm flesh, although there may be here and there a disposition to obesity. Experience has, indeed, proved this. Here follows a list of the principal symptoms which all these drugs have in common:

Irritability; *disposition to get angry;* a sort of internal concentrated mania, in some cases; aversion to company; apathy; resignation, (secondary effects).

Rush of blood to the head, even to the point of causing one to faint, (at the commencement of the action); pulsative and distensive headache; cold or warm sweat on the forehead.

Heat in the face; partial swelling of the face; redness of the face; *yellow complexion;* pressive pullings in one side (generally the left) of the head, face, and even the neck.

Nose-bleed.

Painful swelling of the parotid glands, and of the other glands of the upper half of the body; blueish swelling of the lips.

White coated tongue; *flow of saliva* after every meal, especially after supper, sometimes even without having eaten anything; sticky and bitter mouth; *sensation as if a bitter liquid were constantly rising to the œsophagus and mouth, even though no nausea is felt.*

Sense of swelling, roughness or excoriation in the pharynx, with secretion of profuse viscous saliva.

Deficient appetite; *excessive aversion to animal food,* and sometimes to any kind of food; *loathing and nausea even at the sight of food,* (primary symptoms which may continue for weeks and months, and sometimes does continue this length of time in the case of digitalis.)

Sense of hunger without appetite; increase of appetite, (secondary effect).

Desire for cold water only; any kind of nourishing drink,

[1] Digitalis succeeds in *chronic cases,* when the patients are not of very strong constitutions; but before denying my statement, I ask the reader to trace the origin of the disease with which such patients, whether scrofulous or troubled with worms, are affected, and it will appear that they were *great eaters.*

like beer, (except, in some cases, cold milk,) excites a loathing and nausea.

Vomiting of the solid food, not of drinks, (cool water).

Bilious vomiting, (primary effect).

Pressure, cutting or stinging pains in the pit of the stomach, especially when moving about.

Tearing pains in the abdomen; sense of fulness and bearing-down in the hypogastrium; ascites.

Borborygmi; *painful distension of the abdomen by gas;* seated pains in the abdomen and as far as the ribs, here and there, (occasioned by incarceration of wind,) inguinal hernia; frequent emission of flatulence.

Cutting colic as after a cold, *with urging to stool, which is generally ineffectual;* painful and exhausting diarrhœa; diarrhœa with discharge of ascarides; *diarrhœa with tenesmus*, as in dysentery, (immediate effects, which, frequently, do not exist).

Constipation which is often obstinate and painful, (secondary effect,) but which seems most generally came on at once, and is a leading symptom of bryonia and its analogues on their action upon the alimentary canal.

Tenesmus of the bladder; scanty and burning urine, with frequent desire to urinate; retention of urine; (primary symptoms, which may, however, likewise succeed copious emissions of a clear and light-colored urine); *considerable increase of the urinary secretion, as in diabetes*, (secondary symptoms).

Coryza, which is rather dry than fluent.

Cough with mucous expectoration of more or less duration, but with tendency to become a dry cough; acute stitches in both sides of the chest; tightness at the base of the chest, as if the diaphragm could not descend during an inspiration; pulsative pain at the base of the right lung.

Stitches in the region of the heart; painful palpitations of the heart; serous effusions in the chest.

Pressive, distensive pains in the parts where the muscular system is most powerfully developed, such as the nape of the neck, back, the neighborhood of the moveable joints.

Pulsative pains here and there.

Hot swelling of the affected parts, (primary symptom,) and after a lapse of time, atrophy of the same parts, (secondary symptom).

Aggravation of the pains in the parts on which one had not been lying, with predominance of these pains, as a general rule, in the whole right side of the body.

Infiltration of the extremities.

Aggravation of the largest number of symptoms, by exercise, open air, or by entering a warm room, on coming out of the open air.

Febrile phenomena, which may present three distinct phases in succession, namely :—

1. Frequency of the pulse; increase of the general temperature, (these symptoms are generally very short-lasting when perceptible.)

2. *Slowness of the pulse, which is sometimes excessive; with or* (less frequently,) *without irregularity; whence arise shiverings, a considerable decrease of the temperature of the body, fainting fits, lipothymia*, etc. These symptoms, which, in spite of the preceding ones, seem to constitute primary effects of the drugs of this group, may last a long while, at least, so far as digitalis is concerned.

3. Lastly, a last period characterized by a pungent heat of the skin, great frequency of the pulse, atrophy, etc. Page 68, I have pointed out the relations existing between the drugs of the *Bryonia*, and those of the *Arnica group*.

CORRESPONDING DISEASES.

Headache, (occasioned by moral emotions or excesses at table.)—Acute and chronic gastritis.—Dysentery.—Typhoid fever.—Worms in the bowels.—Dropsy, (not encysted dropsy.) — Dysuria. — Diabetes. — Angina.—Pulmonary catarrh. — Pneumonia. — Pleurisy. — Carditis. — Pericarditis. — Aneurism of the aorta.—Pleurodynia.—Galactorrhœa.—Acute rheumatism.—Scrophula.—Œdema of the extremities, etc.

Bryonia alba, in common parlance in France, *navet du diable, bryony.*—Genus Bryonia, family cucurbitaceæ, class monœcia syngenesia. It is an herbaceous, climbing, perennial plant, a native of the north of Europe, and growing abundantly in the hedges of our eastern departments. According to some authors, it is the *ampelos leuke,* (*white vine,*) of Dioscorides. The stem of the bryonia is smooth and glabrous, and sometimes rises to from six to eight feet in height. Its leaves are large, palmate, with five lobes, the middle one of which is trifid; rough and callous on both sides, and accompanied by long axillary tendrils. The flowers, which are arranged in tufts, monœcious or diœcious, are supported by long pedicles. The berries which grow out of the blossoms, are rounded and black when ripe, and contain each, from four to six ovoïd seeds. The root, which is the only part that is used in medicine, is fusiform, white, fleshy, filled with a milky juice; when cut through, it exhibits concentric yellowish streaks, and bears sufficient resemblance to a thick turnip, to have given rise to very alarming mistakes. The peasants of Lorraine and Franche-Comté, who know this root under the name of *navet du diable* (devil's turnip,) use it fresh as a purgative, and, when dried in an oven and cut in pieces, as a *specific* remedy for *hernia.* This practice gives rise now and then to more or less unpleasant accidents. I have related one of some interest to homœopathic physicians, in the *Journal de la Sociétè gallic. de med. homœop.*[1]

The root of bryonia contains a large proportion of starch, and like the roots of manioca and arum, becomes eatable

[1] *Answer to a note of Dr. Peschier,* (Aug. number, 1851.)

after having been freed from its acrid principle, (*bryonine*,) to which it owes its poisonous properties.[1]

Empirical Applications.—The medicinal history of bryonia is very short. Murray scarcely devotes two pages to it in his *appar. medic.*, 1, Vol. I., p. 920. Modern authors scarcely know any thing else of it than the name, and even this is confounded by Trousseau and Pidoux with the *bryonia dioica*, which, is, however, totally distinct from the bryonia alba. Allœopathic physicians look upon it as a *drastic*, and as a substitute for colocynth, elaterium, etc. Nevertheless, bryonia, howsoever despised or neglected it may be by these physicians, has rendered good service to some of them. *Cataplasms containing the fresh root of this plant*, are known to have scattered *an inflammatory swelling of the joints, œdema of the legs*, etc., (van Helmont, Tissot, etc.) The ancients often employed it internally for *dropsy*, and more particularly for *hydrothorax*, where it must undoubtedly have effected more than one cure. Sydenham recommended it in *intermittent fevers*, accompanied with *mania*, and Arnaud de Villeneuve in *epilepsy*, for which he supposed it to be a specific; this hypothesis, however, was never received with much favor, and Murray (*loc. cit.*) attacks it very justly. Finally, towards the end of the last century, Dr. Harmand de Montgarny fancied that bryonia contained all the therapeutic properties of ipecac. and he proposed, for the benefit of the people in the country, to substitute it for ipecac. in all cases where the use of this exotic root was acknowledged to be proper. Harmand de Montgarny declared having frequently cured with bryonia *bilious fevers, vomiting, colic, diarrhœa* and *dysentery*.[2] This was homœopathic treatment. But, in spite of all these cures, *this emetic which cured vomiting, this drastic which stopped colic and diarrhœa*, was soon

[1] Galien (*de simpl.*, lib. XI.) was acquainted with the alimentary properties of bryonia.

[2] See *Nouv. traité des maladies dysentériques*, par Harmand de Montgarny. Verdun, in 4to., 1783.

forgotten again, until the genius of Hahnemann restored it to a place in the Materia Medica.[1]

Homœopathic Applications.—Dolæus, who practised towards the end of the 17th century, and who sometimes employed bryonia in *hydrothorax, saburral dysentery*, etc., offers the following striking remark about bryonia: "It is much more suitable for robust individuals than for weak persons."[2] There are exceptions to this rule, but, generally speaking, it has been confirmed by homœopathic experience.

When bryonia is indicated by the totality of the symptoms, it is particularly suitable to persons (of either sex, children, adults or old people,) accustomed to rich living, with rich blood, firm and resisting flesh. Like pulsatilla, silicea and lime, it may sometimes be adapted to plethora, but which is very different from that which requires the employment of medicines. The fleshy fibre, in other words the solid element, prevails over the adipose tissue in the constitutions to which bryonia is particularly adapted. I am sure that all experienced practitioners will agree with me in this respect.

The digestive canal, and more particularly the stomach, seem to constitute the principal seat of the action of Bryonia, which we have already named, on this account, among the analogues of *Ars.* and *Ipec.*, which will reappear hereafter among the analogues of *lycop.* and *Bellad.* The following morbid conditions are the principal indications for Bryonia:—

Irritability; disposition to uneasiness, fear, *anger;* deficient memory; disturbance of the mental faculties; so that one does not know any more what one is saying, doing, or where one is; syncope, with red face, sweat on the forehead, staring look and dilated pupils, preceded by bilious vomiting, (in certain forms of indigestion, especially among children, or at the commencement of typhus); *vertigo on rising from a chair, or while sitting up in bed; vertigo when standing* or walking, with disposition *to fall backwards* or sideways; headache on waking in the morning, as after an indigestion;

[1] See the pathogenesis of bryonia in Hahnemann's Mat. Med. Pur., vol. I.

[2] Dolæi *opera omnia*, Francfort, 1703, in fol. p. 280.

headache after every meal; heaviness of the head, which is sometimes enormous; pulsative headache at the occiput, at the forehead, *temples;* stitches from the forehead to the occiput; dull beatings in the right half of the brain; *distensive headache,* as if the skull were too narrow for the brain, especially *at the forehead;* ulcerative pains at the occiput, commencing at the nape of the neck, and extending to the shoulders, in the morning, while lying on the back; smarting gnawing at the hairy scalp; greasy hair, even without the head being sweaty; burning heat at the concha of the ear; *buzzing or ringing in the ears;* hæmorrhage from the ears; pressure, itching and redness in the eyes; swelling of the lids; agglutination of the lids; swelling of the left half of the nose; *nose-bleed; nose-bleed waking one at three in the morning; nose-bleed when rising in the morning;* yellow complexion of the face; *redness of the face;* tension of the face; swelling of one cheek; *pulling in the jaws, from above downwards or from below upwards;* red spots on the neck and in the face; *dry and cracked lips;* pulling, wrenching toothache, *increased* or *diminished by chewing,* but almost always *increased by the contact of warm drinks;* looseness of all the teeth; *bad breath,* (as of foul flesh or spoiled teeth); dry mouth and throat; *flow of saliva* after every meal, but more particularly *after supper and during the first part of the night;* flat, sweetish, sticky, nauseous taste in the mouth; bitter mouth in the morning or after eating; *coated tongue;* aversion to food; *a good deal of hunger, without appetite;* no thirst; *burning thirst,* (which is increased by drinking beer;[1]) loss of taste; roughness in the throat; sensation as if a foreign body had lodged in the throat, (owing to the swelling of the mucous membrane); difficult and painful deglutition; desire for wine and coffee; bitterness ascending from the stomach to the mouth, without nausea; *nausea in the morning;* nausea which is felt even as far as the chest, (in the œsophagus); hiccough after eating, or even with an empty

[1] The gastric derangement caused by bryonia, absolutely requires water as a *dissolvent.*

stomach; *eructations with rising of food*, and a foul taste in the throat; *bitter eructations* after every meal, and even at night; sour eructations; rising of food or bile, almost without straining, and without any violent contractions of the stomach; vomiting of the solid food, *not of the beverages; vomiting of a greenish substance*, generally in the morning, (at the commencement of the disease); *unpleasant consequences of an indigestion caused by meat, mush-room*, or other substantial aliments; scraping in the throat, and hacking cough after eating; heaviness at the stomach after every meal; painful pressure at the stomach, which soon after extends to the bladder and perinæum, becomes intolerable, and ceases entirely after sitting down; *cutting stitches at the stomach*, while walking, *making a wrong step*, or even, in some cases, on performing the least motion; swelling of the umbilicus and hypochondria; constrictive pain at the stomach and in the abdomen; frequent borborygmi; *painful stitches in the abdomen, here and there*, and which are felt as far as below the false ribs; unpleasant gurgling in the lower abdomen, as from some purgative; *cutting colic and horrible stomach-ache, not followed by stool as when dysentery is about setting in;* sudden ascites; colic after a cold; diarrhœic stools at night, or in the morning after rising; discharge of ascarides and lumbrici; *retention of stool;* sensation as of a foreign body in the bottom of the abdomen; *obstinate and painful constipation;*[1] piles; *nephritic colic; frequent urging to urinate, although there is but little urine in the bladder;* burning, and cutting colic in the lower abdomen, before, during and after the emission of urine; involuntary emission of a few drops of urine when coughing, walking, or after having done urinating as one supposes; *incontinence of urine; diabetes; red sediment in the urine;* itching and itching red spots at

[1] The bryonia-constipation is not merely a passive symptom, consisting solely in inertia of the bowels. It depends, on the contrary, upon a more or less marked antiperistaltic movement of the rectum: hence the pains and the ataxic phenomena that accompany it sometimes, as is the case, for example, in the period of constipation of low typhoid fevers, etc.

the vulva; swelling of one of the labia majora; premature menses; metrorrhagia.

Coryza, preceded by frontal headache; *hoarseness; angina*, with swelling of the cervical glands, during which the whole front portion of the neck, and even the whole neck, are sensitive to contact, and sometimes so painful that it is almost impossible to move the head or to eat even; a quantity of plastic mucus in the larynx and trachea, (see Croup, page 367); *acute bronchitis; hæmoptysis*, (vermilion-colored blood and discharged in large coagula); *pulmonary catarrh*, of several months' duration, not preceded by coryza, sometimes without headache, without any marked alteration of the appetite or pulse, which becomes a little quicker only during the paroxysm of oppression. The cough, which is excited by a tickling in the larynx, comes on in violent paroxysms which are always followed by a profuse expectoration of mucus that is either transparent or yellowish, tasteless or slightly saltish, and generally of a sufficient degree of consistence. The least trace of smoke in the room, tobacco smoke, (even among smokers,) laughter, walking, especially up a hill, and even the act of swallowing when eating any thing, are sufficient to excite these paroxysms, which come on more particularly about three in the morning, or between breakfast and dinner, especially in the open air, and lastly, and principally during or after a meal. *Rapid and spasmodic inspirations when coughing; nausea* and retching, caused by the cough; constrictive pain at the base of the chest, which oppresses the breathing; burning pain in the right side of the chest; *pulsative stitches at the base and in the right side of the chest; acute and frequent stitches under the shoulder-blades and pectoral muscles*, worse during the cough, and scarcely allowing one to breathe; pleurisy; *pleurodynia;* asthma; seated pain in the præcordial region; stitches in the region of the heart; *palpitations* on moving the body ever so little; painful swelling of the breasts in nursing females, after weaning the infant; *rheumatic swelling of the nape of the neck and of the sides of the neck*, worse when touching the part; spasms between the shoulders; *painful tension of the back and lumbar regions*, compelling one to walk crooked; luxation-pains in the shoulder-joints, wrist-joints, hip or tarsal-joints; *acute rheumatism, with heat, tension, and more or less marked swelling*, aggravated by the least contact, especially at one or the other shoulder, at the arm or elbow (commonly the right elbow); *sensation of extreme lassitude and general painful lameness and weariness*, with shuddering and coldness, especially towards evening, and even in bed; weakness of the lower limbs and particularly of the knees, which is so great that one is scarcely able to go up or down stairs; pain in the feet as after having made a wrong step; swelling of the feet; heat and sweat of the extremities, the remainder of the body being cold; fever, with chilliness prevailing; coldness of one side only (right side); painful pulsations here and there; yawning and drowsiness in the day-time; restlessness with dry heat on the skin, the first part of the night; constant desire to change one's position in the bed, or to uncover one's self, with coldness as soon as one is uncovered; startings when on the point of falling asleep; *loud dreaming during sleep;* miliary eruptions and dry tetters here and there over the body; pressure at every part of the body; heaviness all over; *plethora sanguinea;* emaciation.

The symptoms of bryonia are generally aggravated by motion, although the reverse may be the case. They are principally felt in the evening, at twilight, about three in the morning, and after rising from bed in the morning. Most of the pains increase in the open air, but some on passing out of the open air, and entering a warm room. Bryonia generally acts upon the right side first, and it is here that the pains it excites, are most violent. I have been led by a purely accidental discovery to look upon *Ferrum muriaticum*, which is as yet little known, as the best antidote of bryonia; since then, regular trials have confirmed me in my opinion.

Allium Sativum, *garlick*. A well known species of allium, family liliaceæ, class hexandria monogynia.

This native of Sicily, and which is cultivated in our gardens, is used very extensively for domestic purposes. It is a spice which, according to Mérat and Delens, *dict. univ. de mat. méd.*, vol. I., p. 189, "sharpens the appetite, stimulates the stomach, facilitates the digestion and expels flatulence," supposing, of course, that the appetite is failing, the digestion difficult, and that there is flatulence. The same authors admit that garlick is endowed with undeniable and pretty strong medicinal properties. According to them it is an excellent remedy for *phlegm*. Why should not garlick, when introduced into the alimentary canal, modify the functions of the organism, if it produces such a marked, and sometimes intense action when applied to the skin? Mérat and Delens admit that it does. "Pounded garlick has been applied to the skin, on account of its acrid properties *in paralytic or rheumatic diseases*, and in about two hours after its application, it draws a blister, like a mustard-plaster. A salve is also made of it, by pounding it together with oil or grease, a compound which is known by the name of *moutarde du diable*, (devil's mustard,) or *huile d'ail*, (oil of garlick); this last-named mixture is a powerful resolvent of *cold swellings*. It is said that it removes corns, cures *scaldhead*, the *itch*, etc., (this is a mistake); that it destroys the worms of children by applying it to the navel, (which is perfectly correct). "Mérat and Delens add, that these applications are not without danger; that beside the blisters they draw, they cause fever, etc.; in spite of which they call garlick a harmless spice.

But it is especially after reading Murray's important and well authenticated statements concerning the therapeutic properties of garlick, that it seems impossible to comprehend how it could ever have disappeared from the materia medica. Murray furnishes the following sketch of the empirical uses of this drug:

The *anthelmintic* and *febrifuge* properties of garlick were known even at the time of Plinius and Dioscorides, and have since been verified by a number of physicians of the highest rank. Rosenstein, Taube, and the English physician Bisset, have even expelled *tænia* with garlick. According to Laurembergius and Lind, garlick is not only a preventive of scurvy, but a real specific for this disease. Forestier, Barthole, and, after them, Sydenham, recommend it as an excellent *diuretic* in *dropsy*. Sydenham especially has seen incipient dropsy arrested by a few doses of this drug, which Duncan, and other physicians of that period praised as a remedy for *nephritic colic* and *vesical calculi*. In certain affections of the air-passages, garlick has been very useful. Celsus and Dioscorides recommended it in *old cough, accompanied by dyspnœa*, and a *profuse expectoration of ropy phlegm*. In accordance with this recommendation it was several times used with success by Mead, Rosenstein, and even Murray.[1] Rosenstein relates even that, by means of garlick, he succeeded in stopping *a chronic cough*, with general prostration and excessive emaciation. I am not astonished at this, for twelve years ago, before I was a homœopath, I cured three similar cases by giving twice a day a clove of garlick crushed in olive oil.

Homœopathic applications.—Allium is scarcely yet known to homœopathic physicians. Some months ago Petroz read a pathogenesis of garlick before the *Gallican Société*, which, although incomplete, bears nevertheless the stamp of the author's intuitive genius of observation. I insert it here together with the symptoms which I have obtained in my own experiments with this drug.

Pathogenesis of Allium Sativum. Anxiety of feeling; impatience; susceptibility; sadness when alone; vagueness of ideas; fear lest one should never get well; *fear lest one should not be able to bear any medicine;* fear of being poisoned; desire to escape;[2] general lassitude, but especially in the

[1] *Pituita in pectore collecta, si difficultatem spirandi vel tussim excitat, egregie ab allio resolvitur,* etc. (*App. Med.*, vol. V., p. 122.)

[2] Compare symptom 767 of Bryonia, in Hahnemann.

lower limbs, so that one dreads the fatigue of ascending a few steps only; lassitude, especially in the morning; catarrhal fever, with predominance of coldness; shiverings from day to day; shiverings sometimes on one side of the body;[1] coldness all over, with heat in the face; *horripilations before noon, and in the evening;* general heat, with malaise, *thirst*, tense pulse, stitches in the extremities; sweat after twelve o'clock in the day-time;[2] sweat with itching; sour sweat; fetid sweat; vomiting during the fever; drowsiness after eating; restless sleep, at night; *oppression of the chest* during sleep; *coldness during sleep*, which occasions frequent waking; thirst, at night, preventing sleep; twitching in the muscles, and shocks in the feet, at night, on falling asleep; stitches in the chest, or weight at the stomach, preventing sleep; dreams which continue after waking.[3] Flaccid skin; formication; excessive sensitiveness of the skin; *tension of the skin in the joints;*[4] dry skin; white spots which afterwards turn yellow, and are accompanied with a stinging itching; red spots on the back, hands,[5] *on the inner surface of the thighs, and at the genital organs;* pain in the glands.

Vertigo in steadily looking at a thing for a long time; short-lasting vertigo, and only on rising from a chair; *weight in the head; dull pain at the occiput, in the morning*, when lying on the back;[6] heaviness in the head, which ceases during the menses, and reappears afterwards; throbbing in the temples; heaviness at the forehead, which scarcely allows one to open one's eyes; buzzing in the ears; pressive transitory pullings, (before twelve o'clock in the day-time), in both jaws, and in the superior molares of the right side; stitches in one side of the face.

Hot taste in the mouth, coming from the throat, exactly like the taste of garlick, immediately after taking the drug; it continues the whole morning, and returns after the second

[1] Com. 707, id. id. [2] Compare with the bryonia fever.

[3] Compare with symptoms 671 and 679 of *Bryonia.*

[4] Characteristic symptom of *Bryonia.*

[5] Compare with the symptom 503 of *Bryonia.*

[6] See symptoms 32, 50, and 61, id.

breakfast so strongly that it causes a flow of saliva;[1] dryness of the lips and palate; *profuse flow of sweetish saliva in the mouth, before noon, after eating, more particularly after supper and at night;* swelling of the lower gums; sense of titillation at the lower teeth; sensation at night and in the evening, as of a hair on the tongue; the mouth-symptoms are aggravated by reading; eructations, (immediately); sensation as if something cold were rising to the throat; nausea and aversion to food, (an immediate and short-lasting symptom); sensation of violent hunger, faint feeling at the stomach, but no increase of appetite; *voracious appetite; burning eructations* after eating; eructations causing a profuse flow of saliva; straining to vomit with retraction of the abdomen; burning in the stomach which is not painful when not touched, but which is otherwise sensitive to the slightest pressure; stitches at the stomach; twisting and pinching around the navel; dull pain at the epigastric region, which is felt only on drawing a long breath, but which, finally, embarrasses the breathing;[2] borborygmi in the morning; incomplete emission of fetid flatulence, as if part of it were retained in the bowels; heaviness in the lower abdomen, immediately after eating, without urging to stool or pressure on the bladder;[3] (natural) stool, immediately after eating, (contrary to habit); several soft, but not diarrhœic stools, in twenty-four hours, for three days in succession; diarrhœa; involuntary stool; diarrhœic stool (after thirty hours) about three o'clock in the morning, preceded, accompanied and succeeded by cutting pains in the abdomen and loins; *constipation, with dull pain in the abdomen, which continues almost all the time*, for eight days, (particularly before noon); sensation in the bladder and urethra as if one had to void

[1] This symptom was so well marked that, on a certain day when I was proving alumina on myself, and had taken by mistake a few globules of the 6th dil. of garlick instead of alumina, *the simple taste of the drug* was sufficient to acquaint me with my mistake. I could not help discovering it, for the vial containing the allium had not yet been replaced in the chest.

[2] See symptoms 420 and 425 of Bryonia.

[3] See symptoms 312, 329 and 330, id.

urine, which is, however, not the case;[1] scanty and dark-colored urine; *profuse, whitish urine, which is rendered cloudy by the addition of nitric acid; sort of diabetes;* the menses come on five days sooner; during the menses, pimples at the vulva and extensive excoriations at the internal surface of the thighs, *spots of a bright-red color, and accompanied by itching and smarting, at the inner surface of the labia majora and the orifice of the vagina.*

Coryza, which is rather dry than fluent, with pressive pain above the root of the nose; increase of the nasal mucus, accompanied with a slight stuffing of both nostrils; discharge of blood from the nose, when blowing it, at night; accumulation of phlegm in the throat, in the morning, with heaviness of the head; insensibility of the anterior portion of the neck, when touching it; scraping in the larynx which excites a dry cough, without any other symptom; violent and sudden paroxysm of a dry cough while smoking, and which obliges him to stop smoking; dry cough after eating; cough which seems to proceed from the stomach;[2] deep cough; cough with fetid breath; cough with painful irritation in the windpipe; *difficult expectoration of a glutinous mucus; cough in the morning, after going out of his room, with profuse expectoration of mucus; almost continual rattling of mucus in the bronchia;* expectoration of a thin, yellowish, apparently purulent, blood-streaked and foul-smelling mucus; stitches in one side of the chest; stitches under the shoulder-blades and pectoral muscles, increased while coughing and drawing a long breath; this deep breathing becomes spasmodic when it is attempted several times in succession, and it obliges one irresistibly to cough; embarrassed respiration, as if the sternum were pressed upon. The chest-symptoms are worse in the open air, after eating, and when stooping. Jerking beating of the heart; red spots between the breasts and around the nipples; dull stitches in the right breast; swelling of the mammæ, which become sensitive to contact (in

[1] See symptoms 661, 666 and 667, id.

[2] See sympt. 398 of *Bryonia.*

twenty-four hours); pulling pains in the neck; itching between the shoulders; stitches in the back; red spots on the back, apparently like tetter;[1] tearing at the sacrum; incisive pain at the sacrum, in the morning; simple pain at the coccyx; painful sense of contraction in the arms; tension and heat at the right elbow, which is painful during the motion of the arm;[2] tearing pain in the fingers, which is felt as far as under the nails; heat, followed by moisture, in the hollow of the hands; tearing pain in the hip; intolerable pain in the united tendon of the iliac and psoas muscles; this pain is not felt much during rest, in the day-time, but is excited by the least motion; it becomes so violent on attempting to place the right over the left thigh, that it extorts a cry; but the pain is scarcely felt when the thigh is gently raised with the hands, and laid across the other thigh, instead of being carried forward by the muscles of the pelvis and thigh; the pain is not excessive during a walk, although it obliges one to limp; it becomes worse in bed, towards eleven o'clock in the evening, when it is impossible to change one's position and fall asleep.[3] Painful lameness in the thighs; boil on the thigh; weakness of the lower limbs; digging pain at the tibio-tarsal articulation (all these symptoms are aggravated by walking); feeling of stiffness in the feet; tearing pain in the feet; digging pain in the toe-joints;[4] formication in the feet; burning at the soles of the feet; these last symptoms are especially unpleasant during rest, especially if the foot is not supported by anything.

The pains caused by *allium* are mostly pressive pains from within outwards, (that is to say *distensive* like those of bryonia); stinging, or at the same time stinging and burn-

[1] See symptoms 490, 491 and 492 of *Bryonia*.

[2] See symptoms 605, 609, 610, and particularly 611, id.

[3] This symptom reminds one of symptom 168 of *Colocynth*, (in Hahnemann's Mat. Med. Pur.) which is as follows: "*Pain in the right thigh, as if the psoas-muscle were too short, only when walking; it ceased when standing still, but recommenced after resuming the walk.*" I have cured this symptom in one case, where Colocynth had no effect, and where *allium* effected a cure.

[4] See symptoms 574, 576, 581 and 589 of *Bryonia*.

ing, or stinging with paralytic weakness, or lastly, tearing and crampy, (the latter much less frequently); sometimes they increase gradually to a high degree, and decrease again in the same manner.

I do not exactly know under what circumstances garlick has been successfully used by Petroz. My own experience with garlick is limited to the following affections: 1st, certain forms of *dyspepsia of long standing*, in old, fleshy persons, whose bowels were deranged by the slightest deviation from the regular diet; they complained of a flow of saliva after eating, of eructations and other gastric symptoms characteristic of garlick, and likewise of great weakness in the lower limbs, and particularly the knees; 2d, *erythematous angina*, not preceded by coryza, occasioned by a cold or by excesses at table, and consisting as yet only of a sticky feeling in the throat, with dryness, tickling, heat and a sense of rawness at the larynx, roughness of voice, hollow, dry and not very frequent cough, dry heat on the back of the hands, and slight moisture in the palms, all of which symptoms generally come on in the evening; 3d, *chronic bronchial catarrh, with profuse mucous expectoration*, without any very acute pains in the chest, (especially in fat individuals); 4th, several cases of *periodical asthma*, (in company with *Capsicum*, *bryonia* and various other drugs); 5th, a case of *permanent dyspnœa* of very long standing, and which was attributed, by mistake, I suppose, to emphysema of the lungs or mediastinum; 6th, three or four cases of *rheumatism of the hip*, (once after *Coloc.*, and in the other cases without any other drug); 7th, *swelling of the breasts*, after weaning the child, (together with *alumina*); 8th, *diabetes mellitus*, which it does not cure entirely, but diminishes to such a degree that I cannot refrain from strongly recommending this drug for this distressing affection.

As a general rule, when indicated, garlick suits persons of either sex who are used to good living, *eat a good deal more than they drink*, or are inclined rather to gourmandizing than gluttony; at any rate, such conditions seemed to prevail in every case where garlick had good results.

Numerous experiments have shown me that Lycopodium is one of the best antidotes of allium.

Nux Vomica, see page 227.

Lycopodium Clavatum. See the group of which this drug is the type.

Colocynthis, see page 234.

Digitalis Purpurea, *foxglove.* A bisannual, native plant of the genus *digitalis*, family *scrofulariæ*, class didynamia angiospermia. This pretty plant which is frequently cultivated in our gardens, on account of its beautiful, purple-colored, bell-shaped flowers which are disposed in long clusters, grows spontaneously, and in great abundance, on dry hills, in sandy woods, along roads, etc. Although it is quite common in Greece and Italy, yet it is not at all sure that the ancients ever used it in medicine. Some authors fancy that it is the plant to which Dioscorides gives the name *baccharis*, and the juice of which was used in the preparation of the *baccharion*, a salve prescribed by Hippocrates.[1] The blossoms and leaves of Digitalis are inodorous until they are crushed. Then they exhale an unpleasant, nauseous odor, of little duration however; they have a bitter and slightly acrid taste.

Every part of this plant is essentially poisonous. But like nux vomica, bryonia and other drugs, it affects carnivorous animals much more violently than graminivorous. Pigeons and hens have swallowed *whole pounds* of the tincture of Digitalis, without being destroyed by the poison,[2] whereas dogs were killed by small quantities. These animals, says Giacomini,[3] after having taken the poison, became sad, lost their spirits; most of them lost also their appetite; some, on the contrary, were tormented by a sort of voraciousness. The excrements were fluid and profuse; the animals sought to be alone; when compelled to walk, they staggered; some experienced slight convulsions, and died in a state of

[1] See Dioscorides, Mat. Med., cap. 51, lib. III.

[2] Giacomini, *Trait. phil. de mat. méd.*, p. 609.

[3] Id. id.

marasmus after a shorter or longer interval, according to the dose that had been taken."

As regards the physiological action of *digitalis*, it is described by some allœopathic authorities in a very general and, therefore, unsatisfactory manner; their knowledge of the therapeutic properties of the drug is derived exclusively from observation at the sick bed.

According to Murray, or rather, according to Boerhaave, Schiemann and Withering, whose opinions Murray records in his *apparatus*, digitalis, if taken uncautiously, and in too large doses, excoriates the mouth, throat, œsophagus and stomach; occasions nausea, vomiting, looseness of the bowels, vertigo, a mist before the eyes, which imparts to objects a particular (greenish) color; flow of saliva, considerable increase of the urinary secretion, cold sweat, lipothymia, great anxiety, cardialgia, hiccough, convulsions, slowness of the pulse, even down to 30 beats in the minute; and, in some cases, even death.[1] This picture is drawn with tolerable correctness.

"Digitalis," say Mérat and Delens, "causes nausea, vertigo, malaise, *sadness*,[2] a flow of saliva, vomiting, looseness of the bowels, acceleration of the pulse, etc. After these phenomena, another more remarkable phenomenon shows itself, which Cullen has been the first to point out, and which con sists in a slowness of the pulse. Sometimes the nervous system is likewise affected, and not seldom do we see drowsiness, delirium, optical illusions, blindness, etc."[3] The same authors state (but incorrectly) that digitalis always produces a flow of urine, and sometimes sweat.

Cullen, who is quoted by Mérat and Delens, was one of the first who pointed out the slowness and irregularity of the pulse caused by digitalis, which he termed, very improperly, the *opium of the heart*.[4] But, what Cullen did not notice, and what was afterwards proven by Sanders, Jœrg and

[1] *Apparat. Medic.*, vol. I., p. 493.

[2] This symptom has been observed even on animals, by the observers of every school.

[3] *Dict. univ. de mat. med.*, vol. II., p. 690.

[4] *Mat. Méd.*, vol. VI., p. 179.

Maclean, was this, that the slowness of the pulse is generally a secondary effect of the drug, and that, at the commencement of its action, digitalis produces almost constantly an opposite phenomenon, namely, a marked increase of the frequency and intensity of the beats of the heart. Saunders in particular, insists strongly on this point. "Two thousand experiments which I have either performed myself, or at which I have been present, have all produced this result, namely, quickness and strength of the pulse (during the first twenty-nine hours)."[1] This author tells us that he has seen the pulse rise, under these circumstances, to 70, 90, 100, 110, 120, and even more beats in the minute, "so that an inflammatory fever, according to his own statement, becomes imminent, and would undoubtedly develop itself, if the physician were unable to arrest the action of the poison."

Rasori, Tommasini, Fanzago, etc., who make of the digitalis their principal cardiac depressor (*hyposthenisans cardiacus*) take no notice whatever of Saunders' statements. According to them, digitalis is exclusively and essentially suitable to hypersthenic diseases of the vascular apparatus, and, this principle being once established, all their efforts were directed towards proving that *tuberculous phthisis*,[2]

[1] *Essay on digitalis purpurea*, by Doctor Saunders, President of the Medical Society of Edinburgh. It has to be remarked that these pretended experiments of Saunders, except one which he made on himself, are *clinical observations*. Saunders gave digitalis in small doses, and this is the reason why the pulse rose from the first, which is in reality, contrary to Saunders' opinion, a *secondary* effect of digitalis. Indeed, as soon as these small doses had been multiplied sufficiently to intoxicate the organism, the *primary* effect, that is to say, the slowness of the pulse, speedily became manifest. If given in high doses, digitalis almost always produces a quick pulse from the commencement.

[2] It is indeed proven that digitalis has even cured tuberculous phthisis, or has arrested for a certain period, say for three years, this disease which is generally set down as incurable. I confess that I am still in doubt about this. I am willing to admit, however, that the affections which have been described by Drake, Mossman, MacLean, Magennis, etc., as tubercular phthisis, and which were cured with digitalis, bear all the characteristics of this malady. On the other hand, chronic catarrh of the bronchia, with expectoration of pus, has been so often confounded with phthisis, (espe-

dropsy, *scrofula* and other affections in which the foxglove has been found efficacious, were in fact *hypersthenix*, or, to use their own expression, *subacute arterial inflammations.* This shows that Rasori's and Broussais' pathological principles rest upon the same basis. It is true, however, that the numerous essays on digitalis which have been published during the last forty years in Italy, contain some very correct appreciations of the physiological effects of this drug, but always too general to be interesting.[1] According to the partisans of Rasori, the effects of digitalis on the healthy organism are: a general lassitude, paleness of the face, sadness, tendency to falling asleep, and to incoherent dreams disturbing the sleep, vertigo, dilatation of the pupils, obscuration of sight, optical illusions, an apparently yellow or green coloring of all things, flow of saliva, a feeling of emptiness at the stomach, (especially if the drug is taken in small doses,) vomiting and diarrhœa, a dark color and cloudiness of the urine, increase of the urinary and all other secretions, an intense coldness over the whole body, or only of one limb or of the vertebral column, fainting fits, paralysis, and lastly, and above all, a retarded circulation, etc.[2]

cially previous to the new method of diagnosing these diseases by auscultation and percussion,) that the authority of these authors, in this matter at least, does not seem to be a sufficient guaranty. When speaking of lycopodium, the doubts which I here express with reference to digitalis, will be again brought forward.

[1] The same remark applies to the recent works on digitalis published by the physicians of the *Ecole de Paris*, and particularly to two memoirs of Messrs. Homolle and Quevenne on *digitaline*, concerning which memoirs two long reports have been made in the Academy of Medicine, which are of very little interest to homœopathic physicians. In reviewing the opinions of his predecessors, Professor Bouillaud, the author of these reports, seems to be shocked at Saunders' statement, that digitalis is possessed of the two opposite properties, of accelerating and moderating the pulse. Now, if Bouillaud were better acquainted with the therapeutic properties of the drugs he uses, (it must be said, however, that he uses very few,) Saunders' observation would not astonish him, for it is based upon a general fact which invariably characterises the physiological action of every drug. See, for these two reports, the *bullet. de l'Académie de méd.*, vol. XV., p. 332, and vol. XVI., p. 383 and foll.

[2] See Fanzago's memoir: *Sulle virtû della digit. med.*, in 8vo., Padova, 1810,

Empirical applications.—Bayle, whose very praiseworthy bibliographical researches I have had occasion to mention more than once, has collected,[1] partly synoptically and partly literally, all the clinical observations concerning digitalis, which had been published in France as well as in other countries, from the period when digitalis was first admitted into the London pharmacopœia, namely, from 1722 to 1835.[2] We cannot even afford room for a simple analysis of this compilation, which comprises no less than 476 facts of a more or less detailed description. The following list is a résumé of these cases:

Diseases treated with Digitalis.	Cured.	Improved.	Not cured.	Total.
Pulmonary phthisis,	83	35	33	155
Dropsies,	65	15	11	92
Dropsies without the results being mentioned,	...	...	...	163
Scrofula,	9	2	...	11
Mental derangement,	3	1	5	9
Headache,	1	...	...	1
Continuous petechial fever,	1	...	...	1
Eruption, not characterised,	...	...	...	1
Pulmonary affection, vaguely described,	...	...	...	1
Chlorosis,	1	...	...	1
Pneumonia,	3	...	1	4
Pleurisy,	2	...	2	4
Whooping-cough,	...	...	...	1
Hæmorrhage,	...	...	...	2
Ulcerated tetter,	...	1	...	1
Pulmonary emphysema,	...	...	3	3
Aneurism of the aorta,	5	4	7	16
Papuliform itch,	1	...	...	1
Strangulated hernia,	1	...	...	1
Bronchitis,	1	...	1	2
Epilepsy,	1	1	...	2
Cerebral congestion,	...	...	1	1
Chronic rheumatism,	...	...	1	1
Chronic gastritis,	...	...	1	1
Asthma,	...	...	1	1
Total,	177	59	64	476

and also a memoir by Rasori, entitled: *della operazione della digit. sul corpo vivo*, in 8vo., Milano, 1811.

[1] *Bibliot. de Thérap.*, vol. III.

[2] Digit. was struck from the list of medicines in the London Pharmacop. of 1746, and was not definitively restored again until the year 1788. At that time there prevailed the same doubts and apprehensions concerning digitalis that exist among allœopaths now-a-days concerning arsenic.

This list shows that the diseases for which digitalis has been used with the greatest efficacy, are *pulmonary phthisis, dropsies, scrofula* and *aneurisms of the aorta.* But we ought not to take the number of the cases reported in this list for an indication of the true proportion of either the cures or failures attributable to this drug in these various diseases. We know but too well that most authors have the deplorable habit of hiding their failures, and only publishing their cures. It is absurd to suppose that digitalis has cured 83 cases of pulmonary phthisis out of 155, 65 cases of dropsy out of 92, 9 cases of scrofula out of 11, etc. All that can be admitted, is that digitalis has actually succeeded in curing some cases of phthisis, dropsy, scrofula, aneurism. This, at least, seems to me to be incontestably true, after reading Bayle's cases. Now, if we consider that, in all these cases *frequency of the pulse* was a constant symptom, we are obliged to admit that Hahnemann has gone too far when he says that digitalis could not, in any case, be successfully opposed to this symptom, inasmuch as, "a few days after having rendered the pulse slower (primary effect) it renders it permanently quicker and smaller (secondary effect)." This statement is contained in a note to digitalis, in the second volume of the Chronic Diseases. But if this doctrine were true, we must never combat constipation with arsenic, neuralgia with coffee, etc., etc.; for constipation is only a *secondary* effect of arsenic, and neuralgia, according to Hahnemann's own doctrine in his memoir on coffee, is only a *secondary effect* of coffee. The suggestions which I have offered in the *introduction* to this work (see page 49,) explain how digitalis, as well as any other drug, if used empirically, may have been homœopathic to diseases of apparently antagonistic symptoms.[1]

[1] Excessive frequency of the pulse is mentioned as a permanent symptom in all cases of phthisis that have been cured with digitalis. G. L. Bayle, uncle of A. L. T. Bayle, author of the *bibliothéque de thérapeutique,* makes the same remark in his *researches on pulmonary phthisis,* Paris, 1810, in 8vo. This extreme frequency of the pulse is indeed one of the *secondary* effects of digitalis, as it was, in all probability, a secondary symptom in all cases

Homœopathic applications. Digitalis is principally indicated in the diseases that are characterized by one or more of the following affections.

Anxious and concentrated sadness, with *sleeplessness at night*, owing to pains at the heart, for instance, *an unhappy love*, especially in women of brown complexions, firm and obstinate dispositions;[1] deficient memory, and difficulty of thinking on a subject; excessive taste for being alone; a sort of taciturn mania; vertigo on rising from one's chair, or in a recumbent posture; pressive headache from one temple to the other, or to the forehead; tearing stitches, sometimes at the vertex, sometimes in one or both temples, most frequently in the left; *pullings in the left side of the head and face, extending even to the side of the neck;* painful throbbing at the bottom of the orbits; ophthalmia; dilatation or contraction of the pupils; *weakness of sight;* objects seem paler than they really are, and have a greenish look; *nose-bleed; bloating and paleness of the face;* partial swelling of the face (for instance of the lower eyelids, or of one cheek;) *blueish swelling of the lips;* the tongue is coated white in the morning; *profuse flow of a frothy saliva* which oblige one to spit all the time; foul taste in the mouth; stitch or smarting pain in the throat, with sense of swelling in the pharynx, or at the root of the tongue; deficient appetite; *anorexia, to such a degree that even the mere sight or smell of food excites violent nausea, with clean tongue, thirst for water and absence of all fever, a condition which has been known to last for months;* increase of appetite; *constant tendency to nausea, without any real nausea;* yawning, hiccough, drowsiness, heaviness at the stomach, sour or tasteless regurgitations after eating; heart-burn, in the afternoon or evening; mucous or bilious vomiting, especially at night or in the morning; constrictive pain mingled with stitches, in the pit of the stomach, aggravated sometimes (when one happens to

where Bayle had seen the foxglove effect a cure. See the pathogenesis of Digitalis in Hahnemann's Chronic Diseases, Vol. II.

[1] In such a case *Digitalis* is by far preferable to *Ignatia*.

be standing, not when sitting) even by a slight pressure on the epigastrium; *dull, continuous stitches in the hypochondria,* with sense of numbness in the surrounding parts; tearings in the abdomen, sometimes followed by a diarrhœic stool, afterwards tenesmus; *tension of the abdomen; ascites;* several soft stools in twenty-four hours; *paiuful and exhausting diarrhœa, with coldness* all over and tenesmus; involuntary stools; quantity of *ascarides* in the stool, (primary symptom); painful borborygmi; *constipation which is sometimes so obstinate that it lasts for several weeks* (secondary symptom); dull pressure on the bladder; *painful and frequent emissions of a small quantity of burning urine, of a dark color and cloudy; complete retention of urine; frequent and profuse emission of a whitish or clear urine,* (a symptom which generally succeeds the former); diabetes; inflammation of the neck of the bladder; sexual excitement; frequent emissions; contusive pain in the testicles (especially the right); *hydrocele;* œdema of the scrotum.

Coryza which is at first dry, afterwards fluent; *fluent coryza only in the day-time, with stuffing of the nose in the evening and at night;* frequent hoarseness; constant secretion of mucus in the larynx and wind-pipe; dry cough after a meal; short and dry cough excited by a tickling in the larynx; obstinate cough with profuse mucous expectoration; *blood-spitting;* difficult, slow, deep breathing; *short, hurried breathing,* (secondary symptom); tensive pain on both sides of the chest; acute stitches in the chest, especially at the base of the right lung; *pleurisy; phthisis* (with frequency of pulse, and excessively irritable disposition); *palpitation of the heart; slowness of the beats of the heart, which is extraordinary in some cases, with lipothymia, cold sweat on the forehead, anorexia;* coldness all over; complete loss of strength, (primary symptom); irregular and intermittent beating of the heart; *frightful stitches in the region of the heart, coming on every fifteen minutes, lasting only five or six seconds each time, with regular pulse, normal temperature, excessive anorexia, com-*

plete retention of stool, and dysuria;[1] *extreme frequency of the pulse, with stinging heat of the skin,* (secondary symptom); general lassitudes but particularly of the lower limbs; incised or tensive pain at the nape of the neck, compelling one to carry the head backwards; rheumatism, with pressive and tearing pain in the shoulder blades, shoulders and arms, (especially of the right side); dull stitches in the shoulder blades; pulling or laming pain in the lumbar region; sometimes alleviated by applying the hand to the part, but aggravated by motion, such as rising from one's chair; paralytic numbness of the left arm; itching and miliary eruption on the back of the hands; *dry, arid heat of the skin* (secondary symptom); tension of the skin of the extremities in the joints; engorgement of the glands, (particularly of the parotid and cervical glands); *œdema of the feet, legs* and (less frequently) of the hands; emaciation bordering on marasmus.

The primary symptoms of digitalis may last a long while; the secondary symptoms ought, of course, to last so much longer; digitalis seems, therefore, to be most suitable for chronic affections.

Opium, I think, is the most certain antidote of the dynamised drug.

Ignatia amara, see page 378.

[1] These symptoms were observed on a sick lady, whose case I have published in the Journ. de la Soc. gallic. de méd. homœop., vol. II., p. 15 and foll.

GROUP X.

TYPE: DULCAMARA.
ANALOGUES: SULPHUR.
CORALLIA RUBRA.
BRYONIA ALBA.
CALCAREA CARBONICA.
CHELIDONIUM MAJUS.
PULSATILLA.
SILICEA.

COMMON CHARACTERISTICS.

Fever with coldness; shiverings in the back; horripilations towards evening or at night, similar to those caused by the suppression of sweat in cold and damp weather.

Coldness, followed by dry heat of the skin; lastly, profuse sweat; red spots or small phlyctænæ surrounded by red areolæ; red, moist tetters.

Congestion of blood to the head; distensive headache, with buzzing in the ears; tendency to delirium and hallucinations; difficulty of speech, as if the tongue were paralyzed.

Coated tongue; flow of saliva; bellyache as after a cold.

Catarrhal affections, similar to those which are caused by a cold.

Engorgement of the lymphatic glands; rheumatic pains at the nape of the neck, shoulders, back, and in the extremities, with dryness of the skin.

These symptoms belong to dulcamara more particularly than to any other drug; it affects man precisely in the same manner as *damp and cold weather;* but there is no doubt that the drugs which I have assigned to it as its analogues, may, in some cases, and with certain temperaments, produce the same effects.

All the analogues of dulcamara, except *chelid. majus*, having already been mentioned and fully described, we have only to speak here of *dulcamara.*

CORRESPONDING DISEASES.

Catarrhal and rheumatic fever.—Diarrhœa.—Catarrh of the bladder.—Fluent coryza.—Angina.—Acute and chronic bronchitis.—Humid asthma.—Scrofula.—Rheumatism.—Humid tetters, etc.

Dulcamara, or rather *solanum dulcamara*, *bitter-sweet*, etc. Bush of the genus *solanum*, family solaneæ, class pentandria monogynia.

The bitter-sweet which is believed to be the *ampelos agria* or wild vine of Dioscorides, is a perennial plant, with branchy and pendulous stems, ligneous at their base, but, except this, herbaceous throughout the remainder of their growth, and generally provided with two kinds of leaves, some of which are oval, cordiform, entire, and others trilobate or lance-shaped, and sometimes at the extremity of the branches, fringed or jagged; with flowers in clusters, of a beautiful violet, giving place, towards the end of the summer, to oblong, fleshy berries, with two or three compartments, and being green at first, afterwards turning yellow, and lastly, when ripe, red and transparent like currants. Dioscorides, and Matthiolus, his commentator, state that these berries are eatable;[1] the truth is, they are insipid or slightly acid, and not very palatable. But are they poisonous, as some botanists pretend? Bye and bye we shall have an opportunity of referring to this point.

Bitter-sweet, which is cultivated in some gardens for ornamental purposes, and for the purpose of arranging it into bowers, grows spontaneously almost all over Europe. It is, especially, found among hedges, along the borders of *damp* woods, in the neighbourhood of dwellings, fields and méadows, principally in clayey and fertile soil.[2] The roots, stems and fresh branches of this plant spread, especially when rubbed between the fingers, a nauseous odor, which at first, somewhat resembles the odor of cat's urine, and afterwards becomes like that of the green substance of most other barks. Its leaves sometimes exhale an odor of musk, similar to that of the *gera-*

[1] *Mat. Med.*, lib. IV., cap. 175. [2] Guersant, *dict. des sc. méd.*, vol. X., p. 161.

nium moschatum; but when dried, all these various parts of the plant, are almost all of them inodorous. Finally, the ligneous portion of the stems, especially of the dry ones, has at first, when chewed, a bitter taste, which afterwards becomes sweetish, or like the taste of honey or liquorice, from which property the plant has derived its name.

A chemist of Besançon, Desforses, has been the first to extract from the bitter-sweet an alkaloid similar to that of delphine, to which he has given the name *solanine.* It is a white, amorphous, opaque powder, sometimes having the lustre of mother-of-pearl, inodorous, slightly bitter and nauseous, and leaves a harsh impression in the throat; it fuses at 100°, and is decomposed at a higher temperature; is scarcely soluble in water and fixed oils, but very soluble in alcohol; with acids it forms bitter salts, which do not crystallize, and are of a gum-like appearance.[1] This alkaloid cannot be considered as the only medicinal constituent of dulcamara. Since the experiments of Desforses, this alkaloid has been discovered in belladonna, Solanum ferox, and in various other solaneæ, whose medicinal properties are doubtless very different from those of our drug. It is more than probable, that solanine produces a small number of phenomena which are common to all poisonous solaneæ.

Bitter-sweet has been tried on animals with contradictory results, from which it is, therefore, impossible to draw any conclusions. A physician of the last century, Floyer, stated[2] that a dog who had been made to swallow thirty berries of bitter-sweet, died in three hours. Haller, Linné, Bergius, Murray, and all other authors of Materia Medica, relate this fact as an unequivocal proof of the deleterious action of the berries of dulcamara. Since then, Floyer's experiment has been repeated several times by Duval, not only on dogs, but upon a cock, without these animals being incommoded in the

[1] *Journal de Pharm.*, Paris, 1820, vol. VI., p. 374; vol. VII., p. 414.

[2] *Pharmacologie*, London, 1687, p. 86.

[3] *Hist. méd. et économ. des Solanum*, etc., Montpelier, 1813, in 4to., pages 70, 73 and 99.

least.[1] It is, therefore, probable that Floyer's experiment implies a mistake. This is the rather probable that the poisonous principle of *solanum dulcamara* seems exclusively concentrated in the bark of its ligneous branches. At any rate, this part of the plant is the only one, which, when chewed, has the bitter taste which I mentioned before, and which is discovered in solanine. Solanine, which was first experimented with by Desforses, and afterwards by Magendie, is said to have vomited dogs and cats, when given in doses of from eight to ten centigrammes, and, after the vomiting, to have produced a more or less prolonged coma. Nevertheless, the action of solanine and that of dulcamara, must not be confounded. According to Giacomini, "it is admitted after the experiments of Bruschi, that an extract of the leaves of bitter-sweet, causes symptoms of poisoning in animals."[1] But *what* symptoms of poisoning, and in *what animals?* This is not stated by Giacomini, and I am not able to say, not having as yet been able to procure Bruschi's work.[2]

The poisonous effects of bitter-sweet on man, although never fatal, or very violent, cannot be denied. This results clearly from the statements of Linné,[3] de Haën, Schlegel, and more particularly from those of J. B. Carrère, from whom Hahnemann has taken many of his symptoms in the pathogenesis of dulcamara.[4]

[1] *Traité philos. et expérim.* de mat. méd., etc., p. 301.

[2] *Instit. de mat. med.* It is conceivable that I should attach some importance to Bruschi's experiments, and whether they were made on dogs or cats. From the physiological action of dulcamara on men, and still more from the constitution of those who were most easily cured by bitter-sweet, I infer that it equally affects carnivorous and herbivorous animals, but with particular violence to the latter; this seems likewise to be true with regard to sulphur, the principal analogue of Dulcamara.

[3] *Dissert. de dulcam.*, etc., Upsal, 1771, in 8vo.

[4] *Traité des propriétés, usages et effects de la douce-amère*, ou *Solanum scandens*, *dans le traitement de plusieurs maladies, et surtout des maladies dartreuses*, in 8vo., Paris, 1781, by Jos. Barthél. Franc. Carrère. This interesting monograph was first published in 1780 under another title, (*mémoire sur la douce-amère*, etc.) and reprinted twice since, (in 1789, and in the year VII.,) translated into German by Molinie, with a preface, notes and additions by J. C.

Empirical applications.—Like most other drugs, dulcamara was first employed externally only. Its leaves, which had the reputation of being possessed of calming, dissolvent, and detergent properties, were applied locally to the head in cases of headache, to tumors in the breasts, to inflamed and erysipelatous surfaces, to hæmorrhoidal tumors, atonic ulcers, etc. The internal use of this plant does not seem to be traceable further back than Bœrhaave. At any rate, it was spread by him and his school. Bœrhaave recommends bitter-sweet for *pneumonia, pleurisy*, and even *phthisis*, provided that, in this last-named disease, the night-sweats are not excessive;[1] Linné recommends it for various kinds of *rheumatism, scurvy, jaundice, bone-pains, suppression of the menses and lochia;* de Haën for *spasms* and *convulsions*, although he ascribes to bitter-sweet, the property of producing these symptoms in certain cases;[2] Sauvages, Rayoux, and several others, praise it against *leucorrhœa* and *constitutional syphilis*.[3] But, say Mérat and Delens, it is especially in *tetters, scald-head, milk-crust, strangles, chronic itch*, etc., or in affections arising from the retrocession of these affections, such as *asthma*, various *nervous diseases, serous effusions, ophthalmia, amaurosis, deafness*, etc.,[4] that dulcamara has been used most frequently." Many cases reported by Carrère, Rayoux, Bertrand de la Grésic, and several other physicians, says Guersant, leave no doubt concerning the efficacy of this *excitant* in various forms of atonic tetters, etc.[5] The same author adds, a little further on: "I have observed, that several kinds of *scaly or crusty tetter, which are spread over a large portion of the surface of the body*, sometimes yield readily to the use of bitter-sweet, whereas, simple furfuraceous tetters, scattered indolently over single parts,

Storke. From this latter publication Hahnemann took about sixty of the most important symptoms of Dulcamara.

[1] See Murray, app. med., vol. I., p. 425.

[2] Rat. medend., vol. IV., p. 228.

[3] See *Ancien. Journ. de Médec.*, vol. XXII., p. 236 and foll.

[4] *Dict. de mat. med.*, vol. VI., p. 412.

[5] *Dict. des sc. méd.*, vol. X., p. 166.

resist the strongest doses of this drug." Doctor Crichton, of Edinburgh, looks upon bitter-sweet as the specific remedy for *lepra*, and asserts that, with this remedy alone, he has cured twenty-one leprous patients out of twenty-two.[1] Gardner thinks that it is particularly adapted to cutaneous diseases characterised by intense irritation, such as *prurigo*, *ichthyosis* and *psoriasis*.[2]

All this shows, that the affinity of dulcamara in tetters, or, at any rate, in affections of this character, is generally admitted among allœopathic physicians. How do they reconcile this fact with the cutaneous affections which bitter-sweet, according to Carrère's own observations, is capable of producing, namely :—

Violent itching all over the body.
Elevated red spots, like flea-bites.
Red spots all over.
Tetter eruption on the back of the hands.
Tetter eruption on the labia majora.
Tetter crusts all over the body.[3]

But, since bitter-sweet produces on a healthy person other affections beside tetters, it must, of necessity, be capable of curing other beside cutaneous diseases. This has been, indeed, abundantly proven by Hahnemann and his disciples.

According to Mérat and Delens, it is especially in *tetters*, *scald-head*, *milk-crust*, *strangles*, *chronic itch*, etc., or in affections which arise from the suppression of these exanthemata, such as *asthma*, various *nervous derangements*, *serous effusions*, *ophthalmia*, *amaurosis*, *deafness*, etc., that dulcamara has been most frequently employed.[4]

Homœopathic applications.—Bitter-sweet is particularly

[1] *Journ. de méd. d'Edinbourg*, vol. II., p. 65.

[2] *Bullet. des sc. méd. de Férussac*, vol. XXXI., p. 439.

[3] *Oper. Cit.*—Carrère is not the only one who has seen such accidents result from the improperly prolonged use of Dulcamara ; Linné, (loc. cit.) Storke, (according to Hahnemann,) Schlegel, (according to Giacomini,) etc., have related similar examples.

[4] *Dict. univ. de mat. méd.*, vol. VI., p. 412. See the pathogenesis of Dulcamara in Hahnemann's Mat. Med., vol. II., p. 198.

27

suitable to persons with fair complexions, red hair, white, freckled skins,[1] leuco-phlegmatic, of mild dispositions, and disposed to contract catarrhal affections in a draught of air, or when exposed to a cold and damp temperature. This herb seems, therefore, as was said above, best adapted to diseases that prevail among the inhabitants of low and damp regions, where it grows spontaneously.

According to Hahnemann, dulcamara has always been found efficacious in diseases characterised by one or more of the following symptoms: "Boring and heat at the forehead; sensation at the forehead, as if it were pressed against by a board; scrofulous ophthalmia; incipient amaurosis; milk-crust; cough, with hoarseness; catarrh of the bladder with difficulty of urinating; sort of whooping-cough after a cold; suppurating, humid tetters; tettery eruptions, with glandular swellings, etc. It is a specific, says Hahnemann, in certain epidemic fevers, and in various acute diseases caused by a cold."[2]

Dryness of the skin, which is at first cold and afterwards becomes hot, is, in acute and catarrhal affections one of the general indications of dulcamara. This suppression of the cutaneous exhalations, similar to what is occasioned by a cold draught of air, is indeed one of the primary symptoms of this drug. This symptom, which may continue for a long time in certain cases, generally exists in persons afflicted with humid asthma or pulmonary catarrh of old standing, in which diseases it is not to be wondered that *dulc.* should have been found efficacious. It frequently happens, however, that dulcamara has cured coryza, angina, bellyache, rheumatism, etc., when perspiration had broken out upon the skin, which is a secondary effect of dulcamara, and sometimes follows the dryness of the skin after a considerable lapse of time. The selection of the drug, in all such cases, which are not very frequent, however, is necessarily very uncertain, according

[1] Matthiolus relates that, in former times, the ladies of Toscana used the juice of bitter-sweet as a cosmetic, for the removal of freckles. (Comment. de Dioscor.)

[2] *Loc. Cit.*

to the unanimous opinion of the most skilful practitioners. It is to be remarked, that *Puls.* and *Chelid. majus*, if improperly given in the place of dulcamara, have no other bad effect than to leave things as they are. At any rate, I have never noticed an aggravation of the disease after a mistake of this kind occurred.

According to the statement of Hahnemann, the tetters which are cured by bitter-sweet, are *moist.* This *morbid moisture* of the skin constitutes one of the principal secondary effects of dulcamara. It is for this reason that bitter-sweet is scarcely ever successful in *furfuraceous tetter*, *pityriasis*, etc., after having assumed the chronic form, no matter how trifling the eruption may seem.

The tetters which dulcamara causes, and is, therefore, capable of curing, show themselves principally on the forehead, cheeks, upper lip, chin, breasts, labia majora, inner and upper surface of the thigh, (where I have seen them come out in the shape of a purple-colored spot, of twice the size of the hand, and resembling altogether an *humid nævus;*) finally, on the arms, back of the hands and legs. At times they break out in the shape of pustules, which soon become covered with a yellowish crust, (like milk-crust;) at times in the shape of simple spots of a brown-red color, from the surface of which exudes a viscous liquid of a nauseous smell, and more or less profusely.

If this exudation takes place slowly at single spots, in the face, on the hands, *warts* arise from it; these are often cured by dulcamara, especially in persons of fair complexions, lymphatic, and with habitually dry skins.

Between the action of bitter-sweet and that of sulphur, there exists a sort of antagonism which I have noticed several times when prescribing these two drugs, one after the other, in the same case. I have uniformly remarked, in all such cases, that, whereas dulcamara produced a marked improvement, in cutaneous diseases, for example, sulphur would aggravate the case by the development of such symptoms as itching, etc. This accounts for the fact, that the unpleasant effects of sulphur have often been removed by dulcamara. Nevertheless, I do not dare to assert that sulphur is the antidote of dulcamara; for I believe I have observed that, if sulphur be given immediately after dulcamara, it will produce its own specific effects, which it could not do, if it first neutralised the bitter-sweet. *Camphor* removes the headache caused by dulcamara, and *capsicum* neutralises its unpleasant effects on the air-passages. Capsicum, especially, seems to me to be the best antidote of this drug.

GROUP XI.

TYPE: CHELIDONIUM MAJUS.

ANALOGUES:		
	CAPSICUM ANNUUM.	VIOLA ODORATA.
	HEPAR SULPHURIS.	CORALLIA RUBRA.
	ALLIUM SATIVUM.	CANNABIS INDICA.
	DULCAMARA.	CINA.
	BRYONIA ALBA.	PULSATILLA.
	SILICEA.	

THE arrangement of this group is based upon such imperfect data, that I do not consider it as definitely settled. Nevertheless, whatever changes it may undergo, I am satisfied that *Chelidonium majus* will remain the type of this group, and that *Capsicum* and *viola* will remain among its analogues. I shall, therefore, content myself with describing these three remedies, which I have too often alternated with success in the same disease, not to be certain of the relations they hold to each other.

For the present I can only name the following as the maladies to which they correspond: *ophthalmia; amaurosis; specks on the cornea; spasmodic angina,* (*endemic, and in some cases, epidemic whooping-cough*;) *pneumonia,* (at the commencement of the disease;) *pulmonary phthisis; acute hepatitis.*

Chelidonium majus.—*Chelidonion miga of the Greeks, great celandine.*—Herbaceous, perennial plant, a native of Europe, genus *Chelidonium;* family, papaveraceæ; class, polyandria monogynia.

The great celandine, whose ramose, glabrous or hairy stem attains a height of from one to one foot and a-half, prefers damp, mountainous and covered districts, shady ruins, old walls, etc., and is known by its winged and deeply indented leaves of a delicate green color above, and blueish underneath; by its flowers of a dazzling yellow, axillary or terminal, pedunculated and umbelliform. The fruit of this plant consists of small, thin, elongated, polypetalous and unilocular pods. Its root has a reddish-brown color, which, when dried, changes to black.

What distinguishes the great celandine from all other plants of our climate is the juice, which is of a bright yellow color, a little sticky, bitter, acrid and even caustic, abounds in every part of the plant and flows out of the least crack or cut. When exposed to the air, this juice becomes thick, passes from a bright yellow to an orange color, finally turns brown, and then loses almost entirely its solubility in water.[1]

The juice of *stalagmitis guttifera*, or *gummi gutta*, when exposed to the air, undergoes the same kind of change. But this is not the only analogy existing between these two kinds of juices, for several chemists, and principally Thompson, affirm having found gummi-gutta in the juice of chelidonium.[2] It is not, therefore, surprising, that the leaves and stems of *chelid.* should be possessed of purgative and even drastic properties, and that some allœopathic physicians should have proposed to substitute it as a *hydragogue* for the exotic gummi-gutta.[3]

Empirical applications.—The fresh juice of celandine was recommended among the ancient Greeks, as an external application in affections of the eyes. "If applied with caution," says Biett, "it may have doubtless succeeded in scattering a few specks on the cornea, or arresting the progress of a pterygion; but the good effects in incipient cataract which Fabricius of Hilden attributes to it, are more than doubtful."[4] It is not only Fabricius of Hilden that mentions such effects. They have been confirmed by several cases related by a German physician, Schallern, in his inaugural thesis.[5] The same

[1] Biett, *dict. des sc. méd.*, vol. V., p. 18.

[2] *Botan. du drog.*, p. 286.

[3] *Mérat and Delens, dict. univ. de mat. méd.*, vol. II., p. 220.

[4] *Loc. Cit.*

[5] Dissert. qua chelid. maj. virt. medic. novis observat. firmatur., Erlangæ, 1790, in 4to.

practitioner mentions, moreover, several cases of *amaurosis*, which were improved or cured by the use of chelidonium majus.

Blankard relates similar cases, and makes particular mention of *specks on the cornea*, which he had seen dissipated by the dry powder of *celandine* introduced into the eye.[1] Be all this as it may, Biett adds the following: "*Chronic old ulcers*, which had resisted every means of treatment, *have been known to have been healed by applying the juice of chelidonium*, or by means of frequent lotions with strong decoctions of the root, etc. I scarcely need mention the use of this plant in destroying *warts*, etc." But why should not this *acrid, irritating, caustic plant*, (these are Biett's own expressions,) and in spite of which properties it will remove specks on the cornea, arrest the developement of pterygion, and bring about the cicatrization of inveterate ulcers, be likewise capable of scattering an incipient cataract? One of the great errors of allœopathic physicians, consists in rejecting as false and illusory, every fact which does not harmonize with their preconceived theories and prejudices.

The internal as well as external use of the great celandine, appears to be traceable to the remotest antiquity.

In *jaundice*, a vinous decoction of this plant was recommended by Galenus and Dioscorides.[2] Was this merely one of those fancies which have been termed *signatures?* It is certainly true that Forestus, Lentilius, Lange and Sennert, quoted by Murray,[3] declare having successfully repeated the experiments of these two celebrated physicians, which had already been confirmed by Lazare Rivierè, whose name has a good deal of weight with me. Schallern relates two cases of jaundice that had been cured by means of the internal use of chelidonium majus.[4] Creuzbauer attributes to it, a faculty of dissolving biliary calculi.[5] Gilibert and the late Récamier,

[1] Collect. medic. phys., etc., CVI., observ. 18. [2] Mat. Med., lib. II., c. 211.

[3] Appar. Med., vol. II., p. 361. [4] *Dissert. Cit.*

[5] *Dissert. inaug. medic. de rad. chelid. maj.* ad solvendos pellendosque cholelitos efficacia, etc., Argentoreti, 1785, in 4to.

have seen good effects from the celandine, not only in icterus, but also in indolent *engorgement of the liver* and *spleen, with or without intermittent fever.* Lange has seen this drug succeed in *pulmonary catarrh* and *chlorosis.*[1] Lisdenfort in *caries.*[2] According to an observation in the *Ephemerides des curieux de la nature,*[3] Chelidonium majus is not without some curative virtues in *cancerous affections.* Murray states, without much believing it, however, that some cases of *dropsy* (occasioned by the abuse of spirits,) *gout* and *gravel,* have been cured or alleviated by the same drug.[4] "Chelidonium," say Mérat and Delens, "is said to possess antiscrofulous virtues. It appears to modify the lymphatic system in an unequivocal manner, etc."[5] And in proof of their assertion, these authors relate cases taken from the Journal of Hufeland, (1813,) and from the *Journal général de médicine,* (vol. XXVI.) which show that chelidonium, when taken internally, has cured *glandular affections, chronic ophthalmia, old ulcers at the neck,* etc.; facts that go to confirm one of the allegations of the late Biett, which we had occasion to mention before. By some modern German physicians the plant before us had been recommended as an *antisyphilitic,* and quite recently, a Paris physician, Doctor Boniface, has made of it a sort of panacea for *pulmonary phthisis;* I know from my own observation that his method, which is undoubtedly much too exclusive, is crowned with success in some cases.

Homœopathic Applications—Hahnemann has given us a very incomplete pathogenesis of Chelidonium, in the second volume of his Mat. Med. My own provings of this drug, although not very definite, have seemed to me of sufficient importance to be published for future use in perfecting the pathogenesis of this drug. I have endeavored to conduct my provings agreeably to the method which I have pointed out in the introduction to my work; a circumstance which has at least the merit of novelty. The provings have been instituted

[1] *De remedies domesticis,* p. 123 and 124.

[2] *Manuscript notes communicated by Petroz.*

[3] *Vol. V., p.* 59. [4] *Loc. Cit.* [5] *Loc. Cit.*

with a solution of globules of the sixth dilution, at the rate of one globule in a table-spoonful of water; first a table-spoonful was taken in the morning, for two or three days; afterwards, the doses were repeated more frequently by the various provers, and the result obtained will be found annexed.

First proving.—Mr. A., 37 years old, tall, not very fat, having a pale and wornout countenance; brown hair; nervous and irritable; subject to muscular pains, intestinal irritations and leucophlegmasia; generally very sensitive to medicinal action.

First Day.—Ten minutes after taking the first dose, profuse emission of a yellow and foaming urine, like beer.

In half an hour, dull deep-seated pain, on both sides of the lumbar region, where the kidneys are situated.

In one hour, pain at the right shoulder as after a cold.

Sore throat as from a cold.

Pressure on the rectum; urging to stool, which was unusual with him at this hour, and a good deal of appetite at the same time.

In three hours: itching of the eyes; lachrymation at the open air, and oppression of the chest when walking.

In four hours: another emission of foaming urine.

Neuralgic pain at the left eyebrow.

Trembling of the head and hands.

Tension in the abdomen, in the iliac fossæ, which is the same on both sides; itching at the hips, as if sweat would break out, in walking, although the temperature is pretty cool.

In nine hours: burning pain at the tip of the left elbow; numbness of both hands.

About two o'clock in the afternoon, or about six hours after the first dose: sort of general numbness, with somnolence; intolerable aversion to motion; confusion of ideas, as if one were half asleep, without shuddering or increase of temperature on the skin, or any other unpleasant sensation. These symptoms disappear gradually towards three o'clock, and nothing remains but the dull pain in the lumbar region, which continues until night; lachrymation in the open air, without any other sensation in the eyes; lastly, but only now and then, itching, and a slight smarting at the orifice of the urethra, as if one had to urinate all the time, which is not the case, however.

First Night.—In the evening, in bed, before falling asleep: beating in both temples, which is isochronous with the pulse, and at the same time, a sensation as if the blood were violently rising to the throat and upper portion of the chest; a few dull beatings in these parts followed by cutting pains in the lower abdomen; the sleep is quieter and sets in more speedily than usual (curative effect?)

Second Day.—Vague sensations; the urine is less copious than the day before, has again its normal color, and foams no longer.

Several small and thin stools in the day-time, preceded, but not followed, by a few slight cutting pains.

Slight irritation at the throat, which is not felt when swallowing.

Small, not frequent paroxysms of cough, more in the room than in the open air, with spasm of the glottis during an expiration.

Burning, continuous pain at one spot of the skin, on the left side of the sternum, four fingers' breadth below the clavicle; the spot where the pain was felt, was at most of the size of a dollar; there is no redness; the skin, at this spot, feels as if it had been burnt by rapidly rubbing it with a piece of woollen.

About two o'clock in the afternoon: another paroxysm of sleepiness, but not so long or intense as that of the previous day.

All day long: tranquillity of mind and even cheerfulness, *in spite of unpleasant thoughts which were uppermost in his mind*, (curative effect?)

In the evening, in bed, for some moments: pressive pain in the upper teeth of the right side.

Third Day.—In the morning, on waking: the eyes are swollen; the lids are agglutinated with dry gum; the tongue is natural; urine likewise; slight rheumatic or contusive pain at the nape of the neck, at the front part of the neck, in the shoulders and arms; here and there a few red indolent pimples on these parts; the pulse is fuller, stronger, but not more frequent than usual; remarkable cheerfulness of spirits.

Towards the middle of the day; a red spot, resembling herpes, makes its appearance in the sternal region, at the place where only a burning pain was felt on the day previous; this pain has become more intense, without changing its character; a little while later, similar sensations, but without redness, are felt at various circumscribed points of the shoulders, trunk, arms, (very unpleasant symptoms which continued all the following days, until the end of the proving.)

Drowsiness, like the first and second day before, about two o'clock in the afternoon.

Two light-colored, tape-shaped stools, without colic, and at unusual hours.

A small indolent pimple in the thickness of the lower lip.

Towards evening, slight irritation of the throat, and a little scraping at the larynx, causing a few paroxysms of cough.

Pressive stitch at the right temple (in bed) which ceases when lying on the affected part, reappears immediately as soon as one turns to the other side, and disappears for good after the lapse of half an hour.

Quiet night, deep sleep, and no dreams.

Fourth day.—In the morning, the throat feels sore; involuntary snorting (although awake); the velum feels as if it would descend into the throat; a few paroxysms of dry cough; dry skin, and as if bruised, on the chest and at the neck.

About half-past one in the afternoon: *Dull and heavy, deep-seated pain in the whole right side of the chest and right shoulder, without cough, but with embarrassed respiration. This pain, which is at times accompanied with dull beatings in the chest, does not allow him to draw a long breath; it is not perceptibly aggravated by the motion of the arm. The pain is particularly felt in the axilla and under the shoulder blade; a sort of numbness of the muscles in the region of the liver, and in the whole right side of the neck, face and head; apprehension of threatening pneumonia; great anxiety; constant desire to stir and change one's place.* This painful state lasts an hour, and decreases gradually.

Natural stool about three o'clock.

Heaviness at the forehead about half-past four.

At half-past six in the evening, immediately after a good dinner, which he relished, he felt some vertigo; after that, return of the chest-symptoms; violent dyspnœa, without shuddering or acceleration of the pulse, which is only a little fuller than usual; anxiety and trembling of the extremities.

Quiet night.

Sixth day.—Not many new symptoms; slight paroxysm of dyspnœa, about two o'clock; red rounded spots on the palmar side of the forearms, of the size of a dime, and accompanied with burning pain.

No stool.

Lachrymation in the open air, without any other sensation.

Quiet night.

Seventh day.—Irritation in the throat on waking; hollow and not frequent cough; prostration; no appetite.

Intolerable pain in the heels as if these parts had been wounded by too narrow and too short shoes;[1] red, indolent pimples, here and there, on the thighs and buttocks. The other cutaneous symptoms become more and more intolerable.

At one in the afternoon: The chest is again affected; deep-seated pain in the right side as from an abscess; pulsations under the upper part of the sternum, which are synchronous with the pulse; the respiration is embarrassed as if the air-passages were filled with a foreign substance; dry skin without any increase of heat; pulse 85; no cough; less anxiety than the day before, but more prostration.

The region of the liver is slightly painful to pressure.

Painful numbness at the right hip and knee.

[1] This symptom had existed for three or four days previous, but indistinctly.

From this period the experiment was occasionally interrupted for a couple of days, and, being carried on very irregularly, gave rise to very vague results only. The previous symptoms disappeared almost immediately.

During the whole period of this proving, the moral condition, except the few chest-symptoms, remained undisturbed. The appetite remained about the same, except the last two or three days, when it was a little less than usual. There was neither any uncommon sweat, nor any fever properly speaking. From the fourth to the fifth day there was a slight acceleration of the pulse, weariness in the extremities, and a little prostration.

SECOND PROVING.—Mrs. A., 27 years, sanguine temperament, delicate constitution, and sensitive to any kind of impressions; disposed to sanguineous congestions and inflammation of the mucous membranes; lively and playful, very sensitive to the action of drugs.

First day.—Eight o'clock in the morning, (a quarter of an hour after the first dose). Vague, pressive pain in the right shoulder.

Extremely profuse emission of a whitish and foaming urine.

Half-past eight.—Dull, sometimes throbbing pain in the loins.

Painful pressure in the outer parts of the tibio-tarsal articulation (immediately below the ankle, on the right side).

The same kind of pain in the right heel, which renders walking painful. It feels as if this part had been bruised by hard and tight shoes; but not the least relief is obtained by taking off the shoes.

Eleven o'clock.—Sore throat, as from taking cold; another emission of a foaming urine.

About two o'clock in the afternoon.—Drowsiness, which is so marked, even in the open air, that she is near falling asleep while walking; this continues for about half an hour.

Half-past four.—Heaviness in the forehead.

Five o'clock.—Unusual and marked aversion to cold things,

at dinner; she does not drink on this account, although she is moderately thirsty.

After dinner.—Luxation-pain in the left hip, which scarcely allows her to walk.

The pain in the tibio-tarsal articulation likewise changes to a pain as from a sprain.

About eight o'clock, while walking, the pain in the hip extends to the knee, which is so painfully affected by it that the whole joint feels as if it were dislocated.

During the whole of the first day the appetite and taste remain unaltered; no stool; no particular changes in the functions of the skin and the vascular apparatus; *extraordinary tranquillity of mind.*

Slight oppression on the chest, in the evening, in bed; the irritation of the throat continues; a few strange spasmodic sensations in the glottis, without cough, before falling asleep; quiet night; no dreams.

Second day.—Sore throat on waking; lassitude in the extremities; white-coated tongue; *not much appetite;* slight drowsiness about two o'clock in the afternoon; half-liquid stool about the middle of the day; slight itching at the vulva; a little oppression and loose cough about six o'clock; the luxation-pain in the knee and foot continues; pulse and skin are natural; peevish.

Third day.—Sore throat worse than the day before, without stoppage of the nose, and with a little cough now and then; coated tongue; not much appetite; dull or rather benumbing pain *in the whole right side of the chest;* a red, flat, not very apparent spot between the breasts, with burning itching.

Difficulty in the chest, which embarrasses the breathing from an hour and a half to two hours.

Apathy the remainder of the day; at dinner every thing she eats seems to taste badly.

The night is less quiet than the previous one; a little dry heat on the skin.

Fourth day.—Mistiness of sight on the right eye, in the

morning on waking; acute neuralgic pain at the right temple (before taking the dose); two insufficient and thin-shaped evacuations in the day-time.

An unforeseen journey interrupted this experiment at a period when it commenced to become interesting.

THIRD PROVING.—Miss R., 10 years old, with red hair, white skin which is inclined to dryness, freckled; mild disposition, without being apathetic; sensitive to the action of drugs, (at least when sick.)

After taking the first doses even, a pungent heat is perceived on the skin, the pulse becomes feverish; the tongue is coated white; vertigo while sitting up; rush of blood to the head, throat and upper part of the chest; violent and slightly spasmodic cough, as at the beginning of whooping-cough; dull pulsations at the base of the right lung and at the liver; pulse up to 90 in the evening; sweat at night. The mother of the child became frightened, and the proving was discontinued.

FOURTH PROVING.—Mrs. X., 32 years old, lymphatic, with a white and fine skin; not very sensitive to the action of drugs.

This lady experienced only the following symptoms:

Excessive and continual apathy; a sort of aversion to exercise, but her spirits remained unaltered; neuralgic pain above the right eye, especially while reading at candle-light; a sort of fluttering before this eye, which scarcely permits her to read; *embarrassed respiration, especially while reading, without coughing;* the pulse is perceptibly more frequent than commonly (it is commonly small and incompressible); cool and dry skin.

The symptoms which I have related, are neither sufficiently numerous, nor sufficiently precise, to give us a complete image of the Chelidonium disease. Nevertheless, they seem to furnish the means of drawing the following sketch of the morbid conditions to which Chelidonium seems best adapted:

1. Excessive secretion of urine, without any perceptible acceleration of the pulse.

2. After the second day, the urine resumes its natural quantity and color.

3. Angina and swelling of the pharyngeal mucous membrane, not preceded by coryza; no cough or a little loose cough, from the first; spasmodic cough (1st and 2d proving.)

4. Paroxysms of drowsiness, without any other unpleasant sensation, coming on periodically at half-past one or two o'clock in the afternoon, (proving 1 and 2,) and changing on the following days to asthma, (proving 1,) with sensation of a violent engorgement of the right lung, and at the same time of the liver, dull pulsations in the chest, anguish, etc.

5. Acute bronchial catarrh, from the commencement, (proving 3,) with a dull and heavy pain at the upper part of the chest; coated tongue; frequent pulse, with slight vertigo; warm and dry skin at first, which is afterwards covered with perspiration.

6. Dull distress in the chest, (proving 4,) embarrassed respiration when walking, small and constantly frequent pulse, prostration, chilliness without shuddering, extreme apathy, aversion to exercise, etc.

7. Eruption (provings 1 and 2,) of red, flat, somewhat uneven, dry spots (the dryness would probably have given place to dampness in the long run), preceded and accompanied by a burning pain at the sternal region, at other parts of the chest and on the arms.

8. Slight vertigo in the evening, but only on the third day, and in one case. (Prov. 2.)

9. Neuralgic pain at the right temple, or at the right eyebrow. (Prov. 2 and 4.)

10. Amaurotic dimness of the right eye. (Prov. 4.)

11. Pain as from a sprain in the left hip, (prov. 2,) as if sprained and bruised in the knee, in the tibio-tarsal articulation, (prov. 2,) and lastly in the right heel, (a very marked symptom.) (Prov. 1 and 2.)

12. Slight itching at the vulva; ephemeral symptom, on the third day. (Prov. 2.)

13. Remarkable tranquillity of mind for two or three days (prov. 1 and 3), succeeded after a while by ill-humor. (Prov. 2.)

14. Vaguely defined derangements of the digestive functions; as a general rule, the nights are quiet and the sleep sound.

These are the bare outlines of the pathogenesis of Chelidonium. But are they not sufficient to account for the cures which this agent has effected in cases of *angina, pulmonary catarrh, hepatitis, intermittent fevers, ophthalmia, amaurosis,* etc. Supported by undoubted clinical facts, I have recommended chelidonium more particularly at the commencement of whooping-cough and pneumonia, especially among children, and with still greater success in the case of fair-complexioned pale children, with mild dispositions, anxiety, a feverish pulse, and marked symptoms of derangement of the air-passages, the skin remained dry, with a loose and somewhat spasmodic cough from the commencement of the disease. Since then, I have employed the same drug for a sort of tetters, coming out on the back and front part of the chest, and the appearance of which on these parts was preceded by cough for a couple of days. Hereafter celandine will probably enjoy a much more extensive sphere of action. Camphor antidotes this drug.

Capsicum annuum, *Spanish Pepper.* — Genus capsicum, family solaneæ, a native of India, which was known even to the Romans, for Plinius makes mention of it, and is now known to every body.

Pepper which is used to excess in England, the United States, and even in France, is a spice whose burning and even corroding taste is, however, not without a certain pleasantness. Common people, and even physicians, imagine that it excites the appetite; hence, according to their notions, it is naturally indicated whenever the appetite is failing.

Empirical applications.—They are scarcely deserving of mention. The juice of pepper, like that of chelidonium majus, diluted with water, appears to have been employed externally, and as a collyrium, with a certain success, *in some cases of chronic ophthalmia.*[1] Chapman says, that the inter-

[1] *Coxe, Americ. disp.*, p. 156.

nal use of pepper has done him great service in *angina tonsillaris*, and even in *malignant angina*,[1] which is quite probable. Wright says he cured with pepper, *passive dropsies*, and Bergius, *old intermittent fevers which he does not describe more particularly*. In most of these cases, pepper was given in combination with iron, cinchona, laurocerasus, etc.

Homœopathic applications.—According to Hahnemann, individuals with a rigid fibre, are less than others liable to being advantageously acted upon by pepper.

Homœopathic physicians have not yet derived from pepper all the good it is undoubtedly able to accomplish. Until now it has only been employed in certain forms of *intermittent fevers*, which have resisted the action of cinchona or were caused by the abuse of this drug; also, in *pyrosis*, *dysentery*, *dysuria*, *gonorrhœa* and *impotence*. So far as my own experience goes, the diseases in which *Capsicum* proves efficacious, are very similar to those to which *Chelidonium majus* is adapted, namely: whooping-cough as long as the cough preserves its normal form, that is to say, its spasmodic character, and especially when it is more frequent in the day-time than at night; *periodical asthma* (in fair-complexioned and sanguine individuals;) *chronic bronchial catarrh*, with spasmodic cough, ropy expectoration, absence of fever and headache, and habitual pain in the loins. In several of these cases, *capsicum* has helped after *Silicea* had failed or caused a headache.

Viola odorata, *violet.*—Genus *viola*, family cysticæ according to Jussieu, and having, since then, been made the type of a particular family, violariæ.

This pretty flower is so well known that I need not describe it. Its medicinal history is devoid of interest. The root is an *emetic* and a *mild purgative;* an infusion of its flowers is a *calming* medicine, a *pectoral*, an *expectorant*, etc. This is all the authors say about it.

Stapf's pathogenesis of the violet, which is very incomplete and published in his Archives, is reprinted in Jahr's Manual.

[1] *Bull. des sc. méd.* de Férussac, vol. XI., p. 302.

The few provings of viola which I have made, and which I intend to publish as soon as they are completed, have shown me so far a striking analogy between the action of *viola* and that of *chelid. majus.*

I use viola quite frequently in my practice. Here is the result of my observations.

Viola is particularly suitable to persons of a lymphatico-nervous temperament, a mild disposition, dry and cool skin. I have employed it with advantage in the following cases:

1st. *Hoarseness*, followed, but not preceded by, coryza, with cough every now and then; slight dyspnœa, and absence of all moisture on the skin, without any other perceptible symptoms (caused by having staid for several hours in succession in a cold room, in the fall season.) 2d. *dyspnœa*, without cough, *more violent in the day time than at night*, with a dry skin, distention of the abdomen, natural stool, no headache, slight trembling of the upper extremities; these symptoms had existed for some three or four days (without any apparent cause, in a hysteric female;) 3d. *dyspnœa* day and night, *more violent in the day time*, with cough now and then, not dry but with very scanty expectoration (in the case of a pregnant female of twenty-nine years, fair complexion, white and dry skin, slender make, mild disposition, and apparently tuberculous.) 4th. *violent cough*, having lasted three weeks, recurring in long, lasting paroxysms somewhat similar to whooping-cough, that is to say with spasmodic expectoration *in the day time, not at night*, with profuse expectoration of jelly-like, clear and ropy mucus; dyspnœa, chilly disposition, apathy, melancholy mood (in a woman of twenty-seven years, pale, tall and slender, sensitive to impressions, and at the same time of a mild disposition;) the cough ceases to be spasmodic after the very first few doses of the drug; the dyspnœa disappeared and *corallia rubra* completed the cure. 5th. *Violent dyspnœa*, with occasional turns of catarrhal cough, which is sometimes wanting for days; *the dyspnœa had continued day and night*, for a week, with marked increase every afternoon, and irregular paroxysms, without fever or heat of the skin (in a young girl of fair complexion, mild disposition, whose right lung was studded with crude tubercles, and whose mother had died of consumption.) 6th. *Whooping-cough*, in the case of several little girls, nervous, thin, and who had been treated allœopathically for some months past. 7th. *Measles* from the start, (in cases where the cough had a spasmodic character.) 8th. *Measles* running an irregular course (in the case of a girl of four years, weakly, slender and tall, extremely intelligent, her mother had died of consumption.) This was a serious case. The eruption, after having come out on the arms and in the face, disappeared quite suddenly. *Puls.*, *bryon.*, and afterwards *sulph.*, could not bring it back. The cough lasted uninterruptedly, was dry, shrill, violent, with considerable dyspnœa; skin warm, dry, except the palms of the hands which were moist; the patient was very restless, talked a good deal, her hands trembled. I hesitated between *causticum* and *viola*, and finally, happily for the patient, selected *viola*. The effect of this drug was as speedy as it was satisfactory. Almost as soon as she had taken the first dose, a little moisture on the wrist showed itself; towards evening, four or five hours after the drug had been first given, (it was administered every two hours,) the eruption reappeared in the face, and next morning the whole body was covered with it. Cough and oppression which had decreased one-half since the first day of the treatment, ceased almost entirely on the third or fourth day after *viola* had been given, which was continued to the end, until the patient was quite well again.[1]

[1] Petroz informed me that he has used *viola* with success in various rheumatic affections of the upper limbs. Several symptoms of viola account for these successes. But in what cases of rheumatism is viola preferable to *Bry.*, *Spig.*, *Colch.*, etc.? I am unable to decide this point.

GROUP XII.

TYPE: ACIDUM MURIATICUM.
ANALOGUES: VITEX AGNUS CASTUS. HYOSCYAMUS NIGER.

COMMON CHARACTERISTICS.

Stupefying, pressive, sometimes stinging, but not throbbing headache, similar to the one which is often noticed at the commencement of low fevers, such as typhus.

Vertigo, as if things were turning about, with staggering gait.

Dullness of mind; deficient memory; delirium.

Whizzing, noises, ringing, buzzing in the ears; *hardness of hearing.*

Dilatation or contraction of the pupils; myopia or presbyopia; obscuration of sight; diplopia; hemiopia; *optical illusions.*

Dryness of the nostrils; *nosebleed; loss of smell.*

Redness and bloating of the face, with or without heat; earthy paleness of the face.

Rough and cracked lips; foul breath; ulcers at the gums or tongue; *scurvy of the mouth;* flow of saliva; tongue covered with a tenacious white or brownish fur; *paralysis of the tongue;* roughness in the throat; *loss of taste.*

Deficient appetite, with feeling of hunger; bulimy.

Dull, pressive pains at the stomach; deep, cutting pains in the bowels; *pricking in the abdomen which is distended and sensitive to pressure; contusive pain in the abdominal muscles.*

Retention of stool, *followed by serous diarrhœa, which is sometimes very fetid and not very painful;* involuntary stool; *fluent piles.*

Numbness of the bladder; frequent and profuse emissions of urine; paralysis of the bladder.

Excited sexual desire; premature menses; retarded or suppressed menses; *impotence.*

Hoarseness; spasmodic cough, especially at night; stitches in the chest and region of the heart.

Blackish and badly-looking pustules on various parts; foul ulcers.

Fever with stinging heat, frequent, small and intermittent pulse; small and frequent pulse, with deficient animal heat; earthy or livid color of the skin.

CORRESPONDING DISEASES.

Typhus and typhoid fever.—Cachexia.—Scurvy.—Stomacace.—Paralysis, (of the organs of sense, speech, etc.)—Cataract.—Various kinds of neuralgia or nervous derangements, etc.

Acidum Muriaticum.—*Muriatic acid, hydrochloric acid.*

This acid was discovered by Glauber, towards the middle of the last century.

In its native state it is an invisible grey, but, in contact with the air, the humidity of which it absorbs, it forms a white vapor. Composed of equal volumes of chlorine and hydrogen, it is essentially unfit for combustion and respiration. The presence of a very small quantity of this gas in the air, is sufficient to communicate to this latter agent such irritating properties that it causes instantaneously lachrymation, coryza, and a suffocative cough. Water dissolves about three-fourths of its weight of hydrochloric gas, in other words 464 times its volume. It is this more or less concentrated dissolution, that is called in chemistry and the arts *liquid hydrochloric acid,* or simply *hydrochloric acid.* Like all other mineral acids, it is a violent poison, which, to judge from its immediate effects, acts as a caustic. But it is not only by disorganizing the tissues that hydrochloric acid is capable of causing unpleasant symptoms, and even death.

This is admitted even by allœopathic physicians. Destouches tells us, for instance, that he has seen the accidental inhalation of this acid in the form of a gas, cause the following symptoms; stickiness of the mouth, headache, anorexia, violent colic from time to time, griping, and diarrhœa, a series of accidents which did not result from an immediate contact of the poison, and could only have arisen from its absorption.[1]

Empirical applications.—On the recommendation of Guyton-Morveau it was first employed as a disinfecting agent, but has since been superseded by chlore for such purposes. In medicine it is still this day employed internally as well as externally, in numerous cases.

Externally, it has been recommended for *scald-head, tetters, the itch, cancer of the face, aphthæ, chancres, inveterate ulcers, gangrenous ulcers of the mouth and throat, diphtheritis, malignant fevers, petechial fevers, scurvy, scrofula, spasms, epilepsy, mania,* and various other nervous derangements.[2]

But it is principally in putrid and petechial fevers, ulcerations of the mouth and throat, and finally diphtheritis, that the efficacy of muriatic acid has been most emphatically shown, for in these affections it is most evidently homœopathic to the disease. This is so true that an allœopathic physician, Doctor Bange, has attempted to cast a doubt over the success which Bretonneau obtained with muriatic acid in the treatment of diphtheritis, because the experiments of Dr. Bange proved that muriatic acid *caused a croupy inflammation,* whence the Doctor concluded that such a disease could not possibly be cured by means of it.[3] But what says Dr. Bange to the well-authenticated fact that muriatic acid cures, with marvellous felicity, certain fetid ulcers of the gums, and that it is nevertheless capable of causing a similar ulceration if applied to the gums?[4]

Homœopathic applications—According to Hahnemann, this acid has been useful in the following affections: vertical

[1] *Bull. de pharm.*, vol. III., p. 268.

[2] See Gmelin, *appar. medic.*, vol. I., p. 53.

[3] Trousseau and Pidoux, *traité de thérap.*, vol. I., p. 347.

[4] See the pathog. of mur. ac. in Hahnemann's Chronic Diseases, vol. II.

hemiopia; insensibility of the meatus auditorius; beating in the ears; deafness; pimples in the face; freckles; sore throat; eructations; *aversion to meat;* swelling and fulness of the abdomen; abdominal spasms; stools that are too thin in size; stoppage of the nose; pressive pulling in the arms and knees; cold feet; sensitiveness to damp weather. These indications, although perfectly correct, only refer to the use of hydrochloric acid in chronic diseases. But there are many chronic diseases, in which this agent cannot be replaced by any other, especially in the following: *mercurial ulcerations* of the mouth and throat, *aphthæ of the* mouth and intestines, and above all in *typhus.* In respect to this latter disease, it must not be supposed that vague notions about the antiseptic virtues of the acid have led me to its use in typhus. I could easily compose a striking and almost complete image of typhus out of some of the pure symptoms of the drug. The following series, for instance, belongs to typhus full as well as to muriatic acid: intense headache, which is rather dull and heavy than pulsative, with dulness of the senses, dilatation of the pupils, tendency to coma, etc., long-continued bleeding of the nose, roughness and cracking of the lips, flow of viscous saliva, foul breath, heaviness of speech as if the tongue were paralysed, an extreme aversion to every kind of food, dull and pressive pains in the stomach and abdomen, even before breakfast; afterwards, ulcerative and burning pains in the right hypochondrium and right iliac fossa, meteorism, gurgling, torpor of the bowels, alternate constipation and diarrhœa, and finally a serous and fetid diarrhœa; general prostration and collapse of the vital functions, frequent and irregular pulse, unusual snorting during sleep, ominous dreams, a strange tendency to lie on the back and to glide downwards in bed; vague sensation, from the commencement of the disease, that some serious malady is impending, etc.

On the other hand, the promptitude with which I had, on former occasions, seen the muriatic acid change and cure bad-looking ulcers of the gums or throat, must naturally lead me to think, that it would affect ulcers of the lesser intestines in the same manner.

This conjecture seems to be fully justified now-a-days by experience,—not only my own, but that of several colleagues whose statements no one will doubt.

Chanet, for instance, who uses the muriatic acid in the diarrhœic stage of typhus, in accordance with my indications, has frequently obtained with it the finest effects. The almost constant and frequently immediate effect of this drug is to modify the character of the intestinal secretions, and to take away their foul smell; and, after this result is accomplished, almost all the other symptoms improve, and the course of the malady is considerably shortened.

I do not mean to say, however, that the muriatic acid is indicated in every case of typhus. It is with this disease as with all others; according as the circumstances of the case alter, different medicines may be required; but I am convinced that muriatic acid is, under any circumstances, the leading remedy in typhus. If the cerebral symptoms require it, I generally give *Belladonna* before I give the acid. I have given it, however, in some cases, from the very commencement, and long before any diarrhœa had set in. In such a case, the disease ran its course; the diarrhœa set in a few days after the constipation; in one word, the totality and the succession of the general symptoms were sufficiently characteristic, to convince me of the correctness of my diagnosis; but, whether this was to be the natural course of the disease, or whether the result was owing to the peculiar method of treatment I had pursued: the truth is, that cases of typhus which had commenced with an intense fierceness of the symptoms, scarcely ever lasted longer than a week. As a general rule, I think that in typhus, muriatic acid is principally suitable to persons whose blood had been impoverished by the long-continued use of unwholesome and insufficient food, or vitiated by over-eating. To wind up, I will state that I have used muriatic acid successfully in one or two cases of *impotence* resulting from deficient erections, in young men, and caused by the premature abuse of the sexual passion; 2d, in some cases of *cacochymia*, the patients being children, characterised by a small and frequent pulse, without heat of the skin, a livid and greenish complexion, peevishness, dull and slow comprehension, habitual foulness of breath, and good appetite; whitish and spongy gums; soft, thin stool without being diarrhœic, but frequent, (two or three a-day,) irregular and fetid; a dry, hacking cough every now and then; 3d, in a case of *chorea*;[1] 4th, for pulling and paralytic pains of long-standing, and co-existing with indurated ganglia at the left elbow, fore-arm, knee and instep, in a lady of forty, presenting very nearly the previously described symptoms of cacochymia.

The surest antidote of muriatic acid is ipecacuanha; camphor and bryonia have also been recommended as such.

Vitex agnus castus, *chaste-tree.*—Genus *vitex*, family verbenaceæ, class didynamia angiospermia.—This bush, which is very common all along the coast of the Mediterranean, is cultivated in some gardens on account of the elegant shape of its lanceolate leaves, and particularly on account of its beautiful flowers of a violet-blue color, and growing in clusters. The fruit of this bush consists of small blackish berries, which, by their shape, consistence and smarting taste, resemble cayenne-pepper, whence the French name *petit poivre*, *poivre de moine*, etc.

Empirical applications.—In ancient times, the berries of agnus-castus were used for medicinal purposes; but the physicians of the middle ages, and even of our time, seem to have paid little attention to the indications which Hippocrates, Dioscorides and Galenus have furnished concerning the use of this drug, which has now fallen into disuse. Dioscorides, who may be called the Murray of his age, relates in a few

[1] The following symptoms induced me to try this drug in a case of chorea, where other remedies had been given in vain: 398, violent intermittent convulsions of some muscles of the right arm.—434. Twitching in the muscles of the thighs.—491. Twitching at all the extremities, etc.

lines, the internal and external use that was then made in Greece, of the leaves of *agnus castus*, which, according to the statement of Matthiolus, his commentator, is frequently confounded by Dioscorides, with the eleagnus angustifolia, the wild olive tree of Bohemia. If we may believe the statement of Dioscorides, a decoction of the berries of *agnus castus*, is useful in *engorgements of the spleen, dropsy, metritis, indurations of the testicles and fissures of the anus; it increases the milk in the breasts, hastens the appearance of the menses, cures the bites of insects, and even of venomous serpents.*[1] The same author adds, that such a decoction *causes drowsiness*, and *occasions a headache;* this, however, does not prevent him from recommending it for headache.

The provings of this drug seem to have confirmed some of these statements, as well as a belief in the antiphrodisiac properties of the leaves of this plant, upon which they slept during the festival of Ceres, in order to strengthen their chastity. This tradition has undoubtedly given rise to the syrup of agnus castus, which was used by the monks in the middle ages, and was afterwards replaced by the syrup of *Nymphea* now fallen into disuse.[2]

Homœopathic applications. Doctor Roth has published the most complete pathogenesis of Agnus castus of any we possess.[3] Homœopaths that will take the trouble to read it attentively, and to compare it to that of muriatic acid, will see in the former a dim image, as it were, of the latter. But the chaste-tree does not, by any means, possess the powerful action of muriatic acid. Some homœopathic physicians, however, fancy having derived some good from agnus castus

[1] *Mat. Med.*, lib. I., cap. CXVI.

[2] Pitet's experiments with the *nymphea lutea*, published in the *Journal de la Société gallic.*, vol. III., p. 129 and foll., show that the common notion concerning the antiaphrodisiac virtues of this plant, were not without foundation. I should like much to verify the results of Pitet's provings. It is more than probable that the *nymphea lutea* will some day be ranged among the analogues of muriatic acid.

[3] Belon, *singularités*, p. 270.

in the treatment of *impotence*, *gonorrhœa*, *amenorrhœa*, *agalactia*, *ulcers in the mouth*, etc. The provings which I have instituted with agnus castus on my own person, lead me to consider it as a drug of so little importance that it seems to me we might blot it out from our Materia Medica, without losing any thing. This, however, is a purely personal opinion, which I am perfectly willing to correct.

Hyoscyamus Niger, *henbane.* A native plant, of the genus *Hyoscyamus*, family solaneæ, class pentandria monogynia.

Henbane is an herbaceous plant, bisannual, very common in uncultivated places, along the border of roads, in the neighbourhood of farms, villages, etc. Its stem is ramose, cylindrical, hairy, downy at the top, and is from 15 to 18 inches high. The leaves are sessile; with wavy borders, of a dark-green color, and hairy like the stems. The flowers are of a dirty yellow color, with claret-colored streaks, paniculated, almost sessile, composed of a bell-shaped chalice, with five sharp lobes, and of an infundibuliform corol with five unequal divisions, inclosing five inclined stamens and a style overtopped by a stigma. The fruit consists of operculate capsules with two compartments, containing greenish, pointed and irregularly-shaped seeds from which a fat oil was formerly extracted in Egypt, and used for lighting purposes.[1] Every part of this plant, which has a dreary and repulsive look, has a viscous feel, and exhales a fetid and nauseous odor. The taste of its leaves is at first insipid and mucilaginous, but afterwards changes to an acrid and unpleasant taste.

Pigs, oxen, sheep and goats eat the leaves of this plant with impunity, and without repugnance. According to Matthiolus, they are fatal to deer and the gallinaceous species; this, however, requires verification. Although this plant does not affect man as powerfully as belladonna, and some other solaneæ, it is nevertheless true that every part of it has a poisonous effect on man, and there is no doubt, that

[1] *Comment. de la mat. méd.* de Dioscorides, lib. VI., cap. 36.

it has destroyed human life. These poisonings were characterized by the following symptoms; vertigo; merry and calm delirium; paroxysms of craziness, with strange hallucinations, and strange gesticulations; panic fright; comatose sleep; syncope followed by lethargy; dizziness; dilated pupils; diplopia; illusions of sight; bloated face; excessive dryness of the mouth and throat; pain at the stomach, accompanied with anxiety; burning pain in the bowels; diarrhœa; constriction of the larynx; aphonia, as if the tongue were paralyzed; general sinking of the temperature of the body; cold extremities; excessive weakness; altered color of the skin; cold sweat; small and unequal pulse; trembling of the limbs; tonic and clonic spasms; diminished sensibility; paralysis of the extremities.[1]

Empirical applications. In the works of ancient physicians little mention is made of the black hyoscyamus. It is named, however, in Dioscorides and Celsus.[2] The former recommends it internally for *neuralgia;* the latter used the juice diluted with water, in the form of injections into the ear, in cases of *purulent otorrhœa.* According to some authors, the recent leaves of hyoscyamus, if locally applied, have a faculty of quieting neuralgia of the pericranium, especially when it can be alleviated by pressure.[3] Tabernæmontanus relates that these leaves, when boiled in milk and applied to the breasts, possess the power of scattering milky engorgements; this fact is confirmed by Ferrein.[4] It was not, however, until towards the end of the 18th century, when Stork drew the attention of the profession to Hyoscyamus, that it commenced to take an important rank in the Materia Medica.[5] In spite of the vehement opposition of Greding, who failed to perform cures with this drug, the physicians of the School of

[1] See Wepfer, *historia cicutæ aquaticæ,* p. 230, history of the poisoning of the benedictin monks of Rinhow by the roots of hyoscyamus, mistaken for parsnip, and eaten as such by these fathers.

[2] Lib. VI., cap. 6.

[3] Mérat and Delens, *dict. de mat. méd.,* vol. II., p. 466.

[4] *Mat. Med.,* vol. II., p. 646.

[5] See Storck, lib. *de stramonio, hyoscyamo,* etc., p. 28 and foll.

Vienna used it a good deal, to their satisfaction, in the following diseases: *pressive headache without congestion; acute meningitis; mania; epilepsy; convulsions; tetanus; delirium tremens; chorea; spasmodic contraction of the pupil; iritis; incipient cataract; dysentery; acute pneumonia; spasmodic cough; croup; whooping-cough; asthma; acute hæmoptysis; nervous palpitations; induration* (Schirrus ?) *of the breasts; arthritis; nervous diseases.*[1]

Most modern authors of Materia Medica, look upon hyoscyamus simply as a *stupefying* agent, that is to say, a drug whose action on the organism is exactly like that of belladonna, stramonium, tobacco, mandrake, etc.[2] This amounts to the same thing as if one would assert that all poisons act precisely alike, simply because they all lead to the same result: death.

It is true, however, that there is a good deal of similarity between the action of hyoscyamus, and that of the drugs constituting the *belladonna* group; we shall, therefore, give it a place among the members of this series.[3]

Homœopathic applications. — The pathogenesis of hyoscyamus seems to confirm the almost intuitive use which Stœrck and his disciples formerly made of this plant. This is the reason why homœopathic physicians use it with more precision, of course, for the same diseases in which this great practitioner employed it, such as *typhus,* (period of delirium,) some forms of *mental derangement* of recent date, or caused by fright or some contrary event; certain forms of *chorea; spasmodic affections of pregnant or parturient women; paralysis of the tongue, sphincter and bladder; nocturnal spasmodic cough; impotence,* etc.

Camphor is one of the antidotes of this drug.

[1] Murray, *app. med.*, vol. I., p. 144, and Giacomini, *tr. de thérap.*, p. 546.

[2] Trousseau and Pidoux, *trait. de thérap.*, vol. II., p. 93.

[3] See the pathog. of Hyoscyam. in Hahnemann's *Mat. Med. Pur.*, vol. II., p. 503.

GROUP XIII.

TYPE: LYCOPODIUM CLAVATUM.
ANALOGUES: NATRUM MURIATICUM, ANTIMONIUM CRUDUM, VIOLA TRICOLOR.[1]

COMMON CHARACTERISTICS.

THE drugs composing this important group, are very similar to each other. They seem to act primarily on the digestive organs and the adjoining glands; on the lesser and larger intestines more particularly than on the stomach.[2] The immediate and consecutive symptoms produced by these drugs resemble a good deal the unpleasant effects caused by the habitually or accidentally excessive use of feculent or glutinous food. This is the reason why most of them, and probably all, cause an instinctive aversion to *bread*, and, more generally, to aliments made of fermented or fermentable dough; a kind of food that is supposed to be very nourishing, but is, nevertheless, rejected by carnivorous animals, because their alimentary canal is not sufficiently developed to digest such aliments with suitable ease.[3]

In accordance with the previous remarks, the following symptoms may be set down as common to lycopodium and its analogues:—

Gas in the stomach, and especially the bowels, during the digestion, and even before breakfast.

Aversion to food.

[1] *Indigo*, probably constitutes one of the analogues of this drug.

[2] In this respect the action of *lycopod.* differs more particularly from that of *bryon.* These two drugs have a good many points of contact. Hence lycop. is found mentioned among the analogues of *bryon.* The preference which is given by physicians to one or the other of these drugs, frequently depends upon etiological considerations.

[3] It is well known that the digestive canal is the larger in size, the greater the changes which the food has to undergo in order to be assimilated.

Frequent and painful eructations.

Sour eructations.

Nausea, which seldom increases to vomiting.

Vomiting of sour food.

Painful spots in the bowels, here and there, as from incarcerated wind.

Swelling of the abdomen.

Alternate diarrhœa and constipation, or, in some cases, constipation of long duration.

During the action or under the influence of these drugs, there seems to prevail a tendency to humoral congestion of the lower abdomen; hence

Pressure on the bladder, uterus, rectum, as if everything would fall out at the perinæum.

Frequent and profuse emission of urine.

Pains in the loins.

Pale, whitish, cloudy urine, full of mucus, and exhaling, in some cases, a putrid odor.

Premature and profuse menses, or premature, but pale and scanty, or (which is a secondary effect,) delaying, without much color, scanty, and even suppressed.

Sexual excitement, generally followed by aversion to sexual intercourse in the female, and impotence in the male.

Acrid leucorrhœa.

Among the other symptoms of the drugs of this group, and which follow with more or less regularity the gastric symptoms, we distinguish :—

Peevish, rather than irritable mood; difficulty of thinking; loathing of life.

Rush of blood to the head; vertigo when stooping, and with tendency to fall forward.

Tearing in the forehead or towards the top of the head.

Falling of the hair; gnawing itching at the hairy scalp; obstinate, crusty eruptions on the hairy scalp and in the face.

Inflammation of the eyes, sometimes periodical; *blepharophthalmia of long standing.*

Angina of long standing, with sensation as of a foreign body in the throat; *obstinate* cough, either dry or loose; beating of the *heart*, at night.

Pulling pains at the nape of the neck, in the loins and extremities, especially in the elbow-joints and lower extremities.

Contraction of the tendons, especially *the hamstrings.*

Deficiency of vital heat.

Anxious sleep, *with frequent and long waking, and full of disagreeable dreams.*

Quotidian *intermittent fever*, (with afternoon paroxysms,) or tertian intermittent.

Obesity; *emaciation*, which sometimes increases to *marasmus.*

CORRESPONDING DISEASES.

Indigestion, (caused by heavy dough.)—Acute and chronic gastro-enteritis.—Hepatitis.—Tympanitis.—Cystitis.—Metritis.—Prolapsus of the uterus, (in one case caused by a fall on the seat.)—Coryza.—Chronic angina.—Pulmonary catarrh.—Acute and especially chronic pneumonia—Pleurisy.—Pleurodynia.—Rheumatic headache.—Impetigo.—Acne rosacea.—Plica polonica.(?)—Acute and chronic ophthalmia.—Iritis.—Amaurosis.—Blepharophthalmia.—Rheumatism of the trunk and extremities.—Contraction of the tendons, (especially the hamstrings.)—Scrofula.—General or partial atrophy.

Lycopodium clavatum, *wolf's-foot.*— Genus, *lycopodium*, ranged among the mosses by Linné and Jussieu, but transformed by modern botanists into a distinct family of plants. This cryptogamous and creeping plant, like all the other plants of the same family, grows in the north of Europe, in stony, mountainous and covered regions. It has its name from the shape of its root, which reminds one of a wolf's foot, (from the Greek words *pous*, foot, and *lycos*, wolf.) It has the appearance of a tall moss. It bears long club-shaped spikes, which drop, towards the end of fall, a yellow, granular, light, inodorous, insipid, inflammable powder, which is known to fire-workers under the name of *vegetable sulphur*, and is considered by botanists as the pollen of the plant under consideration; it is this powder that is used in medicine.

"Until recently," says Hahnemann, "it had only been used for the purpose of imitating lightning, (in theatres,) because it catches fire when a burning body comes near it; of wrapping up pills composed of substances that would adhere to each other without such a precaution; and for the purpose of preventing the painful effects of friction on the excoriated or chapped parts of the body. Lycopodium floats on top of liquids without dissolving, etc. In its gross, natural condition, it has scarcely any medicinal effect on man; at any rate, the statements of ancient authors concerning the effects of lycopodium have not been confirmed by modern experience; on the contrary, modern pathologists doubt the truth thereof."[1]

But of how many other drugs have the medicinal properties been doubted by modern authors? Does this show that the medicinal history of these drugs is without any interest for us, and that all the clinical indications of the ancients should be rejected as fables? I do not believe that this opinion would be shared by many homœopaths devoted to serious studies. Lycopodium has, therefore, like most other therapeutic agents, its traditional history, which seems to me the rather curious that it confirms the results of our physiological provings of this drug.

Empirical applications.—According to Welshand Vicat, quoted by Murray,[2] a decoction of *lycopodium causes vomiting*. It is true, this is said of the entire plant, not merely its pollen; but we know from our provings that the dynamised pollen likewise has this effect.[3] As regards the external use

[1] *Chronic Diseases*, vol. III. [2] *Appar. Med.*, vol. V., p. 49.

[3] The powder of lycop. is not as inert as is believed. Thirty grammes of it have caused nausea, borborygmi, with slight colic and a soft stool. Dr. Arnaud prescribed dynamised lycop. to one of his patients, who went to an allœopathic druggist to have his prescription put up. The druggist gave him the crude lycopodium mixed in water. Strange, however, this mixture, with the crude lycop. in it, produced a striking amelioration in the condition of the patient, who was troubled with a gastric affection.

of the powder of lycopodium in *intertrigo* of children or fat individuals, it is known to every body. But does lycopodium, in such a case, simply exercise, as is generally believed, a desiccative, purely mechanical action, not possessing any specific relation whatsoever to the disease? I do not think so. Indeed, Rosenstein found, that after having mixed the powder with lard, and making a sort of ointment of it, it still preserved, in spite of this alteration of its physical properties, its efficacy against *intertrigo* and the *chapping* of children. He even employed the same ointment for serpiginous ulcerations of the hairy scalp, legs, etc., sometimes with the most satisfactory results. This shows that the powder of lycopodium modifies and cures certain affections of the skin. Internally, this powder has been praised by Wedel, Lentilius, Gesner, and several other practitioners, 1st, for the *cardialgia* and *flatulent colic* of children and young girls; 2d, for the *dysuria* of children; 3d, for *nephritic colic* and *calculi.* What homœopathic physician does not see that this mode of treatment was not founded upon some of the real properties of lycop.? "Internally," say Mérat and Delens, "lycopodium has been given for *rheumatism, retention of urine, nephritis, epilepsy;* it was regarded as an anti-spasmodic, and as a useful remedy in pulmonary diseases, whence the name *pulmonaria* or *poumonaria,* that was formerly given to this plant."[1] According to the same authors, the Polish physicians powder with lycopodium the hair of those who are afflicted with *plica* polonica, and obtain good effects from this process. This is not entirely correct; for it is a decoction of the entire plant, to be employed internally, and also externally as a lotion; this has been recommended for plica. According to Vicat, no treatment is more serviceable in this horrible affection than the use of lycopodium.[2] We pray the Polish homœopaths to enlighten us concerning this important matter.[3]

[1] *Dict. de mat. méd.*, vol. IV., p. 168.

[2] *Mém. sur la plique polonaise*, Lausanne, 1775, p. 58.

[3] See the pathogenesis of lycop. in Hahnemann's Chronic Diseases, vol. II.

Homœopathic applications.—Lycop. seems to be particularly suitable for the affections of females, or rather of persons of mild disposition, leuco-phlegmatic, and given to melancholy. It seems to act primarily on the digestive organs, and not so much on the stomach as on the larger and smaller intestines. As Bryonia seems to correspond more particularly to acute and chronic affections resulting from the excessive use of a strong and exclusively animal diet, so the lycopodium seems to represent by the totality of its symptoms the series of functional disorders, and of the organic alterations arising from them, which are caused by the abuse of *heavy farinaceous* and *fermentable food.* As a general rule, no drug is better adapted to *indigestions caused by fresh or half-baked bread, or by the abominable pies, cakes, butter-crackers*, etc., with which so many adults and children stuff themselves. Such indigestions are characterised by redness and bloating of the face, succeeded at intervals by excessive paleness; syncope; vomiting, first of phlegm, afterwards of the ingesta, followed by cutting colic and several sour-smelling stools, and a good deal of flatulence; lastly, shuddering, mingled with heat and sweat. The constipation which often follows a violent, though short-lasting diarrhœa in these affections, is likewise a well-known and characteristic symptom of lycopodium. In some very *acute diarrhœas* of children, this agent, which is generally given for constipation, has likewise proved very efficacious.

But it is principally in chronic affections that lycopodium is useful; Hahnemann recommends it for the following conditions:

Melancholy; *chagrin;* anxiety, with desire to weep; dread of being left alone; *irritability;* extreme sensitiveness; capricious mood; difficulty of thinking and attending to mental labor; vertigo, especially when stooping; headache as from a deranged stomach; when walking, every step rebounds in the head, as if the head would split; headache caused by adverse events; pressive, tensive headache; paroxysms of tearing pain at the top of the head, at the forehead, temples, eyes, nose; tearing in the forehead every afternoon; headache at night, at the outer head; heaviness of the head; rush of blood to the head, in the morning, when rising, followed by headache; gnawing itching and *profusely suppurating eruption on the hairy scalp;* baldness; *smarting in the eyes;* stitches in the eyes, especially in the evening, at candle-light; itching heat at the upper lid; *ophthalmia; blepharophthalmia;* myopia; presbyopia; dimness of sight, as from feather-dust; *flickering and dark spots before the eyes;* buzzing in the ears; *hardness of hearing;* crusts in the nostrils; nosebleed; swelling and tension of the face; frequent flashes of heat in the face; itching eruption in the face; freckles; toothache, with rheumatic catarrh of the face; toothache after eating; *dry mouth,* without thirst, hindering the motion of the tongue and embarrassing the speech; coated tongue; chronic sore throat; mercurial ulcers in the throat; dry throat; heat in the throat, with thirst at night; phlegm in the throat; slimy taste in the mouth, early in the morning; bad taste in the mouth; loss of taste; *bitter mouth,* in the morning, with nausea; excessive hunger; loss of appetite after eating the first mouthful; *deficient appetite; canine hunger; aversion to boiled and warm food; aversion to rye bread and meat;* marked taste for sweet things; indigestion caused by heavy food, (pastry, etc.,) difficult digestion of the milk, it causes diarrhœa; malaise during a meal, with sweat on the forehead; acid mouth after eating; hiccough, sour or fat eructations; dull beating of the heart during the digestion; violent eructations in the afternoon; malaise at the stomach, in the morning; frequent, continual nausea; nausea when riding in a carriage; *weight at the stomach,* before breakfast and after eating; swelling of the epigastrium, which is painful to the touch; circumscribed and seated pains, similar to those which are caused by flatulence, that is incarcerated under the false ribs; pain above the navel, when touching the part; *fulness in the stomach and lower abdomen;* tightness in the hypochondria; *dull and stitching pain in the liver, after eating;* pain, when walking, in the upper part of the right hypochondrium, *as if the suspensor ligament of the liver would tear;*[1] *painful meteoristic distension* of the abdomen; induration in the abdomen; pinching pain in the hypogastrium, cutting off the respiration; lancinating, pinching pain in the hypogastrium, which seems to be seated in the region of the bladder, and descends to the urethra, in the evening, in bed; *pinching in the abdomen; pinching in the right side of the abdomen;* cutting colic; cutting colic in the upper part of the abdomen, (especially after drinking wine, even when mixing it with a good deal of water); tearing in the sides of the epigastrium and in the groins as far as the thighs; burning in the lower abdomen; *deficient emission of flatulence;* gurgling in the left side of the abdomen; *borborygmi* in the abdomen; serous diarrhœa, with frequent and scanty evacuations, hot fever and distension of the bowels, in children at the breast; unsuccessful urging to stool; hard stool with straining; *constipation lasting several days; chronic constipation;* lumbrici; pin-worms in the rectum; pain at the anus after eating and after stool; itching at the anus; tension at the anus; incisive pain in the rectum and bladder; *urging to urinate;* frequent urging to urinate; *gravel;* hæmorrhage from the urethra; itching in the urethra during and after the emission of urine; feeble erections; absence of all involuntary emissions; swelling of the testicle of long standing; *excessive nocturnal emissions;* deficient sexual desire; impotence of several years' standing; aversion to sexual intercourse; excessive desire for sexual intercourse; immoderate desire for sexual intercourse every night; too sudden ejaculation of semen; *profuse menses, which last too long;* suppression of the menses by fright; *melancholy and sadness* previous to the menses; itching, heat, gnawing at the vulva; expulsive pressure in the genital organs, when stooping; stinging pain in the labia majora, when lying down; discharge of flatulence from the vagina; *leucorrhœa;* leucorrhœa preceded by cutting pains in the epigastrium.

[1] In proving lycopodium, I experienced this pain for more than eight days, so violently that I had to discontinue the proving.

Fluent coryza; coryza with cough and hoarseness; *stuffing and obstruction of the nostrils;* formication in the wind-pipe, at night; dry cough in the morning for years; dry cough day and night; cough after drinking; painful cough; cough which affects the chest; loose cough; cough with spitting of pus; phthisis pulmonalis; *short breathing of children; constant oppression, with suffocation on doing the least work;* stitches in the left side of the chest; contusive pain at the chest; beating of the heart (in the evening, in bed); hepatic spots on the chest; stitches in the sacrum, on raising one's-self after stooping; pain in the loins, at night; tearing in the shoulders; pulling in the nape of the neck, as far as the occiput, day and night; stiffness of the nape of the neck; stiffness of one side of the neck; swelling of the sub-maxillary glands; *pulling pain in the arms;* twitchings in the arms during sleep, in the afternoon; nocturnal bone-pain in the arms; numbness of the arms on raising them, or at night; *deficiency of strength in the arms;* nightly pain in the bones of the arms; arthritic stiffness of the wrist; numbness of the hands; dryness of the skin of the hands; cracks in the finger joints; redness, swelling and arthritic tearing at the finger-joints; stiffness of the fingers caused by arthritic nodosities; stiffness of the fingers while engaged at work; numbness of the little finger; tearing in the hips, knees or insteps, most frequently in the evening and at night; rheumatic pains in the legs, at night; rheumatic pains in the bend of the knee, in the evening; *stiffness of the knee;* swelling of the knee; burning and smarting itching at the bend of the knee; burning at the legs; *contractive pain in the calves, when walking;* former ulcers at the legs, with tearing pain at night, itching and burning swelling of the ankle; cold feet; cramps in the feet; cold sweat at the feet; profuse sweat at the feet; swelling of the sole of the feet; pain at the sole of the feet, when walking; turning over the toes, when walking; cramps in the toes; corns; pain in the corns; *dry skin;* cracking of the skin; itching when getting warm, in the day-time; itching before going to bed, in the evening; painful eruption on the neck and chest; gnawing itching on the arms and legs; *boils and varices of pregnant women;* disposition to straining parts, which brings on a painful stiffness of the nape of the neck; twitching in the extremities and the whole body, when sleeping or waking; difficulty of lying on the left side, on account of beating and stinging at the heart; tendency to take cold; after a short walk lassitude of the legs, and burning heat at the sole of the feet; *languor;* lassitude in the limbs, even in the morning, on waking; frequent yawning, and sleepiness in the day-time; late falling asleep, in the evening, owing to a crowd of ideas; restless sleep, full of dreams and with frequent waking; *frightful dreams; startings during sleep;* habitual deficiency of animal heat; flashes of heat; tertian fever with sour vomiting after the chill, and bloating of the face and hands; fever-sweat in the day-time; *sweat in the day-time,* especially in the face, on taking the least exercise; general emaciation, increasing even to marasmus.

Has lycopodium ever cured pulmonary phthisis, as some homœopathic physicians assert? I doubt it, but it has often been found wonderfully efficient in *chronic pneumonia,* with purulent, foul-smelling expectoration, even when one of the lungs, (especially the left,) had become partially hepatised. Under such circumstances, lycopodium acts the more advantageously, the more it is adapted to the constitution and the moral state of the patient. When given to northern men, (especially such as come from England,) tall, of gentle dispositions, but phlegmatic and taciturn, I have seen it produce the best effects in this disease, which had almost always been falsely diagnosed as tuberculous phthisis. I ought to add, that, according to my experience, *lycopodium,* as well as most other drugs, however, *is much more efficacious* in the higher than the lower attenuations, and more especially when administered in the form of Jenichen's preparations, the one-thousandth, two-thousandth, three-thousandth, etc., potencies.

Camphor, pulsatilla and causticum, have been named by

Hahnemann as the antidotes of lycopodium. I am sure that causticum neutralises most of the effects of this drug. The same is true of coffee; but *lachesis* seems to be the most comprehensive antidote of lycopodium. This, however, depends upon the character of the symptoms that require to be antidoted.

Natrum muriaticum, *common salt.*—"We scarcely possess a single genuine fact relative to the curative action of sea-salt in human diseases, and if, in some diseases, such as blood-spitting, and other kinds of hæmorrhage, it has really done good, it is evident that, owing to the enormous quantities (table-spoonfuls,) which were given at a time, it acted as a derivative on the stomach and intestines; in the same way as the mustard-plasters which are applied to the calves, sometimes quiet toothache for a time, and quite speedily."[1]

Howsoever founded this opinion may be in general, it seems to me, however, that it is liable to objections. Indeed, because common salt, when administered in massive doses, produces vomiting and diarrhœa, it does not follow, in my estimation, that it must necessarily lose, on this account, all its specific properties. Why should there be a difference, in this respect, between salt and tartar emetic? This latter agent, even when taken in enormous quantities, say one-half of a gramme, or a whole gramme, or even several grammes in the twenty-four hours, has undoubtedly cured pneumonia and articular rheumatism. Will it be said, that these results depended upon its derivative action on the digestive canal? This supposition is the rather unfounded, and, I should say, the rather untenable that we know, by positive experience, that the good effects of massive doses of tartar emetic in pneumonia and acute gout, are the more striking and rapid, the more easily the poison is supported by the digestive organs, without exciting vomiting or diarrhœa. I have seen more than one case of pneumonia cured by massive doses of tartar emetic, although a diarrhœa set in after the first dose

[1] See *Chronic Diseases*, Vol. III.

of the drug had been taken, and continued all the time that the drug was administered. Were such cures the result of a derivative action, or of a special action of the medicine on the pulmonary apparatus? I unhesitatingly decide in favor of the latter, which has been productive of too many brilliant and important results to admit of any doubt. What is true of tartar emetic, is likewise true of common salt. It is not as a derivative, but as a homœopathic agent that salt even when administered in massive doses, but not rejected by the organism, has cured diseases of the throat, bronchia, lungs, etc. I admit, however, with Hahnemann, that facts here leave us in the lurch, and that allœopathic testimony, in respect to salt, is not, by any means, conclusive. But this is principally owing to the fact, that, in medical works, salt is scarcely ever recommended alone, but always in combination with some other drug. We find it stated by authors, that *sea-water*, if drank by the tumblerful, causes vomiting, and more particularly diarrhœa, *except in lymphatic individuals*, who generally bear it without feeling any ill effects from it; that, if taken in less quantity, it becomes a *dissolvent;* that, in its quality as a *dissolvent*, it is capable of curing a number of maladies, such as *scrofula*, *engorgements of the liver*, *biliary concretions*, *phthisis*, *white swellings*, etc.[1] But can we rightfully consider *sea-water* and the *chloride of sodium* identical? It is certainly true that, independently of this agent, which is undoubtedly the principal constituent of sea-water, this liquid contains still other ingredients.

In his old age, Stahl, it is said, frequently prescribed small doses of sea-salt; but this system of medication which, in the mind of this celebrated physician, was purely negative, simply showed the extent of the scepticism into which he had fallen concerning the uses of drugs; towards the end of his career, he doubted the curative virtues of every one of them.

"If taken in small doses," say Mérat and Delens, "sea-

[1] See Plinius, lib. II., cap. 12, and lib. XXXI., cap. 6; Celsus, lib. III. cap. 24; *Ancien. Journ. de Méd.*, vol. XLII., p. 250; new *Journ. de Méd.*, vol. XV., p. 41, etc.

salt gently stimulates the digestive organs, excites the appetite, favors the digestion; for most men its use has become absolutely necessary. Formerly it was regarded as an incisive, antipituitous remedy, and as a powerful dissolvent of visceral or glandular engorgements. Dr. Wezener has even recommended it for schirrus of the stomach, of which disease Pittschaft related a few cases of cure in 1822."[1]

According to Gmelin,[2] Herschel, Hunczowsky and Rondelet, praise the curative virtues of sea-salt in *engorgements of the spleen* consequent on intermittent fevers, and in scrofulous diseases in general. Rondelet, whose opinion in this respect was shared by almost all the English physicians, ascribed exclusively to the chloride of sodium contained in sea-water, the efficacy of this liquid in the treatment of scrofula, whereas formerly this efficacy had been attributed to the water itself and to roast-sponge; but this hypothesis was very much shaken by the discovery of iodine, the presence of which in sponge was fully demonstrated.

On the fourth of May, 1835, Dr. Munaret read before the Academy of Sciences a memoir, in which he extolled the febrifuge properties of salt, and, in the same sitting, Ysenbach and Brailou affirmed having employed salt, at the rate of two tablespoonsful in six ounces of water, in *Asiatic cholera*, with so much success that, of fifty patients, they only lost one! "It is by using simple remedies," says Hippocrates, "that great physicians distinguish themselves from lesser ones." I confess I should never have thought of combatting cholera with common salt; but I am willing to believe that, in some districts, salt may have a good effect in the forms of cholera which there prevail.

In 1841 or 42, Dr. Amedée Latour published a memoir, entitled, *Du traitement préservatif et curatif de la phthisie pulmonaire,*[3] in which the author expresses the hope, that salt may become a specific remedy for tubercular phthisis. Unfortunately, the facts upon which this hope is based, are not suf-

[1] *Oper. Cit.*, vol. I., p. 420. [2] *Appar. Med.*, vol. I., p. 80.

[3] This memoir has been reprinted in 1844.

ficiently conclusive, to justify such exaggerated inferences. Nevertheless his observations show that salt is possessed of a certain efficacy in chronic, and, perhaps, tubercular affections of the lungs.

To resume, the notions which alloeopathic physicians possess, concerning the curative properties of salt, are very vague.[1]

Homœopathic applications.—The more we study the pathogenesis of Natrum muriaticum with reference to that of Lycop., the more we find that these two drugs are related to each other; indeed, both frequently correspond to diseases of the same species, and they are frequently employed alternately in the same diseases.

It is important to state in this place, that the daily use of salt for culinary purposes does, in no respect, prejudice the medicinal action of the dynamised salt; I know this from experience.

Although salt is sometimes indicated in acute affections, it is generally used in chronic maladies. Hahnemann recommends salt for the following morbid conditions which embody an exact picture of the curative sphere of this agent, agreeing perfectly with my own experience on this point. If the reader will take the trouble to compare the following list of symptoms with the symptoms for which Lycopodium has been recommended, he will find that Natrum mur. and Lycop. are strikingly similar to each other, even in the details of their respective action upon the organism.

"Sadness; chagrin and anxiety for the future; anxiety; tendency to start; *tendency to ill-humor;* violent temper; vertigo, as if he would fall forward; *weak memory;* impossibility to think; *headache, with dizziness; heaviness of the head all day*, especially at the occiput, and obliging him to close his eyelids; headache in the morning; pressure in the head and temples; *headache, in the morning on waking;* headache as if the skull would split; tearing, lancinating headache, which obliges one to lie down; stitches above the

[1] See the pathogenesis of natrum mur. in Hahnemann's *Chronic Diseases*, vol. III.

eyes; pressive pain above the eyes; stitches in the parietal bone; beating and pulling in the forehead; beating in the head; hammering in the head; beating in the head when moving the body; crusts on the hairy scalp; pimples on the forehead; smarting in the eyes; ophthalmia; gum in the outer canthi; agglutination of the lids, at night; lachrymation; acrid tears; closing of the lids, in the evening; sudden obscuration of sight, on the breaking out of a tearing and stinging headache; dimness of sight, as from a gauze; obscuration of sight in walking or stooping; presbyopia; diplopia; *the letters look blurred while reading;* black points before the eyes; incipient amaurosis; stitches in the ears; ringing in the ears; noise in the ears; *buzzing in the ears;* hardness of hearing; anosmia; smarting pain in the malar bones when eating; itching in the face; pimples in the face; tetters around the mouth; swelling of the upper lip; *chapping of the upper lip;* painful vesicles to contact, at the inner surface of the upper lip; frequent swelling of the sub-maxillary glands; fistula dentalis; vesicles on the tongue; chronic sore throat, with sensation as if one ought to swallow something; phlegm in the throat; spitting up of mucus in the morning; foul taste in the mouth, before breakfast; sour taste in the mouth; bitterness in the mouth; eructations; *sour eructations;* repulsive eructations after eating fat food or milk; heartburn; burning ascending from the stomach; deficient appetite; *no appetite for bread; excessive hunger at noon and in the evening; canine hunger*, with satiety after eating but little; great desire for bitter things; aversion to fat food; constant thirst; sweat in the face when eating; *eructation after eating;* heartburn after eating; *nausea* after eating; *desire to vomit*, with twisting sensation at the stomach; desire to vomit, followed by vomiting of sour food; *vomiting of food; heaviness at the stomach;* pressure at the stomach, in the morning; pressure at the stomach, with nausea and sudden prostration of strength; pressure at the pit of the stomach; spasm of the stomach; pain at the pit of the stomach; swelling at the pit of the stomach, with smarting pain when pressing upon it with the hand; *griping pain at the pit of the stomach;* shocks in the pit of the stomach; cramp in the diaphragm when stooping; stitches in the hepatic region; stitches under the left elbow; pain in the region of the spleen; pressive pain in the left side of the hypogastrium; *swelling of the abdomen;* bloating of the bowels; pain in the left side of the abdomen; *cutting pain in the day time; shifting of flatulence;* borborygmi; *gurgling* in the abdomen; constipation every other day; chronic constipation; *difficult stool,* with tearing and stitching pain at the anus and rectum; smarting and beating in the rectum; piles; pain at the hæmorrhoidal protrusion; involuntary discharge of urine when walking, coughing, sneezing; *emission of urine, at night;* discharge of mucus from the male urethra; blennorrhœa; excessive excitation of the private parts; excessive desire for an embrace; *impotence; the menses last too long; profuse menses; too early menses;* retarded menses; *retarded and scanty menses;* headache before, during and after the menses; ill-humor before the menses; *melancholy before the menses;* sadness at the appearance of the menses; *itching at the vulva;* aversion to sexual intercourse in the female; *leucorrhœa;* acrid leucorrhœa.

"*Stoppage of the nostrils; stuffing of the nose; dryness of the nose;* coryza and sneezing; incomplete sneezing; *hoarseness;* phlegm on the chest, with cough; rattling in the chest; cough every morning; cough with tickling, when walking, drawing a long breath; chronic hacking cough; spasmodic cough in the evening, in bed; headache when coughing, as if the forehead would split; *asthma* during a rapid walk; asthma when attending to manual labor; embarrassed respiration, in the evening, in bed; oppression on the chest; tensive pain in the chest; stitches in the chest when coughing and drawing a long breath; *beating of the heart,* with anxiety; beating of the heart whenever the body is moved; stitches in the breast; stitches in the hips and sacrum; cutting pain in the sacrum; contusive, paralytic pain in the sacrum; pulling pressure in the back; tensive pain in the back; lassitude in the back: pressure at the nape of the neck; goïtre; crusts in the axilla; paralytic heaviness in the arm; lassitude in the arms; digging pain in the arm; stitches in the wrist-joint; *numbness and formication in the fingers;* luxation-pain in the hip; pulling pain in the legs; *painful contraction of the hamstrings;* tetters in the bends of the knees; lassitude in the knees and calves; smarting pain at the ankle when touching it and pressing the foot to the ground; heaviness in the feet; burning at the feet; swelling of the feet; pressive pulling in the extremities; weariness after talking; anger is followed by unpleasant consequences; sour food is hurtful; *bread is hurtful;* disposition to straining or spraining a part; varices; corns; *emaciation;* disposition to take cold; physical prostration; laziness on rising in the morning; *lassitude;* hysterical lassitude; drowsiness in the day-time; *sleep full of dreams; disturbing dreams*, with tears; waking at night, with inability to fall asleep again for hours; thirst at night; pain in the back, at night; nervous trembling, at night; discharge of urine, every hour of the night; internal chilliness, frequently; restlessness with shuddering; *deficiency of vital heat;* cold hands and feet; sweat in walking; sudden and profuse sweat during motion; morning-sweat; alteration of the fever and ague by abuse of quinine."

Smelling of nitric ether is, according to Hahnemann, the surest means of neutralising the effects of salt.

Antimonium crudum, *crude antimony, protosulphuret of antimony.* This mineral exists in great abundance in nature; it is the principal constituent of the gangue from which the metallic antimony is extracted. It is of a dark blueish-gray color, crystallises in long needles that are united in compact masses, and is less shining, lighter and weaker than antimony. Fire decomposes it by disengaging from it sulphurous vapors, and reducing it to the condition of an oxyde. With water, it forms a fire-colored hydrate.

It is this native sulphuret that was formerly employed in

medicine under the name of antimony. But, inasmuch as it is only imperfectly purified by melting, (for after melting it twice, traces of arsenic are still found in it,) it is best to use for medicinal purposes, the artificial protosulphuret of antimony, which is obtained directly, by melting together two parts and a-half of antimony, and one of sulphur.

Empirical applications.—Few drugs have made as much noise in the medical world as antimony. It was known in the remotest antiquity. Hippocrates, Galenus, Plinius and Dioscorides mention it;[1] Basile-Valentin, ranks it among the heroic drugs[2] in the fifteenth century.

From the arcana of Paracelsus, it was afterwards transferred into common use as an almost universal panacea, and, during the fifteenth and sixteenth centuries, became the object of such violent disputes among doctors, that parliament was obliged to interfere, and to interdict the use of this drug.

This interdiction remained in force from the year 1566, until the 16th of April, 1666, when it was revoked at the instance of the Medical Faculty of Paris, one hundred and two members of which, at last united to give their assent to the use of antimonial preparations.[3]

[1] Plinius, vol. XXXIII., c. 6, calls it stibium, Dioscorides describes its properties and calls it Stimmi. Hippocrates and Dioscorides ascribed to it astringent, desiccative properties, etc., and employed it only externally, especially in chronic ophthalmia.

[2] Basile Valentin is said to have discovered metallic antimony, or to be the first who separated it from its native sulphur.

[3] See these decrees in *Lettres de Gui-Patin,* new ed., by Dr. J. H. Reveillé-Parise, Paris, 1846, vol. I., p. 191; vol. III., p. 609. This was the period of *la Fronde.* The discussion concerning crude antimony was so vehement, that it diverted public attention from the grave political events of the time. One of the most vehement opponents of this drug was the celebrated Gui-Patin, distinguished by the force of his style, as well as by his erudition and bitterness; I judge so at least from his Lettres, some of which are models of elegance and sound sense, but all of which reveal a bitter and fierce disposition, and are filled with statements dictated by blind passion, and fanatical adherence to dogmatism and preconceived theories. Gui-Patin treats with equal violence Mazarin, the partisans of antimony and the immortal Van Helmont, whom he calls, in one of his letters, a "*méchant pendard*

It is to be remarked, that the idle and noisy discussions which were carried on at this period on the subject of antimony, did not throw any light on the therapeutic properties of this drug. The only result was, that it was registered as a purgative in the Codex of 1677. At a later period, it was transformed into a *stomach-strengthening* drug, a *sudorific, a cleansing medicine, a dissolvent,* and lastly, an *emetic,* although the chemical physiologists of our time, only account for the power which this sulphuret possesses, of exciting vomiting, upon the ground that the crude antimony is decomposed by the gastric fluids.

Crude antimony has been lauded in *scrofula and glandular obstructions, intermittent fevers, convulsions,* certain *chronic affections of the skin,* such as *favus, lichen, scald-head, ulcers in the face, metastatic ophthalmia, bronchial catarrh, gastric derangement, colic, dropsy, worm-affections, dysentery, gonorrhœa,* etc.[1] A number of authors, among whom I may mention Kunckel, Hermann and Fr. Hoffmann,[2] consider crude antimony an heroic remedy for *rheumatic pains* and *gout.*

According to Mérat and Delens, crude antimony is endowed with a faculty of making people fat; this, at least, is the effect which they say it produces in animals, especially swine, which it cures of the measles. The same authors relate, without guaranteeing the correctness of their statement, that Kunckel cured himself of marasmus which had reached the highest point of development, by means of the tablets that bear his name, and of which the sulphuret of antimony constitutes the principal ingredient.[3] Modern allœopaths have abandoned the use of crude antimony almost completely.[4]

flammand," who died crazy for having refused "to allow himself to be bled." It is not astonishing that such a man who was unjust towards every thing that did not emanate from him, should have overlooked the good effects of antimony amid the frightful evils which were undoubtedly inflicted with it at that period.

[1] Gmelin, appar. med., vol. I., p. 177.

[2] Medic. ration. system., vol. IV., part 2, p. 442.

[3] *Dict. de mat. méd.*, vol. I., p. 343.

[4] See the pathog. of crude antimony in Hahnemann's *Chronic Diseases*, Vol. I.

Homœopathic applications.—Antimony is particularly indicated by the following symptoms.

Loathing of life; sadness, with weeping and impressibility; rush of blood to the head; gnawing pain on the top of the head, apparently in the periosteum; fatiguing itching of the head, with falling off of the hair; *redness and inflammation of the eyelids; chronic blepharophthalmia,* (of children;) crusts and cracks of the nostrils; *suppurating and long-lasting eruption on the cheeks;* cracks at the corners of the mouth; *gnawing pain in the carious teeth,* after every meal; loss of appetite, for a long time; habitual sensation in the stomach, as if over-loaded; *eructations, tasting of the ingesta; loathing, nausea and desire to vomit;* cutting colic, with loss of appetite; *bread and pastry particularly occasion nausea and cutting colic;* aggravation of gastric symptoms by wine, even when diluted with water; *constant discharge of flatulence by the mouth and rectum, which is reproduced as soon as discharged, for years;* alternate diarrhœa and constipation; hard, difficult stool; constant secretion of a yellowish-white mucus at the anus; frequent and profuse emission of urine; chronic catarrh of the bladder.

Stuffing of the nose; *chronic angina,* with sensation as if a foreign body had lodged in the throat, which gives rise to a constant desire of swallowing empty; cough and oppression on the chest; rheumatic pains at the nape of the neck and loins; painful inflammation of the tendons, elbow, with intense redness, and contraction of the arm; *arthritic pains in the fingers;* numbness of the legs during rest and while sitting; pulling pains in the lower limbs; *callosities at the soles of the feet;* sensitiveness to cold; quotidian or tertian intermittent fever, with loathing, nausea, vomiting, cutting in the bowels and diarrhœa; obesity; emaciation.

Hep. sulph., Calc. and *Merc. sol.* are said to antidote *Antim. crud.*

Viola tricolor, *pansy.*—This drug, an incomplete pathogenesis of which has been published in Stapf's Archives, and republished in Jahr's Manual, is as yet little known to homœopathic physicians. I have only used it empirically, but the results which I have obtained with this drug, show that it is analogous in its general action to lycop., and that it certainly deserves to have its physiological properties more carefully investigated.

The ancient physicians used pansy a good deal in *asthma* and *epilepsy*, with occasional success; in these diseases its virtues are uncertain, *but in chronic and obstinate cutaneous diseases*, it was recommended as very efficacious.[1]

The use of this drug had been completely abandoned, when a physician of the past century, Starck, of Mentz, undertook to restore it.[2] Some years after, Haase published a series of observations on the therapeutic effects of pansy, completely justifying the views of Starck.[3] Other physicians, such as Melzer, Veckoskrift and Murray,[4] added their observations to those of Starck and Haase.

The knowledge which these various practitioners had of the curative virtues of pansy, was limited to the following facts: 1st, that a decoction of its recent stem stimulated the intestinal functions, especially in children, and even excited nausea;[5] 2d, that this same stem, when dry and pulverised, was a *cathartic*, capable of exciting nausea in some persons, but never any real vomiting, according to Haase; 3d, and lastly, that, as a decoction, or in powder form, it communicated to the urine of patients who used it, a penetrating and disagreeable odor, like that of cat's urine. In regard to the pathological conditions of pansy, all physicians agree in regard to them, except Mursinna, Achermann, Henning, and some others quoted by Murray, who deny to pansy all medicinal virtues with about the same show of reason that Cullen denied to sulphur the medicinal properties that all nations and ages

[1] See Matthiolus, *Comment. in Diosc.*, p. 822.—Fuchsius, *histor. stirp.*, p. 804.—Bauhin, *hist. plant.*, vol. III., p. 545, etc.

[2] De crusta lactea infant., ejusdemque remed. dissert., Mœn. 1779.

[3] Specim. inaugur. de viol. tricol., in 4to., 1782.

[4] Appar. Med., vol. VI., p. 33.

[5] Bergius, Mat. Med., p. 709.

have conceded to it. Pansy has been found wonderfully efficacious in the following affections: *Milk-crust in children at the breast, recently weaned,* (Starck, Haase, and most practitioners of their time;) *milk-crust,* with violent cough and excessive oppression, (Haase, *op. cit.*, observ. 4;) *impetigo of the hairy scalp and face,* in children of seven years, and even in adult females, (*id.*, observ. 1, 4, 12, 13 and 21;) *acne rosacea at the chin,* (id. id., observ. 12;) *favus and various exanthemata of the hairy scalp,* such as *serpiginous crusts,* etc., in children and adults, with swelling and induration of the cervical glands, etc., (Murray, Veckoskrift and Melzer, quoted by Murray;) *large boils* all over the body, in a scrofulous child, (Haase, *loc. cit.*, obs. 4;) *pustulous and ichorous exanthems at the feet,* (id. id., obs. 17;) *squammous spots on the skin,* (id. id., obs. 19;) *rheumatism* and *gout,* (id. id., obs. 8 and 9;) *articular rheumatism, with itch-like eruption*[1] *around the joints,* (id. obs. 9;) *impetiginous exanthem at the forehead,* consequent on suppression of gonorrhœa by astringents, in a man of twenty years, (id. id., obs. 10;) induration of a testicle, consequent on a gonorrhœa, by applying the leaves of pansy boiled in milk, (id. id., p. 32;) *epilepsy,* in a child of seven months (id. id., obs. 15.) According to Murray, pansy does no good in *lichen,* but it increases the itching in this disease;[2] but according to the same author, it is almost always useful, internally and externally, in *ichorous ulcers,* with violent itching.

In Russia a decoction of pansy is a popular remedy for *scrofula.* In 1805, Schlegel, of Moscow, asserted having used it with great effect in *syphilitic affections,* especially *venereal ulcers.*[3] In 1813, Fauvergne prescribed it for a young girl who was subject to nervous paroxysms, which he thought had been caused by the suppression of milk-crust, and whom he cured by this means. Such facts assuredly render a complete pathogenesis of *viola tr.* desirable.

[1] I have already stated in a previous part of this work, that, formerly, authors designated by the name *itch,* diseases which would be termed quite differently now-a-days.

[2] *Loc. Cit.*, p. 35.

[3] *Journn. univ. des sc. méd.*, vol. XIV., p. 264.

GROUP XIV.

TYPE: ZINCUM METALLICUM.

ANALOGUES: PLUMBUM.
SAMBUCUS NIGRA.
DROSERA ROTUNDIFOLIA.
FERRUM METALLICUM.
CORROSIVUS.
COLCHICUM AUTUMNALE.
ARSENICUM ALBUM.
NITRI ACIDUM.
MERCURIUS.
PLATINA.[1]

COMMON CHARACTERISTICS.

APART from the properties which are peculiar to such drugs of this group, as have already been classified, or have to be studied further on, it seems to me that their physiological action as well as the nature of the diseases for which they have been given with the best effect, show, that they act especially on the nervous system, and more particularly on the plexuses of the chest and lower abdomen, and likewise on the larger trunks and nervous branches which impart mobility and sensibility to the organs of locomotion. It is a characteristic feature of these drugs, to be able to excite the most acute pains or the most violent derangements in the nervous functions, without the other organic functions being at all sensibly altered. All affect likewise the circulation in a marked manner. Nothing is more frequent than to see *zinc* and its analogues moderate or accelerate the beats of the heart; but, after all, this kind of derangement is only a secondary effect of the drugs of this group, and then only in case the nervous network, which, so to say, envelopes the heart, happens to be the elective seat of their action. As a general rule, the diseases which they call forth, and which they are, for this reason, capable of curing, are diseases without fever, unless they come under the category of what are generally termed *nervous fevers*.

[1] *Menyanthes* ought perhaps to be added to this list.

The *Zincum*-group is related to the *Arnica*-group; but it differs from the latter in this, that the diseases to which it corresponds do not arise from mechanical causes.[1] Nevertheless, *zincum* and its analogues are frequently indicated, (especially in *neuralgia* and the so termed *rheumatic pains*,) after the drugs of the *Arnica*-group. Zincum, for instance, is frequently useful after *Spigelia; Colchicum* after *Arnica* or *Rhus; Mercurius corrosivus* likewise after *Rhus*, (less frequently after *Arnica*,) particularly in *chronic rheumatism and gout*, with nodosities of the joints, etc. Let me add, that in the nervous affections of the heart and of the air-passages, such as *whooping-cough*, *suffocative catarrh*, etc., *arnica* and its analogues have frequently shown a remarkable efficacy, which serves to corroborate my statements concerning the relations existing between the *Zincum* and *Arnica*-groups.

The similarities existing between the drugs of the zincum-group themselves, must become evident to any one who will take the trouble to study them with becoming attention.

CORRESPONDING DISEASES.

Nervous derangements of the viscera, (epilepsy, asthma, whooping-cough, angina pectoris, hysteria, nymphomania, etc.)—Amaurosis.—Neuralgia of the head.—Neuralgia of the trunk and extremities.—Chorea.—Chronic rheumatism.—Chronic gout.—Distortion of joints by soft tumors or tophi.—Quotidian intermittent fever, etc.

Zincum, *zinc*.—A solid metal, of a blueish-white color, scaly, ductile, having a feeble, but perceptible odor and taste, changeable in the air, especially in damp air, where it oxydises, and loses its lustre in consequence; it is very brittle, and can be easily pulverised at a temperature of 250° centigr.; it fuses at 360°, beyond which, it volatilises; when melted and very hot, it burns in the open air with a shining flame of a bright violet color, and spreading in the air, small light flakes of the oxyde of zinc (the *lana philosophica* of the

[1] It does not seem clear to me why these drugs should be excluded from the treatment of purely surgical diseases. It will be seen further on that I have employed *Colchicum* in *burns* with the greatest success.

ancient chemists); it is very common in nature, but it is generally found only in the shape of an oxyde, sulphuret, sulphate, carbonate, silicate, etc., and is much used in the arts.[1] The ancients do not seem to have known metallic zinc. It is said, that it was first discovered in the thirteenth century, and mentioned under the name of Marcassite of gold; Paracelsus afterwards gave it its present name.[2]

Empirical applications.—Until Hahnemann, this metal was scarcely used at all in medicine. At most, a few practitioners employed it as a mechanical means for tænia, by making their patients swallow small shot made of zinc. But if zinc was not considered a drug, properly speaking, the *oxyde*, (*flowers of zinc*, *nihil album* of the alchimists,) and the salts of zinc were. Perhaps it would be too great a stretch of analogy to suppose that the medicinal properties of the salts are all contained in the metallic zinc. But the analogy between the empirical applications of the oxyde, and those which the pure provings of the metallic zinc, authorize us to make, is so striking, that it almost borders on identity.[3] A few facts from the precious work of Gmelin, show us in what diseases the oxyde has been used with success.[4] Here is a synopsis of its empirical use.

Externally; 1st, *for chancrous and fetid ulcers*, (Glauber, Justamond); 2d, *inveterate ulcers on the legs*, (Theden, Bell); 3d, for *rhagades of the lips and nipples*, (Crell); 4th, *soreness of children*, caused by the contact of urine, (Rosenstein); 5th, *soreness of the sacral region*, from lying on it for a long time, (Glauber); 6th, *chronic ophthalmia*, (Glauber, Gaubius, Monro, de Haën, Lommer); 7th, for certain *derangements of sight*, (Van Swieten). After the publication of the apparatus medic., the flowers of zinc were used for *zona* and *confluent*

[1] See Memoir on *white-zink paint*, by Dr. Bouchat, in the *Annales d'hygiène*, Paris, 1852, vol. XLVII., p. 5, etc.

[2] Mérat and Delens, op. cit., vol. VI., p. 990.

[3] The pathogenesis of the oxyde, published in Jahr's Manual, does not show any great difference between the pure effects of zink and those of the oxyde.

[4] *Appar. Medic.*, part 2d., vol. I., p. 279 and foll.

small-pox, to prevent the suppuration and ulceration of the pustules;[1] lastly, it has been used in *gonorrhœa* as an astringent, although the sulphate is generally preferred for this disease.

Internally, the oxyde of zinc has been used for many diseases, sometimes with great success, especially for the following: *Nervous fevers; intermittent fevers; typhus with spasms; nervous excitement and spasms, in eruptive fevers,* such as *variola and scarlatina; convulsions of children,* either in consequence of difficult teething, or fright, or worms in the bowels; *epilepsy* of adults, but particularly of children; *hysterical spasms and various nervous derangements which were sometimes very violent,* (Gmelin says, *atrocissimæ convulsione,*) in young girls caused by a fright; *palpitation* of the heart, with *difficulty of speaking and swallowing; spasmodic cough; asthma; whooping-cough; facial neuralgia; arthritic pain in the joints; tetanus.* Hirschel, Lieutaud, Pallas, Crell, Delaroche, Odier, Munsen, Nicolaï, and many others, are the principal physicians, quoted by Gmelin, who have performed the best cures with the oxyde of zinc in the above-mentioned maladies. It is true, that, according to Rahlwes, Duroi, Herz and Cullen, the oxyde has been given without any effect in the above-mentioned affections. But this apparent contradiction simply shows the looseness of allœopathic diagnosis, and the unreliability of the statements of allœopathic physicians, who content themselves with naming the disease, without attaching any definite meaning to the appellation.

Be this as it may, in consequence of the contradictory statements concerning the virtues of the oxyde of zinc, to which Glauber attributed, not without reason, emetic, cathartic and sudorific properties, that have been denied to it since,[2] it is now-a-days *an antispasmodic agent* of a doubtful character. This, at any rate, is the statement of Trousseau and Pidoux, who scarcely devote a page to this great agent.[3]

[1] Mérat and Delens, *loc. cit.* [2] Gmelin, *loc. cit.*

[3] See Hahnemann's pathogenesis of Zink, *Chronic Diseases*, vol. III., and Trousseau and Pidoux's traité de thérap., vol. II., p. 271.

Homœopathic applications.—According to Hahnemann, zinc cures the following symptoms:—

"No desire to work or walk; thoughts about death; weakness of memory; constant headache; dizziness; smarting pain in the head; buzzing in the head; pain at the hairy scalp; baldness; dryness of the eyes; amaurosis with contraction of the pupils; paralysis and falling of the eyelids; buzzing in the ears; looseness of the teeth; sensitiveness of the teeth when eating; smarting toothache; salt taste in the mouth; heaviness at the stomach, with nausea, after eating bread; tensive pain in the sides of the abdomen; inguinal hernia; constipation; soft and liquid stools; involuntary stools; itching at the anus; retention of urine at the moment when it is to be passed; involuntary discharge of urine while walking; inability to retain the urine, when coughing, sneezing or walking; prolonged erections in the night; too sudden ejaculation of the semen during an embrace; premature menses; pain during the menses; swelling of the abdomen during the menses; leucorrhœa. Coryza; cough; tensive pain in the sternum; beating of the heart; shocks of the heart that cut off the breathing; pain in the loins; pain in the back; old rheumatism in the arm; sense of dryness in the hands, in the morning; numbness in the fingers, in the morning on rising; stiffness of the tarsal joint, after sitting; painful chilblains at the feet; insensibility of the body; sense of coldness in the bones; ganglion; drowsiness in the morning; desire to sleep after dinner; reveries at night; frightful dreams; talking and shrieking during sleep; tendency to sweat in the day-time; night-sweat."

It seems to me that these morbid conditions are not described with the same distinction and precision that characterized the cases in which the oxyde of zinc is known to have acted with good effect. I have employed, with the best results, the metallic zinc in cases for which the oxyde used to be recommended, especially in nervous affections of the heart, air-passages, and the organs of locomotion, in chronic spasms, and in various kinds of obstinate nervous derangements with tearing or burning pains.[1] I have recommended it, after the example of Odier in Gmelin, (*loc. cit.*) at the commencement of *variola*, as a means of preventing the eruption; several of my colleagues have used it under such circumstances with success.

The neuralgic or arthritic pains, to which zinc corresponds, seem to have their seat, most generally, in the sub-cutaneous nervous branches, or round the joints, (especially the elbow-joints;) or, finally, in the cavity of the long bones. They are more perceptibly felt during rest than during motion.

Wine, coffee, chamomilla and the vomic-nut aggravate the effects of zinc. I happen to know that *lobelia inflata* moderates them very much.

Plumbum. See page 125.

Colchicum autumnale, *meadow-saffron.* Genus colchicum, family colchicaceæ. This plant, which is very common in damp meadows, is known by its large, dark-green, smooth, fleshy, lanceolate leaves; by its flowers, which are of a pale rose-color, generally solitary, forming long tubes, and coming out in the fall only for a day or two. The root of the meadow-saffron is a bulb of the thickness of a hen's egg; it is reproduced every year. Externally it is of a red-brown, internally of a white color. This bulb, which is the only part of the plant that is used in medicine, is almost inodorous; but it has a bitter, acrid, warm taste, and benumbs the tongue. Mélandri and Moretti were the first who discovered in it a peculiar extractive principle which Messrs. Pelletier and Caventou have recognized as being analogous to the extractive principle contained in the veratrum and sabadilla, and which they term *veratrine.* It appears that in the root of colchicum this alkaloïd exists in combination with gallic acid, with which it forms a soluble gallate, so that this bulb, which is so hurtful when it is first gathered and even after it is dried in an oven, is changed, by being immersed into boiling water for a suffi-

[1] See my treatise *on the diseases of children*, p. 192.

cient length of time, to an eatable fecula resembling that of wheat.[1] In its natural state colchicum is a poison, alike deleterious to herbivorous and carnivorous animals. Herds do not touch it in the meadows, and, if the animals eat it in stables, dried and mixed up with other food, they never fail to be incommoded by it. Tympanitis, hæmorrhage from the bowels, inflammation and gangrene of the lesser intestines, have been known, from post-mortem examinations, to precede death in such cases.[2] The dogs upon which Stœrck,[3] Roques,[4] and E. Home,[5] made experiments with colchicum, in very large doses it is true, (from 8 to 12 grammes of the root,) perished, all of them in 24 hours. Trembling of the limbs; spasms of the abdominal muscles, with retraction of the pit of the stomach; unceasing vomiting; extremely frequent alvine evacuations; profuse discharges of urine, and finally a quiet death, which did not seem to be preceded by any considerable derangement of the cerebral functions; these were the symptoms which were almost uniformly observed by these three provers. Similar phenomena have generally been produced in cases of poisoning of men, except that, in such cases, frightful pains, spasms, convulsions, tetanus, preceded death, although the consciousness and understanding remained undisturbed to the end.[6]

Empirical applications.—Wolffgang Wedel, a German physician of the eighteenth century, speaks of the root of colchicum as being endowed with wonderful prophylactic virtues against epidemic diseases, such as the plague, dysentery, eruptive and malignant fevers. He recommends that, during the prevalence of such an epidemic, a root be worn, tied in a little bag, round the neck.[7] Christ. Wilhelm, a physician of the same period, shares this opinion so far as

[1] Fée says that in Carniola, (Austria,) the bulbs of Colchicum are eaten without any ill effects, (*Cours d'histoire naturelle pharm.*, vol. I., p. 315.)

[2] Giacomini, *traité de thérap.*, p. 184.

[3] *Libel. de rad. colch. aut.*

[4] *Phys. graph. med.*, vol. I., p. 88.

[5] Méret and Delens, *oper. cit.*, vol. II., p. 358.

[6] See in Roth's *mat. med. pur.*, the toxicological observations of Caffé, Faraday, etc.

[7] *Comm. de colch. venen. et alexipharm.*, 1718.

the plague is concerned. But, according to this latter writer, the root has to be made into a plaster, and be worn at the anus; in this form only does it show all its efficiency as a prophylactic; (a strange mode of application, which he says was revealed to him in a dream.)[1] Hasenet tells us, that he and several other physicians, who were not too proud to use the same precaution, were saved from a murderous epidemic fever by wearing a bulb of the colchicum suspended round their necks on their bare chests.[2] Murray looks upon all such statements, although made in good faith, as childish superstition, and he merely adds: "*Si quid in hisce effecerit radix, vix alia ratione quam animam erigendo fiducia in imbelle auxilium profita profuit. Metus enim vim in contigiis fovendis, quis nesciat.*"[3] So far as we are concerned, knowing that, in epidemic diseases, the nervous system, upon which the colchicum exercises such a marked action, is always first affected, we are strongly reminded by these apparently strange and fanciful conjectures of the German physicians of the prophylactic virtues of zinc in variola, the reality of which we have become convinced of by experience . . . *nihil contemnere*, says the father of medicine.

Stoerck, who was one of the first that experimented with colchicum on dogs, and introduced it in the school of Vienna, recommended it for *passive dropsy*, doubtless for no other reason than because he had seen it produce serous stools and diuresis. Stoerck and his disciples effected cures with colchicum in cases where squills had failed, namely, *anasarca* of the extremities and head; *ascites* consequent on intermittent and *eruptive* fevers; *hydrothorax*. All the dropsical patients that were cured by Stoerck or the physicians of his school, appear to have suffered with some kind of derangement of the chest, such as *chronic cough*, with expectoration; habitual *dyspnœa*, with or without palpitation of the heart; *asthma* of a distinct character. It follows, however, from

[1] Murray, *appar. medic.*, vol. V., p. 203.
[2] *Id. Id.*
[3] *Id. Id.*

Stoerck's own observations, that colchicum, in the manner he employed it, did not cure dropsy by virtue of a specific action on the heart or air-passages, for Stoerck relates the case of a young girl who was affected with *ulcerative phthisis* and *ascites;* the latter was cured, but the former remained unchanged.

Murray, after having named the physicians who pretend to have cured dropsy with colchicum after the example of Stoerck, then quotes a not less numerous list of physicians, who have failed in curing the same disease with this drug. But as we do not belong to the specific school, we do not consider it worth our while to mention these facts in detail.

In the last forty years colchicum has lost a good deal of its influence with alloeopathic physicians. As an *hydragogue* it has been superseded by gummi gutta, and the other drastics; as a *diuretic* by *squills*, *digitalis*, etc. Now-a-days, it is used as the principal specific for gout. J. Want and Everard Home, in England; Locker and Balber in Switzerland, and Lobstein, in France, have done the most to give it this reputation, which, for that matter, it deserves as much as quinine deserves to be looked upon as a specific for fever and ague. It is perfectly true, that the *wine of colchicum*, even when administered in feeble (alloeopathic) doses, has arrested paroxysms of *acute gout*, reduced *arthritic swellings*, and has resolved and scattered *articular nodosities*.[1] The authors of the *Dictionaire universel de Matière Médicale*, declare, indeed, that it is not correct to say, that "there is no remedy for gout, etc., that colchicum ought to be employed more and more and more against this cruel disease,[2] etc." Alas, what gouty patient has not taken colchicum once in his life-time! But we will not be unjust, and although we do say, that colchicum is far from curing every case of gout, yet it does cure a great many.

Colchicum has been found useful in various diseases which do not seem to be related to gout, apparently at least. Apart

[1] Kunh, *dissert. sur les colchiacées*, (thèse de Strasburg, 1827, p. 25.)

[2] Vol. II., p. 360.

from acute and chronic *articular rheumatism*, which is not exactly the gout, these diseases are: *ophthalmia*,[1] *chorea*,[2] *hysteria*,[3] various kinds of *neuralgia*, of the most obstinate kind,[4] *contractions* or rather a *contracted* condition of the uterus,[5] *leucorrhœa*,[6] *prurigo*,[7] and *erysipelas*,[8] for most of which affections the oxide of zinc used to be praised formerly.

Homœopathic applications. The proving of colchicum, which is as yet very incomplete, justifies most of the empirical uses of colchicum, without, however, shedding any great light upon them.[9] This pathogenesis contains, nevertheless, most of the morbid effects of colchicum, and, of course, shows what diseases it is capable of curing. The *arthritic pains* to which it corresponds, are generally *tearing*. In warm weather they are principally felt at the surface of the body; as the air grows cooler these pains seem to penetrate the deeper tissues and bones. Noise, light, contact and mental labor aggravate these pains like those of arnica, which I have often found indicated previous to giving *colchicum*. I have found this remedy useful after rhus, and, in some cases, from the first, for engorgements of the subcutaneous glands, especially on the neck, on which colchicum exercises a very marked action. It is, therefore, one of the principal remedies for rheumatism of the neck brought on by a cold or a twist or strain, (*torticollis*.) I have seen it succeed in a few very severe cases of this kind, where the pains in the neck were complicated with

[1] *Révue Méd.*, vol. III., p. 131.

[2] *Bibliot. Méd.*, vol. LVIII., p. 392.

[3] *Id.*, vol., LX., p. 124.

[4] *Gaz. Méd.*, 8th January, 1833.

[5] Filiatre sebario, mai, 1643.

[6] *Journ. de chim. méd.*, 1835, p. 29.

[7] *Archives génév. de méd.*, vol. XVI., p. 290.

[8] In erysipelas colchicum acts like rhus tox., with which drug it has more than one point of contact. A saying which is current in my native place, has even induced me, in one case, to use it externally (15th atten. diluted with a quantity of water, and employed as a wash for some minutes at a time, several times a day,) in a case of burn at the forehead, after *Arnica* and *Rhus*. The result was extraordinary and most satisfactory. The cicatrisation which had remained stationary for some weeks, in spite of Arnica and Rhus, took place in a few days.

[9] See its pathogenesis in Roth's Mat. Med., vol. II., p. 290.

paroxysms of anguish, dyspnœa, beating of the heart, especially at night. Whenever one of the diseases mentioned at the commencement of this group, is named, the pathogenesis of colchicum should be carefully studied, for it has shades of analogy with every member of this group.

Colchicum is antidoted by camphor; it antidotes thuya and all its analogues.

Sambucus nigra, *elder.*—Genus *sambucus,* family caprifoliaceæ, class pentandria monogynia. This tree is very common in France and almost every part of Europe, where it is generally grown for the purpose of forming and supporting the hedges. It prefers good, rather damp soil, and attains a height of from 20 to 25 feet. Its blossoms, the berries which grow out of them, the second bark of its stems and its root, are endowed with more or less toxical properties. Beasts and even caterpillars avoid its leaves. Its berries have destroyed chickens and even peacocks. The juice of its leaves, in dogs, has caused vomiting and diarrhœa. There are several cases of poisoning by elder on record in some authors,[1] with the following symptoms: vomiting, serous diarrhœa, great weakness, sweat (especially at the forehead,) paleness, altered features, a sort of coma (on the third day,) and finally considerable emaciation.

Empirical applications.—Allœopathic physicians have used one after the other and separately, the flowers of elder, the berries, and also the second bark of its stems. The bark was praised as a *hydragogue,* first by Hippocrates, and afterwards by Sydenham and Boerhaave. Hippocrates recommends the *berries* in some *uterine affections.* The flowers, as is well known by every body, possess *sudorific* properties.[2] Cullen seems the only one of old school physicians who pronounces them inert.[3] "They enjoy," say Mérat and Delens, "an universal reputation as sudorifics. They are given in the

[1] Bartholin, *Act. Hafn.*, vol. I., p. 164. *Ephem. nat. cur.* déc. II., year 9, p. 48, etc.

[2] Murray, *appar. med.*, vol. IV., p. 19.

[3] *Mat. Med.*, vol. II., p. 559.

shape of an infusion sweetened with honey or sugar, in all cases where sweat is to be excited, especially in cutaneous eruptions that come out slowly, such as measles, variola and other exanthems, in diseases consequent upon the suppression of sweat, such as rheumatism, gout, neuralgia, etc. This infusion is also prescribed to prevent the development of certain morbid conditions, such as coryza, influenza, catarrh, angina, and even pleurisy, peripneumonia, etc. It is given with still better effect in suppression of cutaneous eruptions, in the last period of phlegmasiæ of the mucous membranes, etc.

"But it is principally when dried that they cause sweat, and exercise a remedial action upon the surface of the body: the recent flowers retain some of the purgative and vomiting properties of the bark and leaves. The flowers are also used as fomentations, either entire or tied up in bags, and are applied to cold swellings, local pains, œdematous parts, etc., for the purpose of scattering and dissolving the tumors."[1] Fomentations with the flowers of elder have also been praised, and not without a show of reason, for *erysipelas*, *acute inflammation*, *acute rheumatism*, *gout*,[2] and also for *uterine cutting pains* and *spasms of the bladder*. The facts that bear upon these last symptoms are, however, scarce, and not very conclusive.

Homœopathic applications.[3] The pathogenesis of Sambucus is still more incomplete than that of colchicum. From experiments on myself and others I feel able, however, to offer a few general hints concerning the therapeutic uses of this agent.

The mother-tincture of Sambucus, which is used in homœopathic practice, probably contains all the medicinal properties of the plant, it being made of the flowers and leaves together. This preparation develops on a healthy person several symptoms resembling those of ipecac. For this reason I stated above that Sambucus ought perhaps to be added to the

[1] *Dict. univ. de mat. méd.*, vol. VI., p. 198.

[2] Quarin, *math. medendi inf.*, p. 219.

[3] Pathogenesis of Sambucus in Roth's Mat. Med. Pura, vol. I., p. 259.

ipecac. group, although it should be placed at the end of it. Upon the whole, however, it is more nearly related to *Colchicum* than to *Ipecac.*

According to my own observations, Sambucus is most suitable to weakly and nervous children that perspire readily, are sensitive to currents of air, liable to stoppage of the nose, suffocative angina (*spurious croup*) and to œdema of the scrotum. Among adults, it is particularly suitable to bilious, lymphatico-nervous individuals, pale, thin, tall and slender, subject to night-sweats with adypsia, and to rheumatism, with a frequent and thin pulse, and constitutionally predisposed for dropsy, or rather œdema of the extremities. The rheumatic or neuralgic pains which it cures, are seated in the arms, especially the elbows, and in the anterior surface of the fore arms, and at the ends of the fingers rather than in the lower extremities. These pains, which are of a burning character at the elbows, benumbing at the forearms, and cutting at the ends of the fingers, follow the tract of nerves, are worse during rest and towards eleven o'clock in the evening. Continual motion of the affected part, dissipates them momentarily; but pressure does not quiet them much. Cold, or excessive eating and drinking excites them most readily: artificial heat has no effect of any kind upon them. When very acute, or after having lasted for a time, they are accompanied with partial, circumscribed and indolent infiltrations of the skin, whence result resisting, rose-colored, flat and itching swellings at the wrist-joint, forearm, and sometimes at the scrotum, buttocks, etc. I have frequently removed such a train of symptoms with *Sambucus* in one or two days.

As regards the efficiency of this drug in *ascites*, it seems to me very dubious, although I am not disposed to deny it altogether. I have never seen it act favorably in this disease, although I have tried it in many cases. In a case of *albuminuria* with œdema of the ankles and scrotum, *Sambucus* seemed to produce a disagreeable complication of symptoms, such as suffocation and pains in the arms, without improving any of the former symptoms. In some cases

Sambucus can be advantageously alternated with *Zinc.* and *Colch. Camph.* seems to be its antidote. But the action of Sambucus is so short, that we need not trouble ourselves much about antidotes.

Arsenicum Album. See page 193.

Drosera Rotundifolia, *sun-dew.* Genus *drosera*, ranged by Jussieu among the family of the Capparideæ, but which has since been made a particular family of plants, the Drosereæ, of the class pentandria trigynia.

Drosera is a small annual plant, very common around Paris. It has no stems, leaves radical, covered with glandular down or hairs, each of which secretes and constantly bears at its summit a little drop of a sticky and clear liquid, (whence the name *ros solis* or *sun-dew*), which was much sought after by alchymists who believed it possessed of marvellous virtues. This plant is inodorous; but the juice which is expressed from its recent leaves, is acrid, smarting, sufficiently sour to set the teeth on edge and turn the milk,[1] and sufficiently irritating to be used as an epispastic.[2] The sun-dew grows in damp prairies, along the border of marshes.[3] Animals do not touch it, because they have an instinctive knowledge of its deleterious properties. According to Barrich, it gives sheep a cough that is fatal to them, a circumstance which ought to have excited the attention of allœopathic physicians, for, as we shall see presently, it is precisely in affections of the air-passages that the therapeutic properties of drosera have been found most useful in old-school practice.

Empirical applications. Drosera has been recommended for *ophthalmia, gutta serena, neuralgia, intermittent fevers and dropsies.*[4] But it has been particularly useful in *angina with spasmodic cough* and *roughness of voice* in *asthma* and *old catarrhal affections of the larynx and bronchia.* Two

[1] Murray, *appar. med.*, vol. III., p. 501.

[2] Mérat and Delens, *dict. de mat. méd.*, vol. II., p. 690.

[3] *Act. Hafn.*, vol. IV., p. 162.

[4] Bulliard, *plantes vénéneuses*, Paris, 1798, p. 365.

German physicians of the last century, Heerman and Siegesbeck, have been its chief panegyrists. The former[1] who used it as a panacea for chest-affections, even tubercular phthisis, deserves but little confidence. Siegesbeck's indications for the use of drosera, seem to imply a sort of intuitive perception of the true curative virtues of this drug. How did he find, for example, that drosera is particularly useful in epidemic *catarrhal* fevers, *with spasmodic cough?* in certain forms of *bronchial catarrh* and *malignant fever.*[2] These catarrhal epidemic fevers of Siegesbeck are nothing else than our influenza and whooping-cough, of which I shall say a few words when speaking of the clinical indications furnished by Hahnemann for the use of drosera.

Homœopathic applications. Although still incomplete, yet the pathogenesis which Hahnemann has given us of drosera in the second volume of his Materia med. pur., is sufficiently comprehensive to enable us to determine the specific therapeutic uses of the drug. Symptoms 9, 10, 11 and 12, furnished by Hahnemann, and symptoms 26, 27, and 28, furnished by his disciples, explain to us how this agent has been able to cure *amaurosis*, even when caused by mercury; certain *muscular*, *stinging*, *gnawing* or *crampy pains* seem to be seated in some cases in the cavity of the long bones, and come on principally at night; these may have yielded to the action of drosera in virtue of the homœopathicity of symptoms 71, 72, 74, 75, 77, 78, 79, 80, 81, 82, 83, 84, 85, 86, 87, 88, 89, 94, 96, 99, 101, etc., furnished by Hahnemann, and of symptoms 21, 22, 43, 47, 48, 91, 92, 93, 94, 97, 98, 99, 107, 110, 111, 113, 114, 120, 122, 123, 124, 125 furnished by his disciples. A species of *quotidian intermittent fever* is represented by symptoms 118, 119, 120, 121, 122 and 126, and also by symptoms 135, 136, 137, etc.

But it is especially *whooping-cough* that the symptoms of drosera seem to correspond to in the most marked manner. Hahnemann tells us, that a single dose of drosera is sufficient

[1] *Dissert. de rosa solis,* Erfurth, 1715.

[2] *Dissert. de rorella,* Vittenberg, 1716.

to cure epidemic whooping-cough within eight or nine days, "provided," adds he in a foot note, "that no second dose is given immediately after the first, nor any other medicine is administered; for this would neutralise the good effects of the former dose, and might even cause serious accidents, as experience has shown me." It is well known that since the publication of his Mat. Med. Hahnemann modified his views concerning the repetition of the dose. All homœopaths, now-a-days, give one or more doses of drosera in whooping-cough. But in whatever form or mode drosera be given, it is now an universally admitted fact, that it cures in one, and fails in another case, and that other remedies have frequently to be resorted to. What is the cause of this antagonism? One cause may be a difference of temperament, some constitutional idiosyncrasy. But the principal reason of this apparent antagonism in the effects of one and the same drug, in the same disease, is, in my estimation, the fact that the supposed identity of this malady is illusory. Thus, apart from the sporadic affections due to the roughness of the weather, and so frequently confounded with whooping-cough, in consequence of the spasmodic nature of the irritation, who assures us that whooping-cough is always the same in character, and arising from the same cause? All good observers, with Rosenstein at their head, admit that every new whooping-cough epidemic is distinguished by some particular type, and varies in intensity, obstinacy, and even in its course and symptoms. An hypothesis which seems to me very plausible, will help to explain these differences.

What is true of the plague, of Asiatic cholera, yellow fever, and, indeed, of any epidemic, is likewise true of whooping-cough; it has its focus, or probably its foci, somewhere in Europe, perhaps in France. The miasm which produces it is nothing else than the effluvia of some decaying or still living vegetable substance, which, owing to changes of weather and climate, are more or less abundant every year, and like all other epidemic miasms, are carried to distant parts by atmospheric currents. This miasmatic principle, which is generally carried onward in an inverse direction to the rotation of the earth, that is to say, from east to west, and at the same time from north to south, (agreeably to the course of the trade-winds,) occupies most probably the superior strata of the atmospheric air, and descends only at certain distances, according as the mercury falls in the barometer; whence it follows, that it may follow the course we have pointed out, and yet let itself down, like the *cholera-cloud* (*nuée cholérique*,) at various points of its progress, leaving the intermediate regions untouched. I repeat that, as the cholera-miasm comes to us from the borders of the Ganges, so the whooping-cough-miasm developes itself in our immediate neighborhood. This, at any rate, is my belief. As regards the marshy character of the whooping-cough miasm, I am so much the more disposed to believe in it, that drosera, which is the principal remedial agent in a majority of whooping-cough epidemics, is principally found in marshy regions. And it is a law of Providence, that the remedies should be generally found in the very parts that give rise to the diseases which decimate humanity; the reverse of this proposition needs scarcely to be demonstrated as true.

But if we admit that whooping-cough not only originates in a marsh-miasm, but in marsh-miasms of different natures, how can it be supposed that the same remedy can cure all the various forms of this disease? This, however, is the real question at issue.

If I should be asked to define the shades of symptoms which distinguish the whooping-cough that will yield to drosera from the kind of cough that will resist it, I should have to confess my inability to solve a question that escaped even the wonderful sagacity of Hahnemann.

Whooping-cough is not the only affection of the air-passages that has been cured by drosera. *Angina of the throat and chest*, *chronic angina*, and even *pharyngeal phthisis*, have been successfully treated with this drug.

Camphor destroys the too violent effects of drosera.[1]

[1] According to my own experience, Menyanthes is most closely analogous

Nitri acidum. See page 145.

Ferrum metallicum. See the group of which this drug is the type.

Mercurius corrosivus. See page 138.

Platina. This drug being more intimately related to thuya than to zinc, we defer our remarks concerning it until we come to a description of the *thuya-group.*

to drosera, except that the effects of drosera are more intense than those of Menyanthes. *Obscuration of sight,* which is one of the first symptoms of these drugs, developes itself alike under the influence of one or the other. It is a sort of *white mist,* or *vibrations,* which are sometimes so violent that they prevent sight, come on irregularly, of varied durations, *especially in the open air, during a walk,* and without any other sensation. I experienced this symptom from either drug so violently, while walking on the Boulevard, that I dared not cross it lest I should be crushed by the carriages. The pains of drosera and menyanthes are likewise alike. In their action on the air-passages they only differ in the degree of intensity. Menyanthes is little used, and never will be used much. I have used it with success in a case of amaurosis; but there are few diseases where menyanthes is indicated that could not be cured much better with drosera. This opinion, however, is founded on my own impressions, which I am always willing to mistrust.

GROUP XV.

TYPE: ACONITUM NAPELLUS.

ANALOGUES: COCCULUS. CHAMOMILLA VULGARIS. DULCAMARA. CANNABIS INDICA. CONIUM MACULATUM.

THE five drugs which I mention here as the analogues of Aconite, have only a very vague relatiou to it. Properly speaking, Aconite has no analogues. Cocculus, hemp, chamomilla, etc., indeed exercise an action on the brain, the sensual organs, the organs of locomotion and the skin, that seems to be, in very many respects, very much like the action of Aconite; but none of them affects even approximatively the heart and vascular apparatus as *Aconite;* the *inflammatory fever* is a phenomenon that belongs exclusively to this great agent.[1]

We shall therefore only mention Aconite, leaving out the other members of this group, which have either been already described in previous groups, or will be described hereafter.

This is a sufficient explanation why I refrain from mentioning the diseases corresponding to the *Aconite-group.* All these diseases yield to Aconite, and will therefore be mentioned in giving a description of the drugs.

Aconitum Napellus, *wolf's-bane.* Genus Aconitum, family ranunculaceæ, section helleboraceæ, which has since been arranged into a distinct family,[2] of the class polyandria

[1] *Actæa spicata* seems to approximate to the action of Aconite, and to possess likewise the property of arresting inflammatory fever. The actæa is a native of Europe, and belongs to the family of the ranunculaceæ. I shall publish some time hence a list of symptoms which I have obtained of this drug that was only known to homœopathic physicians through a miserable imposition that had been practised upon them.

[2] Spach, *hist. des plantes phanérogames,* Paris, 1839, vol. VII., p. 336.

trigynia. Aconite is a perennial plant, herbaceous, the stem of which is ramose, glabrous, cylindrical, and attains to a height of from two to three feet. Its leaves are green, shining, petiolate, deeply incised so as to form five or six lobes, linear, expanding at the upper extremity, and marked with a line; beautiful blue flowers in long terminal spikes; the seeds consist of three winged capsules. Its root is a rhizoma which, by its volume and shape, resembles a small turnip, (*napus*) whence its name *napellus*, which is a diminutive of napus.

On account of its beautiful flowers, and in spite of its poisonous properties, *aconite* is cultivated in some gardens as an ornamented plant. Its Greek name, which is derived from the noun *akony*, rock, shows that it is essentially a mountainous plant. It grows spontaneously in the damp and covered parts of almost every mountainous country in the north or middle of Europe, especially in the Jura, Switzerland, Germany, Sweden, where Murray says he found it in the neighborhood of Fahlun.[1]

Aconite has little odor; but its leaves, stem, and especially its root, have, when chewed, a slight taste at first, which soon changes to an acrid and stinging taste. Slight prickings are at first felt at the tip of the tongue; the mouth becomes filled with saliva; afterwards the lips, gums and palate as far as the root of the tongue become numb.[2] An almost similar impression is felt in the hand after handling the recent leaves and roots of Aconite for a time. According to Bichat the skin becomes burning, red, and, if the contact lasts long enough, becomes covered with vesicles.[3]

Aconite has been analysed by several chemists, but with varied and not very conclusive results. Trutten, Steinacher, Trommsdorff and Pallas have found in it a green fecula, hydrochlorate of ammonia,[4] phosphate and carbonate of lime,

[1] *Appar. Med.*, vol. III., p. 5.

[2] Reinhold, *de acon. napel. dissert.* 1779, *silloge selectiorum opusculorum* de Baklinger, Gœttinguæ, 1779, vol. II.

[3] *Cours manuscrit de mat. méd.*, quoted by Mérat and Delens.

[4] *Journ. général de méd.*, vol. XXXI., p. 467.

potash, and finally a gaseous, odorous substance which was at first taken for the active principle of this plant. Since then, Geiger and Hesse have discovered in it an alkaloïd which had already been pointed out by Brandes, and to which these chemists gave the name *aconitine*. It is a white, granulous substance, looking like delphine or veratrine, unchangeable by exposure to the air, uncrystallisable, fixed, and therefore inodorous, not very soluble in water, on the contrary very soluble in ether and alcohol, of a bitter taste, but not acrid, and not causing in the mouth the sensation of numbness which the chewed leaves or root of aconite produce.[1] Except the experiments of Dr. Turnbull of London, who praises the tincture of Aconitine, when used externally, for neuralgia, and for certain affections of the eyes and ears, this drug has not yet been used.

Aconite is supposed to be fatal to every species of animals. If given to wolves, dogs, cats and rats, even in small quantities, it destroys them in a few days, and sometimes in a few hours.[2] According to Scopoli, a decoction of its root kills bedbugs, and, if mixed with butter or milk, destroys the flies as effectually as an arsenic-solution could do.[3] I do not think that it affects herbivorous animals as much as carnivorous. It is true, some authors, among whom Courten who is quoted by Murray,[4] pretend having seen oxen and goats poisoned by the fresh leaves of this plant. On the other hand, Linné affirms that horses eat the leaves when dried and mixed with other food, without any inconvenience,[5] which explains to some extent the contradictory and somewhat hazardous assertions of Professor Giacomini. "Animals," says he, "avoid aconite when they find it on pasture-grounds. It acts like a

[1] *Journ. de pharm.*, vol. XX., p. 165.

[2] *On the medic. propert. of the natur. order ranunculaceæ*, London, 1835. *Bull. de thérap.*, vol. XX., p. 19.

[3] See Wepfer, *hist. de cic.*, cap. II., p. 176 and 180. Larrey, *mém. de chir. mil.*, vol. III., p. 126. Orfila, méd. lég., vol. II., p. 54. Pereira, arch. génév. de méd., June, 1832, etc.

[4] *Flora Carniolica*, p. 550.

[5] *Loc. Cit.*, p. 9.

[6] *Flora Suecica*, p. 186.

violent poison on every species of animals. It is said, however, (Giacomini does not tell us by whom) that "*horses, goats* and *sheep eat it without hurt.*"[1] Upon the whole, I believe, more however in conformity with speculative theories than real facts, that aconite affects graminivorous animals less violently than it does carnivorous.

As regards the poisonous effects of this drug on man, they are generally admitted. A good many cases of poisoning by aconite, followed by death or some very serious derangements, are recorded in the annals of science. In the 16th century, this poison was several times given to persons condemned to death, with a view of discovering its physiological action upon the organism, and determining its therapeutic virtues. Matthiolus relates two cases of this kind, in one of which he administered the poison himself. In 1524, the commentator of Dioscorides accepted the office proffered by pope Clement VII., of administering the poison to two individuals condemned to death, for the purpose of observing its effects. An hour and a half after one of the two thieves had swallowed a drachm of the root, and no effects whatsoever became yet visible, the experimenter was on the point of administering another dose, when all at once the following symptoms manifested themselves: Extreme prostration, cold sweat in the face, embarrassed respiration, dyspnœa, imminent suffocation, convulsive movements of the extremities, bilious vomiting, involuntary stools, stupor, cadaverous coldness, bloating of the face, and lastly . . . death by apoplexy. The other criminal was more fortunate: whether his constitution was stronger or weaker than that of his fellow-sufferer, or whether he was more speedily relieved by the vomiting, he was only attacked with vertigo, delirium, spasms in the face, an obscure paralysis of the extremities, etc., and with these sufferings purchased the right to live.[2]

These strange experiments, which did not shock the morals of that period, were renewed in Prague, in 1561, by order of

[1] *Traité phil. et exper. de mat. méd.*, etc., p. 286.

[2] *Comm. in Diosc.*, vol. I., p. 408.

the reigning emperor, under the same circumstances and with the same results. But science gained nothing by these trials. For the therapeutic value of Aconite was almost null until the period when Hahnemann revealed by careful provings the true properties of this drug, or, at any rate, until the time when Stœrck used it empirically. In examining after death the bodies of those who had been poisoned with Aconite, it was found that the ventricles of the brain were filled with serum, the lungs and the right heart were engorged with blood, the stomach and the bowels were more or less inflamed, but never ulcerated; whence the conclusion was drawn, that Aconite acted after the manner of *acrid poisons*, inasmuch as narcotics do not inflame the stomach, and corrosive poisons cause an ulceration of this viscus."[1]

Empirical applications. Theophrastus, Dioscorides, Plinius, and several other writers of old, make mention of aconite, and recommend it in different diseases. But inasmuch as it is not exactly known what kind of a plant they mean,[2] it follows that the medicinal history of our aconite can scarcely be traced further back than the experiments and clinical cases which Stœrck published in 1762.

This publication, which gave rise to similar works on the same subject by Manghin, Reinhold, Collin, Razona, etc., could not fail, in consideration of the renown of its author, to create a sensation in the medical world. This little work was very interesting in itself. A terrible poison which it would have been considered criminal to prescribe even in the most desperate cases, became all at once an harmless remedy for all kinds of *patients, provided it was prescribed in small doses;* it was transformed into a precious, heroïc, invaluable remedy when properly administered, if we may judge from the almost wonderful results which the celebrated Vienna professor affirmed having obtained with it.

[1] Mérat and Delens, op. cit., vol. I., p. 59.

[2] See Encontre's and de Candolle's memoir *on the aconit of the ancients,* 1813, in 8vo.

[3] *Exper. et observ. circausum internum Stramonii, Hyoscyami, et Aconiti,* Vindebonæ, in 8vo.

After having assured himself, by various experiments, that the powder of Aconite, whether applied to the skin, to the surface of fungous ulcers, or between the eyelids and the ball of the eye, was not near as *caustic* a drug as had been supposed, Stœrck determined to try it internally, first on himself. For this purpose he procured a certain quantity of the extract of aconite triturated with pulverized sugar in the proportion of two grains of the extract to two drachms of sugar; he assures us that he experienced no sort of change from 6 grains of this mixture taken the first day, in the morning before breakfast, or from 8 grains on the second, and 10 on the third day.[1] On the fourth day he doubled the dose, and a general perspiration broke out. This sweat had to be attributed to the drug, for it ceased invariably after the drug was discontinued for a day or two, and broke out again so soon as it was resumed, whence the experimenter concluded that *aconite* being a *sudorific*, it must act best in diseases that disappeared after the breaking out of critical sweat. This theory was illusory, but it happened to lead to true results.

In this way Stœrck, this great seeker after specifics, and who neither troubled himself about the inmost principle of the disease, nor the inmost active forces of the drugs, was induced to try aconite first in *rheumatism*, and afterwards in *tumors* which he calls *schirrous*, but concerning the nature of which I truly believe he was mistaken.

Be this as it may, at the period when Stœrck published his work, he had administered aconite to fourteen patients, eight of whom were radically cured, and the remaining six recovering. Unfortunately all his cases are curtailed, incomplete, more or less tainted with polypharmacy, and, therefore, unreliable. What is interesting to us homœopaths in

[1] This is not to be wondered at. All homœopaths know that the action of drugs is perceived the more rapidly, the higher the dilution at which they are taken. It is not strange that an extract grossly triturated with sugar, should not have had any immediate effect. Moreover, we do not know whether Stœrck watched the action of the drug with sufficient care and attention.

these cases is, that the patients, while taking the aconite, presented many of the symptoms of this drug, which can, of course, be accounted for by the enormity of the doses. In almost all his patients Stœrck noticed, 1st, *sweat all over, and continually*, which he considered a good symptom; this sweat ceased to break out in proportion as the patients grew better; 2d, in two patients (cases 2 and 4), an *itching* all over the body, especially at the genital organs, followed by the breaking out of red spots and pustules accompanied with burning pains, and terminating in desquamation, etc. All his patients recovered pretty rapidly, nor can this recovery be attributed to a few cathartics which were given during the treatment for reasons which it is difficult to understand; for cathartics had been administered to some of them previous to the administration of aconite without any benefit whatsoever.

Here follows a synopsis of these eight cases:

1st. A man of some thirty odd years: *rheumatism in the whole right side*, after a tertian fever which had been cured quite recently; the patient was unable, from the pain, to move hand or foot; all sorts of remedies had been tried in vain; shortly after the exhibition of aconite he began to perspire profusely, but the sweat diminished as he grew better; perfect recovery in five weeks.

2d. A man of 27 years, had been troubled for six weeks with *acute sciatica;* the pain had invaded the arm without leaving the thigh. Itching in the neighborhood of the genital organs; red pustules filled with an acrid fluid; gentle moisture all the time; cured in five weeks.

3d. A young man of 19 years, who had had a *quartan fever* for three years past, which had resisted the action of quinine; cachectic looks; during all the time that the fever had lasted, the extremities, joints and the dorsal spine were the seat of an exceedingly violent pain, which was accompanied with a burning sensation in the extremities; under the influence of aconite sweats and copious stools set in; he was cured in one month.

4th. A woman of forty-three years experienced such *violent pains* in the right arm and foot that she screamed day and night; she was *purged* by the extract; on the sixth day large red itching pustules broke out, and the pains ceased completely and permanently.

5th. A man of thirty odd years had been suffering with the most *distressing gout* for nine months; all his joints were red, swollen, excessively painful; a number of remedies had been tried in vain; the first doses of aconite produced a marked improvement; the swellings decreased in a fortnight; complete cure in three months.

6th. A woman of forty-three years: wandering pains in the extremities and joints, which finally became seated in the articulations of the hands and feet that were actually deformed by nodosities and *earthy concretions* (is this appellation correct?) preventing motion and flexion of the joints; the pains ceased under the use of aconite, and the swellings disappeared; complete cure in three months.

7th. A man of forty odd years; *ankylosis of the left elbow* (? ?); the joint formed a considerable swelling, and was the seat of acute pains; the tumor was scattered, the pains ceased, and the mobility of the joint was completely restored; cure in a fortnight.

8th. A woman of thirty-four years; acute rheumatic pains in the right thigh and foot; cured in three weeks.

The other six patients who still were under treatment when Stœrck published his work, were affected with *tumors* of various kinds, and which had been treated without result with various kinds of extract, especially with the extract of hemlock; the extract of aconite had already effected a considerable reduction of the tumors, and it was supposed, would scatter them entirely.

"I infer from these trials," says Stœrck, "that aconite is a drug that does not do any harm, and *yet is very powerful* (a strange assertion which, at that period, was not contrary to any theory!) It produces results that the most active drugs fail in producing. If some acrid matter settles in the joints, tendons or bones, and irritates the nerves and causes great pain, this agent renders it fluid, puts it in motion, and drives it out of the body by the urine, stools, sweat, or an *insensible perspiration.*"

Stœrck was so much attached to the humoral doctrine that, when a cure took place without the peccant matter being ostensibly expelled by loose stools, urine, sweat, he fell back upon the theory of an *imperceptible perspiration.* "Aconite," continues he, "softens *schirrous tumors,* (an hazardous assertion,) *nodes, articular concretions,* and sometimes it scatters them entirely; it quiets and puts a stop to the most violent pains, etc." Stœrck admits, however, that he employed aconite without success in some cases of tumor that were afterwards cured with hemlock; this is not surprising.

The conclusions which were most generally drawn and accepted, from these experiments of the Viennese physicians, were, that aconite is an excellent remedy for some kinds of undefined tumors, and for *acute, articular rheumatism;* although, even in this latter disease, Rode accuses it of not always preventing the formation of crudities,[1] and Stoll has seen it fail completely in epidemic articular rheumatism.[2]

Be this as it may, on the strength of his recommendations, a number of German, Swedish and French physicians employed aconite in the cases for which Stœrck praised it, or in cases similar to his, and they frequently found it useful, especially in the following affections: *Articular pains,* sometimes with *nodosities* or *contractions of the flexor muscles, general febrile heat and coldness in the affected parts;*[3] *rheumatism of the head; hemicrania,* (of eleven years standing, and having resisted every kind of treatment;)[4] *rheumatic fever;*[5]

[1] *Med. chir. bibl.,* vol. II., p. 120.

[2] *Ratio medendi,* part III., p. 167.

[3] Collin, *Observat.,* part II., cases 2, 3, 5 & 7. Rosenstein, *litt. in Haller. Epist.,* vol. V., p. 174. Rode, *loc. cit.* Razoux, *dissert. epistol. de Cicut., Stram., Hyoscyam.* et *Aconit.,* Nîmes, 1781, in 8vo., p. 319. Reinhold, *dis. cit.,* p. 37, etc.

[4] Vogel, in Murray, *op. cit.,* vol. III., p. 18.

[5] Guérin et Ehrhart, in Reinhold, *dis. cit.*

tumor (on the left side of the neck, and in which hemlock had failed;)[1] *large tumor at the neck*, (hindering respiration and deglutition;)[2] *paraplegia*, (after fright;)[3] *paralysis of the right arm and leg*, (preceded by convulsions;)[4] *epilepsy*, (in the case of a woman whose cranium was so distorted that it was difficult to understand how this patient was able to live;)[5] *cough*, *asthma*, *gout* and *paralysis of the left arm*, (in the same patient;)[6] *facial neuralgia; sciatica;*[7] *œdema*, (consequent on certain intermittent fevers;)[8] and lastly, *ascites*.

At the commencement of this century, aconite was recommended for other diseases. Drs. *Busch*, of Strasburgh,[10] and *Baumes*,[11] praised its good effects in the first period of *pulmonary phthisis;* Quadri gave it in *pleurisy;* Borda, Tommasini, and several others praised it in *pneumonia* and other *inflammatory affections*.[12]

The modern partisans of Rasori, who, I suspect, have derived their doctrine concerning the curative virtues of aconite from the numerous successes which the homœopaths have obtained with this drug, number it among their *arterial vascular hyposthenisants*. "The ancients," says Giacomini, "who were guided simply by observation, (which was certainly full as well as to be guided by the speculations of Rasori,) placed aconite among the frigid poisons, and, in this respect, they saw more clearly than their successors, who allowed themselves to be carried away by theories. All theories and systems that are not based upon a strict observation of

[1] Collin, *loc. cit.*, case 6.
[2] Guérin, in Murray, *loc. cit.*
[3] Collin, *loc. cit.*, p. 143.
[4] *Id.*, *id.*, p. 186.
[5] Guding, in Murray, *loc. cit.*
[6] *Id.*, *id.*
[7] Bergius, *Mat. Med.*, vol. II., p. 509; Murray, *op. cit.*, p. 16.
[8] Guding, in Murray, *loc. cit.*
[9] A curious case of this kind is related in Plutarch's Biography of Marcus Crassus: "Irodes having been attacked with dropsy, Froates, his son, who wished to get rid of his father, gave him aconite; but the poison took hold of the disease, and the patient was relieved. Froates then choked him." Was the aconite which Froates gave his father the same as we use?
[10] *Recherches sur le traitem. de la phthis. pulm.*, Strasburg, year IX.
[11] *Traité de la phthis. pulm.*, 2d edit. 1805, 2 vol. in 8vo., vol. II., p. 115.
[12] *Giorn. della Soc. med. di Parma.*, vol. VII., p. 200.

facts and the most rigorous logic, lead to such results." System-makers always talk so. "It is an experience of several centuries and carried on in various countries that authorises us to look upon *aconite* as a powerful depressor of the circulation. Its effects on animals and man in health, (shocking antagonism of truths!) the efficacy of our hyposthenisant agents in neutralising them, (another error!) the discouraging results of an antiphlogistic treatment in all such cases; and lastly, the hypersthenic nature of the diseases that have been cured or alleviated with aconite, without any sort of evacuation taking place, all this is to us a peremptory proof, which will doubtless be accepted by all unbiassed and enlightened minds, as it had indeed been accepted at former periods by transcendent practitioners."[1] These were doubtless Stœrck, Van Swieten and Barthez, who, relying upon the *ab usu in morbis*, inferred from their observations, that in phlegmasiæ, aconite acted like an *antiphlogistic*, a more or less judicious remark on the part of these practitioners. But to draw with Giacomini the same conclusions from the action of aconite on animals or men, seems to be proof of a good deal of ignorance concerning the physiological action of this drug.[2]

Homœopathic Applications.—Of all medicines used by homœopathic physicians, aconite is undoubtedly the one which they use most frequently. Without disputing the extraordinary utility of this therapeutic agent, it is, however, my belief that most practitioners abuse it every day. Bye and bye I shall state my reasons for this belief, and the facts upon which it is based.

According to Jahr, who has given us a detailed account of all the clinical facts published by the disciples of Hahnemann, aconite has cured or relieved the following diseases:

"*Acute local inflammation;* rheumatic and arthritic inflammations with swellings; *affections of plethoric persons, of a*

[1] *Trait. de mat. méd. et de thérap.*, p. 289.

[2] See the pathog. of Aconite in Hahnemann's *Mat. Med. Pura*, vol. I., and in Roth's, vol. I., p. 355.

lively disposition, bilious and nervous constitution, brown or black eyes and hairs, deep color in the face, etc. *Active, sanguineous congestions,* neuralgia and spasmodic attacks, especially in young persons, (particularly girls,) of *sanguine temperament,* and leading a sedentary life; *unpleasant consequences of a cold,* contracted by exposure to dry and cold weather (keen north-wester,) or to a draught of air; *affections resulting from fright* or anger; convulsions; tetanus; trismus;[1] *fainting;* catalepsy; burns; miliary eruptions; *purple-rash; rubeola; measles;* eruptive period of variola; *erysipelatous inflammations;* urticaria; *inflammatory fevers,* even with bilious or nervous symptoms; catarrhal fever, with inflammatory character; somnambulism; comatose drowsiness; *mental derangement, with fixed ideas about approaching death; cerebral congestions with vertigo;* sanguineous apoplexy; *congestive,* catarrhal, nervous headache; megrim; *encephalitis;* acute hydrocephalus; *acute ophthalmia,* also traumatic, *congestive* and nervous prosopalgia and toothache; *acute angina,* phlegmonous or catarrhal; angina; scarlatina; difficult dentition, with fever; *bilious ailments;* vomiting of pregnant or hysterical females; various kinds of vomiting; hæmatemesis; jaundice; *hepatitis;* enteritis; peritonitis; metrorrhagia and profuse menstruation, in plethoric females; puerperal peritonitis; metritis; *leucorrhœa; incarcerated hernia;* inflammatory period of ordinary catarrh and influenza; *croup, first period;* asthma Millari; acute laryngitis and bronchitis; *pleurisy;* pneumonia; hæmoptysis; affections of the heart; *palpitations,* etc."[2]

These are, according to Jahr, all the morbid conditions which yield more or less to the specific action of aconite. This list contains several errors, which I desire to point out without, of course, meaning to hurt the feelings of the author, who has simply made it his business to point out, with the

[1] It seems to me that the interrogation-point might have been left out without risk.

[2] Jahr's Symptomen-codex, translated by Dr. Chs. J. Hempel, New York, 1851.

most scrupulous conscientiousness, all the legitimate deductions that might be drawn from the precepts of Hahnemann, or from the clinical observations published in Germany or France, and which do not always seem to rest upon a correct diagnosis, but which it was beyond the province of the compiler to modify, and from which he had to draw such inferences as were in accordance with the given premises.

At the head of all the affections which aconite is said to cure, *provided it is indicated by the totality of the symptoms*, Jahr mentions *acute local inflammations:* a strange, obscure, and very vague indication, not altogether compatible with the homœopathic doctrine, as I understand it, and which seems, nevertheless, to be derived from this passage in Hahnemann: "Aconite is the first and most powerful of all curative means in croup, in various forms of angina (we shall return to these two points bye and bye), and *also in acute local inflammations of other parts*, especially when, with the thirst and the hurried pulse, we notice an anxiety and restlessness that cannot be quieted by any thing we may do, and a constant tossing about as if the patient were in great agony."[1]

We infer from the very text of this passage that the thirst, the frequency of the pulse, the restlessness, and so forth, are not indispensable indications for the use of aconite, for Hahnemann says expressly that it is *especially suitable* in cases where these conditions exist, which undoubtedly implies that it may likewise be indicated in cases where such indications are wanting. This passage, therefore, simply means that "*aconite is the most powerful of all curative agents in acute local inflammations.*" But what is an acute local inflammation? The ideas which I have derived from the writings of Hahnemann concerning the dynamic nature and INHERENT FORCE of diseases, render this question rather embarrassing. If the author of homœopathy had taken the trouble to answer this question for us, how many errors would he have saved us! Not finding the solution of this question

[1] See Hahnemann's Mat. Med. Pur., vol. I., art. Aconite.

in the works of their master, they had to substitute a solution of their own, and were frequently ruled in their efforts by their adherence to former prejudices. With Broussais some supposed that any kind of disease is an inflammation. Aconite was, therefore, the antiphlogistic *par excellence.* It had to be given in all cases where the Broussaists resort to sanguineous depletions, that is to say in all sorts of diseases. Upon such grounds, I am sure, rests the great popularity that aconite enjoys now-a-days, and the great abuse which is made of it every day.

Nevertheless I admit with Hahnemann, and with the physicians of every school that there are affections which, for want of a more exact appellation, we may call *inflammatory*, the rather that an inflammatory condition is undoubtedly their most striking character. Such are on the one hand traumatic lesions, and, on the other, phlegmasiæ, such as develope themselves every day under the influence of modifying physical agents (heat, cold, draughts of air, etc.), without their apparent development giving, in any way, rise to the suspicion that it depends either upon an internally or externally acting force.

Violent traumatic lesions very speedily give rise to symptoms which cannot be considered purely local. On the other hand, the so-called local inflammations which result from the disturbing action of physical agents, are at first general disturbances, and preserve this character even after the disease had concentrated itself in some particular locality of the organism.

Here we have two pretty distinct forms of so-called *local inflammations.* Which of these was meant by Hahnemann in his recommendation of aconite as the most powerful remedy for local inflammations? of course of those of the second class, for, although Jahr mentions *burns* as a condition that can be cured with aconite, yet we know very well that this agent is not essentially useful in traumatic lesions.

It is in phlegmasiæ that were primarily general, and became secondarily local, or *localised*, that we may have to use aconite. This follows, from Hahnemann's own, and extremely correct suggestions concerning the use of this drug.

"It is precisely in those cases, where alloeopathic physicians boast most pompously of their method, and imagine that homœopathy must lower her head before the frequent and excessive depletions of her alloeopathic opponents; it is *in acute inflammatory fevers* that aconite exercises its greatest curative power. Here homœopathy displays her immense superiority over the opposite practice; for she does not shed a single drop of blood; this precious vital fluid which alloeopathy wastes in torrents without sometimes being able to repair the loss; and yet, in spite of this absolute avoidance of all depletions, homœopathy triumphs of these fevers, and frequently restores the patient's health in as many days as the fashionable bleeding method requires months to restore those whom such debilitating proceedings have not brought into their graves, and who frequently have to suffer, during the remainder of their lives, the effects of these destructive means of treatment."[1]

But, because aconite possesses the power of staying *acute inflammatory fevers*, does it follow that it must necessarily be the most powerful remedy for acute local inflammations, preceded or accompanied by the fever? This seems to me very problematical. Indeed, Jahr, in spite of his general proposition concerning the homœopathicity of aconite to acute local inflammations, seems to have deemed it proper to specify the particular kinds of inflammations to which aconite is most appropriate. He mentions first *encephalitis*, *ophthalmia*, *angina*, *hepatitis*, *pleurisy*, etc., and in the second rank he places *enteritis*, *peritonitis*, *metritis*, *pneumonia*, etc. According to Jahr, aconite is not, it seems, equally efficacious in all local inflammations; and, in this respect, I think that all homœopathic physicians will agree with Jahr.

But, before continuing, let us state the question frankly:

Is it true that in all local affections where the totality of

[1] Hahnemann's Mat. Med. *loc. cit.*

the pathognomonic signs, namely pain, heat, redness and swelling, point to what is usually termed inflammation, the best means of combating them, is invariably aconite? I unhesitatingly answer: no.

I am disposed to believe that, if aconite could be given in the very commencement, before the disease has had time to develope a local inflammation, this localisation might be prevented in many cases; but I believe likewise that, when the local inflammation has already acquired a certain degree of intensity, many other drugs may, by virtue of constitutional idiosyncrasies, or with respect to the organ which has become the local focus of the disease, be preferable to aconite which, in such cases, could not be administered without involving a precious loss of time.

As a general rule it seems to me, that, even in acute inflammations, aconite is only indicated when the inflammatory fever is the ruling symptom. Wurmb and Gaspar, of the homœopathic hospital of Leopoldstadt at Vienna, seems to have thought so, when they express themselves as follows, relatively to acute bronchial catarrh:

"The febrile reaction that accompanies acute catarrh, is frequently similar to that which aconite produces on a healthy person. When the fever is so violent *that it becomes the leading symptom*, we must not hesitate to give aconite, although an irritation of the mucous membrane is not one of its characteristic effects.

"We have not seen any drug more frequently indicated in acute catarrh than aconite. After giving aconite, the fever was subdued next morning, and the catarrhal symptoms did not last more than two or three days." And, speaking still more in the sense which I have expressed, Wurmb and Gaspar add: "It is scarcely necessary to mention that the catarrh which is cured by aconite, is never very intense."[1]

What the Viennese physicians have said with regard to aconite in the acute bronchial catarrh, has been verified by

[1] *Clinical observations*, by Drs. Wurmb and Gaspar, published in vol. III. of the Journ. de la Soc. gall. de méd. hom., p. 425.

Tessier so much the more strikingly in the treatment of pneumonia. Carried away by the authority of Hahnemann, this skilful practitioner considered it his duty to commence the treatment of every case of pneumonia with a few doses of aconite; but he soon became aware of the insufficiency of aconite in such cases. We read the following reflection following the report of the first case of pneumonia mentioned in his work. "In this case the aconite had no other effect than to depress the pulse from 120 to 100. *When at its height*, I have scarcely ever seen any other result from aconite. It is said that this drug is capable of suppressing pneumonia in its incipiency. I have never witnessed any such results. We ought to add, however, that, in hospitals, an incipient pneumonia is a very rare occurrence."

This shows that pneumonia and bronchitis are diseases which when fully developed, are very little modified by aconite. I maintain that the same remark applies to pleurisy, enteritis, hepatitis, and most other acute local inflammations, for which aconite is generally lauded as the grand remedy.

Is *croup* which is likewise an acute local inflammation, exempt from this criticism? Hahnemann recommends aconite as the most powerful remedy for croup, and some homœopathic physicians still believe that it is; I am not one of them. Let us look at the pathogenesis of aconite. There is doubtless a certain analogy between the general effects of aconite and the symptoms of croup. And I am willing to admit, although I am not convinced of this fact, that aconite, if given previous to the formation of the false membrane, is capable of preventing the development of the disease. But we shall be bitterly disappointed if we still rely upon the antiphlogistic virtues of aconite after the false membrane is formed; for this is not one of the symptoms of our drug. I go even so far as to assert, that, to commence the treatment with aconite, after the membrane is formed, would be to lose time in a disease where every moment is precious, and where an hour of fruitless expectation may lead to fatal results.

[1] Récherches cliniques sur le traitement de la pneumonie et du choléra, in 8vo., Paris, 1850, p. 11.

Is croup, as is still supposed by some homœopathic physicians who have not been able to relinquish their allœopathic prejudices, simply an acute inflammation of the mucous membrane of the pharynx, larynx and trachea? The true disciples of Hahnemann think not. On the contrary, all think with me, that croup, as well as epidemic whooping-cough, scarlatina, measles, etc., is a disease *sui generis*, characterised by a leading symptom that is independent of the ordinary results of a simple, even very acute inflammation, and which can only be combated by special remedies, the inherent power of which corresponds to the inherent force of the morbid affection.

This is so true, that in one case I have seen croup, that is to say, the formation of a false membrane at the pharynx, develope itself without any initial or concomitant fever. In such a case, I do not believe that aconite would have arrested the disease.

This does not mean that aconite may not have cured croup. Even depletions have effected cures. I do not deny that aconite has a certain action on the air-passages, and I am willing to admit that, by moderating the fever, quieting the anxiety of the patient, and arresting the spasmodic contractions of the glottis, it may frequently have facilitated the resolution of the membrane and lessened the danger so as to save the patient's life; nevertheless, relying upon our provings and clinical experience, I assert that, when the disease is at its height, aconite is an insufficient agent, and that, at this stage, its use is improper. This is, at any rate, my conviction, in spite of my unlimited respect for Hahnemann's opinions.

As regards the affection, known by the name of *spurious croup* or *asthma Millari*, it is well known that it is neither a simple nor special kind of inflammation, but a nervous disease, which, it is true, is sometimes complicated by congestive symptoms. The asthma Millari attacks weakly, nervous children with bad humors, rather than strong, plethoric children, disposed to inflammatory congestions. On this account, such remedies as *Caust.*, *Coral rub.*, *Coff.*, *Opium*, etc., are preferable to *aconite* in the incipiency of this disease.

I do not deny, however, that aconite has cured some cases of dyspnœa, with or without cough, but without a trace of fever, in the same manner as it has cured purely nervous affections, without the presence of a single symptom denoting vascular irritation; they were seated in the head, face, nape of the neck, pectoral muscles, arms, thighs, (sciatica,) etc., and almost always owed their origin to exposure of some keen, dry and cold wind. Among the facts in my possession, that bear upon this point, I beg leave to relate the following case, which seems to me to be peculiarly interesting.

Mr. X——, 42 years old, tall, athletic, of a sanguine temperament, mild disposition, possessed of the most perfect equanimity, without anxiety about any thing, and endowed with an adventurous spirit. He had been all over the world. His life had been full of incidents, and, therefore, a series of emotions. For the last two years he had been treated for *aneurism of the heart;* such, at any rate, his disease had been pronounced by several medical celebrities of Russia, Germany and England.

His disease set in in 1850, in consequence of a journey in a sleigh, which my patient had been obliged to take in mid-winter, in the north of Russia, when the thermometer was from 30 to 35° below zero, and during which, trusting only to his own skill for the management of his team in the snows, he remained with the upper part of his body exposed to the wind for several weeks, night and day, although he was covered with the thickest kind of fur. But, in spite of this precaution, he was not able to resist such a hard exposure. It brought on, in his opinion and my own, the sad condition in which he now found himself, and which I shall endeavor to describe.

Mr. X—— looked as if he enjoyed the most perfect health: calm features, a natural complexion, easy speech, normal color of the lips which are not, by any means, bloated; in one word, there was not a single symptom that might lead one to believe in the existence of an organic affection of the heart. Nevertheless, he experienced acute stitches in the region of this organ, which alternated with violent palpitations, accompanied with an intense anxiety, a good deal of dryness at the throat, and a noise in the head, which was particularly distressing in the left ear. During the most violent paroxysms he seemed even threatened with cerebral apoplexy, and lost his consciousness; these symptoms were only slowly and incompletely relieved by bleeding, for they came on again after a certain interval. The whole left side of the chest, including the back and shoulders, were so painful, that they could not be touched. For some months past, the patient, who had lost his sleep, dared not sleep any longer in his bed, and spent his nights in an easy chair.

It is to be observed, (and this point is of great importance,) that during the seven months that the patient spent in Egypt, which has a warm climate, all the morbid symptoms which have been related above, gradually disappeared, so that Mr. X. believed himself cured; but they all returned as soon as he again exposed himself to the climate of northern Europe.

When I saw him for the first time, his pains, which were intense, were not at their height. After listening to a recital of his sorrow, I thought his case over in my accustomed manner, and the result of my investigations was as follows:

In placing my hand on the left anterior and superior portion of the thorax, over the nipple, I perceived in this region an irregular, tumultuous beating, which came on at momentary intervals, separated by short and rare intermissions. This beating was so violent that it raised and agitated the clothes, so that it could be seen, and the intervals distinctly noticed at a distance of several paces. The sensation of a rush of blood to the head was proportionate, according to the declaration of the patient, to the intensity of the beating. If the hand was applied below the costal insertions of the pectoralis major muscle, that is to say, on the præcordial region proper, the beats of the heart seemed perfectly normal and regular. Auscultation at these two points led to the same results, namely, a dull friction-sound above, and a spasmodic sensation perceptible to the touch, which shocked the ear; below, the normal sounds of the heart. Finally, while applying one hand to the pectoralis major, and with the other feeling the pulse, either at the wrist, or at the carotid artery, or heart, it is at once seen that there is no sort of simultaneity between the pretended *palpitations*, mentioned by the patient, and perceived by the former hand, and the real beats of the heart and the arteries.

There was no doubt, therefore, that these ten celebrated allœopathic physicians, among whom, I read to my amazement, the name of Dr. Clarke, physician to the Queen of England, and who gave a similar diagnosis as the rest of them, had made a mistake. It was not an *aneurism of the heart*, but a simple *neurosis*, or, in other words, a *spasm of the pectoralis major muscle*. The only physician who was of my opinion, was Dr. Bouillaud, but I did not become aware of this fact until after I had established my own diagnosis.

This disease was certainly much less serious than an aneurism, but was I any the surer to cure it? What was the character of the disease? It was, if I may use this vague expression, a *rheumatic* affection of a muscle, produced by the influence of a keen and icy-cold wind on a strong and plethoric organization. The muscles of the shoulder, chest, and of that portion of the back which corresponds to the heart; the intercostal muscles of the upper part of the left side; and lastly, the heart itself, although in a much less marked manner, were the parts involved. The spasm of the pectoralis muscle, did not seem to me to furnish a particular indication; it was not a fixed symptom, but came and went at short intervals. As to the rush of blood to the left brain, without any derangement of the rhythm of the pulse, which was 65 a minute, I explained it by the fact that either the arteries or the large venous trunks of the neck were pressed upon at every spasmodic contraction of the muscles which covered these vessels.

The pathological condition which I have here described is

undoubtedly of sufficient interest to merit a detailed account, and there probably never was such a case before. I hesitated what remedy I should give. First, I hit upon *Spigelia*. This stopped the stitches, but the spasm remained; he slept a few hours the first night (which he had not done for six months); but there was prostration, loss of appetite, bitterness of mouth, and a slight headache with dizziness in the morning. Three days after Spigelia, I gave *Colchicum*, which had a little better effect. There was less dryness in the throat; no headache; six or seven hours good sleep at night; no stitches of any kind; for some hours the spasm ceased; but the pain in the shoulder continued, nor did the appetite return; nevertheless Mr. X. felt very much encouraged. He looked upon homœopathy as his sheet-anchor, whereas the old school practice had never afforded him a quarter of an hour's relief, and left him no other prospect than a life of suffering, which death alone, so often desired by him, could terminate.

On the fifth or sixth day of the treatment, Mr. X. received some bad news, and all the symptoms, spasms, stitches, congestion, noises,) became worse again. The colchicum remained powerless. Fortunately my opinion concerning the true remedy in this case had become settled. The nature of the disease, its cause (exposure to a keen and icy-cold wind), the constitution of the patient (sanguine and athletic), every symptom, except the non-existence of fever, pointed to *aconite*. It acted like magic. The morning after the medicine had been taken, Dr. Clarke and his colleagues, who so often and so gratuitously accuse us of ignorance as diagnosticians, would have vainly sought any traces of the aneurism of the heart, with which they had said Mr. X. was afflicted.

At present Mr. X. is in London; I do not consider him cured, and he may have a relapse; but I am persuaded that the continued use of aconite, with perhaps an occasional intercurrent remedy, such as *Lycopodium*, and the substitution of a milder climate for that of England, will completely restore the health of this patient.

This case and a number of others of a similar nature, show that aconite may effect cures even when no fever is present, just as well as when there is fever. This indication is moreover founded on the pathogenesis of aconite. The 1344 symptoms of aconite collected by Dr. Roth, from forty-one observers, and arbitrarily arranged by regions and organs, do not furnish a precise image of the maladies which this agent is capable of curing. On reading this shapeless pathogenesis with due attention, we must see that, although inflammatory fever is one of its leading phenomena, yet there are other morbid conditions that seem to be independent of the fever, and even precede it in chronological order; the whole of these constitute the real sphere of action of the inherent principle of our drug. Among these conditions we have a tendency to start, a desire to be alone, a false estimation of the length of time, etc., which manifest themselves sometimes as soon as the poison has been swallowed; almost all the symptoms of the head and senses; some symptoms of the nasal fossa, mouth, throat, stomach, rectum, anus, bladder, genital organs, lumbar region, shoulder, lower limbs, etc.[1]

It is not to be wondered that this agent should have proved curative in certain cases of *mental derangement*, in persons to whose constitution it was adapted, especially in cases of recent date, and occasioned by fright; in the *delirium* which precedes or accompanies certain *acute* fevers; in recent cases of congestive ophthalmia and deafness; in *amenorrhœa*, or, rather, in sudden suppression of the menses by fright, etc., etc.

Hahnemann recommends it expressly for *measles* and

[1] See in Roth's pathogenesis of Aconite, which of course comprises Hahnemann's symptoms, the 26, 27, 28, 34, 38, 55, 63, 89, 101, 102, 106, 107, 114, 125, 134, 135, 138, 149, 154, 164, 165, 170, 212, 220, 226, 228, 234, 244, 252, 261, 265, 268, 305, 334, 340, 342, 349, 359, 406, 427, 434, 463, 468, 484, 491, 538, 608, 632, 649, 666, 688, 689, 693, 698, 932, 1043, 1119. Most of these symptoms were felt three hours after taking the poison, whereas the symptoms of the heart and the febrile symptoms were only perceived on the second and third day, in most provers, including Stœrck. This fact merits attention, though no more than its nature demands.

purple-rash, in which diseases it frequently exhibits, according to him, a "marvellous efficacy." This may or may not be true, so far as the purple-rash is concerned, my experience, in this respect, is too limited to enable me to express an opinion, but as regards measles, I am prepared to affirm that, in most cases, *Pulsatilla* deserves a preference over aconite.

Inflammatory affections of the heart and arteries, and probably of the circulatory apparatus generally, belong more particularly to the curative sphere of aconite.

Jahr's general indication: "Unpleasant consequences of a cold contracted by exposure to keen and dry cold weather, (north-west wind)" appears to me perfectly correct; yes, the keen and cold wind that prevails on the mountain-ranges where aconite grows.

"Vegetable acids and wine," says Hahnemann, "destroy the effects of this substance. The same result is produced by other drugs that correspond palliatively or homœopathically to the unpleasant symptoms which an excessive or improperly selected dose of aconite, sometimes develops."[1]

[1] Hahnemann's Mat. Med. Pura, vol. I., art. Aconite.

GROUP XVI.

TYPE: CONIUM MACULATUM.
ANALOGUES: CHAMOMILLA VULGARIS. PHOSPHORIS ACIDUM. SENEGA, CANTHARIS.[1]

COMMON CHARACTERISTICS.

THIS group forms, so to say, a sort of transition-link between the one that precedes, and the one that follows it. This will appear the more logical, the more attentively the general action of the drugs of which it is composed, is compared, on the one hand, to that of aconite and its analogues, among which *Conium* and *Chamomilla* belong, which must not be forgotten; and, on the other hand, to that of *thuja*, and its group. *Aconite* represents the acute, phlegmonous inflammation; *Conium*, the chronic or sub-acute inflammation, with sanguineous engorgement of the parenchyma, induration and even subsequent ulceration of the tissues; and *Thuja* represents, I will not say, the degeneration, but the slow and progressive hypertrophy of certain tissues, certain constituents of our organs.

Conium and its analogues, whose modifying powers seem proportionate to the degree of vitality they meet with in the different individuals, are particularly suitable in affections that were primarily *inflammatory*, and are principally adapted to persons primarily endowed with a certain vital activity, individuals with sanguine and nervous constitutions, lively, impressible, irritable, communicative, sensitive to pain, which they bear impatiently. To complete this list of general indications, (which are founded upon facts,) I ought to add, that conium is particularly useful to those who, beside the above-

[1] I fancy that *Jatropha Curcas* and *Solanum nigrum* will hereafter have to be added to the analogues of Conium.

mentioned conditions, have certain glandular organs, especially the testicles and the mammary glands, largely developed.

CORRESPONDING MALADIES.

Chronic inflammations of the vascular system.—Parotitis.—Orchitis, mastitis.—Ovaritis, (sub-acute, with circumscribed or diffuse swelling, induration, and even ulceration of the affected organs, generally consequent upon a contusion.)—Chronic ulcers, (with red borders and extensive indurations.) — Caries. — Cataract, (traumatic). — Glaucoma. — Passive hæmorrhages.—Chronic catarrh, (of the nostrils, bronchia, urethra, vagina.)—Hypostatic pneumonia.—Convulsive cough.—Inflammatory or nervous symptoms consequent on the bite of venomous reptiles.(?)—Hysteria.—Tetanus.—Various nervous diseases.

Conium maculatum, *the cicuta major* of Lamarck, *common hemlock*. Genius *conium*, family umbelliferæ, class pentandria digynia. This is an herbaceous, bisannual plant, known by the following signs; fleshy root, having the shape and size of a small turnip, hairy, white, marked with circular streaks, discharging, when cut into, a white, milky, bitter, acrid juice, the contact of which makes the tongue sore, and causes it to swell. Stem from two to four feet high, hollow interiorly, smooth, branchy, dotted with numerous brown-red spots towards the base, which are the more apparent the younger the plant, (hence its name *maculatum*). Leaves bipinnate, with oval folioles, somewhat distant from one another, pinnatifid at their summit, glabrous, of a dark-green color, especially on the upper side; umbels furnished with little sheaths, (composed of from three to five reflexed folioles, and the little umbels having involucra, composed of from three to five pointed folioles. Flowers white, with unequal petals, and borders reflexed from without inwards. Seeds globular, with rugose borders, tuberculous.

It is important to be acquainted with these characteristics of *Conium maculatum*, for the reason that this plant has sometimes been confounded with parsley, from which more or less distressing accidents have resulted. Being rubbed between the fingers, conium emits a fetid, musty, disagreeable odor, which is sufficient to distinguish it from parsley, the odor of which is aromatic; parsley has no spotted stems, nor hollow petioles, nor are the leaves of such a sombre hue; the leaves of parsley are oval, trifid, incised and indented; those of hemlock oval-oblong, or lanceolate, deep pennafid, the lobes incised or serrated. The flowers of parsley have no involucra, nor are the seeds rugose; the stems of parsley expand at the joints, the leaves are hairy, the seeds are elongated, not globular.

Hemlock, which is found in almost every country, prefers fat and strong soil, amidst ruins, along the borders of empty ditches, woods, etc. It grows in great abundance in Spain, the South of France, Sicily, Greece, especially between Megaræ and Athens, which removes all doubt relatively to the identity of this plant with the hemlock that was used by the Athenians for the purpose of destroying their criminals.

Every part of the plant exhales a fetid odor, that has been compared to that of copper, or the odor of cat's urine, and which is increased rather than diminished by drying the plant.

A comparative view of the experiments that have been made with this poison on animals of different species, seems to show that it acts with more destructive force in carnivorous than upon graminivorous animals. Although Linné states, that it destroys oxen,[1] (which is not proven, by any means,) it is admitted, now-a-days, that rabbits, horses, sheep, and goats, eat it with impunity;[2] whereas, small quantities of the poison were sufficient to kill dogs and wolves.[3] As regards the fatal effects of the poison on man, the deaths of Socrates and Phocion suffice to prove it. It is well known that the poisonous or medicinal properties of conium are the less active, the colder the climate where the plant was gathered. This is the reason why some experimenters of the North of Europe, where the plant is almost deprived of its poisonous properties, have imagined, that it was not poisonous any where.

[1] Wœstgola resd., p. 98.

[2] Gmelin, *Flora sibirica*, Petropoli, 1747, vol. I., p. 203.

[3] Giacomini, *traité de mat. méd.*, p. 471.

Empirical applications.—The medicinal use of hemlock is traceable to the remotest antiquity. It is this plant, according to Ehrhart,[1] contrary to the opinion of Haller, it is true;[2] which Hippocrates, Dioscorides and Galenus, designate by the name of *Koneion.* Aretæus,[3] and other physicians after him, have recommended its use externally to depress the *sexual instinct.* Plinius attributes to it the property of curing *pains, tumors, abscesses,* and *ulcers of a bad character.*[4] Avicennæ[5] and Serapion proposed a plaster of hemlock, to scatter *tumors of the breasts and testicles,* and to *prevent a too copious secretion of milk.*

In the fifteenth century, several practitioners, among whom, Ehrhart[6] mentions Ettmueller, Paré, Ray and Lemery, recommended hemlock, externally, for *glandular swellings, indurated, schirrous or carcinomatous tumors, lupiæ and visceral obstructions.* Reneaulme, a physician of Blois, employed it internally for scirrhous *enlargements of the liver, spleen* and *pancreas.*[7] Jean Wier lauded it, internally, for *scald-head, tetters* and *suppressed itch.*[8]

In spite of these authors, and several others, among whom, Sprengel[9] mentions H. de Heers, Nathlauw, etc., Con. macul. had fallen into complete disuse, until Stœrck[10] restored it in the latter half of the past century to great celebrity.

Guided by the suggestions of the authors whom we have named, and particularly by the remarks of Wier, Stœrck first tried conium externally. He applied it to the affected part in bags, having previously dipped them for a moment in

[1] *Dissert. medic. de cicuta,* Strasb., 1763.

[2] Histor. stirp. helv., n. 966, note a.

[3] *De morbis acutis,* lib. II., cap. 11.

[4] Lib. XXVI., cap. 22 and 24.

[5] Lib. II., tract. 2, cap. 671.

[6] *Dissert. Cit.*

[7] *Curationes,* obs. 3 et 4.

[8] Journ. gén. de méd., vol. XXXVIII., p. 439.

[9] Hist. de la méd., Paris, 1815, vol. V., p. 477.

[10] See Stœrck's three memoirs, namely: *libellus quo* demonstratur cicutana non solum usu interno, tutissime exhiberi posse sed esse semel remedium valde utile in multis morbis, etc., Vindebonæ, 1760, in 8vo; libellus secundus, quo confirmatur, etc., Vind., 1761, in 8vo; libellus quo confirmatur, etc., Vind., 1765, in 8vo.

warm water or milk, to soften them; and he assures us that, by this means, he succeeded in arresting gangrene, quieting the pains of gouty patients, suffering arthritic nodosities (in a man of 60 years,) alleviating the most inveterate rheumatisms, and finally, in scattering scrofulous tumors, glandular indurations of the mammæ, and curing even the most malignant cancers.[1] Encouraged by these successful results, Stœrck prepared an extract of conium in the same manner that he employed afterwards in making an extract of aconite (see page 490.) He first tried it on a little dog, then on himself; and having assured himself that this drug was not so deleterious that it might not be taken without danger in small quantities, he made it into pills and gave them, in progressive doses, to such of his patients as seemed to require them. Stœrck asserts that, by this means, he cured 1st, a *schirrus of the parotid gland*, against which all the dissolvents, even corrosive sublimate, had been used without any success; 2d, two cases of *cancerous ulceration* of the right breast, with hardness of the axillary and inguinal glands; 3d, two cases of *schirrus* of the right breast, one of which changed to an abscess during the treatment, but healed nevertheless; 4th, an unyielding, hard tumor of the breast, coming on six weeks after confinement; 5th, a case of *cancer*, extending from the corner of the mouth to the ear (in a man who, after having got much better, had not patience enough to persevere in the treatment, and died under the hands of an empirical quack;) 6th, a *tumor* of the breast caused by a contusion; 7th, an *enormous induration* of the left breast, red, livid, etc., with short breathing and dry cough (in the case of a lady who, when almost well, drank wine and died of an apoplectic fit in consequence;) 8th, open *schirrus* of the neck, with profuse secretion of fetid ichor; 9th, two *schirri* of the sublingual

[1] See the first memoir. Stœrck likewise tried on himself the juice of the fresh root; but having placed two drops of it on his tongue, it became swollen, stiff and painful, so that he was unable to articulate. All these symptoms passed off in a few hours, by washing the mouth with lemon-water, (the juice of lemon antidotes both *Conium* and *Aconite*.)

glands, in the same individual; 10th, a case of *cancer* of the left breast, extending from the border of the lower jaw to the abdomen (in a female who, when on the point of recovering, according to all appearances, *exposed herself to a draught of air*, (sic!) and was taken with acute pain in the bowels and a diarrhœa that nothing could stop, in consequence of which she died;[1]) 11th, *schirrous glands* at the neck, in the axillæ, groins, and likewise an *ulcerated schirrus* of the left breast; discharging an acrid, corrosive ichor; 12th, a case of *schirrous induration and ulceration* of the sublingual and cervical glands, accompanied with a schirrous tumor on the clavicle, which was so hard that it was supposed to be cartilage; 13th, a recent *schirrus* of the breast; 14th, a case of *schirrous induration* of the left testicle, accompanied by three *carcinomatous excrescences* on the penis and an enormous swelling of this organ, (the cure was completed with mercury;) 15th, two *fistulous ulcers* of the neck, running to the tongue, sternum, between the œsophagus and the wind-pipe, to the xiphoid cartilage and the lumbar-vertebræ, in a female of 32 years (cured in three weeks by the combined use of the conium pills, and fomentations of conium;) 16th, a *schirrous induration* (?) *of the liver*, accompanied with icterus; 17th, several *abdominal tumors*, consequent on paroxysms of quartan fever;[1] 18th, two cases of compound cataract; 19th, *scrofulous swellings* (to which Stœrck adds the adjective *schirrous*,) and a scrofulous ulcer on the left thigh, in the case of a female of 25 years.

In the two memoirs which Stœrck published after this first pamphlet (from 1761 to 1765) we find a considerable number of cases of a different nature from those to which the conium was first applied; such as, 1st, *schirrous tubercles* in the vagina, with acrid leucorrhœa; 2d, an *horrible ulcer* on the face, that had resisted all known means until then; 3d, a

[1] Ought this result to have been charged on the current of air?

[2] Ehrhart (*dis. cit.*) mentions several cases of abdominal tumors consequent on paroxysms of quartan fever, and which were cured with conium; this fact is worth remembering.

case of acrid, corrosive leucorrhœa of ten years' standing, with sleeplessness and hardness near the anus; 4th, a case of *tetter*, with itching, stinging heat, and discharge of an acrid serum; 5th, a case of *asthma*, with cough, anguish, dyspnœa, etc.; 6th, a case of general *scurvy;* 7th, two cases of *cataract;* 8th, two cases of *amaurosis*, one of one, the other of four years' standing; 9th, two cases of *amenorrhœa*, with intermittent pulse, vertigo, etc.; 10th, a case of *epilepsy*, the paroxysms coming on every five or six weeks.

The celebrated de Hæn was one of Stœrck's most vehement opponents. This writer says that he administered conium to upwards of one hundred and twenty women afflicted with cancer, but without any success.[1] His testimony, however, is rather suspicious, owing to his bitter opposition to Stœrck. Whereas Stœrck's disciples, Ehrhart, Collin and others, were perhaps guilty of silently passing over their reverses, de Hæn, governed by petty rancor, took care to publish his own to the world.[2]

Be this as it may, if conium had violent opponents, it had, on the other hand, zealous partizans, among whom we may mention Locher,[3] Fred. Hoffmann,[4] Collin,[5] Cullen,[6] Quarin,[7] Ehrhart,[8] Decotes,[9] Marteau,[10] Vincent,[11] Dupuy de la Porcherie,[12] Gase,[13] Hufeland,[14] Hallé,[15] Valentin,[16] Bridault,[17]

[1] *Ratio medendi*, vol. VIII., part II., epist. de cicut.

[2] Alibert (see *Elém. de Thérap.*) likewise pretends having treated upwards of one hundred females for cancer; but I attach no sort of importance to the testimony of this writer, whose celebrity I have never been able to account for.

[3] *Observationes practicæ*, published in French at Hague, 1764, p. 195.

[4] *Usage des bains de cigue*, Hague, 1764.

[5] *Annus medicus.*

[6] *Mat. Med.*, art. *Conium.*

[7] *Tentamen de Cicuta.* Francofurti, 1799.

[8] *Diss. Cit.*

[9] Anc. *Journ. de Méd.*, vol. XVI., p. 35.

[10] Anc. *Journ. de Méd.*, vol. XIV., p. 121.

[11] *Id.*, vol. XV., p. 522.

[12] *Id.*, vol. XXII., p. 219.

[13] *Récueil pér.* de la Soc. de Méd. de Paris, vol. XXIII.

[14] *Traité de la mal. Scrof.*, p. 236.

[15] Nouv. *Journ. de Méd.*, vol. VIII., p. 106.

[16] *Ann. de la Soc. de Med. prat. de Montpellier*, vol. IV.

[17] Id., vol. VI.

Lespine,[1] Récamier,[2] etc. This shows that the number of those who have used conium after the manner of Stœrck, is quite considerable. I have read the reports of some three or four hundred cases, and I have no doubt there are many more; but most of them are so vaguely stated that it is difficult to derive from them a clear knowledge of the true pathological conditions for which conium is the appropriate remedy. In the following diseases conium has at times been found useful, at others inefficacious, without, however, the cause of its efficacy or failures having been enquired into; *cancerous and scrofulous affections, various tumors,* (most generally at the neck, breasts, in the axillæ, groins, hypogastrium, at the feet;) *obstructions; ulcers that were not cancerous,* (in the face, on the thigh, etc.;) affections that were *considered syphilitic* (which I deem unfounded;) *tetters; fevers; pulmonary phthisis; asthma; leucorrhœa; scurvy; cataract* (occasioned by contusions of the eye-ball;) *ophthalmia,* termed *serous; hemeralopia; amaurosis; dropsy; amenorrhœa; epilepsy; rickets; piles; nasal polypus; vomiting; various kinds of neuralgia; deafness; gout, chronic cystitis* with strangury.[3] Latterly some allœopathic physicians have tried conium for *influenza* and *whooping-cough,* and pretend to have made successful cures in both diseases, which is very probable.

The physicians of the School of Paris, consider conium a *stupefying* drug, the Rasorians place it among their *lymphatico-glandular hyposthenisants.*

Homœopathic applications.—Hahnemann has left us a pathogenesis of conium in both the Materia Med. Pura and the Chronic Diseases; but the latter is much more complete, and it is this one that ought to be studied. It is contained in the second volume, and contains the results of all his new experiments, and more extensive bibliographical researches.

[1] Journ. gén. de méd., vol. XXXVIII., p. 437.

[2] *Recherches sur le traitement du cancer* par la compression. Paris, 1829, two vol. in 8vo.

[3] The order in which these affections are here stated, has reference to the proportionate number of the cases treated with conium.

Contrary to the doctrine of Rasori, the primary action of conium upon the healthy organism, in its general tendency, is stimulating; hence, as a pathological agent, it is depressing, at least, in certain affections, of an essentially inflammatory character. This property, however, is possessed by all poisonous substances, which, like conium, grow in southern countries, and, like it, act more powerfully on carnivorous than herbivorous animals. With his accustomed and wonderful sagacity, Hahnemann seems to have deduced from simple physiological and clinical observations, the general law which I have here stated. The following suggestions are certainly very remarkable: "Conium is one of those drugs," says Hahnemann, "of which it is exceedingly difficult to distinguish the primary and secondary effects. Among its symptoms there are several of an opposite character, that can only be considered as alternate, or rather, consecutive and transitory effects, suspended for a time by a new assault of the remedial force. As regards the sad results of the continued use of massive doses of conium, and which are revealed to us by the failures of the mode of treatment that Stœrck, Lange, Andrea, Ehrhart, Greding, Baylies, Reismann, Collin and Tartreux had rendered fashionable; such results ought to be looked upon as true secondary phenomena developed by the vital reaction that had been so deeply and violently injured by the frequent repetition of these massive doses of the poison. They imply a dissolution of the cohesion of the fibres, accompanied with asthenic inflammation, and a very painful sensitiveness. The contrary effect seems to take place during the primary action of conium, which seems to be characterised by a *rigidity*, *condensation* and *constriction of the fibres*, *with swelling of the glands* and diminution of the senses; indeed, such action is confirmed by the homœopathic treatment and cure, under my hands, of various cases of glandular engorgements of the breasts and lips, occasioned by contusions, and of cataract resulting from blows on the eye."[1]

[1] Mat. Med. Pur., vol. II., art. Conium.

This shows that Hahnemann thinks as I do, that, in order to be used rationally, that is to say, homœopathically in the real sense of the term, the employment of conium in disease, must be indicated by a certain primary rigidity of the fibre; 2d, by a primarily inflammatory character of the disease. This is the reason why conium is particularly suitable to persons of a lively, quick, sanguine disposition, with a marked development of the glandular system; and is characteristically adapted to painful glandular affections, principally such as result from a strain, blow, but the precise cause of which may have escaped our recollection.

It is very probable that in affections of long standing, of which the secondary symptoms have alone remained, conium may be, and probably ought to be, indicated by symptoms that are opposed to those which I have enumerated. This is the unavoidable result of the contrast that exists between the primary and secondary effects of every natural or medicinal disease, after lasting for a certain length of time.

In general terms my views regarding the action of conium may be expressed as follows:—

This drug is to the glands and the capillary system, what aconite is to the heart and the arterial system. In many cases, therefore, we may look upon *conium* as the *aconite of chronic diseases.*—It is not, without sound reflection, that I have placed conium at the head of the analogues of aconite, albeit these two drugs are distinguished from each other by radical differences.

The following symptoms, according to Hahnemann, indicate more specially the use of conium:—

Sadness; hypochondria; anxiety; ill-humor and peevishness; depressed spirits; irritability; tendency to start; disposition to feel out of humor; *aversion to work;* tendency to forget, with weakness of the head; vertigo in looking around, as if the patient would fall on his head; heaviness of the head; paroxysms of tearing headache, obliging one to lie down; stitches at the top of the head; chronic lancinating headache; *falling off of the hair;* itching under the eyes, and after rubbing them; smarting heat; sense of coldness in the eyes, during a walk in the open air; stye; myopia; presbyopia; dark points and colored lines before the eyes; the eyes are dazzled by the light of day; stitches in the ear, during a walk in the open air; tearing and stitches in the ears and the adjoining parts; pulling stitches in the ear, with swelling of the parotids; accumulation of ear-wax; *noise in the ears;* buzzing and *ringing in the ears;* discharge of pus from the nose; itching in the face; itching pimples in the face; tetters in the face; gnawing ulcers in the face; *heat in the face;* dryness and peeling off of the lips; pulling pains in the sound teeth, during a walk in the open air; lancinating pain in the teeth; involuntary deglutition; scraping in the throat; hawking and sense of fulness in the throat; *frequent eructations all day;* noisy eructations tasting of the food; heart-burn; canine hunger; the bread is tasteless; burning in the throat after eating; nausea of pregnant females; acidity of the stomach; weight at the stomach, when eating; constrictive pain at the stomach; spasm of the stomach; stitches in the left hypochondrium; fulness in the lower abdomen, in the morning on waking; constriction of the hypogastrium; twisting and digging in the umbilical region; sense of smarting in the abdomen; gurgling in the abdomen; cutting colic, with emission of flatulence; *constipation, with ineffectual urging to stool; hard stool;* every other day; diarrhœa; blood-streaked stools; the stream of urine suddenly stops, and then flows again in a few minutes; pressure on the bladder, as if the urine would be voided at once; white, cloudy, *thick* urine; *cutting pain in the urethra, when urinating;* insufficient and short-lasting erections; impotence and absence of erections; feeble erection during sexual intercourse; exhaustion after an embrace; *uterine spasms;* pinching in the uterus; pressure from above downwards, and stitches in the vagina; stitches in the labia majora; *itching at the pudendum;* scanty menses;[1] during the menses, pres-

[1] Aconite causes profuse menstruation, metrorrhagia; but this condition

sure downwards, and pulling in the thighs; acrid, excoriating leucorrhœa.

Frequent sneezing; stoppage of the nostrils; stoppage of the nose, in the morning; stuffing of the nose, which had lasted for years; painful feeling of dryness in the nose; *cough*, especially in scrofulous subjects; asthma when walking; asthma on waking in the morning; *asthma during the morning-hours;* stitches in the sternum; shocks in the chest; pressure above the hips; tension at the nape of the neck; smarting pain in the lower cervical vertebræ; burning pressure on the shoulders; sweat in the hollow of the hands; pulling pain in the hips; lassitude in the knees; cramps in the calves; *cold feet* and hands; tendency of the feet to feel cold; uneasiness in the legs; itching of the skin; frequent red itching spots on the body; brown spots on the body; urticaria after violent exercise; old humid tetters; restlessness, especially in the legs; paroxysms of hypochondria and hysteria; hypochondria arising from abstemiousness of sexual intercourse; stitches in the whole body, here and there; *malaise in the open air;* sudden weakness when walking; painful weariness in the extremities; painful sensitiveness of the skin; general lassitude, especially in the extremities; lassitude in the morning, in bed; sense of malaise in the extremities, as after extreme fatigue; drowsiness in the daytime; drowsiness in the evening, with closing of the eyelids; falling asleep late in the evening, in bed; sleep disturbed by dreams; a number of dreams, at night; unrefreshing sleep; nocturnal pains.

On comparing this list of symptoms to those of aconite, it becomes evident that they are distinguished from the aconite symptoms only in this, that the latter represent the acute form of the former; indeed, conium is frequently indicated when aconite has exhausted its action, that is to say when the inflammatory fever has ceased. In some cases *Conium* might be suitable after arnica; but this is a mere hypothesis which I offer.

gradually changes to the opposite, *scanty menstruation*, to which *Conium* corresponds.

All the vegetable acids, such as vinegar and lemon-juice, destroy the effects of dynamised conium so promptly, that a few leaves of salad eaten during the treatment are sufficient to call up again pains that had yielded to recently administered doses of this agent.

Coff. crud. and *Nitri acid.*, have also been mentioned as antidotes of Conium.

Chamomilla Vulgaris. See the group of which this drug is the type.

Phosphori Acidum, *phosphoric acid.* This acid which seems to exist in a free state in some animal substances, constitutes in a great measure, in combination with lime (phosphate of lime) the osseous structure of vertebrated animals. It may be obtained by a direct process, by burning phosphorus in a china saucer, under a glass-jar, resting on Mercury, and filled with air or dry oxygen. It is deposited on the sides of the jar in the shape of flakes of exquisite whiteness, which, when exposed to the open air, rapidly absorb its moisture and are transformed into little drops. This acid is inodorous, but has a very marked taste. When heated in a platina-crucible, it first becomes solid and looks like glass, after which it becomes soft below red heat, fuses at this temperature, and volatilises. In this condition it corrodes glass and earthen vessels by combining with their oxydes. On account of its liability to melting, it can only be preserved in a solid state in hermetically sealed flasks. According to Devergie,[1] phosphoric acid, when given in large doses, exercises on the animal economy the same action, and developes the same symptoms as concentrated sulphuric acid." Baumes, basing himself on the property which this acid enjoys, of dissolving the phosphate of lime in the bones, attributes to excess of this acid *scrofulous caries, rickets,* etc.,[2] an opinion which I should not have mentioned, if it had not been for the remark-

[1] *Médecine légale*, vol. III., p. 294.

[2] *Traité sur le vice scrofuleux*, 2d ed., 1805, p. 32.

able contrast it implies in regard to the known efficacy of phosphoric acid in the very diseases which this author attributes to it.

Empirical applications. This acid has not cured or alleviated many diseases. L. J. Bayle, who had taken care, at the period when his *Bibliothèque de thérapeutique* was published, in 1830, to collect in the second volume of this work, all the cases that had been published until then, only mentions five, namely, three by Lentin,[1] one by Lutzenberger,[2] and one by Wolff.[3] Lentin relates the following cases: A case of *caries of the frontal bone, cured* by the internal and external use of phosphoric acid, the patient using externally conium and asafœtida; a case of *caries of the first false rib*, cured by the internal and external use of phosphoric acid exclusively; a case of pulmonary phthisis, with fetid breath, excessive emaciation, hectic fever, etc., *improved*[4] by the internal use of the same drug. In the case of Lutzenberger we have *complete exhaustion, consequent on puerperal menorrhagia*, with general coldness, cadaverous paleness, hippocratic countenance, tremulous and almost imperceptible pulse, cold and clammy sweat, etc.; his patient was a female who had been confined for six days past, and was naturally very delicate. The acid, which was given in despair, arrested the hæmorrhage that had been going on all the time, although the patient seemed to have literally lost all her blood; the pulse and vital heat were strengthened again, and in a few days the cure which seemed almost miraculous, was completed.[5] Wolff's case is less interesting: it is a case of

[1] *Dissert. de acid. phosph. cariei ossium domitore*, part I., p. 391, (Comment. Gutting., vol. XIII.)

[2] *Journal de Hufeland*, and *Bibliot. Méd.*, vol. XXI., p. 245.

[3] *Hufeland's Journal*, Nov. 1821.

[4] The author says: The patient promptly felt the good effects of this treatment; the breath lost its bad odor, the fever and expectoration became less, and the patient recovered his strength sufficiently to walk about in the city every day; he died, however, of the measles.

[5] Lutzenberger informs us that he used the phosphoric acid with much success in other cases of asthenic hæmorrhage from other parts of the body

whitlow with caries, where external applications of phosphoric acid facilitated in a remarkable manner the reproduction of the ulcerated phalynx, whence the author infers that the action of phosphoric acid is purely chemical, which we cannot admit.

But apart from the facts related by Bayle, there exist a few other documents relating to the empirical use of phosphoric acid, which are worthy of mention. Marles tells us that he has given phosphoric acid with much success in the *serpiginous crust* of the cornea, accompanied with hectic fever;[1] Gœden in *contagious typhus*;[2] Baumes in *angina pectoris*;[3] Sumerling of Stralsund, again recommended it in 1830 for *phthisis, passive hœmorrhage, caries* and *rickets, typhoid fever*, with tendency to prolapsus, and *symptomatic sweat*; finally, another doctor of Stralsund, named Marké, and after him Alphonse Leroyson, administered it dissolved in a large quantity of water, in cancer of the uterus, in the shape of injections. According to *the statement* of these doctors, these injections speedily modified the foul smell of the pus, and gave more relief than all the narcotics together generally do in similar cases.[4]

Homœopathic applications.—According to Hahnemann phosphoric acid is indicated when the following conditions prevail either entirely or in part:

Headache in the morning; inability to bear noise in conversation; crusts on the back of the nose; heaviness of the nose; heat in the cheeks; pimples on the chin; pimples on the forehead and chin; heat at the hypogastrium; urination at night; pain at the liver during the menses; roughness at the larynx; scraping in the larynx which excites cough; short breathing, and inability to talk for any length of time;

[1] Hufeland's Journal.

[2] Mèrat and Delens, *dict. univ. de mat. med.*, vol. V., p. 291, (see Gœden's Work: *Von der Arzneikraft der Phosphorsœure gegen den ansteckanden, Typhus*, Berlin, 1814.)

[3] Ann. Clin., vol. XXII.

[4] Mérat and Delens, *loc. cit.* See the pathogenesis of Phosph. ac. in Hahnemann's Chronic Diseases, Vol. III.

weakness of the chest after talking; pimples on the arms; sweat at the feet; tetters; corns; night-sweat.

Considering the vast array of indications which Hahnemann has placed in front of some of his antipsoric remedies, such as sulphur, calcarea, lycopodium, sepia, carbo vegetabilis, it seems strange, that the indications of phosphoric acid should be so few. Can it be possible that Hahnemann should have been ignorant of the many therapeutic uses of this agent? This is not to be supposed. When Hahnemann published the pathogenesis of phosphoric acid in the chronic diseases, he had been in the habit of using it for a long time agreeably to the provings which we find recorded of this acid in the Mat. Med. pura; hence I infer that the above-mentioned indications are really the only ones to which phosphoric acid corresponds.

It is, however, true that this drug has been used empirically with the greatest success in various diseases to which it seemed adapted, such as *passive hæmorrhages* (of the bronchia or uterus;) *typhoïd fever*, *diseases of the bones*, (especially in old men,) *seminal emissions*, with general prostration, occasioned by masturbation or excessive sexual intercourse. I have used it successfully, 1st, (after *Puls.*) in a case of obstinate *hæmoptysis*, with symptoms of pneumonia at first, in the case of a female of forty years, nervous, of a restless disposition, exhausted by a long disease, during which she had been bled several times, to the great shame of the *throat-cutting method*, for the bleedings had only served to increase the debility without easing the cough; 2nd, in a case of *hypostatic pneumonia*, in a woman of sixty years, which I had despaired of. Acidum phosph. is principally suitable to individuals of originally strong constitutions, but which had become weakened by losses of animal fluids, by excesses, violent acute diseases, chagrin or a long succession of moral emotions.

Camphor and *raw coffee* are said to antidote this drug.

Senega, or rather *polygala senega polygala of Virginia.*—

A perennnial plant, ligneous, genus *polygala*, formerly belonging to the family of the pediculareæ, but recently made the type of a new family, the polygaleæ, class diadelphia octandria. This plant is a native of Virginia, Pennsylvania, Maryland, and of some other states of the American Union. The root is the only part of this plant that has been used in medicine. Externally it is of a reddish-gray color, internally it is white, wrinkled, rugose, strangely twisted, as if composed of a heap of little stumps or simple pieces of the size of a goose-quill. It has a slightly aromatic odor. Its taste is first flat, afterwards acrid, stinging, irritating, when chewed, it causes a heat in the throat, excites cough and a flow of saliva. The cough-symptom, I should think, must seem very strange to the few allœopathic physicians who use it for the chest and bronchial affections characterised by cough. This root is only known in Europe for about a century. Murray tells us that, in his time, the root was yet very scarce, and that it was difficult to procure it.[1]

The effects of senega on animals are not known. Bretonneau says that it makes them vomit, and irritates their mucous membranes; but such vague statements are of no sort of importance to us.

Empirical applications.—The introduction of this root as a therapeutic agent appears to be due to Tennent, a Scotch physician, who inhabited Virginia for a long time, and, from 1735 to '41, published three memoirs on the subject.[2] Tennent having heard that the Indians used this root to neutralise the bad effects of the bite of the rattlesnake, soon had an opportunity of testing these supposed virtues. These effects, apart from the pain inflicted by the bite, consist chiefly of dyspnœa, cough, hæmoptysis, with a hard and frequent pulse, or sometimes frequent and weak, and hence he concluded that the root of senega might perhaps likewise prove useful

[1] *Appar. Medic.*, vol. II., p. 439.

[2] 1. *Physical disquisitions*, Lond., 1735; 2. *Essays on the Pleurisy*, Philad. 1736; 3. *Epistle to Rich. Mead*, concerning the efficacy of the *seneka snake-root*, Edinb. 1772.

in *pneumonia* and *pleurisy* occasioned by other causes. He soon found that it was so. Before, however, giving senega, Tennent first bled his pneumonic and pleuritic patients once; under the influence of senega the sanguineous engorgement in the lungs disappeared, and even the *dropsical effusion in the chest*, where it existed. Be this as it may, he had no sooner addressed his work (*Essays on the pleurisy*) to the Faculty of the Sciences, in Paris, when Leméry, Jussieu, Duhamel, Perceval, and especially Bouvard, adopted his method with success.[1] But the experiments of these practitioners showed that, in spite of the case of Linné, who had cured himself of acute pneumonia with no other remedy than senega,[2] it really was only suitable in cases of sub-acute, chronic inflammation of the lungs. Desbois de Rochefort, however, although of the same opinion and advising the senega root only as a good *expectorant* in *chronic catarrh* of the air-passages, declares having seen this root produce good effects in *acute phthisis*.[3] And lastly, *rheumatic fever*, *dropsies*, *incipient cataract*[4] and *croup*[5] are the affections for which the senega-root was tried with more or less success.

Homœopathic applications.—The provings of this drug seem to justify to some extent the empirical applications that have been made of it.[6] Homœopathic physicians use it in the same affections for which it is recommended by Tennent, Bouvard, etc., namely, for engorgement of the pulmonary parenchyma, chronic catarrh, etc. I do not know how far it antidotes the bites of poisonous serpents; facts of this kind are very rare in Europe. But what seems to me proven beyond a doubt is, that this root, like conium and

[1] See *Mémoires de l'Acad. des sc.* de Paris, year 1777, p. 37 and 135.

[2] *Amœnit. acad.*, vol. IV., p. 35.

[3] *Mat. Med.*, vol. II., p. 4.

[4] See Murray, *appar. med.*, *loc. cit.*

[5] Valentin, Rech. hist. et prat. sur le croup, p. 571, and Bretonneau, *traité de la diphthérite*, p. 241. Bretonneau attributes to senega the faculty of fluidising the mucous secretions, and, by this means, preventing the formation of the false membrane.

[6] See Jahr's Symptomen-codex, Hempel's translation.

phosphoric acid, is essentially adapted to the constitution of persons possessing originally a good deal of physical and moral strength. I have only used senega with advantage in very old affections of the chest, in females of slender and tall make, thin, but having retained a good deal of sprightliness and moral power. For instance, it produced a marked improvement in the case of a lady of forty years, with the following symptoms: Contusive, pressive, sometimes crampy, very old pains in the chest, the anterior wall of which was sensitive to contact, (on both sides;) these pains at times decreased, at others increased in the open air; the respiratory murmur at the top of the lungs was dull, feeble, without rhonchus; the percussion sound had its full resonance; dyspnœa when walking, and especially when going up stairs; paroxysms of vascular agitation in the chest, as if she would faint; catarrhal cough, not very frequent, with ropy, not very profuse expectoration; spitting of red blood, now and then; the pulse varies from 70 to 80 per minute; *paroxysms of palpitations, during which the rhythm of the heart changed to an almost imperceptible tremor, and which, in some cases, lasted all night, and even longer;* the courses were regular, profuse, lasting from six to seven days, (the palpitation generally took place after the courses, or in consequence of some moral emotion;) the stools were generally natural, etc. Senega does not seem to admit of many other applications. According to Jahr, *Arnic.*, *Bellad.*, *Bryon.*, and *Camph.*, are the antidotes of this drug.

Cantharides. *Meloë vesicatorius* of Linné, cantharis *vesicatoria* of Geoffroy; *Spanish fly*, etc.; an insect of the genus *meloë*, family of the epipasticæ of Duméril. This coleoptera, which abounds in the south of Europe, shows itself in France in the months of May and June. The trees on which it is principally seen, are the beach, lilac, elder, privet, etc. It exhales a fetid and dangerous odor, and it is well known that its introduction into the organism is still more dangerous.

These insects have enjoyed a great celebrity in the annals

of Old School medicine, and they do so still. The following diseases are said to have been cured or ameliorated by their internal administration:—*Incontinence of urine, dysuria, stranguria, hæmaturia, dropsy, lepra,* and especially some *nervous diseases,* such as cardialgia, *spasmodic vomiting, hiccough, chorea,* epilepsy, and lastly *rage.*[1] Until now this drug has been very little used by homœopathic physicians;[2] its general action seems to be very much like that of senega.

[1] See the art. *meloë* in Mérat and Delens' *dict. de mat. méd.;* this article is really interesting in an historical point of view.

[2] See the pathogenesis in Jahr's Symptomen-codex, translated by Chs. J. Hempel.

GROUP XVII.

TYPE: THUYA OCCIDENTALIS.

ANALOGUES: PLATINA, BISMUTHUM. CASTOREUM.[1]

COMMON CHARACTERISTICS.

KEEN sensitiveness to the cold.

Fever, with predominance of chilliness; shuddering, emanating from the back and followed by heat in the face, (with or without thirst,) anxious sadness, generally towards evening or at night.

Habitual deficiency of vital heat.

Coldness of the back, all along the vertebral column.

Sleeplessness or waking at night, occasioned by a general coldness, or only coldness of the extremities.

Sleeplessness, without any appreciable cause, or with restlessness.

Starts when on the point of falling asleep; lascivious or frightful dreams.

Depression of spirits; discouragement; difficulty of thinking.

Vertigo.

Sense of fulness in the head.

Compressive, crampy, or ulcerative cephalalgia, especially at the vertex.

Falling off of the hair, on the top of the head.

Semi-lateral, pulling, gnawing, or crampy prosopalgia.

Toothache aggravated by cold drinks, eased by warm water.

Dryness of the mouth and throat; flat taste in the mouth; aphthæ on the tongue and gums; altered appetite; swelling of the sublingual and other salivary glands.

[1] *Scilla marit.* and several resins may hereafter have to be added to this group.

Spasms, or crampy pains at the stomach or in the bowels.

Distention of the lower abdomen.

Benumbing pains in the abdominal viscera.

Violent spasmodic pains, which are seldom followed by copious stools.

Emission of copious flatulence, especially in the morning, most frequently without smell.

Normal or delaying stools, (or, which is less frequent,) diarrhœic stools, or stools inform and bloody.

Frequent urging to urinate, as if the bladder contracted spasmodically, or as if it were prevented by some obstacle from distending.

Spasms of the bladder.

Stitches in the urethra; sycosic gonorrhœa.

Weight in the uterus; spasms of the uterus; induration, prolapsus and deviation of the uterus; polypous or fungous vegetation in the uterus.

Sycosic leucorrhœa.

Too early menses, (or, much less frequently,) retarded, pale, of short duration, with difficult flow of blood, a very marked sensation, as if something were flowing to the womb, by which this organ is pressed down.

Beatings or pullings, (sometimes without cessation,) in the suspensory ligaments of the womb; these symptoms are generally increased, and, in some rare cases, suspended during the menstrual flow.

Uterine hæmorrhages, (only by platina and castoreum.)

No thrill, or very much retarded, during an embrace, (in both sexes.)

Sexual excitement, (much less frequently by thuya than its analogues.)

Sexual desire without erection; impotence; sterility.

Stoppage of the nostrils.

Hoarseness.

Sensation as of a foreign body in the larynx, trachea and chest.

Embarrassed respiration.

Convulsive cough, generally at night, with scanty and difficult expectoration of thick or fungous masses.

Palpitation of the heart.

Benumbing, tensive, gnawing, crampy, twitching pains at the nape of the neck, back, loins, in the shoulders, hips, etc., with habitual predominance of these symptoms in the left side of the body, in a room rather than in the open air, more during rest than during moderate exercise.

Catarrhal affections, ulcers and sycosic excrescences at the genital organs, anus, or, more commonly, over all the mucous surfaces of the skin.

CORRESPONDING DISEASES.

Catarrhal and rheumatic affections.—Boils.—Acne.—Variola.—Ulcerated and vegetating sycosis.—Acne rosacea.(?)—Pimples of Aleppo and Bagdad.(?)—Plica.(?)—Follicular granulations.—Condylomata.—Fungous and fibrous polypi.—Warts.—Corns.—Phlegmasia alba dolens.—Elephantiasis of the Greeks.(?)—Elephantiasis of the Arabs.(?)—Hypertrophy of the papillæ.(?)—Induration and hypertrophy of the testicles, uterus and ovaries.—Horny excrescences.(?) — Onyxis.(?) — Ichthyosis.(?)—Sycosic gonorrhœa and leucorrhœa.—Prolapsus and deviation of the uterus.—Dysmenorrhœa.—Impotence.—Sterility.—Eclampsia.—Hysteria, etc.

The drugs of the thuya group are in special correspondence to the internal and external signs of sycosis. But what is sycosis?

This disease to which only some twenty lines are devoted in the *Dictionary of the Medical Sciences*,[1] only plays an unimportant and obscure part in the ancient systems of pathology. The reason of this is not that sycosis, or the figwart disease, as Hahnemann terms it, is a new disease; it was vaguely known even in the remotest antiquity, and, consequently many centuries previous to the invasion of Europe by the syphilitic disease.

Celsus, speaking of ulcers, expresses himself in this wise: "There is one which has been termed by the Greeks *sycosis*, owing to its resembling a fig in shape; it is a fleshy excrescence, and this is indeed the generic character of this disease,

[1] Vol. LIII., p. 531.

of which we have two species: the former comprises hard and round, the latter moist and irregularly shaped ulcers. From the hard ulcers oozes a sticky humor; the moist ulcers discharge a more profuse quantity of liquid of a fetid odor. Both ulcers show themselves on the hairy parts, the callous and round ulcer principally in the region of the beard, the moist ulcer on the hairy scalp."[1]

Paul of Egina, Ætius, Galenus, etc., apply the name *sycosis* to a tumor on the lids; but each of these authors describes it differently, no doubt guided by the examples which he had before him. It is not certain, therefore, that the sycosis of these authors is the sycosis of Celsus.

Hahnemann gives the name sycosis or sycosic miasm to the principle that generates the excrescences which come out on the skin or mucous membranes, provided these excrescences do not depend upon the psoric or syphilitic miasms; a distinction, however, which the founder of homœopathy does not teach us to establish.

Dr. Petroz, who read an excellent paper on sycosis at the homœopathic Congress of 1852, seems to be of Hahnemann's opinion in reference to this subject, with this difference that he does not believe the syphilitic miasm capable of engendering apparently sycosic ulcers or excrescences without the aid of the sycosic miasm. "Every kind of tumor," says he, "which forms under the epidermis, in the tissue of the dermis, in the papillæ and the rete mucosum of Malpighi, must be considered a product of sycosis, unless variola or the syphilitic virus should be the determining causes; if it should be the syphilitic virus, *it is to its complication with sycosis* that the formation of the excrescence is due."[2]

If this definition be accepted, modern dermatologists who, it must be confessed, observe scarcely any thing more of disease than its cutaneous efflorescence, have frequently described, under different names, the various manifestations

[1] Lib. VI., cap. 3.

[2] *Mémoire sur la sycose*, in the *Journal de la Soc. gall. de méd. homœop.*, vol. II., p. 362.

of one and the same morbid principle. Starting from this hypothesis of an identity of principle, I have mentioned among the corresponding diseases of the thuya group (with a doubt, however, for clinical experience alone can decide in last resorts,) a considerable number of diseases which are considered as distinct affections by dermatologists, which are not even classed by them in the same category, and which, according to my judgment, are simply symptomatic varieties of sycosis.

"Sycosic productions," says Petroz, "are elevations of the epidermis, occasioned by the hypertrophied papillæ that rest upon a point which had become indurated in consequence of a chronic inflammation.[1]

"The form of these excrescences varies; these variations depend upon the degree of density of the tissues where the excrescences become seated. Excrescences that develope themselves on parts exposed to the air, where the dermis is formed of dense laminæ, as on the hands and in some parts of the face, are strikingly different from those that grow on parts with a dermis of less thickness and density, such as the genital organs, the margin of the anus, and the mucous membranes which are immediately acted upon by the atmospheric air.

"When the sycosic miasm acts upon hairy and very vascular parts whose papillæ become easily hypertrophied, as the margin of the lips, the sycosic excrescence assumes a particular form, which frequently causes it to be confounded with a cancerous tubercle; excision of the sycosic tubercle is followed by a cure, whereas the excision of the cancerous tubercle is followed by a relapse."[2]

[1] I am even inclined to think that a chronic inflammation, or a purely mechanical irrition may, after a certain lapse of time, and without the intervention of any miasm, determine the hypertrophy in question. I doubt, therefore, that a corn, a bunion, or even a wart are always sycosic symptoms.

[2] Sycosis being, after all, a general affection, like cancer, it is not impossible that, like cancer, it should reproduce itself; experience, in this respect, has not yet enlightened us altogether.

Further on, Petroz adds:

"Sycosic excrescences vary as regards their shape; it is difficult to class them, and this would, indeed, be useless so far as the treatment is concerned. Nevertheless the sycosic ulcer of Celsus ought to be considered as the sycosic disease in its acute form."[1]

It might perhaps not be quite as useless as Petroz seems to imagine, to class the sycosic excrescences, basing such a classification upon a rigorous observation of the internal or external, general or particular symptoms which precede or accompany each single excrescence. Let us not forget that the miasmatic identity which we suppose exists between these various sycosic excrescences, is as yet an ingenious hypothesis. May not the sycosic, like the psoric miasm, be a multiple principle, or, in other words, may we not have varieties of sycosis as we have, as I firmly believe, varieties of psora? It cannot, therefore, be without some practical interest to distinguish these varieties from each other, the rather that we admit, and Mr. Petroz with us, the existence of *several anti-sycosic remedies*.[2]

Is sycosis, as Hahnemann believes, a syphilitic disease? I think not. It is certain that it can be transmitted by intercourse; it is likewise true that the genital organs are the parts where the disease habitually manifests itself in the most striking manner; and it is a matter of observation that the syphilitic virus excites the sycosic disease, and provokes the development of its cutaneous or mucous symptoms, (which, however, is likewise done by a variety of toxical agents.) But these facts do not imply that the sycosic disease, which was known some dozen centuries prior to the appearance of syphilis, cannot or does not exist independently of all sexual relations, of all sexual intercourse. This

[1] *Mém. Cit.*, p. 362.

[2] *Mém. Cit.*, p. 374. Petroz regards the following medecines as antisycosic: *acidum nitric.*, *silica*, *cuprum acet.*, *secale cornut.*, *sabina* and mugwort. I have not sufficient proofs before me of the existence of a real analogy between these drugs and *Thuya*.

is so true, that sycosis has often been noticed among animals, an instance of which is given by Petroz.[1]

Let us now, before concluding these general remarks, say a word concerning the treatment of sycosis.

If the hypothetic assumption of a sycosic miasm accounts in a plausible manner for a multitude of pathological phenomena that had remained unexplained until then; what an intensity of thought it must have required on the part of Hahnemann to find in thuya the principal remedy, yea the true *specific* for sycosis.

At a period when the doctrine of the *signaturæ rerum* was still the prevailing belief, the resinous callosities of the stems and leaves of the thuya occidentalis might have seemed an indication that this plant was the specific for sycosis and warts; but the age of the signaturæ rerum is passed. And even, if Hahnemann had lived at the time of Serapion and Dioscorides, his genius would have elevated him above the childish prejudices of this first age of medicine. I may, however, ask, whether the assumption, that a substance which, like the rosin that we obtain from various coniferæ, is capable of modifying vegetable juices in a peculiar manner, might perhaps affect the animal fluids in a similar manner, is any thing else than a mere signature. Whatever may be thought of this correlation, to which I attach no more importance than it merits, I have no doubt whatsoever that several rosins must act upon figwarts in the same manner as thuya; a few pages further on (under *Castoreum*), the grounds for this belief will be found explained.

Thuya Occidentalis, *tree of life.* Genus *Thuya,* family coniferæ, class monœcia monadelphia. Thuya is a resinous tree with small imbricate leaves, always green, growing in cool and rather damp regions, in Virginia and Canada, where it seems to originate. In Europe it is cultivated in gardens as an ornamental plant. Its wood is supposed to be inaccessible to decay; for this reason it is frequently used for

[1] *Id.*, p. 368.

coffins. By distillation a sort of essential oil has been obtained from its leaves, similar to the essence of turpentine, very fluid, light, transparent, slightly tinged like ambra, or becoming colorless if distilled over again, of a strong odor similar to that of tansy, of a slightly acrid taste like the taste of camphor. It is said that several Edinburgh and Berlin physicians employ this substance as an *anthelmintic*, a few drops on sugar at a dose.[1]

Empirical applications. They are so trifling that Hahnemann was perfectly justified in saying that nobody, before him, had seriously employed thuya as a drug.[2] Parkinson advises the eating the leaves and the young sprouts on bread and butter, as a means of bringing about the *expectoration of the tenacious and vitiated humors.*[3] According to Herzmann[4] thuya is a *dissolvent*, *desiccative*, *carminative* and *sudorific*, a very vague though not altogether incorrect definition. Kalm tells us that in Canada the pounded leaves are used to quiet *rheumatic pains*, and he adds that a decoction of these leaves is praised for *cough* and *intermittent fevers.*[5] Boerhaave recommends it for dropsy, doubtless founding his recommendation upon the property possessed by thuya of exciting the bladder, and causing frequent discharges of urine.[6]

Homœopathic applications. The discovery of the antisycosic virtues of thuya is so important a fact in therapeutics, that it alone, it seems to me, would have been sufficient to immortalize its author. But among his many claims to the gratitude of humanity, this discovery seems almost to be forgotten.

In Hahnemann's pathogenesis of thuya[7] we have 334 symptoms recorded by himself, and 300 more by his disciples, making in all 634 symptoms; since then, thuya has been re-proved by the Viennese physicians, and we have now

[1] *Journ. de Pharm.*, vol. II., p. 156.
[2] Mat. Med. Pura, vol. III.
[3] Murray, *appar. medic.*, vol. I., p. 31.
[4] Mat. Med., vol. II., p. 565.
[5] *Resa*, vol. III., p. 389.
[6] Element. chem., vol. II., p. 68.
[7] *Loc. Cit.*

a series of 2088 symptoms constituting the complete pathogenesis of this drug.[1]

My otherwise limited experience in regard to the use of this drug, induces me to lay it down as a principle that thuya is particularly suitable to persons of a lymphatico-sanguine, or of a sanguine temperament, with dark complexions, black hair, dry fibre and not very fat. The following symptoms seem to me to require more particularly the exhibition of this agent:

Depression of spirits; lowness of spirits and discouragement even to loathing of life; difficulty of thinking; general prostration, *with coldness*, especially in the afternoon and evening; vertigo when walking, sitting or lying down; *stupefying headache*, worse when stooping, especially *in the morning on waking;* rush of blood to the head; heaviness at the occiput; pressive headache, with boring sensation at the vertex, as if a nail were sticking there; *excessive painfulness of the hairy scalp*, but especially in the left parietal and temporal regions; gnawing itching of the hairy scalp; falling off of the hair *at the vertex; chronic ulcer on the hairy scalp, with flat, but widely indurated borders, grayish bottom, discharging an ichorous and fetid pus;* itching at the eyes; twitching in the eye-balls; pressive pain at the bottom of the orbits; *myopia;* small red tubercles at the free margin of the eyelids; stye; gnawing itching at the eyebrows; *sycosic tubercle in the eyebrow;* stitches with pressure in the ears, in the evening; tearing jerks in the ears; crampy pain at the outer ear; painful crusts in the nose; *stuffing of the nose;* fluent coryza in the air; ulcerations in the nostrils; secretion of thick, greenish, and sometimes fetid mucus in the nasal fossæ; *nose-bleed; polypus in the nose;* heat in the face, with coldness all over the rest of the body; sweat in the face; *digging pain in the malar bones*, momentarily relieved by slight pressure, but aggravated by lying on the affected part; twitching of the lips; small pustules at the lips, readily bleeding when

[1] See this pathogenesis translated and arranged by Doctor Metcalf, in the North American Hom. Journal, No. IV.

touched; sycosic vegetations at the lips; gnawing toothache, in carious teeth, aggravated by the contact of cold drinks; swelling of the salivary glands; *dryness of the mouth;* profuse flow of a flat, sweetish, and sometimes bitter saliva; ulcerations in the mouth; pain in the throat, as if excoriated, with continual desire to swallow; diminished appetite; altered taste; empty eructations; loud eructations; *spasm of the stomach;* exhaustion after eating; stitches in the hypochondria; *constrictive pain on the hypogastrium; copious emission of generally inodorous flatulence, especially in the morning;* movement in the abdomen as of something alive; *beatings in the right iliac fossa, after walking;* delaying and insufficient stool; large-sized, hard, and blood-encircled stools; stitches in the rectum; smarting at the anus, even between the stools; *sycosic vegetations at the anus; frequent desire to urinate; warts on the corona glandis and prepuce; condylomata at the male and female sexual parts; sycosic gonorrhœa,* (see page 314); sexual desire, with erections, and with inability to expel the semen during an embrace; no thrill (in either sex,) during an embrace; *smarting at the female sexual organs when urinating;* tubercles in the mucous membrane of the vagina; *prolapsus and anteversion of the uterus; funguses in the uterus; uterine polypi; sterility;* delaying menses, or *generally too early by seven or eight days,* and, in this case, not very abundant, and only lasting one or two days; *thick leucorrhœa.*

Hoarseness; scraping and formication in the larynx; sensation as of a foreign body in the larynx and trachea; *cough with expectoration of yellowish mucus;* violent, convulsive cough, excited by inspiring cool air, with stupefying headache, copious flatuosities in the bowels, and expectoration of polypus-like fungous masses, which, on being scattered, show *hypertrophied mucous follicles;*[1] embarrassed respiration; stitches in the chest; palpitation of the heart when lying on the left side; blueish tint of the skin on the clavicles; *painful stiffness of the neck and back;* swelling of the cervical

[1] Petroz, *mém. cit.*, case VI.

ganglia; laming pain in the back, in the morning after rising; throbbing tearing in the upper limbs, worse in a warm bed; icy coldness of the hands, or only of the ends of the fingers; *warts on the dorsal surface of the hands;* heaviness of the lower limbs; *cold feet and knees, even at night, in bed;* stitches in the legs; red swelling of the ends of the fingers, toes and insteps; *boils here and there;* excessive sensitiveness of the skin all over the body; *profuse sweat in the axillæ; rounded ulcers, with broad indurated borders, grayish bottom, on the thighs, at the perinæum, or in the neighbourhood of the genital organs;* fever with icy-coldness all along the dorsal spine; shaking shudderings; thirst, or absence of thirst and heat in the face, in the afternoon, and especially towards evening or even at night; restlessness at night, which prevents one from falling asleep; sleeplessness, with coldness of the feet and legs up to the knees; rheumatic or neuralgic, jerking, spasmodic or crampy pains, compelling one to leave the bed; the sleep is disturbed by ominous dreams about battles, blood, death, or by *lascivious dreams;* the pains are worse in the left side of the body.

In 1848, Bœnninghausen published an interesting note on the good effects of thuya in variola.[1] According to this author, whose labors in the cause of homœopathy are so justly valued by homœopathic physicians, the use of this drug, not only moderates the symptoms of small-pox, and abridges the disease, but prevents the pitting, and shortens the duration of the red spots which remain after the scabs come off. *Thuya,* which has already rendered great service to veterinary surgery, appears to be of great service in *farcy.*

I know from repeated observations, that *colchicum* is the best antidote of *thuya.*

Platina.—This metal has the color and lustre of silver, except that it has a little more grayish tint; when perfectly pure, it is softer than silver; almost as tenacious as iron;

[1] See *Journ. of hom. med.,* vol. IV., p. 680.

fusible only in the flame of an explosive mixture of oxygen and hydrogen; it is not altered by exposure to the air, nor does it oxydise at any temperature; specific weight 21, 80, higher than that of any other substance. This metal, which appears to have been discovered towards the end of the sixteenth century, is scarcely ever found pure; it is generally mixed with iridium, omnium, palladium or rhodium. It is found in the sands of the river Pinto, in Choco, Quito, Peru, and especially in the neighbourhood of Carthagena, in South America. Fifteen or sixteen years ago it was discovered in the mines of Siberia and in the auriferous sands of the Ural mountains.

Before Hahnemann, nobody had ever used platina as a drug; nobody could have supposed this metal possessed of medicinal properties which it, indeed, does not seem to acquire except by the process of dynamization. Some of its salts, however, have been used as *alterative* medicines. The *perchloride* of platina has been praised for *melancholy*, but especially for various old *syphilitic affections* which had resisted the action of mercury, and probably were of sycosic origin.[1] Doctor Ferd. Hœfer, who recommends this salt for the last-named affections, and who tried it on himself in massive doses, found, that it acts better in a room than in the open air; a particularity which seems to belong to most of the symptoms of metallic platina.[2]

According to Hahnemann, this metal is particularly indicated by the following symptoms:

"Loss of appetite; loud eructations after eating; constipation when travelling; discharge of the prostatic fluid; induration of the uterus; lassitude in the legs; cold feet; stuffing of the nose."[3]

But it is especially in certain kinds of uterine affections and in neuralgia, that platina has been employed with the greatest success. The more the nature and course of these

[1] See *Dict. des sc. méd.*, vol. XLIII., p. 171, et Coxe, *Amer. disp.*, p. 472.
[2] *Gaz. Med.*, 8 Nov. 1840.
[3] See the pathog. of Platina in Hahnemann's *Chronic Diseases*, vol. III.

diseases are studied, the more we shall find that they are related to the general character of thuya. I base this opinion upon numerous clinical facts, which convince me of its truth. What contributes to fortify me in this belief, is the fact, that Colchicum is the most certain antidote of *Platina* as well as of *Thuya*, *Bismuth* and *Castoreum*.

Bismuthum. See page 249.

Castoreum. A product furnished by the *castor fiber*, a mammiferous amphibious animal, of the genus *Castor*, order of the gnawers. This little quadruped, which is about the size of an ordinary cat, and whose curious manners are well known to every body, used to be quite common all over Europe, and especially in the south of France. But it has been so steadily pursued by our hunters, that it has completely disappeared from our soil, and is only yet found in the uninhabited regions of Siberia and North America. The substance which is known to druggists by the name of *castoreum*, appears to be secreted by a double row of glands agglomerated under the skin of the abdomen, (in the male as well as female;) it is collected in two bladders placed against each other, with thin walls, partitioned off interiorly, and enclosed in a sort of cloaca which communicates with both the anus and the genital organs. It seems to be the particular destination of the glandular secretion to lubricate these parts. It is these two pouches, united by their excretory duct, of unequal size, flat and wrinkled, which, in commerce, go by the name of *castoreum*, although this name applies in reality only to the contents of these pouches.

This substance, when fresh, is yellow, and of the consistence of syrup; when dry, it is red or red-brown, and of the consistence of hard wax. It has a strong, penetrating, fetid, empyreumatic odor, resembling partly the odor of musk and partly that of the goat; its taste is bitter and pungent. Chemists, who have analysed castoreum, generally look upon it as a resinous substance; we shall hereafter see that this circumstance is not without interest for us.

Empirical applications.—Castoreum was known to the physicians of the remotest ages, and has been praised by Galenus, Celsus, Aretæus, Plinius, Alexander of Tralles, Dioscorides, and especially by Ætius. Every writer on Materia Medica has considered it an *anti-spasmodic.* Indeed it seems to have been particularly efficacious in spasmodic affections of the uterus and air-passages. It is said to have been given with advantage in the following affections:—*Hysteria, amenorrhœa, leucorrhœa, suppression of the lochia, blennorrhœa, difficult cutaneous eruptions, slow malignant fevers, adynamic fevers,* (last period,) *sciatica, gouty rheumatism, pityriasis,* (employed externally,) etc.[1] Trousseau and Pidoux furnish two tolerably correct indications concerning the use of this drug:—"It is especially in amenorrhœa, accompanied with painful and tympanitic swelling of the abdomen that we have seen castoreum succeed. We mean the cases where only a few drops of blood escape from the uterus, with a sort of *uterine tenesmus.*" And further on: "The kinds of colic to which castoreum seems to be principally adapted, are of the nervous kind, that seem to be particularly seated in the small intestine. They are accompanied with paleness, cold sweats, a sudden sinking of strength, as if the very principle of life had been struck down. They are without any alvine evacuations, come on suddenly, after lively emotions, a cold on the bowels or by the feet, as after long exposure to a cold rain; they constitute a species of iliac passion, termed by authors *miserere.*"[2] We may add, moreover, that obstetricians, who believed this agent possessed of a special influence on the uterus, have used it as an anti-spasmodic in *eclampsia,* or as a means of hastening the labor by exciting or restoring the uterine contractions, or, finally, for the purpose of expelling by such means the placenta, after the rupture of the umbilical cord.

[1] Mérat and Delens, *dict. de mat. med.,* vol. II., p. 140.

Homœopathic applications.—We have a pathogenesis of castoreum by Hartlaub and Trinks, but so vague that it may be considered of little value. Until recently, this drug has only been used by homœopaths for the *vomiting of pregnant females.* My experiments with castoreum convinced me of the resemblance of its action to that of thuya so fully, that I could not help concluding, that these two drugs must be suitable to the same diseases, in which opinion I was of course confirmed by the history of the empirical uses of castoreum. I seized the first opportunity that presented itself of verifying this analogy. It was evidently a case of sycosis, fungous and pedunculated vegetations at the margin of the anus, and which had resisted the allœopathic use of mercury that had been given on the supposition that they were syphilitic diseases. The result was slow, but full of meaning; apart from a general improvement in the health of the patient, the excrescences shrank in less than three weeks to one half their former size.[1] *Thuya*, which would probably have brought about a change for the better in less time, completed the cure; but the anti-sycosic properties of castoreum were not any the less rendered evident. The natural history of the castor suggested to me the following explanation of this fact:—

The bark of pine and other resinous trees, constitute almost the only food of the castor.[2]

[1] This patient was an hysteric young female, of brown complexion, enthusiastic, fond of sexual pleasures; her menstrution was habitually premature, profuse, and accompanied by cutting pains, abdominal spasms and other nervous symptoms. There had been granulations at the neck of the womb, which had been cauterised once a week; the womb was moreover prolapsed, with anteversion.

[2] This is the opinion of all naturalists. Castoreum, as we said above, is, in a great measure, composed of resin, and may, therefore, be looked upon as the dynamised product of the habitual food of the castor. This is so true that the medicinal and physical properties of the Siberian castoreum differ somewhat from those of the castoreum of America; the cause of this is, that the castors of Siberia feed principally on the bark of birch trees, while those of America make their chief food of the bark of fir-trees. It now remains for us to ascertain whether the *Thuya occident.* is one of the

This discovery was very interesting to me. On the one hand, it afforded a confirmation of the therapeutic virtues which I had believed from the first were inherent in castoreum; and, on the other hand, it gave me a general but very clear view of the medicinal properties of resins, which, in fact, induced me to present these resins, or at least a large number of them, as analogues of thuya.

Colchicum antidotes *castoreum.*

trees that the Canadian castors feed upon. I have not been able to verify this fact. But the chemical identity of the resins with the leading principle of castoreum seems to me indubitable. Indeed, it has been remarked that the *carbolic* acid obtained by Rung from the distillation of tar and resin, had precisely the smell of castoreum, (*Annuaire de Chim.*, Paris, 1845, p. 521.)

GROUP XVIII.

TYPE: CHAMOMILLA VULGARIS.
ANALOGUES: GRATIOLA OFFICINALIS. HELLEBORUS NIGER.
VIOLA TRICOLOR.

COMMON CHARACTERISTICS.

Of these four drugs, chamomilla is the only one that homœopaths seem to have a good knowledge of. The other drugs have only been used in a very small number of cases. By studying the symptoms of these three last-named drugs, my readers will become convinced that the symptoms of each of these represent an affection which is, properly speaking, only a variety of the chamomilla disease.

A particular derangement of the cerebral functions, and even of the whole nervous system; a painful increase of the sentient action, followed by a considerable depression of the vital forces, and a certain disorder of the mental faculties; these are the leading phenomena of this disease, for which nosologists, if they had occupied themselves with it, would have had to organize a separate class, intermediate between organic and purely nervous affections.

CORRESPONDING MALADIES.

Typhus.—Dementia.—Delirium tremens.—Spasms.—Convulsions.—Tetanus.—Odontalgia.—Inflammations of the mucous membranes.—Inflammation and induration of the lymphatic glands.—Gastralgia.—Bilious affections, (consequent on violent moral emotions.)—Flatulent colic.—Metritis.—Metro-peritonitis.—Puerperal fever, etc.

Chamomilla vulgaris, or rather, *matricaria chamomilla, common chamomilla.*—Genus *matricaria*, family radiatæ, class syngenesia polygamia superflua. This plant, which is very common all over Europe, where it is found along roads, in uncultivated fields, stony grounds, etc., is distinguished by its ramose stems, about eighteen inches high; by its leaves, which are of a pale-green color, tripinnate, with capillary indentations, glabrous, like all the other parts of the plant; by its white, numerous flowers, with yellow disks, imbricated, scabiose and naked calices, succeeded by small ovoïd seeds, without tufts. These flowers, whether fresh or dried, exhale a sweet, aromatic odor, somewhat like that of ants, and due to the presence of an essential oil, which not only seems to exist in the other varieties of matricaria, but in all the species belonging to the genus *anthemis;* when chewed, they have a bitter taste.

"Insects and other animals avoid the places where the chamomilla grows. It is even supposed that, with a bundle of chamomilla-flowers in one's hand, one may walk in the very midst of a swarm of wasps without fear of being stung. We are not acquainted with any other facts relative to the action of chamomilla upon animals."[1] We are not any more enlightened on this subject than Giacomini; moreover, it is my impression that he is mistaken in the species of chamomile that is said to keep off insects; this observation does not relate to the common field-chamomile, but to the *matricaria parthenium*, a bisannual plant; this one has, indeed, a much stronger smell than the chamomile that we have described, and which is truly fetid and unpleasant.

Empirical applications.—The therapeutic use of chamomile seems to date from the earliest ages. A number of authors, among whom we may mention Ray, Lange, Morton, Fred. Hoffmann, Hister, Schulz, Pringle and Miller, mention it as a very efficacious remedy, especially in *cardialgia*, *black vomiting*, *flatulent colic*, *suppression of the menses and lochia*, *consequences of confinement*, *hysteria*, *stranguria*, *rheumatism* and *intermittent fevers*. Our uncertainty regarding the peculiar variety of chamomile designated by these various authors, increases, unfortunately for us, the vagueness of their patho-

[1] *Giacomini, Traité de Thérap.*, p. 217.

logical indications. Some, indeed, but by far the smallest number, were in the habit of using the common chamomile, others the matricaria parthenium; most of them used the Roman chamomile (*anthemis nobilis*). Although these different species are undoubtedly very similar as regards their medicinal properties; yet it would be incorrect to attribute to one species exclusively, the results that had been obtained with the other species. This summary mode of proceeding may do for alloeopathic authors of Materia Medica; it cannot be indulged in by homoeopathists.[1] Everybody knows that the common chamomile has been, from time immemorial, a popular medicine, with which old nurses, in every country, drench all recently confined women, new-born children, women whose menses had been stopped by some cause or other, no matter which, (the old ladies do not mind the cause so much, etc.). It is likewise known, that, so far from protesting against these abuses, the consequences of which might be deplorable, alloeopathic physicians tolerate, and even encourage them, as if chamomile were under all circumstances a salutary agent, of no consequence, and unable to do any harm.[2]

Homœopathic applications.—We have seen chamomile assigned to four different groups, among the analogues of pulsatilla, ipecac., aconite and conium maculatum. Indeed, this substance, which is essentially a polychrest, is evidently analogous to each of these four drugs; a comparison of their respective symptoms with each other, will render this analogy perfectly evident. But apart from these analogous effects, chamomilla possesses a perfectly characteristic and exclusive

[1] Even the careful Murray makes this mistake, (app. med., vol. I., p. 143.) In his history of the matricaria, which he calls an annual plant, he mixes up all that the authors which he quotes, have stated of the *matricaria parthenium*, which is a bisannual plant, and of the Roman chamomile, (anthemis nobilis,) a perennial plant, and so distinct from the matricariæ that botanists have made a particular genus of it. Mérat and Delens (in their *dict. de mat. méd.*, art. anthemis and matricaria,) give the history of chamomile more correctly than probably any other modern authors.

[2] See the pathog. of Chamom. in Hahnemann's Mat. Med. Pur., vol. II.

action upon the nervous system, not possessed by either of its above-mentioned analogues; it increases the general nervous sensibility, and stimulates the cerebral functions; a property that seems to give rise secondarily to the various organic alterations that chamomilla is capable of producing, and for which it has so often been given with success.

"Chamomilla," says Hahnemann, "appears to diminish, in a great degree, the excessive sensitiveness to pain,[1] and the violent derangements which pain occasions in the moral condition of the patient. This is the reason why it appeases a multitude of sufferings to which coffee-drinkers, and persons who have been treated with narcotic palliatives are subject. And this is likewise the reason why it ought not to be given to those who bear pain patiently and with resignation. I mention this rule here, for it is of very great importance."[2]

As is very judiciously remarked by Hahnemann, chamomilla is frequently suitable to coffee-drinkers, for the important reason, that the action of coffee is antagonistic to that of chamomilla; a species of negative similarity which merits so much the more to be studied, that it implies a most important question concerning the antidotes.[3] It is interesting to compare the similitudes, and to contrast the dissimilarities existing between *coffee* and *chamomilla*. It is a positive fact, however, that these two drugs, although often employed together in diseases that are reputed as identical, exclude each other rigorously in all diseases that are really the same; this is much more easily comprehended than explained.

"In some cases only, have I been able," says Hahnemann, "to use chamomilla as a curative agent. Generally, when the symptoms pointed to chamomilla, they were not, to judge from the statement made by the patients, the primary symptoms of the disease, but symptoms caused by the excessive

[1] In sick people, of course; for in healthy persons Chamomilla produces the very sensitiveness to pain that it removes in the sick.

[2] *Loc. Cit.*

[3] Chamomilla not only antidotes Coffea, but also *Causticum* and most of its analogues to which Coffea belongs.

use of chamomilla, so that I had only to employ the antidotes of this drug in order to terminate this artifical disease."[1] Notwithstanding this remark by Hahnemann, I believe that the usefulness of chamomilla, as a therapeutic agent, is proportionate to the abundance with which it grows all over Europe, and especially in France, where, however, chamomilla is not near as much abused as in Germany. Be this as it may, all homœopaths are convinced now-a-days, that chamomile is the chief agent in a number of affections peculiar to pregnant females, nurses and little children. Its action being of short duration, it appears to agree principally in recent and acute affections. Nevertheless, there are certain chronic diseases, (of the air-passages and uterus, for instance,) in which chamomilla is capable of exercising a powerful effect. Its principal indication, in such affections, is the moral condition of the patient, a continually gloomy, desponding and irascible disposition. This drug is so well known to homœopathic physicians, that it seems unnecessary to describe the special indications for its employment in disease.

Caust. Cocc., *Nux vom.*, *Ignat. Pulsat.*, are, as the case may be, the antidotes of *Cham.*

Gratiola officinalis, *hedge-hyssop*. Annual species, genus *gratiola*, family scrofulariæ, class decandria monogynia.

The hedge hyssop, which is generally found, in Europe, in wet meadows, along the borders of ponds, on the banks of rivers, etc., is an inodorous plant, but of a bitter taste, and endowed with poisonous properties, which reveal themselves to the instinct of animals, and, in man, cause violent colic, diarrhœa, bloody stools, enteritis, jaundice, trembling of the extremities, convulsions, cramps, excitement and disordered condition of the sexual powers,[2] and, if the dose was considerable, death.

[1] *Loc. Cit.*

[2] Bouvier saw four cases of *nymphomania* in females who had been given by herb-doctors injections made of a decoction of freshly-gathered gratiola. (*Journ. gén. de méd.*, vol. LIV., p. 259.)

Empirical applications.—It is especially in cerebral affections without fever, (*mania*, *hypochondria*, etc.,) and in *delirium tremens* that the hedge-hyssop seems to have been used with the best success.[1] But after having enjoyed for some time a certain celebrity as a *drastic*, *hydragogue*, etc., this plant has so completely fallen into disuse now-a-days, that most allœopathic physicians do not even know of its existence.

Homœopathic applications.—Although we have been, for some time past, in possession of a pathogenesis of this drug, arranged by Hartlaub and Trinks,[2] yet, according to Jahr, it has only been used in *hypochondriac affections*, some cases of *gastralgia* and some kinds of *constipation*. To these few cases I can add a little piece of information, which may not appear uninteresting; that gratiola will be found particularly useful in cases bordering upon such as would, by their symptoms, unequivocally point to chamomilla. Gratiola would seem to be to chronic affections what chamomilla is to acute. In nervous diseases, for example, (such as *mania*, *gastralgia*, *enteralgia*, *nymphomania*, *delirium tremens*, etc.,) and in neuralgic affections, (such as *megrim*, *toothache*, *sciatica*, etc.,) *caused by the prolonged abuse of coffee*, gratiola often renders good service. I have often given it after causticum; this seems to be its antidote.[3]

Helleborus niger, black hellebore.—Native plant, genus *helleborus*, family ranunculaceæ, section helleboraceæ, (which constitutes a separate family according to some botanists,) class polyandria polygynia.—This plant, which blossoms in

[1] See Murray, app. med., vol. I., p. 352. Mérat has taken from Hufeland's Journal a case of delirium tremens cured by Gratiola; it is a case by Dr. Mukebeck, and very interesting.

[2] See Jahr's Symptomen-codex by Hempel.

[3] Gratiola only succeeded after Caust., probably because this remedy had been given in too large a dose or too long. It is difficult, especially, in gastralgic affections, to hit the exact shade of symptoms that determine *Causticum* or *Gratiola*, the rather that, in some persons at least, *Caust.* and *Coff. crud.* remove the ill effects of *Coffea tosta*.

hot-houses, in the month of December, grows spontaneously on the Alps, Pyrenees, the mountains of Auvergne, etc. It does not seem to differ much, either botanically or medicinally, from the helleborus orientalis, which enjoyed a great deal of celebrity among the ancient Greeks. Every part of the black hellebore exhales a disagreeable odor, but not very marked; it has a bitter, pungent, but not lasting taste.

Empirical applications.—On account of the great confusion which prevails in authors concerning the family of the hellebores, it is difficult to apportion to each variety the remarks that belong to it.[1] All that we can say is, that the root of our hellebore, which has been alternately praised as a *drastic*, *hydragogue*, *anthelmintic*, *emmenagogue*, etc., has been found particularly efficacious in *mental diseases*, and in some nervous affections, such as *spasmodic sneezing*, trembling of the extremities, *convulsions*, etc.[2]

Homœopathic applications.—" I conclude from various observations," says Hahnemann, that one of the first effects of black hellebore, is a state of stupor, a dulness of the *sensorium commune*, a condition where, with a sight unimpaired, nothing is seen very fully, and the patient does not pay any attention to any thing; where, with the hearing perfectly sound, nothing is heard distinctly; where, with properly constituted gustatory organs, every thing seems to have lost its genuine taste; where the mind is often or always without ideas; where the past is forgotten or little remembered; where nothing gives one any pleasure; where one's sleep is very light, and a really sound, refreshing sleep is not to be

[1] See in the methodic Encyclopedia of Pinel, the art. *helleborism;* in Murray's *Appar.*, vol. III., p. 43, chap. *Elleborus*, where the author displays as much sagacity as learning; Barbier's Mat. Med., vol. III., p. 135.

[2] This was even the opinion of Dioscorides, (see his Mat. Med., Lib. IV., cap. 151.) But Dioscorides, Galenus, and all the humoralists attribute the good effects of hellebore to the copious evacuations caused by powerful doses, instead of ascribing them to the specific action of this drug upon the nervous centres. See the pathog. of helleb. in Hahnemann's Mat. Med. Pura, vol. II. See Hahnemann's *dissertation on helleborism* in his " Lesser writings," published by Radde, 322 Broadway, New York.

had; and where one desires to work without having the necessary strength or the attention required for it."[1]

The action of black hellebore on the digestive organs, the sexual organs, the air-passages, the organs of locomotion and the skin, is strikingly analogous to the action of chamomile on the same organs. The same analogy exists between the hellebore fever, (frequent alternations of chilliness and dry heat,) and the fever produced by *chamomile.*

It is especially in congenital epilepsy of children at the breast that the pathogenesis of helleborus niger should be consulted. I remember one case which was perfectly cured by means of this drug. The patient was a little girl of five weeks, apparently well formed, nursing very greedily, but habitually constipated since the day she was born. Her mother, a woman of twenty-eight years, of dark complexion, robust appearance, but of an irritable temperament, laid her child's sickness to a fear she had had towards the end of her pregnancy. I do not know how far this explanation was founded; for the previous year this lady had lost a little boy who died in convulsions, and had shown the same symptoms that I now discovered in her daughter. The little patient had every day five or six paroxysms, each of which lasted from one to three minutes, was almost always followed by sleep, and was characterised by the following symptoms:

Sudden inability of the body, without any marked stiffness; the head was slightly thrown backwards; repeated oscillations of the tongue from right to left, which was slightly protruded from the mouth; staring looks, and convulsive rolling of the eyeballs upwards when the paroxysms were very violent; the pulse remained unaltered; a few acute cries followed by drowsiness, when the spasm was near its end. I have to add that, during these paroxysms, the child remained so perfectly sensible, that a slight shock, a noise such as is made by the closing of a door, arrested the paroxysms at once, and thus shortened them a good deal. *Cham.*,

[1] *Loc. Cit.*

which I first prescribed for the nurse, remained without effect. *Hellebore*, on the contrary, which was directly given to the little patient, cured her in two or three days.—According to Hahnemann *camphor* antidotes *hell. nig.*

Viola tricolor.—See p. 449.

GROUP XIX.

TYPE: ATROPA BELLADONNA.

ANALOGUES:

AGARICUS MUSCARIUS.
LACHESIS.
CEDRON.
DATURA STRAMONIUM.
OPIUM.
ARNICA MONTANA.
CLEMATIS ERECTA.
RUTA GRAVEOLENS.
TABACUM.
AURUM.
CAMPHORA.
CANNABIS INDICA.
HYOSCYAMUS NIGER.
BRYONIA ALBA.

COMMON CHARACTERISTICS.

THE action of the drugs that compose this group, seems primarily to bear upon, or, at any rate, to start from, the brain, and more particularly from its periphery. Allœopathic physicians, having been vaguely struck by some of the more striking features of the primary effects of most of these drugs, have brought them all together under the improper appellations of *narcotics, stupefying, narcotico-acrid*, etc. medicines. It is evident that they are analogous to each other. All of them produce the following phenomena, of course with shades of differences, and with a degree of intensity and more particularly with an order of development inherent in, and peculiar to, each of them:

Dulness of the brain; congestion of blood to the brain, with whizzing in the ears; flickering before the eyes, etc.; dull and heavy, distensive headache, with deep stitches as from steel-blades, preceded or followed, according to the nature of the drug and the dose perhaps, by a sort of torpor of the whole brain, with absence of pain in the common acceptation of the term;

Febrile excitement of the intellectual faculties, increasing, in some cases, to a furious delirium, with dulness of the senses and decrease of the irritability and mobility of the voluntary muscles; or the reverse; torpor of the mental faculties, with increase of the muscular irritability;

More or less intense derangement of the cerebral functions, (sadness, delirium, coma, syncope, illusions of the senses, hallucinations, with clonic or tonic spasms, etc.,) coming in paroxysms, by fits and starts, at irregular intervals, but capable of assuming a form of regular periodicity, with absence of fever, or else violent fever (at the moment while the paroxysm is taking place, or afterwards,) profuse sweat, etc.;

Nocturnal sleeplessness, with restlessness, subsultus tendinum, crowding of sad or merry, incoherent, absurd thoughts upon one's mind, that follow each other with an extreme rapidity, fantastic, pleasant or hideous images and visions, etc., at times preceded, at times followed by a state of comatose somnolence, day and night;

Pulse full, large, hard, frequent or of normal regularity, or else small and very frequent (by poisonous doses).

Burning heat all over, or only at the head, with cold extremities; general heat with sweat, preceded or followed by general chilliness.

Breaking out on the skin of red, smooth, scarlet-colored, brownish, and persistent spots (especially by the lachesis), or resembling large freckles, in the face and on the hands (by tobacco, for instance), or of a sort of miliaria with elevated red vesicles, arranged in groups of greater or less extent, itching, but generally passing off soon (especially by camphor).

Eyes red, injected, protruding as if they would start out of their sockets, sometimes convulsed, distorted, with dilated pupils and photophobia; or hollow, with pupils that are contracted and insensible to the light; ophthalmia.

Animated, red, bloated, burning-hot face, or else pale and without any expression.

Burning dryness of the mouth and throat, with bitter taste in the mouth, thirst or else absence of thirst; or, burning thirst with aversion to liquids, as in hydrophobia; or lastly, thirst with inability to drink, in consequence of the contraction of the throat, such as generally takes place in most cerebral diseases.

Inflammatory swelling of the tonsils, the whole throat, and even of the soft parts of the neck, with constant desire to swallow, and a tensive pain extending to the parotid regions.

Unpleasant taste in the mouth; aversion to food; loathing; nausea; desire to vomit; violent vomiting (less frequently); pressure at the stomach; noisy eructations which afford relief; spasmodic hiccough; tension of the epigastric region which is painful to contact.

Distention of the abdomen; painful constipation; constipation as from inertia of the intestines (especially by opium); or else violent, watery, sudden diarrhœa, generally at night, with exceedingly painful cutting colic; copious emissions of flatulence.

Pressure on the bladder; strangury, with emission of drops of a red and cloudy urine; profuse discharge of watery urine (especially during or after the paroxysms; involuntary emission of urine).

Dysmenorrhœa, with pressure in the region of the uterus; *leucorrhœal* or *gonorrhœal discharge* (especially after Clematis, Camphor and Cannabis); painful swelling of the mammæ and other glands.

Paroxysm of dyspnœa at night, with anguish; spasmodic cough.

Trembling of the extremities and of the whole body; cramps; contraction of the muscles; sense of lameness in all the joints, especially after the paroxysms.

CORRESPONDING DISEASES.

Meningitis, (cerebral and of the spinal marrow.)—Encephalitis.—Hydrocephalus.—Febris intermittens perniciosa.—Typhus, (stage of delirium.) —Mental derangements. —Epilepsy. —Hydrophobia. —Convulsions. —Tetanus.—Various accidents caused by bites of venomous serpents.—Congestive or nervous headache.—Otitis.—Otalgia.—Deafness.—Ophthalmia.—Amaurosis.—Cataract.—Parotitis.—Facial neuralgia.—Stomatitis. —Toothache, (with swelling of the gums and cheek.)—Amygdalitis.—Anginæ.—Glossitis.—Stuttering.—Hiccough.—Gastric and intestinal spasms.—Colica saturnina.—Constipation.—Sporadic cholera.—Strangulated hernia.—Dysuria.—Spasm of the uterus.—Metritis.—Nymphomania.—Hysteria.—Dysmenorrhœa.—Sudden suppression of the menses or lochia, (after a fright or some other emotion.)—Metrorrhagia, (active or passive.)—Swelling and induration of the breasts.—Influenza.—Whooping-cough.—Periodical asthma, (with nocturnal paroxysms.)—False croup.—Chorea. — Trembling of drunkards. — Erysipelatous, scarlet-shaped exanthems, etc.

Atropa Belladonna, *solanum maniacum furiosum*, *lethale* of the ancients; *strychnos manikos* of Dioscorides, (though not all authors agree on this point); *deadly nightshade.* Genus *atropa*, family solaneæ, class pentandria monogynia; the generic name is derived from *atropos*, one of the Parcæ who cut the thread of life, and the special name of this plant emanates from a former custom of the Italian ladies, according to Debregne,[1] Mérat and Delens,[2] etc., to wash their faces with the distilled water of this plant, for the purpose of rendering their complexion fairer; or, which is much more probable, for the purpose of procuring an artificial color in their faces. This plant, which is found almost all over Europe, prefers a dry soil, and the slopes of hills. It being of importance to a practitioner to know it well, we will give an exact description of it.[3]

"The root is cylindrical, of a middling thickness, slightly ligneous, bent like a knee, rounded, brownish-yellow on the outside, whitish within, succulent, of a stupefying smell, and

[1] *Des vertus thérapeutiques de la belladone*, 1852.

[2] *Dict. de mat. méd*, vol. I., p. 489.

[3] *Jahr's and Gruner's Pharmacopœia.*

a nauseous, sweetish taste; it transforms the natural saliva into froth; the stem is erect, round, from 3 to 5 feet high, of a reddish-brown color, striated, branching off into three parts; the leaves, which are attached by short foot-stalks to the stem, are in pairs of unequal sizes, longer near the root, and shorter high up, oval, pointed at both extremities, entire, pretty smooth, of a dusky-green color on their upper surfaces, and paler beneath. The flowers, which are supported upon solitary peduncles, and rise from the axils of the leaves, are about an inch long, of a dingy green-yellow color, with brownish veins, violet at the forepart; the fruit is a roundish berry, with a longitudinal furrow on each side, at first green, afterwards red, ultimately of a deep purple color, bearing considerable resemblance to the black cherry, except that it has a nauseous, slightly sweetish taste; it contains numerous kidney-shaped seeds in two distinct cells, and has a sweetish, violet-colored juice. The stems and leaves of this plant exhale a disagreeable, poisonous, but not very marked odor."

The chemical analysis of belladonna has not yet furnished us with very precise and truly interesting results; its deleterious properties are generally attributed to the presence of an alkaloïd which was discovered by Brandes, and to which he has given the name *atropine.* When pure, it exists in the shape of small prisms, with a silky gloss, has a bitter taste, is soluble in five hundred parts its volume of cold water, and, by combination with acids, gives rise to the formation of salts.

Experiments with belladonna have been made on animals of different species, and with various results. "It appears," says Giacomini, "that only goats can eat the leaves of belladonna with impunity; all other animals suffer more or less from them, or are killed by them."[1] This is not so. We read in the "*Journal de pharmacie*,"[2] that a rabbit was fed exclusively on the leaves of belladonna for eight days, without being apparently incommoded by them, and without showing any signs of dilatation of the pupils. Carnivorous

[1] Traité de Thérap., p. 536.

[2] Vol. X., p. 85.

animals (such as dogs and cats) were more sensitive to the action of belladonna. Daries, Rossi, etc.,[1] have seen the pupils of these animals sensibly dilated by the action of belladonna. Dogs to which Orfila had given 15 grammes of the extract, died from it in twenty-four hours.[2] It must be admitted, however, that 15 grammes are an enormous dose, and that men have perished from much smaller quantities. What is the conclusion that we derive from such facts? First, that belladonna is more pernicious to carnivorous than to herbivorous animals, since goats and rabbits eat it with perfect impunity. In such a case, is belladonna, like nux vomica, nothing but a *hypersthenisant poison* so much more frightful in its effects upon animals and men, that they have a harder, more resisting fibre, or, in vulgar parlance but which expresses my idea perfectly, *a harder life?* If this were so, belladonna would destroy carnivorous animals more rapidly, and when given in smaller quantity, than men; which is not the case.[3] The action of this poison is not, therefore, proportional to the degree of resistance offered by the inherent vitality with which every being has been endowed by nature.

The suggestions which I here offer, seem to imply a general law, and it seems to me that I confer a real benefit on the healing art by giving the solution of one of the most important therapeutic problems that have been proposed since the days of Hahnemann; it is as follows:

The deleterious action of belladonna is exactly proportionate, in every species as in every individual, to the degree of development and functional activity of the organ upon which the poison exercises its specific action, namely the brain. This explains to us—

1st. Why, of all animals, man is most accessible to the action of belladonna.

[1] Daries, *de atropa bellad.*, Lipsiæ, 1776, p. 37.

[2] *Toxicologie*, vol. II., p. 231.

[3] Orfila relates (loc. cit.) that a little dog who had swallowed thirty ripe berries of belladonna, had not at all been affected by them. Such a dose is known to have produced in man the most frightful accidents, even death.

2d. Why, among men in a state of health, or to whose diseases (by a legitimate application of the law of similitude) it corresponds most exactly, those are most powerfully affected by belladonna whose cerebral faculties are most liable to becoming irritated by particular causes, or whose physical brains, consequently heads, have the greatest development; these are, of course, children.

In proof of this theory, I will state a fact mentioned by Hufeland,[1] that *idiots* are protected from the deleterious action of belladonna, which they eat with almost the same degree of impunity as animals of an inferior order, by the inertia and incomplete development of their cerebral organ.

Speaking of the deleterious effects of belladonna, we ought to state, that although the annals of medical science are freighted with reports of cases of poisoning by this drug, yet, they seldom terminate fatally, although the effects are more or less serious, or rather more or less alarming.[2]

Debregne has furnished the following list of the toxical effects of belladonna:

"Nausea; vomiting; dryness of the mouth and throat; thirst; dysphagia; anxiety; lipothymia; cardialgia; colic; constipation; dulness of the head; headache; dizziness; vertigo; paleness of the face; dulness of the senses; red, prominent, wandering eyes; immoveable and widely dilated pupils; cloudiness, and even permanent loss of sight; delirium, which is generally of a merry kind, but sometimes assuming a furious character; loquacity; singing; laughing; dancing; stupidity; appearance of drunkenness; mania; craziness; rage; a variety of gesticulations; extraordinary contortions; frequent motions of the arms and hands; convulsive movements; trismus; tetanic stiffness of the spine or

[1] *Journ. Prat.*, 1822.

[2] In the *Hist. de l'Acad. roy. des sc.*, (year 1703, p. 96,) we read of the case of a child of four years, who died in less than 24 hours from the effects of a few berries of belladonna. Several among 180 soldiers who had likewise poisoned themselves with the berries of belladonna, died likewise from the effects of this fruit. (Journ. gén. de méd., vol. XLVIII., p. 53, related by E. Gaultier-Claubry.)

extremities; staggering gait; general muscular weakness; strange hallucinations of various kinds; mental exaltation; difficulty of articulating; thin, hoarse, croupy voice; aphonia; somnolence; coma; lethargy; somnambulism; pulse frequent, excited or slow, feeble and irregular; short, accelerated, or irregular and oppressive, stertorous breathing; profuse sweat; aversion to liquids; cutaneous heat; scarlatinous eruption; gangrenous spots; incontinence of urine; dysuria; ischuria; lastly, syncope, or convulsions; subsultus tendinum; risus sardonicus; swelling and insensibility of the abdomen; small, filiform, wretched pulse; cold extremities; sinking of strength; prostration; death.[1]

Having read most cases of poisoning by belladonna that have been published for the last half century, and having met with two cases in my own practice, I might easily have given a tolerably complete pathogenesis of belladonna, such, at any rate, as would have embodied all the principal effects resulting from poisonous doses; but I have preferred using the text of Debregne. I was anxious to deprive such of the alloeopathic practitioners as might wish to read my work and become more accurately informed in regard to the subject of homoeopathy, of every possible pretext of rejecting my own conclusions, by basing them upon evidence, derived, not from the works of Hahnemann or his disciples, but from facts, cures and modes of treatment related by the best and most authentic writers of the alloeopathic school.

Alloeopathic physicians differ much concerning the best mode of antidoting the poisonous effects of belladonna, as they do concerning most other subjects of therapeutics, large doses of emetics,[2] purgatives, derivatives applied to the lower extremities, water mixed with vinegar,[3] coffee, opium, cold

[1] Op. cit., p. 17.

[2] Baldinger informs us that he has seen a man who had poisoned himself with Belladonna, and was in a fair way of recovery, die an instant after taking a strong dose of tartar-emetic.

[3] Among the 180 soldiers who were poisoned by belladonna, the one who was most speedily restored, was a sergeant who, in order to cool the burning in his throat, took it into his head to eat three or four green apples; but

and tepid baths, and, above all, the customary general and local depletions, have been recommended as antidotes.[1]

"Almost all authors mention vinegar as an antidote to belladonna, but only by way of conjecture, and copying one from the other. But this assertion is entirely unfounded. On the contrary, vinegar aggravates the deleterious effects of belladonna.

"Opium appeases the paralytic symptoms, and the pains caused by belladonna, but only antipathically and palliatively. Small doses of opium probably removed the somnolence caused by belladonna.

"The surest and speediest means of homœopathically arresting the stupor, mental derangement and rage caused by belladonna, are small doses of hyoscyamus; the intoxication yields to wine, as I know from my own experience, and as has already been stated by Tragus and Moibenus."[2]

As regards hyoscyamus, I confess I have never used it as an antidote; but, so far as opium is concerned, I am not entirely of Hahnemann's opinion. I have become too well convinced by experience, that infinitesimal doses of opium and belladonna neutralise each other, to suppose that massive doses can act otherwise than antipathically and palliatively. These two drugs have the same sphere of action, and, if the phenomena which they respectively produce, manifest themselves in an opposite direction, this antagonism takes place simply by virtue of a general law, to which all homœopathic medicines that act as antidotes upon each other are subject. I mean to demonstrate this fact in a special work with which I have been occupied for several months past.

The best antidote of massive doses of belladonna, are perhaps infinitesimal doses of the same drug. This is, indeed, the case with haschish, which is antidoted by the dynamised cannabis; however, the fact remains subject to verification.

this isolated fact, which proves very little in favor of malic acid, proves absolutely nothing in regard to vinegar.

[1] See Debregne, *op. cit.*, p. 19; Trousseau and Pidoux, *traité de thérap.*, vol. II., p. 53, etc.

[2] *Mat. Méd.*, vol. I., p. 491.

In most, if not in all cases of poisoning by belladonna, a strong infusion of coffee is sufficient to neutralise the poison, and remove the drug.[1]

Empirical applications. As it is not proved that the otherwise vague description which Theophraste and Dioscorides have left us of the plant which modern authors have supposed to be belladonna, does not rather apply to the mandrake, the therapeutic history of belladonna, as recorded in the works of ancient authors, is of no interest to us, and does not become invested with a certain character of authenticity until towards the end of the 16th century, or the beginning of the 17th, that is to say about the period when the writings of J. M. Faber,[2] J. J. Mardorf,[3] and Melchior Frick,[4] were published. But, from this period, the therapeutic use of belladonna spread very rapidly, and there are few drugs now-a-days, that have been used as much as this agent. In the following diseases its curative effects have been most marked:

Mania; craziness; epilepsy; chorea; convulsions; tetanus; hydrophobia; scarlatina; ophthalmia; ceratitis; iritis; prolapsus of the iris; staphyloma; central spots; central cataracts; nyctalopia; amaurosis; gastralgia; spasmodic hiccough; spasmodic constriction of the throat and larynx; aphonia; whooping-cough; nervous cough; sternalgia; facial neuralgia; neuralgia in general; spasmodic constriction of the anus, urethra and neck of the womb; incontinence of urine; strangulated hernia; dystocia; hysteria; eclampsia; schirrous (?) engorgement of the breasts and of other glands;

[1] In a case to which I was called, such an infusion produced vomiting, which would probably not have resulted from tickling the throat with a feather; my patient had swallowed half a gramme of the extract of belladonna, in consequence of the mistake made by an apothecary who had read a *gramme* instead of a *grain;* all the poison that had remained in the stomach, was expelled by this means.

[2] J. M. Faber, *Strychnomania, explicans* solani furiosi historiam, etc. Aug. Vindel., 1677.

[3] J. J. Mardorf, *dissert. demaniacis nuperis giessensibus a solano furiosi,* No. 4. Giessæ., 1691.

[4] M. Friccius, *paradoxa de venenis,* Aug. Vindel, 1710.

orchitis; epididymitis; febris perniciosa (with violent headache);[1] and latterly, *ileus* and *colica saturnina.*[2]

It is true, it is only a few years since some of these diseases have been treated with belladonna by allœopathic physicians, most probably in imitation of the homœopaths. But these silent acts of plagiarism not only compromise the sincerity of those who are guilty of them, but they imply at the same time, a more or less voluntary acknowledgment of our doctrine; I have, therefore, no desire to complain of them, the rather that the period approaches when public opinion will do them justice.

It must not be supposed, however, that all allœopathic physicians are acquainted with the good effects of belladonna in the above-mentioned diseases. In two of them, more particularly, the curative or preventive virtues of this drug are considered purely fictitious by the leading men of the allœopathic school. I mean *hydrophobia* and *scarlet fever.*

"During the latter half of the last century," says Trousseau and Pidoux, "belladonna was looked upon as a specific remedy for hydrophobia, and Murray (*appar. med.*, v. I., p. 639,) has informed us of the result of the many trials that were made with this drug. Unfortunately not one of these experiments is conclusive, and most of them are fictitious. In our time, the inadequacy of belladonna to cure this disease, has become a painful certainty."[3]

We will content ourselves with opposing to these sweeping and hazardous assertions on the part of Trousseau and Pidoux the following very discreet reflections of Bayle, suggested by Murray's statements:

"Belladonna was given to one hundred and eighty-two patients, all of whom had been bitten by mad dogs. *One*

[1] The only case of this kind I know of, is one by Ducros of Marseilles, in 1827. In the *Revue Méd.*, Aug. 1838, p. 260, we find an extract from a work of Graves, published in the *Dublin Journ.*, where belladonna is recommended for similar diseases; the homœopaths, however, have nothing to learn, either from the one or the other.

[2] See Debregne, *loc. cit.*

[3] *Tr. de Thérap.*, vol. II., p. 61.

hundred and seventy-six of this number had been bitten recently, and showed no symptom of hydrophobia; in the remaining six the disease had fairly broken out; one of these was attacked with aversion to water, with convulsions and other violent cerebral symptoms. Here are the results of the treatment: The *one hundred and sixteen* recently bitten were preserved (Munch and his sons); of the *six* attacked with the disease four were cured, and two died (Munch, Bucholz, Neimecke). We may, of course, entertain doubts concerning the correctness of all these trials; we may object that the madness of the dogs was not proven; but, unless we take it for granted that Munch was an impostor, I should say that one must be wofully given to scepticism in order to reject all the results stated by this author. Why then, it may be asked, has not this mode of treatment been adopted? For a very simple reason; it is this; that, of the physicians who were called upon to treat the patients that had been bitten by mad dogs, not one has instituted consistent experiments with belladonna, either because he was ignorant of Munch's labors, or because he was carried away by the spirit of system, and rejected beforehand every thing that might seem contrary to his preconceived theory. Consequently it seems to me that it is of the utmost importance to repeat Munch's experiments."[1] This is my opinion likewise. Well, have these experiments been repeated in good earnest? I assert that Messrs. Trousseau and Pidoux could not name any physician who has done it. Except the cauterisation of the wound, which is an useless proceeding (for the absorption of the virus takes place instantaneously), it is not till several paroxysms had broken out, that is to say after the disease had almost become incurable, that alloeopathic physicians brought their more or less absurd means of treatment to bear upon this frightful disorder.[2] And it is upon such a slender

[1] *Bibliothèque de Thérap.*, vol. II., p. 502.

[2] Apart from the instances quoted by Murray, Richter, Hufeland and others, mention several facts of confirmed hydrophobia that were cured by belladonna, and Daniel, Johnston, Buchan, and others, several that were

basis that Trousseau and Pidoux found their conviction regarding the inadequacy of the means that have been so far employed against hydrophobia. Having no reason to doubt the statements of Munch, who was an honorable protestant minister, and enjoyed an excellent reputation in his own country; or of his sons who were respectable physicians, or of such men as Bucholz and Neimecke, I feel obliged to believe in the efficacy of belladonna as a curative, and still more as a prophylactic means against hydrophobia.[1] I will

cured by mercury. See *Journ. gén. de méd.*, vol., LXX. p. 266, and art. *Rage* in the *dict. des sc. méd.*

[1] The following letter was sent to me by one of my patients regarding the prophylactic virtues of belladonna in hydrophobia: the writer is a man of a high order of mind, and a distinguished character, and occupies a very high position in his own country.

"SIR:—

"At your request I send you the following detailed account of a case which shows conclusively, as it seems to me, the prophylactic virtues of belladonna in hydrophobia.

"I spent the summer of 1850 at Oranienbaum, a country-seat which is situated about ten miles from St. Petersburg. On a fine morning, I took a walk with my wife in the pine-grove adjoining the village of Oranienbaum. We were accompanied by our dog, a female of the King Charles breed. Leaving the footpath, she met a sickly-looking dog coming from the village, and running along in a straight line, with his head and tail hanging down. She was bitten by this dog, who then continued on his route without the least change in his features. I conceived the most serious apprehensions, for the poor dog seemed to exhibit all the signs of incipient hydrophobia. A few minutes after, having returned home, I gave our dog a drop of the 3d attenuation of Belladonna. Six weeks after, the dog, who was lying quietly at the feet of my wife, rose precipitately and ran about the room; soon after she stumbled on flower-pots, and swallowed a few flowers, especially reseda. We tried to catch her; but she escaped into the garden, and ran about in every direction, tearing out and eating grass. This paroxysm lasted about five minutes, after which she returned to the room, and remained quiet: this was towards the end of August. At the commencement of October, after our return to the city, the same paroxysm took place; it was in closed rooms. The dog ran through all of them, panting as during the first paroxysm; she again threw herself on the flower-pots, and swallowed all the reseda she could lay hold of. In vain we tried to catch her; she jumped now on the chairs, now on the window-sills. In four or five minutes she became quiet, and has remained well ever since.

"It seems to me that these two paroxysms, which took place, each of add, however, that, after the disease has actually broken out, the characteristic symptoms of the attack, the constitutional idiosyncrasies of the patient, or the nature of the climate may require one of the analogues of belladonna, such as cedron or lachesis, or even mercury and arsenic.[1]

Let us now pass over to scarlet fever.

The idea of administering belladonna in this disease, both as a curative and a prophylactic medicine, was one of the first and most striking applications of the principle of similitude. This discovery was published by Hahnemann in 1801.[2] Forced to admit the evidence of facts, allœopathic physicians took hold of this discovery, without, however, perceiving the general law which was involved in it; in their eyes, belladonna became simply an additional specific. The manner in which this discovery is spoken of by modern allœopathic writers, shows that, if they cannot deny that this discovery

them, in the morning, at the very hour when the dog had been bitten, were symptoms of incipient hydrophobia, the breaking out of which was prevented by the reactive powers of the medicine. It behooves professional men to test the prophylactic virtues of belladonna, and set this hypothesis at rest.

Accept the assurances, etc., etc.

ALEXANDER STCHERBININE,
Conseiller d'Etat of Russia."

Nizza, March 3d, 1853.

[1] It appears that the following proceeding is resorted to in Russia to prevent the development of hydrophobia, and that this proceeding is generally successful, or rather infallible.

When, in a pack of hounds, one is bitten, all the rest are set against him, and he is soon torn to pieces. Several of the pack get bitten, but this is not heeded, provided they have swallowed some of the blood of the dead dog. If any of the dogs should not have liked any of this blood, their fauces are rubbed with the bleeding flesh. Not one of them is attacked with the disease in such a case. The same proceeding is employed in regard to men, with this difference, that it is some of their own blood they drink instead of the dog's, on the same day, or the day after the bite was inflicted.

These facts were related to me by a man of high standing, of high intellect, and worthy of all confidence in the correctness of his statements. Himself was bitten by a mad wolf in the right hand, and it is this very treatment that saved him from the terrible consequences of such an accident. Other intelligent Russians have likewise confirmed these facts.

[2] *On the treatment and prevention of scarlet-fever*, by S. Hahnemann.

is due to the founder of homœopathy, they endeavor, at any rate, to detract from its merit. "We have now to mention," say Trousseau and Pidoux, "the remarkable property possessed by belladonna, of preventing scarlet-fever. Hufeland has done most to spread this idea, which, however, originated with Hahnemann; he affirms, that by giving belladonna to those who were exposed to the scarlet-fever miasm, the disease is effectually prevented. The German Journals are freighted with facts that seem to confirm this strange idea. Howsoever imposing may be the authorities that assert the prophylactic virtues of belladonna in scarlet-fever, we do not by any means accept their inferences, for the simple reason, that we do not know whether the effects of epidemic influences had been correctly appreciated by these practitioners."[1]

The reasons upon which Trousseau and Pidoux base their doubts, seem to me exceedingly obscure; but the following facts, are, on the contrary, perfectly precise:—

"Two thousand and twenty-seven children exposed to more or less severe epidemic scarlet-fever, took belladonna. One thousand nine hundred and forty-eight were protected from the disease, and seventy-nine were attacked."[2]

Such are the facts, which, without speaking of much more numerous similar, and not less conclusive facts which have since been published in Germany and France, *seem* to confirm, according to Trousseau and Pidoux, the prophylactic virtue of belladonna in scarlet-fever.[3] But who are the authors whom our two authors suspect of having failed in correctly estimating the effects of epidemic influences, and

[1] Traité de Thérap., vol. II., p. 72.

[2] A. L. J. Bayle, *bibliot. de thérap.*, vol. II., p. 504.

[3] The property possessed by Belladonna, if a small dose of it be taken every six or seven days, to protect one from genuine scarlet-fever, such as it has been described by Sydenham, Plenenitz and others, and which I was the first to discover, has been laughed at by a number of physicians who, not knowing the true characteristics of this disease peculiar to children, confounded it with the purple-rash that was imported from Belgium in 1801, and necessarily failed in their attempts to apply the Belladonna to this disease as a preventive means, etc. Hahnemann's Mat. Med. Pura, vol. I., art. *Belladonna.*

whose conclusions they reject? They are such men as Hahnemann, Hufeland, Rhodius, Schenk, Masius, Gumpert, Wolf, Benedik, Berndt, Zeuch, Kuntsmann, Genecki, Maisier, Velsen, etc. Have Trousseau and Pidoux monopolised the art of observing, and is their book the only one that is worth preserving and believing in? We pray you, spare Hahnemann! To defy this great practitioner as an observer! Messrs. Trousseau and Pidoux, you have either not read, or not understood a line of his writings.[1]

Homœopathic Applications.—Belladonna is so well known to homœopathic practitioners, that I need not give a lengthy description of its therapeutic uses. The pathogenesis of this drug explains to us, why it should have been such a useful agent in the hands of empirics. But what is particularly evident from the provings of this drug, is, that it exercises specific curative effects on idiopathic or symptomatic cerebral affections, such as typhus, etc., where a state of vital surexcitation (delirium, convulsions, etc.,) is followed by an order of opposite phenomena (coma, paralysis, etc.). All homœopathic physicians agree, concerning the form of cerebral derangements, ophthalmia, angina, etc., to which belladonna corresponds most specifically. Let us recall to mind, moreover, that, in conformity to the physiological law which we have pointed out, page 561, belladonna is particularly suitable to persons whose physical brain and cranium are strikingly developed, namely, to children.

The dynamised belladonna is antidoted by *opium*, *camphor*, and *Hep. sulp.*

Agaricus muscarius, *amanita muscaria* of Persoon, *bug agaric, common toad stool.* — Genus *agaricus*, Linn., or *amanita*, Pers., family fungi, class cryptogamia. This fungus is very common in the north of Europe, where it grows in prairies and damp woods. It offers the following characteristic signs and properties: "On first coming out of

[1] See the pathogenesis of Belladonna in Hahnemann's Mat. Med. Pura, (*loc. cit.*)

the ground, it is oval, and enclosed in a soft, fleshy envelope; the young stem is short and thick, bulbous at the base, generally hollow when old, from four to six inches long, the part above the middle being provided with a white, membranous ring; the cap is at first eminently vaulted, afterwards it becomes flatter, is of a scarlet-red color, furnished with yellowish-white scales, which are sometimes wanting, with a white border, or a border with brown-yellow stripes; pulp, yellowish or white, or reddish, the lamellæ radiate from the middle to the margin; it has a burning acrid taste. It is distinguished from the eatable laseras by the white remains of the vulva, which are scattered over the fully developed cap.

The bug-agaric has very little smell, although it is a common belief that its offensive smell destroys flies and bugs, whence the common name bug agaric.[1] It is poisonous, but a large quantity of it requires to be eaten, in order that its poisonous effects should be fully developed. I recollect a case of this kind, which I witnessed in my youth. A shepherd and his whole family had been poisoned by this fungus. Upon entering his hut, I found him squatting against a ladder, with a red face, his eyes congested, and preaching with a most grotesque emphasis a long sermon, whilst his wife, daughters and sons were dancing and singing at the foot of the ladder; they all got well again.[2]

To some of the Northern tribes, the bug agaric answers the same purposes that the haschisch and opium do to the Orientals; the Samoyedes, Ostiaks, Kamtschadales, etc., produce with it a sort of intoxication, full of fantastical visions, and apparently without any serious inconvenience to them.

Empirical applications.—Agaric has been given with more or less success for *epilepsy*, *trembling of the extremities*, (especially in epileptic individuals,) *spots on the cornea*, *indu-*

[1] Murray, App. Med., vol. V., p. 556.

[2] I dare not affirm that the fungi which had been eaten by these persons were real amanitæ; but this fungus is very frequent in the district where the poisoning took place, (a village of the Haute-Saône,) where it is commonly termed *champignon fou*, (fool's fungus.)

ration of the tonsils and other glands; and, lastly, it has been applied externally to *callous ulcers.*[1]

Homœopathic applications.—Not very numerous. I do not think that I have given agaric to more than five or six patients, and then always after *belladonna*, or before and after *lachesis.* Agaric seems suitable in cases where *bellad.* and *lach.* appear likewise indicated.[2]

Camph. and *Nitr. ac.* antidote it.

Lachesis, *vipera lanceolata* of Daudin, *trigonocephalus lachesis.* This serpent, which has, for some years past, been made the type of a particular genus, (*trigonocephalus*,) is still considered by some naturalists as a variety of the genus *coluber* of Linné, or the *vipera* of modern authors. Although multiplying rapidly in the countries of which it is a native, it appears, so far as we know, to inhabit only three West India Islands, of which it is the scourge, namely, Martinique, Sainte-Lucie, and Becouïa. It is one of the most terrible of all serpents. The general and almost always fatal accidents caused by the bite of this serpent, probably do not essentially differ from those caused by the bite of the European viper, (*coluber berus*, Linn., or *vipera berus*, Daud.;) but they are much more intense, and develope themselves so rapidly that there is scarcely any time left for neutralizing the poison. Latterly, the *cedron* has been considered by the few physicians who are acquainted with this medicine, as an infallible means of neutralizing the effects of the bite of the lachesis.

It is generally admitted now-a-days, that the poison of serpents, like that of variola, syphilis, rabies, the inoculation of which is attended with such disastrous consequences, can be

[1] Murray, (*loc. cit.*) Pathog. of agar. in *Chronic Diseases*, vol. I.

[2] One day when I happened to be in the country with some friends, a young lady, whose physician I was, was suddenly taken with convulsions, partly in consequence of the fatigue of the journey, partly owing to some disappointment. I had seen her in this state more than once, and *bellad.* always relieved her in a few minutes. If left to itself, the attack lasted a long time. This time I happened to be without bellad., and I gave her a few pellets of *agar.;* the result was the same.

be swallowed by animals and men with impunity. This fact confirms the power of dynamisation; for the same poisons, as is well known to all homœopathic physicians, recover their toxical energies, no matter in what manner they are introduced into the animal economy, so soon as they are dynamised in the Hahnemannian fashion.

The empirical applications of the lachesis-poison may be set down as non-existing.[1] The honor of having introduced this powerful agent into our Materia Medica, belongs exclusively to Dr. Hering, who was the first to use it in the treatment of disease after having previously proved it according to Hahnemann's method, and elicited a long list of physiological effects of the poison. This is undoubtedly one of the greatest benefits which this physician has rendered to homœopathy.[2]

Homœopathic applications.—The pathogenesis of lachesis, as all homœopaths must have noticed, embodies most of the symptoms of belladonna, with slight differences in the chronological order of their manifestation, and characterised by a tendency to persistency which makes it to be in chronic diseases what belladonna is in the acute form thereof. More-

[1] Father Labet, (Voyage, vol. I., p. 470, and vol. IV., p. 406,) speaks of the medicinal virtues of the *fat* of Lachesis, which he says is very efficacious in *consumption, neuralgia, rheumatism*, etc. But these vague indications are so much less interesting to us that there is, in reality, no point of contact between the fat and the poison of Lachesis. Still less would it be proper to admit the wonders that used to be attributed to the *broth, jelly, distilled water, fetid oil*, etc., of the viper, for which despicable preparations the viper of Egypt, or the *vipera haja* of Daudin, was formerly used. In connection with this subject it is worth mentioning that several physicians of the last century have proposed the inoculation of the common viper poison by the bite of the animal as a remedy for *confirmed hydrophobia*, a disease to which lachesis corresponds at least partially. Demathis, in the *Anc. Journ. de Méd.*, vol. LXI., p. 365, relates an experiment of this kind which he tried on a mad dog in 1783. The animal died, it is true, but not of rage; this was cured; it died from the effects of the bite, for he saw the dog lap water several times, and without any repugnance. The same experiment was tried on man, without any more success, in the Hospital la Charité, in 1831. (See Rev. Méd., vol. III., p. 394.)

[2] See the pathogenesis of Lachesis in Jahr's Symptomen-codex, translated by Charles J. Hempel, M. D., published by W. Radde, 322 Broadway, New York.

over, it is well known that the physiological conditions which favor the action of these agents, either in the sick or healthy organism, are not the same. "It appears," says Hering, "that lachesis is particularly suitable to melancholic dispositions, (provers with such dispositions, showed the greatest number of symptoms,) next to *choleric* individuals. Phlegmatic and lymphatic persons are likewise suitable subjects for the action of lachesis, but principally when their dispositions border on the *melancholic*, with dark-colored eyes, and tendency to laziness and sadness. As regards persons with sanguine temperaments, a high color, fine, delicate skins, and impressible natures, *lachesis* does not suit such individuals, unless the disease should have imparted to their dispositions a choleric and melancholy tinge. Lachesis is particularly suitable to choleric females, even to such as have red hair and are covered with freckles."[1]

Daily experience seems to me to confirm these statements, and I think, moreover, with this author, 1st, that thin, weakly, exhausted persons have most to hope from lachesis, the symptoms being otherwise similar; 2d, that this drug is particularly suitable to the acute diseases of children, and to the chronic affections of old people. All homœopaths know, moreover, that in many diseases, such as cerebral affections, (meningitis, mental alienation, imbecility, etc.,) in erysipelas, angina, cerebral neuroses, various forms of neuralgia, etc., lachesis can be usefully alternated in the same case with belladonna, agaricus, opium, etc.

Dynamised cedron antidotes lachesis.

Cedron. This is the fruit of a tree that has remained unknown to our French botanists until the present time. This tree grows in America, and according to the statement of Hallert, somewhat resembles our large almond-tree.[2] This

[1] *Journal de la méd. homœop.*, vol. V., p. 760.

[2] *Journ. de la Soc. gall. de méd. hom.*, vol. I., p. 366. Mérat, with whom I conversed on the subject of this fruit in 1850, was unable to give me the least information in reference to the tree that produces it.

fruit, which is about the size of a cashew-nut, has an angular, irregularly prismatic shape, is externally blackish and rough, internally of a dingy yellow color, and so hard that it has to be scraped; it is inodorous, and excessively bitter.

Dr. Petroz had been in possession of some of these nuts for one or more years, and had used the medicine as an *anti-periodic*, when several of them were received by the department of public instruction, from our consul at Panama, accompanied by vague statements concerning their medicinal use. The Academy of Medicine having been consulted on the subject, a committee, composed of Drs. Chevallier, Mérat, Honoré and Duncéril,[1] was named, with a request to examine the properties of this agent.[2] The report of the committee has not yet been published.

Empirical applications.—They are limited to the following fragment, which has been extracted from the minutes of the *Soc. gall. de méd. homœop.*:—"On his arrival at Panama, Mr. Hellert was able to procure the cedron, which had been represented to him as an infallible antidote against the bites of the poisonous serpents of the countries adjoining the equator. He soon was given an opportunity to try the antidote on his own person. In one of his excursions in the cordilleras of Veraguas, while turning over a fragment of rock, he was bitten in the right leg by a *coral-snake*, the most poisonous snake on the isthmus of Panama. During the few seconds which it took him to take the antidote out of the little bag which he wore suspended round his neck, he was seized with violent pains at the heart and throat; but he had scarcely chewed and swallowed a small portion of cedron, of the size of a small bean, when the pains ceased as by magic. An oppression and general prostration remained. He chewed another portion of the same fruit, and applied it to the wound externally, and, in another quarter of an hour, all he felt was a slight colic, which disappeared after eating a little. This

[1] See *Bullet. de l'Acad. de Méd.*, sittings of the 14th of February, 1848, 30th of January, 1849, and 17th February, of the same year.

colic was followed almost immediately by a copious evacuation of a substance that looked like curdled milk, white, with a slightly yellowish tint."[1]

Thirteen months afterwards, six natives, while clearing a piece of ground in the neighborhood of Panama, were likewise bitten by a coral-snake. Two took the antidote and were saved; the other four omitted to take it, and died in about five minutes in the most horrible convulsions.

Hellert tells us that he employed the cedron several times on himself and others for the endemic intermittent fevers of Panama, and always with the best success, whereas quinine frequently remained unattended with any good result under similar circumstances.

It is on the faith of these simple data that Dr. Petroz and myself have given cedron in some cases of intermittent nervous diseases, and have found it to act with wonderful efficacy, whereas a number of medicines had been tried without any effect.

Pathogenesis of Cedron. *First proving.* M. G. B . . . , a native of Wallachia, 24 years old, skin white, hair auburn; not very fat; constitution delicate; enjoyed good health at the time of the trial.

The proving was instituted with ten drops of the sixth dilution in a tumblerful of water, of which the prover took a table-spoonful every morning for four days, and a table-spoonful morning and evening on the fifth day, after which he discontinued the medicine. On the day following, the sixth day of the proving, the following symptoms showed themselves:

30*th of Aug.* 1851. At three o'clock, shuddering all over the body, with malaise and desire to lie down; the shuddering is renewed by motion; hands, feet and nose are cold; flying heat in the face, several times; and lastly, towards six o'clock in the evening, constant heat in the face, which looks animated, with smarting in the eyes, especially when closing

[1] *Journ. de la Soc. gall.* etc., *loc. cit.*

them. Lips dry, with desire to moisten them often. Headache, especially in the bottom of the orbits, compelling him to close the eyes, and extending to the occiput. While this congestion of the head lasts, the shuddering continues all the time; the hands, feet and nose remain cold; urine of a dark-red color.

31st of Aug.—Malaise with much weakness; loss of appetite; red urine; no stool.

1st of Sept.—Same as the day before; in the evening, copious stool.

2d Sept.—Weakness; flatulent colic, in the morning, with discharge of fetid flatulence. After talking, the saliva becomes white and thick like cream. At three o'clock, the paroxysm of the previous day returns again, but much feebler.

3d Sept.—Weakness; the appetite returns; laming, passing pains in the joints, and especially the right elbow.

4th Sept.—All the symptoms disappear.

5th Sept.—Slight shuddering, only towards three o'clock. No symptom of any consequence either on the next or the following days.

Second proving.—Mrs. T., 27 years, sanguine temperament, delicate constitution, disposed to cerebral congestions, although her head is rather small; lively and cheerful; want of decision; very sensitive to the action of drugs. Ten drops of the sixth dilut. in a glass of water; a tablespoonful morning and evening, for two days only.

First day.—At nine o'clock in the morning. Pain at the elbow and right forearm, as from a shock or blow, for a quarter of an hour. Oppressive pain in the chest, extending to the back every now and then, with frequent desire to moan and take a long breath. Pressure at the right temple, causing a dull pain in the whole right side of the head. These symptoms continue part of the morning, but disappear completely towards noon.

Towards six o'clock in the evening (immediately after dinner), cold all over; shuddering in the back; icy coldness of the feet; the hands are burning; sensation in the eyes as if one had wept a good deal.

For a week past she had had a frequent desire to urinate; this ceased on the first day of the proving.

Second day.—Pain in the right arm, as the day before, (at nine o'clock in the morning); distended abdomen; borborygmi in the left side of the abdomen. In the evening, towards half-past six, half an hour after dinner: shuddering in the back and legs; unusual paleness of the hands; red face; heaviness of the head; stretching, towards seven in the evening; general coldness all evening; increase of the headache, in the open air (towards nine o'clock); pressive pain over the eyes as if a band were tied round the parts; no thirst during the shuddering; dry heat at night.

Third day.—(No medicine had been taken since the day previous). No perceptible symptoms in the morning. Towards five in the afternoonn: intolerable prickling itching at the tongue, obliging her to rub this organ incessantly against the palate; at the same time taste as of iron in the mouth, causing a profuse flow of saliva; sour taste, colic at dinner; unsuccessful urging to stool. At half-past six, feverish paroxysm like that of the day previous, but more intense, with smarting in the eyes, which is only stopped for a moment by rubbing; laming and weary pains in the shoulders; profuse emission of watery urine.

Fourth day.—In the morning, pain at the heel, as from an abscess, only when walking, for one hour, after which period the pain ceases entirely.

Towards six o'clock, feverish paroxysm similar to that of the previous day, but less marked.

Fifth day.—Constipation; the evening-paroxysm is much less violent than that of two days previous, but much more so than the paroxysm of the day previous.

Eighth day.—Pains in the loins and back, on rising in the morning. In the evening, towards half past five: pricking at the tongue; itching at the eyes; shuddering, an hour after, with heat in the face; hands pale, feet and tip of the nose cold.

Twenty-second day.—Slight shuddering towards nine o'clock in the evening.

The febrile paroxysm returned, one day stronger, the next weaker, for more than three weeks in succession, and at least for twenty days after discontinuing the drug. Various unpleasant sensations, such as contusive pains at the elbow, or pains as from an abscess at the heel, likewise recurred periodically every morning about nine o'clock, but only the first week. From the second day of the proving, the appetite decreased considerably, the alvine evacuations became less frequent, and the headache, which generally consisted in a pressure at the top of the head, slight in the day-time and somewhat violent, only at the moment when the shuddering commenced, never ceased altogether; the face was generally slightly bloated.

Third proving.—Miss C., 17 years old, lymphatico-nervous; skin fine and white; hair ash-colored; face pale; shape rounded; small; neck and head considerably developed; of an enthusiastic turn of mind; very sensitive to the action of drugs; suffering with a nervous affection of the heart, for which she took cedron, four globules of the sixth dil., dissolved in a table-spoonful of water; this medicine did her no good; on the contrary, it produced the following effects:

First day.—Towards six o'clock in the evening (the medicine had been taken at nine in the morning); shuddering, soon followed by a dull and heavy frontal headache, spreading to both parietal regions, with redness of the eyes, itching of the inner and outer sides of the eyelids; icy coldness of the hands and *the tip of the nose*, even in the midst of the febrile reaction, (the pulse is 80,) the remainder of the face being red and burning; lastly, dimness of sight; dilatation of the pupils; objects look red; mouth dry, with thick, viscous saliva; constriction of the throat, which scarcely allows her to swallow the saliva; anxiety; restlessness, general malaise.

Night restless; no sleep, with a flow of confused ideas

until five in the morning (until then the prover had always slept well at nights).

Second day.—No other symptoms but those of her disease, until half past five in the afternoon, when a paroxysm similar to the previous one, takes place; she took a dose of lachesis, and the paroxysms did not return.

Do these few trials give us an exact idea of the effects of cedron? I am unable to affirm this. They were sufficient to show me its adaptation to certain paroxysmal fevers, with predominance of the cerebral symptoms, and their paroxysms occurring about five or six o'clock in the afternoon. From the latitude and the nature of the climate of the countries that produce the cedron, I inferred that it is particularly suitable to the inhabitants of warm and damp regions, where so-called pernicious fevers resembling the panama fever, are endemic; experience has justified the use of cedron in these diseases.

At the beginning of summer, in 1851, one of my friends, Professor Demler, had to go to Martinique on business. I gave him a vial of the sixth atten. of cedron, with directions for use. Although he had no occasion to use the medicine on himself, he used it on others, until not a single drop was left. My vial, which had no label on it—for the allœopaths would have spit upon it with a label — went through the whole colony, under the mean appellation of a *secret remedy;* this procured for it access to all families, and did such wonders, that a physician of Martinique sent a report on the subject to the *Gazette médicale* of Paris, where I was named, although my name was strangely misspelled, *Peste,* instead of Teste. I am not quite sure, whether the report was contained in the *Gazette médicale*, or in the *Gazette des hôpitaux;* what I am certain of, is, that the *febrifuge* properties of cedron procured for me all this honor. Since then I have been told that several gentlemen of Wallachia, to whom I had sent a few drops of dynamized cedron, have employed it with great success in the intermittent fevers which prevail in their own country, especially around Bucharest, during the heat of summer, and the paroxysms of which are accompanied by violent cerebral symptoms.

Belladonna and lachesis antidote cedron with equal certainty.

Datura stramonium, *thorn-apple*, vulgarly termed stink-weed and *witch-herb*, on account of the fantastic visions which these poor imbeciles procured with it, and which they believed to be real.—Genus *datura*, family solaneæ, class pentandria monogynia. This plant, which some botanists fancy comes from the North of America, is now-a-days found in most European countries, where it grows in sandy soil, along roads, near villages, etc. It is an annual, herbaceous plant, and has the following signs: "Root, spindle-shaped, almost vertical, ligneous, fibrous, whitish; the stem is erect, round, smooth, somewhat shining, simple below, dichotomous above, with numerous spreading branches; the leaves, which stand on short, round footstalks in the forks of the stem, are from five to six inches long, of an ovate, triangular form, irregularly sinuated and toothed at the edges, unequal at the base, of a dark-green color on the upper surface, and pale beneath; the flowers are large, axillary, solitary, peduncled, having a tubular, pentangular, five-toothed calyx, and a funnel-shaped corolla, with a long tube, and a waived, plaited border, terminating in five acuminate teeth; the upper portion of the calyx falls with the deciduous parts of the flower, leaving its base, which becomes reflexed, and remains attached to the fruit, which is a large, fleshy, roundish, ovate, four-valved, four-celled capsule, thickly covered with sharp spines, and containing numerous seeds, attached to a longitudinal receptacle in the centre of each cell; it opens at the summit."[1] Every part of this plant exhales a poisonous and nauseous odor, and has a bitter and acrid taste, which disappears when the plant is dried. Every part, but especially the seeds, is likewise endowed with deleterious properties. The general signs of poisoning by stramonium do not differ much from the

[1] See *Jahr's and Gruner's Pharmacopœia*, page 139.

symptoms of poisoning by belladonna, to judge from the description which authors give of such accidents.[1] It is said, however, that stramonium affects the brain more powerfully than belladonna, and produces a more furibond delirium.[2]

Empirical applications.—Stramonium has been employed with the most marked success for the following diseases; *mental alienation*, *epilepsy*, *asthma*, *neuralgia*. The first use of this poison as a drug, is due to Stœrck. He determined to try it first in mental alienation for this reason, that it was supposed, in his time, to produce a marked and persistent disorder of the mental faculties.[3] Stœrck must have had a perception of the law "*similia similibus*." The mental diseases for which Stœrck, and after him Schematz, Razoun, Reep, Wedenberg, Meza,[4] Maret,[5] Bergius,[6] Greding,[7] Schneider,[8] Bernard,[9] etc., have seen stramonium act with success, were, generally speaking, *mania*, some cases of which occurred among recently-confined women, some cases of *melancholy* and craziness, some of them, though not all, complicated with various symptoms of other kinds of cerebral derangement.

According to Mérat and Delens, professors Elletore and Brera of Pavia, have communicated to Harles facts going to show that Stramonium is a good remedy in hydrophobia.[10]

Homœopathic applications.—"During its primary actions," says Hahnemann, "Stramonium excites no pain properly speaking, for the unpleasant sensations which the prover

[1] See *Ephemer. natur. curios.*, de'c., vol. III., year 3, p. 302. *Annales de litter. méd. e'trangère*, by J. F. Kluyckens, vol. I., p. 381. *Essays and observ., physical and literary*, vol. II., p. 272. *Journ. univ. des sc. méd.*, vol. XLVI., p. 227, etc.

[2] Orfila, *toxicologie*, vol. II., p. 299.

[3] See *libellus quo demonstratur stramonium*, etc.

[4] Murray, *app. med.*, vol. I., p. 456.

[5] *Gazette de Santé*, de 1779, p. 143.

[6] Mat. Med., vol. I., p. 125.

[7] Adversaria medico-practica, vol. I., p. 259.

[8] See Guislain, *traité de l'aliénation*, vol. I., p. 360.

[9] Bullet. des sc. méd., vol. II., p. 340.

[10] *Dict. univ. de mat. méd.*, vol. II., p. 596. See the pathog. of Stramonium in Hahnemann's Mat. Med. Pura, vol. III.

experiences, cannot be called pain. Truly painful sensations are not felt till the secondary symptoms commence to develope themselves; it is then that the organism exhibits signs of vital reaction, and opposes a proportionally increased intensity of its sentient powers to the stupefying dose of the poison. One of the primary effects of stramonium, is to increase the mobility of the voluntary muscles, and to suppress all the secretions and excretions; the secondary action is the opposite of the primary; and consists in paralysis of the muscles and excessive copiousness of the secretions. This is the reason why a suitable dose of stramonium quiets various spasmodic movements of the muscles, and restores the suppressed evacuations in several cases where there is a perfect absence of pain."[1] Whence Hahnemann infers that stramonium being only able to cure such diseases as correspond to its primary effects, is neither suitable in complete paralysis, nor inveterate diarrhœa, nor in cases characterized by excessive pain.

We might, perhaps, apply to stramonium, the suggestions that we have offered in regard to many other drugs; namely, that the primary effects might have ceased in a great measure and the remedy might nevertheless continue to be indicated. The existence of diarrhœa, for instance, is not necessarily a counter-indication of stramonium.

It is well known that an absence of pain properly speaking, and an extreme mobility of the voluntary muscles, frequently co-exist in the case of maniacs, crazy persons, and other mental derangements. "What other drug," says Hahnemann, "is as efficacious as stramonium, in combating mental affections, provided the whole moral condition of the patient points to Stram. as the true curative agent?" Among these diseases we distinguish principally: nymphomania of lying-in women, certain forms of religious monomania, with exaggerated and ridiculous scruples of conscience, fixed notion that some unpardonable sin has been committed, (which the patient

[1] See Hahnemann's Mat. Med. Pura, vol. III., art. Stramonium.

is nevertheless unable to remember,) that he is possessed of the devil, etc.; lastly, hallucinations.

Moreover, the maladies for which Stramonium is employed homœopathically, are pretty much the same as those for which Belladonna is given.[1] These two medicines are frequently given in succession, considering that it is not always easy to distinguish the exact indications requiring either of these respective drugs.

Stramonium is antidoted by the vegetable acids, tobacco, and particularly camphor.

Opium, *laudanum.*—Inspissated juice of several kinds of plant of the genus *papaver*, which has been made the type of the family papaveraceæ, especially the *P. somniferum album*, white poppy, *P. somniferum nigrum*, black or purple poppy, and lastly, *P. orientale*, oriental poppy. These various plants which are supposed to be natives of Asia, are now grown in almost every country of Europe. In the south of France, they are even grown on a large scale, not only for the purpose of extracting the oil from their seeds, but for the sake of obtaining a home-made preparation of opium, which seems, indeed, to be possessed of all the properties of the oriental opium, and is quite current in trade.[2] The oriental opium, the manufacturing which has been for centuries a source of profit to the trade of Smyrna, Constantinople, and Egypt generally, and a source of misfortune to the unhappy beings who consume this poison, is sent to us in masses of several hundred pounds, in various shapes, according to the place where it is

[1] I am not aware that Stramonium has been given in scarlet-fever; but it certainly corresponds to some of the symptoms of this disease. Even alloeopathic physicians note among the effects of poisonous doses *smooth red spots resembling those of scarlet-fever.* See *traité de thérap.* by Trousseau and Pidoux, *dict. de mat. méd.* by Mérat and Delens, etc.

[2] See in the *bullet.* of the *Acad. roy. de méd.*, vol. XIII., p. 278 and 450, the report of Bouchardat on a work of M. Aubergier, entitled: *Mémoire rélatif à la preparation de l'opium indigène.* What a pity that this gentleman should have wasted his time, talent and money on the naturalization of a product which has been so injurious to the world, and which it is to be hoped will soon be rendered useless by the increasing progress of our art.

manufactured. It is brown, blackish or reddish, and when pure, has a shining break; its odor is poisonous, and it has a bitter and nauseous taste. It is readily dissolved in water or alcohol, and burns so readily, with a white and thick smoke, that it can be used as tobacco, which is indeed done in Turkey.

Almost all the oriental nations use opium in the place of alcoholic drinks, which are forbidden by the Koran. It is to them, an agreeable stimulant, which procures pleasant sensations and dreams; exalts their dispositions for the moment, even gives them courage, takes away the fear of death, and sometimes intoxicates them so as to render them furious, and drive them to the perpetration of murders, etc. This intoxication does not last long, however. It is speedily followed by a disastrous reaction. Such patients feel prostrated, chilly, they become livid, bloated, trembling, weak, stupid, and lose their courage. Life would become a burden to them, or they would, at any rate, find it difficult to wait until their health was restored, before they again rush to the opium shop and swallow an additional number of pills to reanimate their drooping spirits.

It is generally believed, and this belief is probably founded upon facts, that a large dose of opium is capable of producing death without pain. This is the reason why it is so frequently resorted to by those who wish to destroy themselves. In such cases, death is generally preceded by the following phenomena: shortly after swallowing the poison, the patient feels sick at the stomach, and wants to vomit, but actual vomiting seldom takes place. He feels prostrated, drowsy, and the sleep is sometimes so deep, that it is impossible to wake him by calling his name or otherwise endeavoring to rouse him. He lies stretched out, immovable, his face pale, skin cold, quiet expression of countenance. When the coma is less intense, then the patient stares, the pupils are more frequently contracted than dilated, (massive doses of belladonna have a contrary effect,) and they are insensible to the light. When spoken to, he does not reply, or only speaks a few words after having been violently roused: the answers are generally correct. The pulse is full, hard, frequent, or small, contracted, and, in such a case, still more frequent. Every now and then, the extremities tremble; at times, as death nears, convulsions and tetanus succeed each other at short intervals, with swelling of the face and neck, staring, protruded eyes, froth at the mouth, tremulous vibrations of the tongue, tension and hardness of the abdomen, blueish color of the skin as in epilepsy, for a few moments. Finally, the pulse begins to flag; the breathing, which is loud, difficult, mingled with long sighs, becomes slower and slower; a viscous substance oozes from the mouth and nostrils; the body becomes cold as in death, and the patient expires. Ipecacuanha, camphor, and especially strong coffee, repeated in quick succession, and, if deglutition be impossible, administered in the shape of injections; frictions on the body, warm baths, such are the general measures to be resorted to in cases of poisoning with opium, which, fortunately, seldom terminates fatally if art interferes in season.

Empirical applications. "There is no drug," say Trousseau and Pidoux, "the effects of which are better and more correctly known than opium."[1] That is to say, in spite of a vast array of the most disastrous results, allœopathic physicians assert that opium soothes pain and procures sleep. Starting from this double falsehood, old-school physicians have abused, and do still abuse opium so frightfully, that the history of this drug alone is the condemnation and shame of the allœopathic system of medicine. Pain and sleeplessness being characteristic symptoms in almost every form of disease, there is scarcely any for which opium has not been recommended, except, of course, such as are characterized by a dulness of the sentient powers, and a comatose sleep, in which diseases opium would have developed the most marvellous, curative effects. Good observers, and there have been some in every age, have found opium particularly efficacious in *dementia*, *epilepsy*, *tetanus*, *chorea*, *delirium tremens* and

[1] *Traité de Thérap.*, vol. II., p. 24.

various other *nervous derangements*, *neuralgia*, *asthma*, *acute diarrhœa*, *dysentery*, *uterine hæmorrhage*,[1] and various other morbid conditions where its good effects probably depended upon the homœopathicity of the remedy to the disease. But, when one beholds even this day unfortunate consumptive patients gorged with opium in the public hospitals of Paris, in the expectation of procuring sleep for these victims of professional ignorance and delusion,[2] common sense and an enlightened conscience rebel against the perpetration of such enormities, and one feels tempted to demand of the constituted authorities to stop such criminal proceedings. The fact is, there exists but one work on opium in old school literature, that deserves to be read, and that is the work of the celebrated Stahl,[3] where the good effects which opium might produce in the hands of a skilful and enlightened physician, are, indeed, not sufficiently recognised, but where the sad consequences of the enormous abuse of opium that had become fashionable even at that time, are depicted in striking but true colors.[4]

Homœopathic applications.—Hahnemann regards opium as a drug, the effects of which it is most difficult to ascertain correctly. This opinion is probably owing to the peculiar manner in which he conducted his experiments.

"The primary effect of weak and small doses," says he, "during the action of which the organism is, so to say, passively affected by the poison, appears to be to exalt for a short space of time the irritability and activity of the voluntary muscles, and to diminish, on the other hand, the irritability of the involuntary ones; to rouse the courage and the imagination, but to blunt and stupefy the external senses, the sensus communis, and the consciousness of one's self. The reverse effect takes place during the vital reaction of the organism; deficient excitability and activity of the

[1] See Murray, *appar. med.*, vol. II., p. 215.

[2] See *Bullet. de l'Acad. de Med.*, vol. XVIII., p. 290.

[3] *Dissert. de impost. opii.*, Halæ, 1707, in 4to.

[4] See the pathogenesis of Op. in Hahnemann's *Mat. Med. Pura*, vol. III., art. Opium. It will be seen, bye and bye, that I do not attach much importance to this record.

voluntary muscles, absence of ideas, dullness of the imagination, with cowardice, and hypersthenia of the sensus communis."[1]

These reflections, which are almost literally the same as those that Hahnemann has offered concerning the general action of stramonium, render more striking some of the analogies existing between this drug and opium, as well as some of the principal differences between opium and those two agents. But by limiting the indications for the use of opium to the absence of pain and the few phenomena which have been detailed before: Hahnemann, I should say, has unnecessarily restricted the curative sphere of this heroic drug. Let us remember, that he considers the primary effects of drugs as the only ones that should be used as indications of the homœopathicity of drugs to diseases. It is, therefore, proper to inquire, for what purpose Hahnemann has swelled his pathogenesis of opium with a long list of secondary symptoms, pure effects, according to his statement, of the reaction of the organism, and which were, therefore, of no use as therapeutic indications. For, either the symptoms of organic reaction mentioned by Hahnemann, are, in reality, primary effects of opium, in which case, the number of diseases to which opium corresponds, at once becomes quite considerable, or else, they are actually secondary symptoms, and, in such a case, the curative action of opium, according to Hahnemann's own statement, is limited to a very small number of diseases. I think, that, in this respect, Hahnemann has made a mistake, and that the diseases which yield to the action of opium, are much more numerous than he seems to think. This list comprises all such affections as exhibit, often for a short and almost imperceptible period, an image of the primary effects of opium, and, after they have run their course, develope likewise the much more numerous secondary symptoms which correspond to the secondary effects of the drug, considered by Hahnemann,

[1] *Loc. Cit.*

correctly or incorrectly, as symptoms of organic reaction, and, so to say, taking place independently of the inherent force of the medicinal agent.

The fact is, that it is with opium, as with coffee, *cannabis indica*, of which we shall speak presently, etc.; these drugs have likewise a short primary action, more or less agreeable, or negative, if one chooses to consider it so; but, in spite of this, they cure homœopathically a number of very *painful affections*, as we know from abundant experience.

Is not Hahnemann's erroneous opinion concerning the physiological and therapeutic action of opium, owing to the fact that he made his experiments with large doses, instead of employing the dilutions? Ask the coffee-drinkers and the haschisch-eaters whether they suspect, at all, the existence of the painful effects which the attenuations of these two drugs are capable of producing, and which we, therefore, do not hesitate, to place among the genuine symptoms of these agents.[1] Now try the attenuated opium, and we shall at once develope the many painful sensations which Hahnemann sets down as symptoms of organic reaction, and which the crude opium is, indeed, incapable of producing. In proof of the truth of my assertions, let me mention the diseases which have been cured with opium.[2]

Stupor; fainting; headache; delirium; sudden trembling of the whole body; vomiting; diarrhœa, with general coldness or stinging heat of the skin; sudden suppression of the menses, etc., in consequence of a violent emotion, fright or disgust; acute fevers, with comatose sleep, day and night, snoring with the mouth open; contortion of the limbs and burning heat of the body, which is covered with perspiration; dull and pressive headache from without inwards, as if the head were strung together by a cord, on a level with the frontal emi-

[1] Are not an anxious sadness, irritability, paroxysms of weeping without any apparent cause, acute neuralgic pains, etc., symptoms which, according to Hahnemann's own statement, indicate more particularly the use of coffee, the *primary effect* of which exhibits symptoms of an entirely opposite nature?

[2] Several of the following symptoms are derived from my own experience; but I can warrant their correctness.

nences, in front of and immediately above the insertion of the ears, on the sides of the head, with constant drowsiness; full, not frequent pulse; face pale, skin slightly hot, digestive functions normal: these symptoms had lasted for some weeks, in a lady of sixty years, fat, with a white skin, covered with freckles. Chronic headache of upwards of six years' standing, pressive, mingled with dull stitches, which continued almost incessantly, and which became intolerable after the patient had remained for a time in a warm room or in company, or had been engaged in some mental labor; the pain was especially seated in the forehead, where the skin exhibited an habitual efflorescence; the face looked old and sickly, the whole body seemed wasting away; heaviness without any real desire to sleep; excessive sadness; pulse slow and regular, sleep almost natural at night, but long spells of wakefulness towards morning; digestive functions normal; the patient was a young man of twenty-six years, who, to judge from his looks, seemed at least forty, (opium was given together with *coffea* and *silicea;*) at the commencement of his illness he had, for several months, suffered with constipation and drowsiness.

Intermittent fever, in the case of a young lady of eighteen years who had had her first child two years ago, small, pale, with brown eyes and ash-colored hair; not very impressible, but endowed with a wonderful activity of mind, and a good deal of energy of character, of a chlorotic habit. Her sickness, which had lasted for about a year, and was attributed to her having stayed for some months in a damp region of country, presented the following symptoms:—Every day, *at noon*, she was attacked with a fainting spell that lasted some minutes, and was followed by a frightful headache, followed in its turn by a violent fever and sweat, which continued until four o'clock, after midnight, and did not cease until the sun had risen. When the fainting spell did not set in, (which was seldom the case,) it was replaced by a short paroxysm of vomiting and diarrhœa; these symptoms were likewise succeeded by the headache, (which lasted an hour, and then decreased until evening,) the febrile symptoms and the night-sweat. Her courses had ceased, and she was troubled with such violent and frequent palpitations on making the least motion, that the greatest care was required in transporting the patient from her room to the entrance of the garden, where she liked to be for the purpose of breathing fresh air. The lower extremities, and even the pelvis, were attacked with considerable œdema, which might have been caused by the enormous doses of iron, cinchona and quinine, with which the patient had been drenched. The paroxysm ceased after the second dose of opium, and in less than a month she was completely cured. Convulsions, preceded by stupor and coma. Chronic epilepsy, especially when the paroxysms are followed by prolonged sleep. Tetanus. Chronic sleeplessness, which had been preceded by a contrary condition of more or less duration. Sleeplessness, with constant crying, in the case of a child of three months old, of a delicate but plethoric constitution, enjoying good health apparently, not constipated, and having suffered with such symptoms ever since it was born. Very painful, intermittent neuralgia, coming on in paroxysms of from one week to one month, seated now in one, then in the other temporal region, with tendency to constipation between the paroxysms, which were generally preceded (one or two days before the attack,) by a movement in the bowels, as if all the abdominal organs had fallen into the pelvis, and by several copious soft stools following each other in rapid succession (opium did not cure her, but ameliorated her condition). Sudden diarrhœa (after an emotion or cold,) accompanied by acute colicky pains which caused the patient to cry out. Chronic inertia of the bowels. Constipation which alternated with diarrhœa, that was so painful that it might have passed for cholera. Uterine discharges, or rather, courses of fifteen days' duration and longer, with scarcely one week's intermission, accompanied with anxious sadness, sleeplessness, etc., in the case of an impressible, thin, chilly, but not hysterical female.

Plumbum antidotes the dynamized opium; this fact may

perhaps help to determine the true action of this latter agent.

Arnica montana.—See page 65.

Clematis erecta or **recta** of the ancient botanists.—**Flammula jovis** of commerce, *upright virgin's bower.*—A perennial plant, sarmentose, growing in hedges, on the hills of the south of France, Switzerland, etc.; genus *clematitis*, family ranunculaceæ, class polyandria polygynia. The recent leaves, and even the flowers of this plant, are acrid, irritating, and, when applied to the skin for a certain length of time, they cause an efflorescence of the skin, and a vesicular eruption; but they lose this property in a great measure, by being dried.

Empirical applications.—Stœrck, who spent a portion of his time in the very worthy endeavor, although without any method, of finding remedies for diseases that were reputed incurable, tried clematitis very nearly in the same cases for which he had given conium, stramonium, aconite, etc. The pamphlet in which he published the result of his clinical observations, (twenty-four cases in all,) made its appearance in 1769, and its object is to show that the extract of clematitis, which he had prepared from the dry plant, when taken internally, may be of great advantage in certain forms of *chronic headache, melancholy, secondary syphilis,* (*venereal ulcers, buboes, bone-pains,*) *fungous tumors, and even ulcerated cancers at the lips and breasts, various fungous excrescences on the dorsal surface of the hands;* and lastly, in cases of chronic humid exanthem, of which he relates an example, (case 13,) but in terms too vague to render it possible for us to designate the disease of which he means to speak. Be this as it may, the pathogenesis of clematitis, although still very incomplete, accounts for the success which Stœrck obtained with this plant in the cases where he prescribed it almost at random.[1]

[1] *Libellus quo demonstratur herbam veteribus dictam flammulam jovis posse tuto et magna cum utilitate,* etc. Vindobonæ, in 8vo. See also the pathogenesis of Clematitis in Hahnemann's *Chronic Diseases,* vol. II.

Homœopathic applications.—Clematitis is a powerful drug, and, on account of its long action, seems particularly suitable to the treatment of chronic diseases; but it is as yet little known, and rarely used by homœopathic physicians. The diseases which, beside the affections that are analogous to the cases for which Stœrck prescribed it, have been most successfully treated with clematitis, are chronic ophthalmia, obstinate, congestive toothache, with nocturnal paroxysms, ancient gonorrhœa, chronic orchitis, and various nervous diseases.

Camphor is said to antidote this drug.

Ruta graveolens, *garden-rue.*—A bush of the genus *ruta*, type of the family rutaceæ, class decandria monogynia, very common in the south of France. This plant, the leaves of which are, like those of clematitis, possessed of irritating and rubefacient properties, and, if applied to the skin for a certain time, producc an efflorescence of the part, formerly enjoyed considerable celebrity as a therapeutic agent; it was used as an excitant, a sedative, a carminative, a vermifuge, an anti-spasmodic, an antiphrodisiac, an emmenagogue, and even an abortive; in one word, it was, according to Murray, an universal antidote;[1] even in our time the Roman ladies imagine that the most odoriferous flowers may be left in their rooms without the least danger, provided a bush of garden-rue is amongst them to neutralise the hurtful emanations of the other flowers.[2]

Empirical applications—Rue, which is almost completely forgotten now-a-days,[3] has been recommended for the following diseases: *Epilepsy, hysteria, hydrophobia,*[4] *weakness of sight,* (from excessive reading,) *ozæna, hæmorrhage from*

[1] *App. Med.*, vol. III., p. 115. Hélie, *de l'action vénéneuse de la ruc, et de son influence sur la grossesse,* (Annales d'Hygiène, 1838, vol. XX., p. 180.)

[2] Mérat and Delens, *dict. de mat. med.*, vol. VI., p. 141.

[3] See the pathog. of ruta in Hahnemann's Mat. Med. Pur., vol. III.

[4] *Bull. des sc. méd. de Ferussac,* vol. XIII., p. 356. In Russia ruta isused against hydrophobia; I am in possession of a few facts in reference to this subject, interesting but not conclusive.

the nose, foul gum-boils, flatulent colic (in hysteric females), *inertia of the bowels*, etc.

Homœopathic applications.—Ruta, the general pathogenesis of which, reminds one obscurely of belladonna, has, indeed, been found serviceable in the diseases for which belladonna seemed, at the first blush, indicated. Ruta has cured, for instance, certain kinds of ophthalmia, or rather, amaurotic amblyopia, with slight congestion of the sclerotica, muscæ volitantes, etc., consequent on straining the eyes by reading or fine work at candle-light. This drug has also rendered some service in cases of intermittent neuralgia, starting from the eyes, and shooting along the tract of the nerves towards the supra-orbital and parietal regions, where the patients experienced the most acute cutting or tearing pains. I have used it with good effect in a case of this kind, after *arnica.* In chronic cases of traumatic lesions, ruta may be found useful after arnica has exhausted its curative influence.

Camphor antidotes the attenuations of ruta.

Tabacum, *tobacco.*—A powerful drug, which undoubtedly corresponds to the diseases for which belladonna is indicated, and has indeed been used more or less in allœopathic practice in most of the affections where belladonna has been found efficacious.[1] In Jahr's symptomen-codex, we have a pathogenesis of this drug, which has as yet been very little used by homœopathic physicians. I have used it in one or two cases of nervous diseases, but without any effect, probably because it was not indicated in these affections. In *lentigo,* I have seen good effects from tobacco in four or five cases. But it has to be continued in small doses for weeks and even months. A country girl had her hands and face covered with freckles, two-thirds of which disappeared completely in summer, when these spots are most frequent and obstinate.

Tabac. is antidoted by *Camph.*, *Coff.*, *Ipecac.*, etc.

[1] See Mérat and Delens, *dict. de mat. med.*, art. *Nicotiana*, where all the facts relating to the therapeutic use of tobacco are very satisfactorily stated.

Aurum metallicum, *rex metallorum,* of the alchymists, *gold.*—"Modern physicians," says Hahnemann, "look upon gold as completely deprived of all medicinal properties. They say that it does not dissolve in our gastric juice. Such is their belief, and it is well known that, at all times, theoretical conjectures have, in medicine, taken the place of positive experience. The ancients likewise shared this view concerning gold, among others, Fabricius, Monardes, Alston, Gmelin, Brassavola, F. Plater, Cardan, Duret, Camerarius, Couring, Lemery, A. Sala, Schrœter, etc. They are all wrong: gold possesses great medicinal virtues, which nothing can replace."[1] Since the period when Hahnemann wrote these lines, the opinions of allœopathic physicians concerning the complete inertia of gold, has been considerably modified.

Empirical applications. The few positive indications on record concerning the internal use of gold in the shape of filings or thin leaves, in a small number of affections, are so precise, or, rather, so rational, that it seems to me they have to be looked upon as results of an intuitive perception of its curative virtues on the part of the illuminated individuals whom patients went to consult in the temple of Esculapius, by the mouth of the priests. Even if we admit that some happy accident led Dioscorides and his cotemporaries to recommend gold as one of the best remedies for the injurious effects of orpiment and realgar, in other words, the *mercurial disease,*[2] how could Serapion the younger, Avicenna, Albucasis, Jean de St. Amand, Zacutus Lusitanus,[3] etc., have known *a priori,* as they did know and show by facts, that gold is a most efficient remedy for *melancholy, hypochondriac affections* (which is probably the same thing), *epilepsy, falling off of the hair, weakness of sight, foul breath, palpitation of the heart, difficulty of breathing?* Does it not seem as though the pathogenesis of gold was the only true means of arriving at this kind of knowledge? However,

[1] *Chronic Diseases,* vol. I., art. *Aurum.*

[2] Dioscorides, *mat. med.,* lib. v., cap. co.

[3] Hahnemann, *Chronic Diseases,* vol. I., art. *Aurum.*

gold and gold-preparations have never played any other than an obscure and secondary part in the therapeutics of the past centuries, and even now they would probably be completely abandoned, if some few conclusive observations had not restored the character of gold as a therapeutic agent. I allude more particularly to the use of the *muriate of gold* in *indurations of the testes and uterus, bone-pains or old cutaneous affections of a syphilitic nature.* In these affections this agent has been used for some twenty-five or thirty years past, first by Chrestien of Montpellier, and afterwards, in imitation of his example, by Professors Caizergues and Lallemand, etc. These physicians have moreover determined by experiment that, in some cases, the simple gold-filings were as efficacious as the chlorides of gold which had been exclusively employed heretofore, so that allœopaths have no longer any pretext of questioning the efficacy of metallic gold.[1]

Homœopathic applications. So far as I am able to judge, gold is particularly suitable to adults of both sexes, with black hair, dark, olive-brown complexion, disposed to constipation, sad, gloomy, taciturn, misanthropic; or to sanguine individuals, with black hair and black eyes, a lively, restless, anxious disposition, always disposed to feel anxious for the future, even when their prospects are ever so bright. Gold has been found efficacious in affections characterized by one or more of the following morbid conditions:

Melancholy which nothing can dispel; hypochondria; loathing of life; tendency to suicide; *rush of blood to the head;* ozæna; chronic stuffing of the nose; caries of the nasal and palatine bones; muscæ volitantes; congestive toothache, especially at night and in the morning, with rush of blood to the head; itching red spots on the face, of an irregular shape; foul breath; induration of the pancreas and liver; obstinate constipation; inguinal hernia; old induration of the prostate gland and testes; prolapsus and induration of the uterus; *rush of blood to the chest;* paroxysms

[1] See Lallemand's case in *Nouv. Bibliot. Med.*, 1827, vol. III., p. 414. See the pathogenesis of gold in Hahnemann's *Chronic Diseases*, vol. I.

of fainting, with blueness of the face; suffocative paroxysm; ill effects of mercury; nocturnal bone-pains; trembling of the whole body every evening, on going to bed (without shuddering or feeling chilly); arthritic nodes.

Bell., *Camph.*, *China*, *Merc.*, are said to antidote *aurum*.

Camphora, *camphor.* A sort of resinous substance, or concrete essential oil, which appears to exist in a large number of vegetables of different families, the quantity being the larger, the warmer the climate in which the plants grow. This substance was unknown to the Greeks and Romans, but it was known to the Arabs under the name of *Kaphur* or *Kanphur*, which has been changed to *Camphor*. Now-a-days a large quantity of this substance is manufactured. It is white, semi-transparent, resembling rock alum with which it is sometimes falsified; lighter than water upon which it floats, turning round in a circle until it has imbibed all the water it can hold; its taste is first cool, afterwards heating, without bitterness, of a strong odor, *sui generis*, known to every body; not very soluble in water, but very much so in alcohol, ether, in the fixed and essential oils; very volatile in all temperatures; it crystallizes in flattened hexaëdræ and octaëdræ, with unequal sides. The camphor of the shops is obtained from the *laurus camphora*, a large tree of the family *laurineæ*, which is very common in the mountainous regions of Japan, Java, Sumatra, etc., where it grows to the size of our tall oak. It is extracted directly either by cutting the trunk of the tree to pieces, in the middle of which it is found in compact masses (this is a very valuable sort of camphor, and is never exported, but consumed entirely in the country where it grows), or by distilling the branches of the tree in various ways and in closed vessels.

Various experiments on all sorts of animals have been instituted with camphor. Graminivorous animals (such as sheep) bear much larger doses of it than carnivorous (dogs and cats). From the same dose, and among animals of the same kind, effects have frequently been obtained that were not only dissimilar but apparently of an opposite character; the cause of this antagonism is simply this, that, owing to individual predispositions, the secondary effects of this drug manifest themselves more or less rapidly after, or even alternately with, its primary symptoms. This is the reason why Menghini,[1] Carminati,[2] have seen camphor produce in dogs now a comatose drowsiness, and then again a sort of rage, having all the appearance of a paroxysm of hydrophobia, at times torpor of the extremities, and at others convulsions, etc. This antagonism of effects likewise takes place in man, on which account the exact determination of the successive phases of the camphor-disease will always be more or less difficult.

Empirical applications. Dwelling exclusively upon the primary, more or less ephemeral effects of camphor, namely the local or general coldness, and the slowness of the circulation, which it momentarily produces, Rasori has made of camphor one of his *cardiaco-vascular hyposthenisants.* The physicians who belong to other branches of the allœopathic school, look upon camphor, according as the case may require, as a *sedative* (although Halle[3] considers it very properly as the *corrective* and antidote of opium, which is the type of all sedatives); as an *antiphrodisiac* (notwithstanding the experiments of Scuderi,[4] who saw it produce sexual excitement and nocturnal emissions); as a *dissolvent*, an *expectorant*, a *vermifuge*, and an *antiseptic;* and lastly, with some show of reason, as an *anti-spasmodic.* The reputation of being an anti-spasmodic agent, was especially procured for it by F. Hoffmann. He recommends it as one of the surest means of calming anxiety, and procuring rest and sleep in *acute fevers.*[5] Pouteau praises it for similar reasons in *puerperal fever.*[6] Murray who ascribes to it the property of

[1] *Comment. Bonon.*, vol. VI., p. 201.

[2] *De animalibus mephitibus interitu*, p. 192.

[3] *Mem. de la Soc. roy. de med.*, 1783, p. 63.

[4] *Opuscoli della Soc. med. chir.* de Bologna, 1827, Gen. p. 85.

[5] Dissert. de usu interno camphoræ, etc., Halæ, 1714, in 4to., sect. 15.

[6] *Melanges de Chirurgie*, p. 180.

arresting the secretion of humors, of quieting spasms, reanimating the strength, promoting sweat, preventing gangrene and *killing worms,*[1] advises it for *ophthalmia, angina and erysipelas.*[2] Collin quotes cases of *rheumatism* or rather *neuralgia,* with partial or general convulsions, starting from the dorsal spine, sacrum, thigh, instep, for which camphor was given with the best success.[3] It is particularly in nervous affections, such as *epilepsy, hypochondria, mania, hysteria, asthma Millari,*[4] that camphor has been found efficacious; this astonishes the alloeopaths, for large doses of camphor produce precisely similar effects, as was seen in the case of Doctor Alexander of Edinburgh, who came near killing himself by his experiments; and it is well known that camphor has, on several occasions, caused real paroxysms of epilepsy.[6]

Among the medicinal properties of camphor, the principal seems to be the prophylactic virtue with which it is endowed in regard to a large number of epidemic diseases, such as *scarlatina,*[7] *measles,*[8] *variola,* and the *plague.*[9] The facts upon which this assumption is based, require undoubtedly a closer examination, but what invests them with a certain authenticity in the eyes of homœopathic physicians is the fact, that camphor either homœopathically or antipathically and palliatively, is the antidote of a number of vegetable poisons. It would not be surprising if it should prove a similar antidote to miasmatic diseases; this hypothesis is so much more probable, that both classes of miasms are undoubtedly, identical in their origins and natures.

Homœopathic applications.—The physiological effects of

[1] *Appar. Med.*, vol. V., p. 485.

[2] *Id. Id.*, p. 495.

[3] *Observ. Pract.*, cases 7, 9, 12, etc.

[4] Fr. Hoffmann, *Op. Cit.*, p. 32. Sennert, *Pract. Med.*, part II., sect. 3, cap. 5, etc.

[5] Alexander's *exper. essays*, p. 227.

[6] *Thèses de la facut.* de Paris, 1824, No. 110, p. 25.

[7] Rosenstein in Murray, *loc. cit.*

[8] Tote, *Bull. des sc. méd. de Ferussac*, vol. XVI., p. 143.

[9] Haller, *opuscul. pathol.*, p. 145.

camphor, and their true order of development, are as yet so little settled, that homœopathic physicians have only used it in some cases of nervous headache, spasms, cramps, ophthalmia and erythema. Its extreme diffusibility, and the consequent suddenness of its otherwise ephemeral action, give us the hope that it may, some time, after it is better known, become useful at the commencement of a large number of acute affections; indeed the use which has been made of camphor in the invasive stage of cholera and influenza, seems to confirm this expectation.

As we said before, camphor antidotes a great many vegetable as well as mineral poisons, the primary action of which, like that of camphor, first affects the brain. This effect is common to the drugs of the group to which it belongs. It is among the drugs of this group that we have to look for prophylactic agents against epidemic or nervous diseases, in the same sense as *Bellad.* is a prophylactic against scarlet-fever, cedron against the bite of the lachesis, etc. We have to add, that all these drugs, possessing as they do the same sphere of action, strengthen or neutralise each other. Thus, *Bellad.* antidotes cedron, lachesis, opium, and vice versa; camphor antidotes opium, ruta, tobacco, and vice versa, etc. It is scarcely ever necessary to antidote the attenuations of camphor, the action of which is exceedingly short-lasting.

Cannabis Indica, *Indian-hemp.* A variety of the ordinary hemp, (*cannabis sativa,*) genus *Cannabis*, family *Urticeæ.* Hahnemann has left us a pathogenesis of this drug in the second volume of Mat. Med. pura.

The *haschisch*, which is abused by the East Indians as the Turks abuse their opium, is prepared in various ways out of the flowering tops of this variety of hemp, which owes its intoxicating properties, it is said, to the presence of a resinous substance which is not found in the common hemp of cold or even temperate climates. I am disposed to believe, however, that the medicinal properties of the attenuated Cannabis indica do not differ very much from those of the Cannabis sativa known to homœopaths. A comparison instituted between a few general inductions, drawn from the effects of haschisch and from those of its attenuations, has induced me to speak of this agent so little used by homœopathic physicians.

Several modern authors have furnished long treatises on the effects of haschisch.[1] Almost all authors have been struck by the resemblance which the effects of haschisch bear to some forms of mental derangement. I have tried it a number of times on myself and some twenty other persons, and have arrived at the following results:

If taken before a meal, the haschisch excites the appetite; if taken during a meal, it promotes digestion without disturbing it. Alcoholic drinks, tobacco-smoke and coffee heighten its effects; vegetable acids, such as lemon-juice and vinegar, weaken them.

The first effects of haschisch are a vague and full feeling in the brain, without pain or malaise; whizzing in the ears, increasing more or less rapidly to the real boiling sensation, that seems to raise the skull-cap, accompanied with flashes of heat and flushes of color in the face, animation and swelling of the eyes. Soon after, the whizzing and the buzzing cease; now the first paroxysm is on the point of setting in. It breaks out suddenly. The prover wants to speak, but the tongue feels heavy; he forgets what he was going to say; the words and the ideas become confused; a burst of laughter cuts short the phrase which had just been commenced; it is in vain that one tries to complete it; the idea has escaped from the memory. One laughs at every thing, at one's-self, in fact, at nothing, and for some minutes this laughter, which induces those present who had taken haschisch, to laugh likewise, continues for some minutes. It gradually ceases, but breaks out afresh in a few moments, without any apparent cause. After a certain interval the symptoms become still

[1] See *the haschisch*, by Lallemand, 1823; *du haschisch et de l'aliénation mentale*, by Dr. Moreau, (of Tours,) 1845; Gastinel, *bull. de l'académ. de méd.*, Paris, 1848, vol. XIII., p. 675, etc.

more striking. Unless a very large dose had been taken, the consciousness remains undisturbed, and one's reason beholds, as it were, the dissolution of its own government. Whilst a sweet languor overpowers you, whilst the muscular power grows torpid, the knees give way under the weight of the body, it seems impossible to move, and one has taken leave of one's body, as it were,[1] every thing around one looks embellished; the commonest faces look like angels' faces; the ideas come and go so rapidly that all notions of time seem to disappear, as though a century and a minute lasted equally long.[2] These illusions are often followed by real hallucinations, and this caps the climax of our bliss.[3] The imagination, however, is no more excited than the other faculties. On the contrary, it is precisely those faculties which, in a state of perfect health are most active, that are most powerfully affected by the haschisch. Hence the mental effects of haschisch may be very different in different provers, and may give rise to many odd extravagances in company. One becomes talkative and noisy, the other quiet and thoughtful; one makes verses, another one sings, calculates, talks about political economy, philosophy, medicine, etc. But all are, as a general rule, satisfied with themselves. All they hear, say, see, were it ever so trifling, seems to them new, marvellous, or exceedingly ludicrous. In a word, they seem as happy as can be, they seem to be absorbed in a fairy dream. In some rare cases, of which not one has come under my notice, the haschisch is said to have produced sadness, despair, and even a furious delirium.[4]

[1] When the intoxication is not very violent, the muscles are not numb, but the sensibility seems diminished.

[2] I have seen the sexual instinct excited by the haschisch; this negative symptom is important, as will be seen bye and bye.

[3] "We have been sitting now at dinner some one hundred and fifty years," said to me a lady who had taken haschisch.

[4] This succession of symptoms occurs in certain acute forms of craziness, in which such hallucinations scarcely ever manifest from the commencement the mental derangement, without being preceded by any other abnormal symptoms.

In a few hours the exultation passess off, and drowsiness takes its place. Sometimes a little nausea, borborygmi, cutting colic, are felt, these symptoms pass off after a copious, half-liquid stool; the prover experiences an irresistible desire to lie down. After a single night's rest, all traces of this intoxication, which has none of the consequences and features of any other intoxication, and which I should call delightful if my reason did not tell me that the continued use of such an intoxicating agent must finally prove injurious, disappear entirely and without leaving the least unpleasant sensations.

These are the principal symptoms of large doses of haschisch. The effects of the attenuations are different. These produce real pains, very similar to those of our hemp as stated by Hahnemann. Here follow some of them:

Painful emptiness of the mind; sadness, anxiety: a sort of spleen, or, if you please, a sort of *negative craziness*,[1] with absence of thought, disposition to despair or suicide, obscuration of sight, griping pain at the top of the head (principally along the sagittal suture); pressure and dull beating at the occiput; pale face; no appetite; dry mouth, or the mouth incessantly filled with sweetish saliva; desire to vomit, with sweat on the forehead and in the hollow of the hands; diarrhœa with cutting colic and tenesmus; pressure on the bladder; continual and painful sexual excitement; nocturnal emissions; burning urine; cough with greenish expectoration, at night; trembling of the hands; uncertainty of one's movements; cramps in the fingers and calves; cracking of the knees, when walking; sleeplessness, anxiety and excessive sadness at night; nightmare and waking as if in affright; small and frequent pulse.[2]

If I had proved haschisch in massive doses only, might I not have said of this drug what Hahnemann says of opium:

[1] Even in massive, but moderate doses, the Indian hemp causes an opposite effect, namely, gloomy sadness, which is of course increased by the mirth and playfulness of the rest

[2] I quote these symptoms from memory; I lost the results of my provings of the atten. haschisch, which I had instituted on myself and others.

that it does not cause any pain? And, in accordance with the law "similia similibus," I should have said that haschisch is only capable of curing certain kinds of *merry craziness* which is a very rare disease, as every body knows. This would certainly have been a double mistake.

But, it may be objected, were not the pains caused by the dynamised haschisch, like the pains caused by opium, secondary effects, or symptoms of vital reaction? If this be so, why should we not as such consider the symptoms of all other drugs that have been proved with attenuations, such as sepia, carbo veg., lycopodium, etc. Evidently this question implies a very delicate point of observation, which the double provings of the crude and attenuated haschisch may help to decide. I am afraid that the distinction between secondary symptoms and symptoms of organic reaction, is gratuitous and unnecessary. An important point, however, would be, to determine the exact order in which the symptoms of our drugs develope themselves in the organism. Unfortunately this whole question has yet to be settled, as I have tried to settle it in regard to haschisch.

It has seemed to me that the dynamised haschisch antidotes the massive doses of this agent, and that the former is antidoted by *belladonna.*

Hyoscyamus niger. See page 442.

Bryonia alba. See page 389.

GROUP XX.

TYPE: FERRUM METALLICUM.
ANALOGUES: PLUMBUM.
PHOSPHORUS.
CARBO ANIMALIS.
PULSATILLA.
ZINCUM.
SECALE CORNUTUM.[1]
MAGNESIA MURIATICA.
RATANIA.
BOVISTA.
CHINA.
BARYTA CARBONICA.

COMMON CHARACTERISTICS.

CHEMICAL analysis has shown that several of the drugs which compose this important but as yet vaguely determined group, such as iron, lead, the muriate of magnesia, phosphorus, carbo and zinc, constitute integral parts of the human blood.[2] Most of them, especially those which I have named, and moreover tannin, an immediate principle which is common to cinchona, ratania, ergot, exercise a very remarkable chemical action on the composition of this fluid, although physiologists have so far endeavored in vain to deduce from it its legitimate conclusions. Physiological experimentation as well as clinical experience show, that all these substances modify by their *dynamic* action the inmost constitution of their blood. This shows that, when Old School physicians affirm that *iron* is the *generating agent of the blood-disk*, they have only expressed a partial truth, and simply stated the most striking of a whole series of facts of the same order, omitting all the rest as non-existing.[3]

[1] It is very probable that a large number of drugs which I have not mentioned among the analogues of iron, are related to it both physiologically and therapeutically; among such remedies I may mention *copper*, *manganese*, *sulphur*, *silex*, and perhaps also *arsenic* and *alumina*.

[2] See J. Mûeller's *manual of physiology*, second ed., revised, with notes by E. Littré, member of the Institute, Paris, 1851; 2 vol., vol. I., p. 102, etc.

[3] This explains to us the reason why the disease termed *chlorosis* may

For all that, however, even if we accept for the sake of argument, and conditionally, the allœopathic hypothesis concerning the influence which iron exercises on the reconstruction of the blood-disk from an abnormal to a normal state; or, even if we attribute to lead, magnesia, phosphorus, tannin, etc., according as the case may be, or to fibrin, albumen, or any other constituent element of the blood, the part which has been exclusively assigned to iron in the formation of the disk: we are, nevertheless, obliged to admit on the other hand, that this first or primary action of the above-mentioned agents, is succeeded by phenomena of an entirely opposite character, which constitute the permanent physiological effect, and the real therapeutic value of these same substances. In other words, if iron and its analogues enjoy, each in its way, the property of re-making the altered blood, or of increasing, for the time being, in a healthy person, the relative amount of hematine, globuline, fibrine, etc.; it is likewise true, that, after a certain lapse of time, the same substances produce opposite results, namely, the impoverishment, discoloration and liquefaction of the sanguineous fluid. From this antagonism emanate all the symptoms which characterise their action, such as, short-lasting, sanguineous congestions, (during the primary effect,) whereas, the secondary action is characterised by discoloration of the tissues; fullness of the veins; torpor of all the functions; dryness of the mucous membranes; mucous or purulent discharges; engorgement of the glands, which are immediately connected with the circulatory apparatus, such as the spleen, liver; passive hæmorrhages; inertia of the involuntary muscles, such as the bowels and uterus; œdema of the extremities; atonic ulcers, etc.; and lastly, more or less obstinate nervous disorders, arising from a derangement of the sympathetic nerve, rather than from a disordered condition of the cerebro-spinal axis.[1]

present a variety of shades of symptoms, and why iron, which is one of our chief remedies for this disease, will not cure every case of chlorosis, but requires to be assisted in its action by other remedies.

[1] Among these disorders we have for instance intermittent fevers. This

CORRESPONDING DISEASES.

Chlorosis.—Anæmia.—General atony, (caused by losses of vital fluids, such as blood, semen, etc., or by acute diseases.)—Dyspepsia.—Gastralgia.—Typhoid fever, cholera, and (last stage of) lienteria.—Diarrhœa.—Hypertrophy of the spleen, liver, etc.—Passive hœmorrhages.—Inertia of the bladder, uterus, etc.—Spermatorrhœa.—Impotence.—Angina, (with swelling of the tonsils.)—Whooping-cough and other affections of the air-passages, (last stage.)—Visceral nervous disorders.—Marsh-intermittents.—Dropsies.—Neuralgia, (in chlorotic or debilitated subjects.)—Chorea —Atonic ulcers.—Œdema.—Herpes.—Circinnatus and other kinds.—Gangrene, etc.

Ferrum, *mars* of the alchymists.—A metal which is found all over the globe, and has been known from time immemorial. When pure, iron is of a blueish-gray color, very hard, malleable, ductile, of a granulous or laminated texture, oxydisable in the damp air at any temperature, of a styptic taste, and slight odor.

Various ferruginous preparations have been tried on animals with almost the same results. The most familiar of these experiments are those conducted by Vincent Menghini; but, in order to become really useful and interesting, they ought to be continued for a long time. Menghini relates as follows:—

"I have made, in various ways, eighteen experiments on animals, which could not have been made on man. I fed *eighteen* of these animals on food impregnated with iron. After such a regime, I always found their blood more charged with iron than before, although at various degrees; six of them seemed to be affected by this diet in a particular manner. Two of them, that were hunting-dogs, were fed on food strongly mixed with iron-filings passed through a sieve; two others, no hunting-dogs, on food, mixed with common iron ore; the fifth was fed on the peroxyde of iron, and the sixth

hypothesis which I give for what it is worth, for I alone am responsible for it, becomes the more plausible, the more we study the functions of the sympathetic nerve. In the above mentioned work of Mûeller, (vol. I., p. 676,) we find a variety of ingenious suggestions that seem to corroborate this view.

on ground iron. For some days they did not seem to like this food; some vomited, others showed by their barking, their anxiety and moaning the internal trouble which the iron caused them, least, however, those that were fed on iron-ore. On the fifth day they seemed to have got used to this kind of food; they seemed to feel hungry, and the excrements looked black. Little by little they swallowed this kind of food with greediness. They became more lively, vigorous, and grew impatient at being shut up. The pulse became more frequent, and in the two hunting-dogs that were fed on iron-filings, whose eyes became more glistening, and which looked wilder, and had grown more voracious and more impatient than all the rest, the pulse had increased sixteen beats a minute. At the termination of this experiment the dogs were weighed, and it was found that their weight had increased several pounds, especially those that had been fed on ore. The one that had been fed on the peroxyde, weighed two pounds less than before the experiments, which was probably owing to the fact, that dirty-looking pustules had broken out on his back while the experiment was going on. The blood of these eighteen dogs was more charged with iron after than before the diet. This effect was least perceptible in those that had been fed on filings, and on the peroxyde; it was more striking in those that had been fed on ground filings, and still more striking in those that had been fed on iron ore."[1]

These experiments, the results of which agree with the primary effects of iron upon man, exhibit these effects in their general outlines. The secondary effects which were slightly developed in only one of the dogs, is diametrically opposed to the former. Physicians having omitted to take any notice of the secondary effects which are, however, the most important, they have, with their usual obstinacy, contented themselves with setting down iron as a *tonic*, a notion that seemed indeed justified by the apparent results which iron produced in disease. Iron, they argued, is not a poison;

[1] *Collect. Acad.*, part. étrang., vol. X., p. 265.

chemistry shows that it is one of the constituent elements of the blood which becomes impoverished and discolored when that element does not exist in sufficient quantity. Even the untimely administration of iron cannot possibly result in any other inconvenience to the patient than the abuse of any other *tonic*. Very well, but these inconveniences are sometimes rather dangerous. "The hygienic condition of those who live near iron-springs might have sufficed to enlighten physicians concerning the powerful action of iron on the human system. In regions of country where all the water is somewhat impregnated with iron, all the inhabitants, with few exceptions, bear traces of its deleterious influence. We find them tainted with chronic diseases more than any where else, even when their mode of life is otherwise unexceptionable. A general or partial debility bordering on paralysis, certain violent pains in the extremities, various affections of the lower abdomen, vomiting of food day and night, pulmonary phthisis, which is often accompanied with a bloody cough, want of animal heat, menstrual suppression, miscarriage, impotence, sterility, jaundice, and many other rare symptoms of cachexia, prevail among them."[1] If iron be capable of producing such disorders, even if they should not result in death, it must certainly be a poisonous agent.[2]

Empirical applications. The therapeutic use of iron is lost in the remotest antiquity. It is one of those agents which, in company with opium, mercury, cinchona, etc., have been most frequently used in medicine. Dioscorides, Plinius, Celsus, Oribasius, Galenus, Actius, Alexander of Tralles, Paulus of Egina, Cœlius Aurelianus, Avicenna, etc., recommend the preparations of iron against *hæmorrhages*, *lienteria*, *diarrhœa*, *engorgements of the spleen*, *amenorrhœa* and *menorrhagia accompanied with general debility;* Etmuller, Sydenham, Van-Swieten, etc., for *cachexia*, *leucophlegmasia* and *chlorosis;* Wepfer and Boerhaave for *dropsy;* Mead for

[1] See Mat. Med. Pura, vol. II., art. Ferrum.

[2] It may be, and is not impossible, that the improper use of iron should have caused cerebral apoplexy.

intermittent fevers,[1] especially in debilitated subjects; Jacobi, for *leucorrhœa*; Zacutus Lusitanus for *hypochondria* and *hysteria*, with atony and laxness of the fibres; Boerhaave, Benevoli, Mellin, Angelus Sala, for *headache*, *vertigo*, *rhachitis* and *prostration occasioned by disease*, *intemperance or venereal excesses*; Barbeyrac for *visceral obstructions*; Wedel for *worm affections*, etc., etc.[2]

In many of these diseases iron is only used now and then by modern allœopathic physicians; on the other hand, when all their remedial resources are exhausted, they use it blindly and extravagantly in *nervous affections*, *chorea*, *hysteria*, *hypochondria*, *gastralgia*, *asthma*, etc., or in *neuralgic affections*, such as *tic doloureux*, *hemicrania*, etc. They look upon it as a certain remedy for *dyspepsia* of any kind. Guersant says[3] that he has cured a case of icterus with iron, which is very probable for the simple reason that icterus is one of the results of the action of iron upon the human organism. Some physicians assert that they have obtained the greatest advantages from the use of iron in *cancerous affections*; this, however, requires to be verified by experience.[4]

But apart from all these diseases, there is one for which allœopathic physicians consider iron as the only, indeed the *specific* remedy, although the specific character of this drug in the disease to which I allude—*chlorosis*, of course,—has been found at fault in numberless cases, and is furthermore

[1] See Mead, *Mon. et præc. med.*, p. 26. Bœrhaave (*de morb. nerv.*, p. 156,) likewise considers iron an *excellent febrifuge*. These two authors, relying upon their own experience as well as upon the statements of Mercatus, Lazare Rivière, etc., affirm that iron possesses, to the same extent as cinchona, the property of dissolving visceral engorgements, especially hypertrophies of the liver and spleen, which are such frequent, if not constant accompaniments of marsh-intermittents. Indeed, Mead and Bœrhaave look upon iron as an equivalent for cinchona.

[2] See F. Gmelin, appar. med., vol. I., p. 303. Bayle's *bibliot. de thérap.*, vol. IV., p. 219, etc.

[3] This case has been quoted by Cruveilhier in the *dict. de méd. et de chir. prat.*, art. *Fer.*

[4] Bibliot. Med., vol. XXIII., p. 449.

rendered more than doubtful by the fact, that chlorosis, which is supposed to result from the absence of iron in the blood, whereas this absence is simply the effect, not the cause of the disease, has been cured in a number of cases by infinitesimal doses of iron. Is it not evident that such a cure, viz.: the normal re-constitution of the blood-disks cannot depend upon the *material* or *chemical* action of the iron?[1]

Homœopathic applications. Ferrum has not as yet been extensively used by homœopaths, probably for no other reason than because its physiological action is not yet well understood. It has been used with advantage in some forms of dyspepsia, diarrhœa, hæmorrhage, etc.; and it has been recommended as a means of counteracting the weakness occasioned by the abuse of tea or Peruvian bark. It seems to me that all the various symptoms which iron is capable of curing, livid complexion, dyspepsia, diarrhœa, amenorrhœa or passive menorrhagia, cough, hæmoptysis, palpitation of the heart, bellows' sound at the heart, loss of breath on making the least motion, neuralgia, etc., depend upon the same general disease, *chlorosis;* but that the shade of chlorosis, to which iron corresponds, is not yet accurately determined. This is the reason why iron is scarcely ever sufficient to cure this disease; nevertheless it is well, in almost all cases of chlorosis, to commence the treatment with iron.

I know from experience that Kreasot antidotes some of the effects of iron; cinchona is another antidote.

Plumbum, See page 125.

Magnesia Muriatica and **Magnesia Carbonica.** These drugs, although Hahnemann has given us their physiological symptoms, are still little known; they have been used for the cure of cachexiæ occasioned by long and painful diseases. I have seen *Magnesia muriatica* produce a very great improvement in a case of hydrarthrosis of the left knee, with emaciation of the left thigh, consequent upon a wandering neuralgia,

[1] See Hahnemann's pathogenesis of iron, Mat. Med. Pura, vol. II.

which, after having commenced in the form of cystitis with (non-venereal) discharge from the urethra, had successively invaded the shoulder, left elbow, eyes, and lastly the knees where it had become seated.[1]

Phosphorus. See page 285.

Ratania. See page 187.

Carbo animalis, *animal charcoal.* This substance was scarcely used at all by Old School physicians, although Kunh, Wagner, Gampert and Giaduron have employed it with success[2] in *scrofulous affections*, and Dr. Schmalz in *cancer of the uterus.*[3] According to Hahnemann, carbo animalis cures the following symptoms:

Tendency to start; vertigo in the morning; pressure in the whole brain; pressure on the head after dinner; eruptions on the head; buzzing in the ears; discharge from the ears; erysipelas in the face; stitches in the malar bones, the lower jaw and teeth; pulling pains in the gums; bleeding of the gums; *purulent pustules* on the gums; dryness of the palate and tongue; *bitterness of the mouth;* painful eructations; sour eructations; hiccough after eating; malaise increasing to fainting; nausea at night; weakness of digestion, so that any kind of food disagrees; heaviness at the stomach; *gastralgia;* heaviness and cutting pains in the hepatic region; gurgling in the pelvis; shifting of flatulence; frequent stools every day; stitches at the anus; fetid urine; *leucorrhœa;* acrid, burning leucorrhœa; stoppage of the nose; stuffing of the nose; painful induration of one breast; heat in the back; induration of the cervical glands, with stinging pain; tetters in the axillæ; arthritic stiffness of the fingers; pain in the hip, causing one to limp; pulling and stitches in the legs; sensitive to the open air; tendency to strains and sprains;

[1] See their pathogenesis in Hahnemann's *Chronic Diseases.*

[2] *Revue Méd.*, 1835, vol. I., p. 247.

[3] Id., 1836, p. 264. See the pathog. in Chronic Diseases, vol. I.

chilblains; sweat during a walk in the open air; profuse and exhausting sweats, especially on the thighs; morning sweat.

Camphor is said to antidote carbo.

Bovista, page 172.

Pulsatilla, page 260.

China, from the Peruvian *kina*, bark, or *kina-kina*, bark of barks, which the French have changed to *quinquina*. This is the bark of several kinds of tall trees, of the genus *cinchona*, family rosaceæ, which grow spontaneously in Brazil, Santa Fé, and Peru, especially in the neighborhood of Loxa, in the deep valleys of the Andes, along the borders of brooks, etc.[1] According to Humboldt, about 500,000 pounds of this bark are annually exported to Europe for the purpose of being converted into sulphate of quinine. Poor patients!

Empirical applications. China is, as is well known, one of the specifics of the allœopathic school. A collection of all the cases and observations referring to this drug, would fill several volumes; if some able writer, free from prejudice, would give us such a book, it would undoubtedly be useful, and show the deplorable consequences of the abuse which old school physicians have made of this drug. Such a book would simply be a display of the blind and still existing infatuation of old school physicians, of mutilated inductions accommodated to absurd theories, dogmatic speculations that are constantly belied by facts which have been separated from their most immediate consequences for the purpose of being invested with specious appearances of truth; and finally of evils of every description, grave, incurable evils produced by a course of medication which is obstinately persevered in as

[1] La Cordamine, *mém. de l'Acad. des sc.*, 1738, p. 226. The natural history of the varieties of cinchona, and of spurious cinchona, has been given with great accuracy by Guibourt, (*hist. nat. des drogues simples*, 4th ed., Paris, vol. III., p. 94, etc.)

innocent and even salutary.[1] There is not a disease for which this drug has not been recommended.[2] The first effect of cinchona being to stimulate the sinking energies of the system, it is quite natural that it should have become the chief *tonic* of the old school. Under the system of Brown, when every affection was made a peculiar form of *asthenia*, this tonic became of course a necessary means of cure in every case. The question was not whether the patients got better on died. The honor of the system required that bark should produce, if only for a moment, a state of excitement; if the patient died, the sophisms of the school were amply sufficient to account for such an event. The Rasorians that came after Brown who, in spite of them, is nevertheless their superior in doctrine, made of bark one of their *vascular hyposthenisants*, in other words a drug capable of combating *acute inflammations, acute and subacute arteritis*, etc.,[3] sophisms that are at any rate fully as absurd as those of the Scotch physician. It is true, since the end of the last century, the sphere of cinchona has been remarkably restricted. It has simply become a *febrifuge*, or, to use the language of modern allœopathy, an *antiperiodic* remedy. As such it is supposed to be infallible. What is the consequence of this doctrine? That in all intermittent fevers, in all intermittent forms of neurosis or neuralgia, cinchona is prescribed in the most extravagant manner. Under this treatment, it is true, the type of the disease becomes altered, the disease seems even repressed, or, which is more frequently the case, changes to

[1] Mérat and Delens, vol. V.: "Bark is never hurtful, at whatever dose it may be taken."

[2] See Murray, *appar. med.*, vol. I., p. 546.

[3] See Giacomini, *traité phil. et expér. de mat. méd.*, p. 336. According to this author, iron is likewise an *hyposthenisant* agent; this is inconceivable, for, in obedience to the rules of his school, he takes no notice of the secondary effects of drugs, and, on the other hand, determines their primary action from their *usu in morbis*. It is assuredly absurd to say that chlorosis is a form of arteritis, and that iron cures it in virtue of its hyposthenitant action. This seems likewise to be the opinion of another partisan of Rasori, Prof. Speranza of Parma. See his memoir, entitled: *Memoria sull' azione terapeut. del ferro*. Venezia, 1840, in 8vo.

a continuous fever. "It is true," says Hahnemann, "the paroxysms do not occur any more as before, on regular days and at regular hours, but behold his livid complexion, his bloated countenance, his languishing looks! Behold, how difficult it is for him to breathe, see his head and distended abdomen, the swelling in his hypochondria, see how his stomach is depressed by every thing he eats, how his appetite is diminished and his taste altered; how loose his bowels are, and how unnatural and contrary to what they should be; hard his sleep is, restless, unrefreshing and full of dreams! behold him weak, out of humor and prostrated, his sensibility morbidly excited, his intellectual faculties weakened; how much more does he suffer now than when he was a prey to his fever!"[1] The fact is, in this unfortunate patient the cinchona disease had taken the place of fever and ague, without, however, curing the latter (what an argument against the famous doctrine of substitution,) for the original disease only stays away as long as the cinchona disease remains in full vigor, but breaks out afresh, as soon as this one becomes extinct. Every day homœopathic physicians are called upon to combat drug diseases of this kind;[2] and, not long ago, homœopathy came very near acquiring an official position as a state doctrine, owing to the cure which a few globules of dynamised arsenic achieved in the case of an illustrious personage whose disease had been horribly complicated and aggravated by massive doses of bark.[3]

Homœopathic applications.—Cinchona appears to be the first drug, the physiological effects of which Hahnemann tried to determine by regular provings. "The first trials on cinchona which I made on myself, and which showed to me that it has the power of exciting an intermittent fever, date as far back as 1790. These provings revealed to me the dawn of a brighter day in therapeutics; for they showed

[1] See Mat. Med., vol. III., art. *China.*

[2] In spite of the pretended harmlessness of cinchona.

[3] See the pathogenesis of cinchona in Hahnemann's Mat. Med. Pura, Vol. III.

to me this great truth, that diseases can only be cured by drugs that are capable of exciting diseases in the healthy organism, the totality of whose symptoms corresponds to the totality of the phenomena that characterise the natural disturbance."[1] This accounts for the great care with which Hahnemann has collected and arrayed the symptoms of bark. What is particularly remarkable in this work, which was something quite novel when it was first published, is the skill with which this great physician rises from apparently disconnected facts to most comprehensive and yet accurate inductions. Nobody, before him, had carried the spirit of observation and analysis on the one, and that of synthesis on the other hand. "In studying the symptoms which cinchona develops in the healthy organism, we shall find that it is in reality suitable only in a small number of cases, but that in these cases its action is so powerful and intense that a single feeble dose is sufficient to cure the disease."[2] This statement is repeated in various places, and, however much it may shock the preconceived opinions of our opponents, I am nevertheless convinced that it is perfectly true in regard to the endemic diseases that prevail in Europe. In regard to the endemic diseases of the countries where the cinchona is a natural product of the soil, the case may be different; in these countries cinchona may be adapted to many diseases which are peculiar to those climates, and are either unknown in our own, or, at any rate, of rare occurrence.

After having stigmatised the monstrous abuse of cinchona as an universal panacea for all sorts of diseases, and especially for those of which prostration is a characteristic symptom, Hahnemann continues:—"It is true, the first doses of cinchona stimulate the strength even of the weakest patient; he rises in his bed as by magic; he wants to get up and dress himself; his voice is stronger, and his looks are more decided and resolute; he tries to walk and wants to eat. But in all these changes the accurate observer discovers a state of artificial stimulation. In a few hours the disease resumes its

[1] Mat. Med. Pura, vol. III., art. *Cinchona*. [2] *Id. Id.*

influence, etc.[1] This sign of sur-excitation, which cinchona produces both in the healthy and sick man, and which could not fail to mislead allœopathic physicians, constitutes, in its general character, the *primary* action of cinchona, which is perfectly analogous to the primary action of iron. Both in a healthy person and in a patient to whom cinchona is improperly administered, the primary action of the drug is speedily and inevitably followed by the opposite condition of debility, except in such patients as were originally affected, with precisely such a state of weakness and general atony as result from the prolonged, improper and untimely use of cinchona. These kinds of cachexia are generally produced by considerable losses of vital fluids, profuse hæmorrhages, copious venesections, loss of milk, saliva, or semen; excessive suppurations, sweats or purgations; abuse of ferruginous preparations, tea, alcoholic drinks, mercury or arsenic. Such cachexias frequently develope themselves after acute diseases, such as acute angina, pneumonia, measles, scarlatina, typhus, cholera. Nothing is more common than to see recently confined women get into such a state of prostration, when the labor was very hard, or the lochia too profuse, long-lasting or purulent. A certain dulness of the head, which embarrasses the flow of ideas; indifference to every thing; lowness of spirits, anxiety; no sleep at night; dry, cracked, brownish lips; a flat taste in the mouth; no thirst, but little appetite; a sort of fulness at the stomach, even before breakfast; engorgements in the hypochondria and lower abdomen; frequent, whitish, loose stools, composed in a great measure of undigested food; inertia of the sexual organs; no desire for an embrace, or absence of thrill during the act; feeble ejaculation of a watery, thin, brownish-yellow semen; prolonged menses; leucorrhœa of a sickly smell and a purulent consistence; tendency to hæmorrhage from the mucous membrane; coldness of the skin all over; febrile, small, soft and frequent pulse; sweat after the least exercise; night-sweats, as soon as one lies down in bed, etc.; such are the leading symptoms in

[1] Mat. Med. Pura, vol. III., art. *China*.

these cachexias, which, although apparently succeeding some other disease, yet, upon the whole, constitute with it one and the same disorder.

Indeed, it is only in patients afflicted with one or more of the above-mentioned symptoms that cinchona has cured diarrhœa, humid gangrene of the outer parts of the body, various neuralgic diseases where the paroxysms were excited by the least contact or motion of the affected part, and gradually rose to a fearful height; and lastly, suppurations of the lungs or some other important viscus, jaundice, hypertrophy of the liver and spleen and intermittent fevers.

"The fever and ague which cinchona is to cure, must resemble the fever that it is capable of producing in a healthy person."[1] Here follow the symptoms of this cinchona fever:

After having suffered for some days with an undefined malaise, dulness of the head, dryness of the mouth, cracking of the lips and tongue, loss of thirst and appetite, or else intense thirst and canine hunger, heaviness at the stomach and hypochondria, the fever paroxysm announces itself with some accessory symptoms, such as palpitation of the heart, sneezing, paroxysms of anxiety, nausea, ete. Like the common marsh-intermittents, it is characterised by three stages, chill, heat and sweat; but, except when the heat is accompanied with a stinging sensation through the whole body, we notice almost constantly *an absence of thirst in the hot stage and during the chill;* this is, generally speaking, the contrary of what takes place when arsenic is the specific remedy. "The cinchona-fever is commonly characterised by rush of blood to the head, with redness and heat of the cheeks, and coldness of the rest of the body."[2] Even during the chill, and before the hot stage has developed itself, we notice a striking swelling of the sub-cutaneous veins.

The type of the cinchona-fever varies, as does likewise the hour when the chill commences; in some individuals the chill may even be wanting, and the paroxysm set in with dry heat.

[1] *Loc. Cit.* [2] *Loc. Cit.*

The paroxysm scarcely ever sets in in the evening or at night; this is generally the period of the sweat. Hypertrophy of the liver, and still more of the spleen, is an almost constant symptom, if not of the cinchona-fever, at least of the natural fever to which cinchona corresponds, and, by means of percussion, we can perceive from day to day a progressive diminution of the volume of the organ, in proportion as the disease disappears under the influence of the drug.

It is quite natural that cinchona will only cure the natural fever to which the effects of the drug corresponds, on condition that the patient should leave, for the time being, the atmosphere where his fever had been engendered." If the patient, says Hahnemann, should remain exposed to the malarious influences that have excited the fever, the disease will not get well, and the remedy will remain ineffectual even if the dose of cinchona should be repeated; in the same way as the ill effects of coffee will rapidly yield to a suitable remedy, provided the use of this beverage is stopped, but will invariably break out anew, if the use of it is resumed."[1]

Ferrum, ipecac., arsenic, bellad., veratrum and arnica, are the principal antidotes of cinchona, by means of which the disorders produced by massive doses of cinchona can be removed, provided they are not incurable.

Zincum, page 471.

Baryta carbonica, *carbonate of barytes*.—This drug is almost unknown to alloeopathic physicians. A small number have recommended it recently for *scrofulous affections*, *white swellings*, etc., as a *depressor of the circulation*, a *deobstruant*, *fluidifying agent*, etc.[2] Trousseau and Pidoux state that it is an ingredient of various secret remedies *for tetters*,[3] which would account for the efficacy that baryta really possesses in some cutaneous affections. I have no doubt that

[1] *Loc. Cit.*

[2] See Mialhe, *art. de formuler*, p. CXXVII., and Payan, *mémoire sur Hydrochlor. de baryt. dans les malad. scroful.*, Ain., 1841, in 8vo.

[3] See the pathogenesis, *traité de thérap.*, vol. I., p. 322.

baryta exercises on the composition of the blood and the other fluids, on the circulation, glands, the ganglionic system, etc. an influence that is analogous to the action of iron, and justifies me in assigning this drug a place in the present group.

Homœopathic applications.—According to Hahnemann, who probably overrates the use of baryta, it has had good effect in the following morbid conditions:—

Disposition to weep; anxiety on account of one's domestic affairs; headache, immediately above the eyes; disposition to taking cold in the head; *baldness;* eruption on and *behind the ears;* pimples behind the ears; eruptions on the lobules of the ear; buzzing and ringing in the ears; pressure in the eyes; inflammation of the eyes and ears, with photophobia; suppuration of the eyelids; cobwebs and muscæ volitantes before the eyes; dimness of sight, that does not allow one to read; dazzling of the light; crusts under the nose; eruption in the face; single shocks in the teeth; burning stitches in a hollow tooth when touched by a warm body; *dryness of the mouth;* continual thirst; eructations after eating; sour eructations; *flow of water in the mouth;* constant nausea; *heaviness at the stomach* after eating; pains in the stomach before breakfast and after a meal; stomach-ache when touching the epigastric region; difficult, knotty stools; hard and insufficient stools; desire to urinate, and frequent discharges of urine; *weakness of the genital faculties;* leucorrhœa immediately after the menses; coryza; fatiguing dryness of the nose; *cough during the night;* mucous engorgement of the chest, with cough, at night; beating of the heart; *pain at the sacrum;* stiffness of the sacrum; *stiffness of the nape of the neck;* stitches in the neck; pain in the deltoid muscle, when raising the arm; numbness of the fingers; pulling and tearing in the legs; *fetid sweat of the feet;* painful swelling of the big toe; jerking of the body in the day-time; heaviness in the whole body; want of strength; general weakness; disposition to take cold; *warts;* talking during sleep; twitching of all the muscles at night; *night-sweat.*[1]

[1] Chronic Diseases, vol. I., art. *Baryta.*

Baryta is of excellent use in *angina of the tonsils*, caused by exposure to damp and cold weather, and characterised by one or more of the above-mentioned affections. I have seen baryta act very favorably in several cases of *herpes circinnatus*, provided all the other symptoms corresponded to the action of the drug.

Merc. sol. is one of the best antidotes of baryta.

Secale cornutum, *ergot; spurred rye.*—This is a very incorrect designation of a substance, concerning which, the opinion of botanists is still divided; some considering it as an amorphous product and the result of a putrid fermentation; others, and these constitute the greatest number, as a real fungus, shooting up, in damp years, from various grains, but most frequently from rye.

Ergot, which is a most celebrated drug in the annals of Old School medicine, and, if properly employed, is really an heroic agent, has scarcely been used by homœopathic physicians, to whom Hartlaub and Trinks have given a pathogenesis of this drug,[1] in any other than those diseases for which it has been recommended by allœopathic practitioners, namely, in *inertia of the uterus* (during labor), *retention of the placenta*, *profuse lochia*, *menorrhagia* and *leucorrhœa*.[2] But there is no doubt that this agent, which is evidently related to iron and cinchona, can be used in other affections than those above mentioned.[3]

[1] See the pathogenesis of Secale in Jahr's Symptomen-codex by Hempel.

[2] See Bayle, *bibliot. de therap.*, Paris, 1835, vol. III., p. 373. Arnal, *de l'action du seigle ergoté et de l'emploi de son extrait dans les cas d'hémorrhagies internes*, (Mém. de l'Acad. de Méd., Paris, 1849, vol. XIV., p. 408, etc.)

[3] Secale is perhaps more than any other drug capable of showing the action of infinitesimal doses. Eight or nine years ago, when I was physician to the baths of Bagnolle, I had charge of a lady of 50 years, fat, with soft flesh, and attacked with flooding that nothing could stop. After several useless attempts I gave her large doses of Secale, without scarcely any effect. The patient being used to homœopathy, desired infinitesimal doses, in which I had no faith at that time. Yielding to her request, I gave her a drop of the sixth dilution, and the flooding ceased *immediately* and permanently. I repeat that three days previous, Secale had been given in large doses without any result.

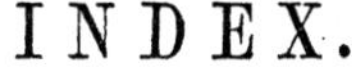

INDEX.

GENERAL INDEX

OF THE

MEDICINES DESCRIBED IN THIS WORK, AND THEIR EMPIRICAL AND HOMŒOPATHIC APPLICATIONS.

A.

B.

C.

D.

E.

F.

G.

H.

I.

L.

P.

R.

S.

Becker, Dr. A. C., On Constipation. Translated from the German, 1848. Bound, 38 cents.

Becker, Dr. A. C., On Consumption. Translated from the German. 1848. Bound, 38 cents.

Becker, Dr. A. C., On Dentition. Translated from the German. 1848. Bound, 38 cents.

Becker, Dr. A. C., On Diseases of the Eye. Translated from the German. 1848. Bound, 38 cents.

☞ The above four works by Dr. A. C. Becker, can be had bound in one volume, at $1 00.

Bœnninghausen's Essay on the Homœopathic Treatment of Intermittent Fevers. Translated and Edited by C. J. Hempel, M. D. 1845. 38 cts.

Bryant, Dr. J., A Pocket Manual or Repertory of Homœopathic Medicine, alphabetically and nosologically arranged; which may be used as the physician's Vade-Mecum, the traveller's Medical Companion, or the Family Physician: containing the principal remedies for the most important diseases, symptoms, sensations, characteristics of diseases, &c.; with the principal pathogenetic effects of the medicines on the most important organs and functions of the body; together with diagnosis, explanation of technical terms, directions for the selection and exhibition of remedies, rules of diet, &c., &c. Compiled from the best homœopathic authorities. 1851. Bound, $1 25.

Caspari's Homœopathic Domestic Physician, edited by F. Hartmann, M. D., "Author of the Acute and Chronic Diseases." Translated from the eighth German edition, and enriched by a Treatise on Anatomy and Physiology, embellished with 30 illustrations by W. P. Esrey, M. D. With additions and a preface by C. Hering, M. D. Containing also a chapter on Mesmerism and Magnetism; directions for patients living some distance from a homœopathic physician, to describe their symptoms; a Tabular Index of the medicines and the diseases in which they are used; and a Sketch of the Biography of Dr. Samuel Hahnemann, the Founder of Homœopathy. 1851. Bound, $1 25.

Chepmell, Dr. E. C., Domestic Homœopathy restricted to its legitimate sphere of practice, together with rules for diet and regimen. First American edition, with additions and improvements by Samuel B. Barlow, M. D. 1849. Bound, 50 cents.

Croserio, Dr. C., Homœopathic Manual of Obstetrics: or a Treatise on the aid the art of Midwifery may derive from Homœopathy. From the French by M. Coté, M. D. 1853. Bound, 75 cents.

Dysentery and its Homœopathic Treatment. Containing also a Repertory and numerous Cases, by Fred. Humphreys, M. D., Professor of Homœopathic Institutes, Pathology and the Practice of Medicine in the Homœopathic Medical College of Pennsylvania. 1853. Bound, 50 cents.

Epitome of Homœopathic Practice. Compiled chiefly from Jahr, Rückert, Beauvais, Bœnninghausen, &c. By J. T. Curtis, M. D., and J. Lillie, M. D. Second enlarged edition. 1850. Bound, 75 cents.

Epps, Dr. J., Affections of the Head and the nervous System. London. Bound, $1 00.

Epps, Dr. J., Domestic Homœopathy; or Rules for the Domestic Treatment of the Maladies of Infants, Children and Adults, and for the conduct and the treatment during Pregnancy, Confinement, and Suckling. Fifth American, from the Fourth London edition. Edited and enlarged by John A. Tarbell, M. D. 1853. Bound, 75 cents.

Esrey, Dr. W. P., Treatise on Anatomy and Physiology. With 30 illustrations. 195 pages. 1851. Bound, 50 cents.

☞ Dr. W. P. Esrey's Treatise on Anatomy and Physiology, is the cheapest book ever published on those subjects, and is particularly of great use to Students of Medicine as a compendium.

Flora Homœopathica; or Illustrations and Descriptions of the Medical Plants used as Homœopathic Remedies. By Edward Hamilton, M. D., F. L. S. The work is illustrated by Henry Sowerby, from Drawings made expressly for the Author. The Flora Homœopathica contains a colored illustration and complete history of every plant generally employed in Homœopathic Pharmacy, arranged in alphabetical order. The drawings are chiefly made from natural specimens, and to ensure correctness, the

Author has secured the services of Mr. Henry Sowerby, the Assistant Curator of the Linnean Society. With a Preface, Glossary of Botanical terms and Index. London, 1853. Price for the whole work, containing sixty-six handsomely colored plates, elegantly bound. $18 00.

Forbes, Dr. J., Homœopathy, Allopathy, and Young Physic. 1846. Paper cover, 19 cents.

Guenther, Dr. E. A., New Manual of Homœopathic Veterinary Medicine; or the Homœopathic Treatment of the Horse, the Ox, the Sheep, the Dog, and other Domestic Animals. 1847. Bound, $1 25.

Guernsey's Homœopathic Domestic Practice. Containing also Chapters on Anatomy, Physiology, Hygiene, and an Abridged Materia Medica. 1853. Bound, $1 50.

Hahnemann, Dr. Samuel, The Lesser Writings of, collected and translated by R. E. Dudgeon, M. D. With a Preface and Notes by E. E. Marcy, M. D. With a beautiful steel engraving of Hahnemann, from the statue by Steinhæuser. Bound, $3 00.

☞ This valuable work contains a large number of Essays of great interest to laymen as well as medical men, upon diet, the prevention of diseases, ventilation of dwellings, etc. As many of these papers were written before the discovery of the Homœopathic theory of cure, the reader will be enabled to peruse in this volume the ideas of a gigantic intellect when directed to subjects of general and practical interest.

Hahnemann, Dr. Samuel, Materia Medica Pura. Translated by C. J. Hempel, M. D. 4 vols. 1846. Bound, $6.

Hahnemann, Dr. Samuel, the Chronic Diseases, their Specific Nature and Homœopathic Treatment. Translated and edited by C. J. Hempel, M. D., with a Preface by C. Hering, M. D., Philadelphia. 5 vols. 1849. $7. Bound,

Hahnemann, Dr. Samuel, Organon of Homœopathic Medicine, third American edition, with improvements and additions from the last German edition, and Dr. C. Hering's introductory remarks. 1848. Bound, $1.

☞ The above four works of Dr. Samuel Hahnemann, are and will forever be the greatest treasures of Homœopathy; they are the most necessary works for Homœopathic Practitioners, and should grace the library of every Homœopathic Physician.

Hamilton, Dr. Edward, Guide to the Practice of Homœopathy; translated and compiled in alphabetical order, from the German of Ruoff, Haas, and Rueckert. With many additions. London, 1844. Bound, $1 50.

Hartmann, Dr. F., Acute and Chronic Diseases, and their Homœopathic Treatment. Third German edition, revised and considerably enlarged by the author. Translated, with additions, and adapted to the use of the American profession, by C. J. Hempel, M. D. 4 vols. $5 75.

Hartmann, Dr. F., Diseases of Children and their Homœopathic Treatment. Translated, with notes, and prepared for the use of the American and English Profession, by Charles J. Hempel, M. D. 1853. Bound, $2.

Hartmann, Dr. F., Practical Observations on some of the chief Homœopathic Remedies. Translated from the German by A. H. Okie, M. D. Two series. Bound, $2.

Hempel, Dr. Charles Julius, A Treatise on the Use of Arnica, in cases of Contusions, Wounds, Sprains, Lacerations of the Solids, Concussions, Paralysis, Rheumatism, Soreness of the Nipples, &c., &c., with a number of cases illustrative of the use of that drug. 1845. 19 cents.

Hempel, Dr. Charles Julius, Complete Repertory of the Homœopathic Materia Medica. Being the Third volume of Jahr's New Manual, or Symptomen-Codex, and the most important and complete work ever published, and indispensable for every Homœopathic Practitioner. 1224 pages. 1853. Bound, $6 00.

Hempel's Bœnninghausen's Therapeutic Pocket Book, for Homœopathic Physicians; to be used at the bedside of the patient, and in studying the Materia Medica Pura. 1 octavo vol., most complete edition, including the Concordance of Homœopathic Remedies. Translated and adapted to the use of the American profession, by C. J. Hempel, M. D. 1847. Stitched, $1 50. Bound, $2 00.

Hempel's Homœopathic Domestic Physician. 1850. Bound, 50 cents.

Henderson, Dr. Wm., Homœopathic Practice. 1846. 50 cents.

Henderson, Dr. Wm., Letter to J. Forbes. 1846. 19 cents.

Hering, Dr. C., Domestic Physician, revised with additions from the author's manuscript of the *Seventh German Edition.* Containing also a Tabular Index of the medicines and the diseases in which they are used. *Fifth American Edition.* 1851. Bound, $2 00.

☞ *Dr. C. Hering's Domestic Physician* is also to be had of the subscribers in *German,* (eighth edition,) *French* (second edition,) and *Spanish.*

Homœopathic Cookery. Second edition, with additions, by the Lady of an American Homœopathic Physician. Designed chiefly for the use of such persons as are under homœopathic treatment. Bound, 50 cents.

Homœopathic Treatment of Diseases of the Sexual System, being a complete Repertory of all the symptoms occurring in the Sexual Systems of the Male and Female. Adapted to the use of physicians and laymen. Translated, arranged and edited, with additions and improvements, by Dr. F. Humphreys. Second thousand, 1854. Bound, 50 cents.

Hooker, Dr. Worthington, Homœopathy: An Examination of its Doctrines and Evidences. Second edition, 1852. Bound, $1 50.

Humphreys, Dr. F., the Cholera and its Homœopathic Treatment. 1849. Bound, 38 cents.

Hydriatics; or Manual of the Water Cure, especially as practised by Vincent Priessnitz in Graefenberg. Compiled and translated from the writings of Dr. Charles Munde, Dr. Aertel, Dr. B. Hirschel, and other eye-witnesses and practitioners. By Francis Græter. 1843. Bound, 50 cts.

Jahr, Dr. G. H. G., Clinical Guide, or Pocket-Repertory for the Treatment of Acute and Chronic Diseases. Translated from the German, by C. J. Hempel, M. D. 1850. Bound, $1 50.

Jahr, Dr. G. H. G., Diseases of the Skin; or Alphabetical Repertory of the Skin-symptoms and external alterations of substance, together with the morbid phenomena observed in the glandular, osseous, mucous, and circulatory systems, arranged with pathological remarks on the diseases of the skin. Edited by C. J. Hempel, M. D. 1850. Bound, $1.

Jahr, Dr. G. H. G., and **Gruner's** New Homœopathic Pharmacopœia and Posology, or the Mode of Preparing Homœopathic Medicine, and the Administration of Doses, compiled and translated from the German works of Buchner, Gruner, and the French work of Jahr, by C. J. Hempel, M. D., 1850. Bound, $2.

Jahr, Dr. G. H. G., and **Possart's** New Manual of the Homœopathic Materia Medica, arranged with reference to well authenticated observations at the sick bed, and accompanied by an alphabetical Repertory, to facilitate and secure the selection of a suitable remedy in any given case. Fourth edition, revised and enlarged by the Author, and translated and edited by Charles J. Hempel, M. D., 1853. Bound, $3 50.

Jahr, Dr. G. H. G., New Manual: originally published under the name of Symptomen-Codex (Digest of Symptoms). This work is intended to facilitate a comparison of the parallel symptoms of the various Homœopathic agents, thereby enabling the practitioner to discover the characteristic symptoms of each drug, and to determine with ease and correctness what remedy is most homœopathic to the existing group of symptoms. Translated, with important and extensive additions from various sources, by Charles Julius Hempel, M. D., assisted by James M. Quin, M. D., with revisions and clinical notes by John F. Gray, M. D.; contributions by Drs. A. Gerard Hull, George W. Cook, and B. F. Joslin of New York; and Drs. C. Hering, J. Jeanes, C. Neidhard, W. Williamson, and J. Kitchen of Phila.; with a Preface by C. Hering, M. D. 2 vols., 1848. Bound, $11.

☞ **Jahr's** New Manual or Symptomen Codex, is published in three volumes, of which the third was issued as a separate work, under the title of Complete Repertory of the Homœopathic Materia Medica. By Charles J. Hempel, M. D., 1224 pages. Price $6 00, or all 3 volumes at $17 00.

Jahr, Dr. G. H. G., New Manual of Homœopathic Practice; edited, with Annotations, by A. Gerard Hull, M. D. From the last Paris edition. This is the fourth American edition of a very celebrated work, written in French by the eminent homœopathic Professor Jahr, and it is considered the best practical compendium of this extraordinary science that has yet been composed. After a very judicious and instructive introduction, the work presents a Table of the Homœopathic Medicines, with their names in Latin, English and German; the order in which they are to be studied, with their most important distinctions, and clinical illustrations of their symptoms and effects upon the various organs and functions of the human system. The second volume embraces an elaborate Analysis of the indications in disease, of the medicines adapted to cure, and a Glossary of the technics used in the work, arranged so luminously as to form an admirable guide to every medical student. The whole system is here displayed with a modesty of pretension, and a scrupulosity in statement, well calculated to bespeak candid investigation. This laborious work is indispensable to the students and practitioners of homœopathy, and highly interesting to medical scientific men of all classes. 2 vols., 1850. $6.

Joslin, Dr. B. F., Homœopathic Treatment of Diarrhœa, Dysentery, Cholera Morbus, and Cholera, with repertory. Bound, 50 cents.

Joslin, Dr. B. F., Principles of Homœopathia. In a series of lectures. 1850. Bound, 75 cents.

Laurie's Homœopathic Domestic, by A. Gerard Hull, M. D. Small edition. 1848. Bound, 75 cents.

Laurie, Dr. J., Elements of Homœopathic Practice of Physic. Second American edition, enlarged and improved, by A. Gerard Hull, M. D., and an Appendix on Intermittent Fever, by J. S. Douglas, A. M., M. D. 1853. 939 large 8vo. pages. Bound, $3 00.

Laurie, Dr. J., Elements of Homœopathic Practice of Physic. An Appendix to Laurie's Domestic, containing also all the Diseases of the *Urinary and Genital Organs.* 1849. Bound, $1 25.

Laurie's Homœopathic Domestic Medicine. Arranged as a practical work for Students. Containing a Glossary of medical terms. Sixth American edition, enlarged and improved, by A. Gerard Hull, M. D. 1853. Bound, $2 00.

Law of Cure. Dr. Joslin's Address before the American Institute of Homœopathy, held at Philadelphia, June 13, 1850. 13 cents.

☞ To physicians wishing the Law of Cure for distribution, we will sell 12 copies for $1.

Madden's Uterine Diseases, with an Appendix containing abstracts of 180 Cases of Uterine Diseases and their Treatment, together with Analytical Tables of Results, Ages, Symptoms, Dose, etc., to which is added a Clinical Record of interesting cases treated in the Manchester Homœopathic Hospital. 1852. Paper cover, 50 cents.

Malan's Family Guide to the Administration of Homœopathic Remedies. Bound, 25 cts.

Marcy, Dr. E. E., Homœopathy and Allœopathy; Reply to an Examination of the Doctrines and Evidences of Homœopathy, by Worthington Hooker, M. D. 1853. Bound, 50 cents.

Marcy, Dr. E. E., the Homœopathic Theory and Practice of Medicine. 1850. Bound, $2.

Mariner's Physician and Surgeon; or, a Guide to the Homœopathic Treatment of those diseases to which Seamen are liable. By Geo. W. Cook, M. D. 1848. Bound, 37½ cents.

Materia Medica of American Provings. By C. Hering, M. D., J. Jeanes, M. D., C. B. Matthews, M. D., W. Williamson, M. D., C. Neidhard, M. D., S. R. Dubs, M. D., C. Bute, M. D. Containing the Provings of: Acidum benzoicum, Acidum fluoricum, Acidum oxalicum, Elaterium, Eupatorium perfoliatum, Kalmia latifolia, Lobelia inflata, Lobelia cardinalis, Podophyllum peltatum, Sanguinaria canadensis and Triosteum perfoliatum. Collected and arranged by the American Institute of Homœopathy. With a Repertory by W. P. Esrey, M.D. Second Thousand. 1853. Bound, $1.

Peters, Dr. John C., A Treatise on the Diseases of Females. Disorders of Menstruation. 1853. Bound, 75 cents.

Pocket-Homœopathist, and Family Guide. By J. A. Tarbell, M. D. 1849. Bound, 25 cents.

Provings of the Apis Mellifica, or Poison of the Honey Bee. By Drs. Bishop, Humphreys and Munger. 1852. Paper cover, 25 cents.

Pulte's Homœopathic Domestic Physician, containing the Treatment of Diseases; with popular explanations of Anatomy, Physiology, Hygiene and Hydropathy; also an abridged Materia Medica. Illustrated with anatomical plates. Fourth edition. 1853. Bound, $1 50.

Pulte's Woman's Medical Guide; containing Essays on the Physical, Moral and Educational development of Females, and the Homœopathic Treatment of their diseases in all periods of Life, together with Directions for the Remedial use of Water and Gymnastics. 1853. Bound, $1 00.

Rapou, Dr. Aug., Treatise on Typhoid Fever, and its Homœopathic Treatment. Translated from the French, by Arthur Alleyn Granville. 1853. Bound, 50 cents.

Rau, Dr. G. L., Organon of the Specific Healing Art of Homœopathy, by C. J. Hempel, M. D. Bound, $1 25.

Rueckert, Dr. Th. J., Apoplexy and Palsy. Successful Homœopathic cures, collected from the best homœopathic periodicals. Translated and edited by J. C. Peters, M. D. With full descriptions of the dose to each single case. 1853. Bound, 75 cents.

Rueckert, Dr. Th. J., Treatise on Headaches; including acute, chronic, nervous, gastric, dyspeptic or sick headaches; also congestive, rheumatic and periodical headaches. Based on clinical experience in Homœopathy. With Introduction, Appendix, Synopsis, Notes, Directions for doses, and 50 additional cases, by John C. Peters, M. D., 1853. Bound, 75 cents.

Rueckert, Dr. Ernest Ferdinand, Therapeutics; or, Successful Homœopathic cures, collected from the best homœopathic periodicals. Translated and edited by C. J. Hempel, M. D. 1 large 8vo. vol. 1846. Bound, $3 50.

Ruoff's Repertory of Homœopathic Medicine, nosologically arranged. Translated from the German by A. H. Okie, M. D., translator of Hartmann's Remedies. Second American edition, with additions and improvements, by G. Humphrey, M. D. 1845. Bound, $1 50.

Simpson, Professor Dr. James Y., Homœopathy: its Tenets and Tendencies, theoretical, theological, and therapeutical. Third edition. Edinburgh, 1853. Bound, $2 25.

Stapf, Dr. E., Addition to the Materia Medica Pura. Translated by C. J. Hempel, M. D. Bound, $1 50.

Tarbell, Dr. J. A., Sources of Health, and the Prevention of Disease. 1850. Bound, 50 cts.

Vanderburgh, Dr. F., an Appeal for Homœopathy; or, Remarks on the Decision of the late Judge Cowan, relative to the legal rights of homœopathic physicians. 1844. 13 cents.

HOMŒOPATHIC JOURNALS.

The Philadelphia Journal of Homœopathy. Edited by William A. Gardiner, M. D., Professor of Anatomy in the Homœopathic Medical College of Pennsylvania, assisted by the following contributors: Drs. B. F. Joslin, A. H. Okie, H. C. Preston, J. P. Dake, P. P. Wells, W. E. Payne. C. Dunham, James Kitchen, W. S. Helmuth, A. E. Small, S. R. Dubs, W. E. Payne. Published Monthly by Rademacher & Sheek, 239 Arch st., Phila. Price per volume of 12 monthly numbers, free of postage, $3 00.

The North American Homœopathic Journal, a quarterly Magazine of Medicine and the Auxiliary Sciences. Conducted by C. Hering, M. D., Philadelphia; E. E. Marcy, M. D., and J. W. Metcalf, M. D., New York. Price per volume of 586 octavo pages, $3.

The British Journal of Homœopathy, edited by J. J. Drysdale, M. D., J. R. Russell, M. D., and R. J. Dudgeon, M. D. Price per volume, $3 00. The numbers of 1849, 1850, 1851, 1852 and 1853, are on hand, at $3 each vol. of four quarterly numbers, with title and index.

The Homœopathic Examiner, Vols. I. and II., new series, by Drs. Gray and Hempel, 1845–1847. Bound, in two vols., with an inoptical index of the two vols., to be used as a manual. $5 00.

Boston Quarterly Homœopathic Journal. Edited by Drs. Joseph Birnstill and B. de Gersdorf. Vol. I., 1849, Vol. II., 1850. Price per Vol. in numbers, $3, bound per Vol., $3 50.

Quarterly Homœopathic Journal. Edited by Drs. J. Birnstill and J. A. Tarbell. Boston. Price per year, $1 00.